Orthopaedic Radiology

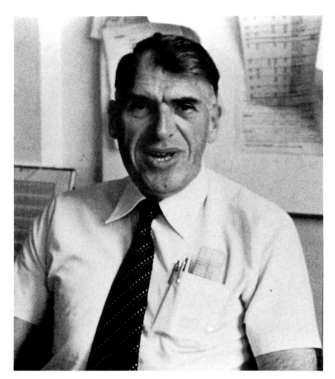

The late Dr William Park
to whom this book is dedicated.

Orthopaedic Radiology

EDITED BY

The late
WILLIAM M. PARK
MB ChB, FRCR, FFR, DMRD
Formerly Consultant Radiologist
Institute of Orthopaedics
The Robert Jones and Agnes Hunt Orthopaedic Hospital
Oswestry

SEAN P. F. HUGHES
MS, FRCS Ed, FRCS, FRCSI, FRCS Ed Orth
Professor of Orthopaedic Surgery
University of Edinburgh

BLACKWELL SCIENTIFIC PUBLICATIONS

OXFORD LONDON EDINBURGH

BOSTON PALO ALTO MELBOURNE

© 1987 by Blackwell Scientific Publications
Editorial offices:
Osney Mead, Oxford, OX2 0EL
8 John Street, London, WC1N 2ES
23 Ainslie Place, Edinburgh, EH3 6AJ
52 Beacon Street, Boston
   Massachusetts 02108, USA
667 Lytton Avenue, Palo Alto
   California 94301, USA
107 Barry Street, Carlton
   Victoria 3053, Australia

First published 1987

Set, printed and bound in
Great Britain by Butler & Tanner Ltd,
Frome and London

DISTRIBUTORS

USA
   Year Book Medical Publishers
   35 East Wacker Drive
   Chicago, Illinois 60601

Canada
   The C.V. Mosby Company
   5240 Finch Avenue East,
   Scarborough, Ontario

Australia
   Blackwell Scientific Publications
      (Australia) Pty Ltd
   107 Barry Street
   Carlton, Victoria 3053

**British Library
Cataloguing in Publication Data**

Orthopaedia radiology.
   1. Radiology in orthopaedia
I. Park, William M.   II. Hughes, Sean
   617'.3   RD734.5.R33

   ISBN 0–632–01191–2

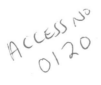

Contents

Contributors, vii

Preface, ix

SECTION I
PRINCIPLES OF DIAGNOSTIC
IMAGING AND INTERPRETATION

1   Standard Radiographic Examination, 3
    W. P. BUTT

2   Contrast Medium Investigations, 45
    I. WATT

3   Radionuclide Imaging of Bones and
    Joints, 105
    H. E. SCHÜTTE

4   Computed Tomography of the
    Musculoskeletal System, 144
    H. K. GENANT

5   Other Advanced Imaging Techniques,
    167
    W. M. PARK

6   Bone and Joint Measurement, 177
    E. HIGGINBOTTOM &
    G. A. EVANS

SECTION II
PRACTICAL CLINICAL PROBLEMS

7   Skeletal Trauma in the Adult, 209
    B. JONES & P. M. ROZING

8   General Orthopaedic Disease, 264
    Z. MATĚJOVSKÝ

9   Common Paediatric Problems, 297
    H. CARTY & J. F. TAYLOR

10 Orthopaedic Problems in the Tropics, 365
    G. F. WALKER

11 The Spine, 388
    I. W. MCCALL

12 The Upper Extremity, 446
    D. W. LAMB & I. M. PROSSOR

13 Pelvic Girdle, 465
    M. F. MACNICOL

14 Knee Joint, 486
    D. H. R. JENKINS

15 Foot and Ankle, 504
    S. P. F. HUGHES & I. M. PROSSOR

Index, 524

Contributors

W. P. BUTT MD, FRCP. Consultant Radiologist, St James's University Hospital, Beckett Street, Leeds, LS9 7TF, U.K.

H. CARTY MD, MRCP, FFR. Consultant Radiologist, Alder Hey Children's Hospital, Eaton Road, Liverpool, L12 2AP, U.K.

G. A. EVANS FRCS, FRCS Ed Orth. Consultant Orthopaedic Surgeon, The Robert Jones and Agnes Hunt Orthopaedic Hospital, Oswestry, Shropshire, SY10 7AG, U.K.

H. K. GENANT MD. Professor of Radiology, School of Medicine, University of California, San Francisco, Ca 94143, U.S.A.

E. HIGGINBOTTOM FCR, HDCR. Superintendent Radiographer, The Robert Jones and Agnes Hunt Orthopaedic Hospital, Oswestry, Shropshire, SY10 7AG, U.K.

S. P. F. HUGHES MS, FRCS Ed, FRCS, FRCSI, FRCS Ed Orth. Professor of Orthopaedic Surgery, University of Edinburgh, Honorary Consultant Orthopaedic Surgeon, Princess Margaret Rose Orthopaedic Hospital, Fairmilehead, Edinburgh, EH10 7ED, U.K.

D. H. R. JENKINS MCh, FRCS. Consultant Orthopaedic Surgeon, Cardiff Royal Infirmary, Newport Road, Cardiff, CF2 1SZ, U.K.

B. JONES FRCR. Consultant Radiologist, Peterborough District Hospital, Thorpe Road, Peterborough, U.K.

D. W. LAMB FRCSE. Consultant Orthopaedic Surgeon and Honorary Senior Lecturer, Princess Margaret Rose Orthopaedic Hospital, Fairmilehead, Edinburgh, EH10 7ED, U.K.

I. W. McCALL FRCR, DMRD. Institute of Orthopaedics, The Robert Jones and Agnes Hunt Orthopaedic Hospital, Oswestry, Shropshire, SY10 7AG, U.K.

M. F. MACNICOL MChOrth, FRCS Ed Orth. Consultant Orthopaedic Surgeon, Princess Margaret Rose Orthopaedic Hospital, Fairmilehead, Edinburgh, EH10 7ED, U.K.

Z. MATĚJOVSKÝ MD. Head of Orthopaedic Oncology, Orthopaedic Clinic, Institute for Postgraduate Studies, Bulovka, 180 81 Prague, Czechoslovakia.

The late W. M. PARK FRCR, FFR, DMRD. Consultant Radiologist, The Robert Jones and Agnes Hunt Orthopaedic Hospital, Oswestry, Shropshire, SY10 7AG, U.K.

I. M. PROSSOR MB, FRCR, FRCS Ed. Department of Radiology, The Royal Infirmary, Edinburgh, EH3 9YW, U.K.

P. M. ROZING MD. Consultant Orthopaedic Surgeon, Academic Teaching Hospital, Laan van Avenstein 13, LS 2341 Oegstgeest, Leiden, Holland.

H. E. SCHÜTTE MD. Department of Radiology, Elizabeth Gasthuis, Boerhaavelaan 22, Haarlem, Holland.

J. F. TAYLOR MD, MChOrth, FRCS, DTM & H. Consultant Orthopaedic Surgeon, Alder Hey Children's Hospital, Eaton Road, Liverpool, L12 2AP, U.K.

G. F. WALKER FRCS. Consultant Orthopaedic Surgeon, Queen Mary's Hospital for Children, Carshalton, Surrey, SM5 4NR, U.K.

I. WATT FRCR. Consultant Radiologist, Bristol Royal Infirmary, Bristol, BS2 8HW, U.K.

Preface

The art of Orthopaedics is long hallowed in tradition; the skills of the bonesetter have been in demand since the days of Hippocrates. However, the scope of clinical coverage has expanded and now encompasses a very wide range of musculoskeletal disorders. In contrast, the practice of radiology was born at the close of the last century. Although it was obvious from the start that medicine would be revolutionized by this facility for recording objective manifestations of disease, rapidly advancing technology, particularly in the last decade, has now made available a bewildering variety of new diagnostic modalities far beyond the wildest dreams of early pioneers.

If these new facilities are to be used with efficiency and efficacy two conditions must be met. First, the orthopaedic surgeon should be aware of the scope of radiology in the definitive demonstration of the disease process, and its natural history and response to treatment. Second, the radiologist should appreciate the clinical problems and management objectives as clearly as possible. In day to day practice this can only be achieved by close clinical cooperation and regular consultation.

This book therefore has two main objectives: first, to indicate the range and scope of different investigative techniques in orthopaedic radiology today, and second, to identify specific regional orthopaedic problems to which radiology can make a useful contribution.

To this end the book has been divided into two sections. Section I, Principles of Diagnostic Imaging and Interpretation, is intended as a guide for clinicians who want to use radiological services and for radiologists who are unfamiliar with orthopaedic problems. As well as describing the technique of each investigation, the indications, contraindications, complications, and value of each method are discussed. Section II, Practical Clinical Problems, discusses the application to clinical problems of the knowledge in Section I. Particular emphasis is placed on common and easily missed disorders to try to establish a logical investigation sequence based on good standard film technique. Especially helpful to junior or inexperienced doctors is the consideration of pitfalls likely to be encountered in interpreting aspects of radiological examination, with useful notes and guidance on how to resolve dilemmas.

Essentially this is a practical book which includes all the aspects of modern radiology and states how these can be used on clinical orthopaedics. There are sections on the use of contrast media: bone scanning, CT scanning and MRI. These chapters are enhanced by a section on the measurement of bone and joints and form the basis of investigatory orthopaedic radiology. For the radiologists there are detailed sections on trauma, children's orthopaedics, general orthopaedics, and separate chapters on important regions of the locomotor system. A section is also provided on orthopaedic problems encountered in the tropics and the place and role of radiology in this area.

Throughout the book there has been close collaboration between authors and editors, with the aim of obtaining an even and uniform presentation of material, which is usually difficult to achieve in a multiauthor book. Although written primarily for radiologists and orthopaedic surgeons, it is hoped that other disciplines in allied spheres, both clinical and para-medical, will find interest, stimulus and illumination on these pages.

This book is dedicated to the memory of the late Bill Park and to his widow Ann Park. It was originally conceived by Bill Park who called on his friends and colleagues around the world, whose reputation and understanding of their subject was renowned and established. As the junior editor it has been my role to put this book together, which was unfortunately unfinished by the time of Bill Park's death.

The contributors have been selected for both their technical knowledge and their clinical experience. I would like to thank all authors for their invaluable help and for giving so freely of their time in the writing of this book, particularly Iain McCall, Iain Watt and Paul Butt. I would also like to thank Mr Per Saugman, Mr Nigel Palmer, Mr Richard Zorab, and Miss Helen Forrest of Blackwell Scientific Publications for their patience and consideration.

Sean P. F. Hughes
Edinburgh, 1987

SECTION I

PRINCIPLES OF
DIAGNOSTIC IMAGING AND INTERPRETATION

Chapter 1
Standard Radiographic Examination

W. P. BUTT

The standard radiographic examinations currently performed were developed to permit the diagnosis 'normal', rather than to demonstrate specific conditions. Special views, on the other hand, were designed to show specific findings. All special views, additional views, and esoteric examinations are complementary to, not substitutes for, a properly performed standard radiographic study. If one accepts these statements several conclusions are inescapable. The diagnosis 'normal', or its synonyms 'grossly normal', 'no abnormality demonstrated', means that an adequate examination has been performed to routine standards, and that areas normally covered by the examination were, in fact, covered and were, in fact, normal. Secondly, the diagnosis 'normal' or its variants cannot be made on inadequate, incomplete or atypical examinations, no matter how tempted one is to do so. Finally, the only solution for an incomplete or inadequate study is to repeat it. To try and compensate for an inadequate study by performing a different one is both ineffecive and hazardous (Fig. 1.1).

Currently, radiation hazard and cost-effectiveness are popular causes whose influence is felt daily in any X-ray department. Ardran (1957) has long emphasized that the best form of radiation protection to the patient, and therefore to the genetic pool, is a properly performed radiographic study which is appropriate for the clinical situation. As far as the hazard to the individual patient is concerned, we must remember that diagnostic radiography as currently practised is the safest of all medical tools, and that more patients have been injured by clinical thermometers than by modern diagnostic radiography. For every patient who has

suffered from too much diagnostic radiation there are thousands who have been gravely mismanaged because of too little. It is clear that radiation dose is not a valid excuse for modifying, altering or cancelling a radiographic study unless there is the possibility of prenatal exposure.

The most cost-effective radiography is an inadequate study performed on a normal patient, and economic pressure, if unchecked, leads to that end result. In radiology, as elsewhere, quality is expensive. Cost-effectiveness is an administrative concept which has no place in the management of the individual patient.

The performance and interpretation of a radiographic investigation cannot be divorced from the patient, and there is no better discussion of this than that given by Edeiken (1981). His *General Radiological Approach to Bone Lesions* should be read by all.

Cardinal signs of bone disorder

DISCONTINUITY

(a) Of cortical integrity
Preservation of the subperiosteal and the endosteal surfaces is the radiological sign of bone health and, conversely, the loss of either is the earliest sign of bone disorder (Figs. 1.2, 1.35). Probably the best-known example of loss of cortical bone is the disappearance of a pedicle (Fig. 1.3), but the principle applies anywhere. The early loss of endosteal cortical bone (Fig. 1.2) is more difficult to appreciate, and the demonstration of either may require meticulous radiography. It is a brave radiologist indeed

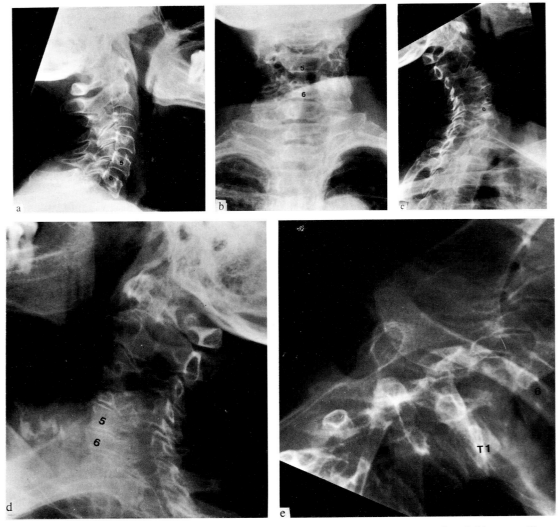

Fig. 1.1. An attempt to compensate for an inadequate examination (a) by a different examination (c and d) is wrong. The original inadequate examination must be repeated (e).

who will declare a bone normal without films of high quality. Careful examination of the subperiosteal cortical integrity in an area of suspected bone disease is often rewarding—for example, in discovering the disappearance of a vertebral body corner (Fig. 1.4). This appearance is more common than is the loss of a pedicle.

The radiological demonstration of intact cortical bone goes a long way to exclude bone disorder provided that one remembers the considerable delay in the appearance of radiographic change in bone after the onset of disease. In adults, overwhelming bone disease may be present for days without the radiographs being abnormal, and it is well known

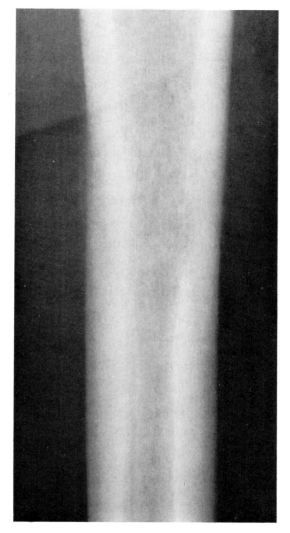

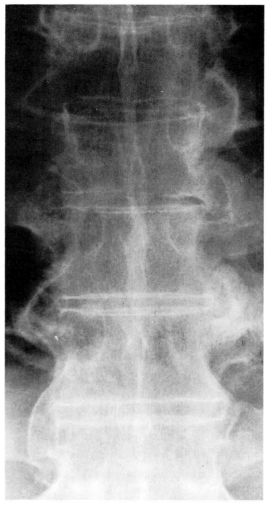

Fig. 1.3. Loss of a pedicle is the best-known example of cortical bone destruction indicating bone disease.

Fig. 1.2. Endosteal cortical bone loss is more difficult to appreciate than is subperiosteal cortical bone loss, but both are equally significant.

that children have died from osteomyelitis before their X-rays have become abnormal. In adults, it may take two weeks before bone atrophy is visible, and although the time is shorter in children the delay is still considerable.

(b) By fracture
Linear fractures of bone are not demonstrable radiographically unless they are displaced, and even then they may not be shown unless the X-ray beam is parallel to the plane of the fracture (Fig. 1.5). The femoral neck (Fig. 1.6) and the scaphoid are two bones commonly affected by undisplaced fractures, and radiographs of the very highest quality taken at the time of the injury may be normal.

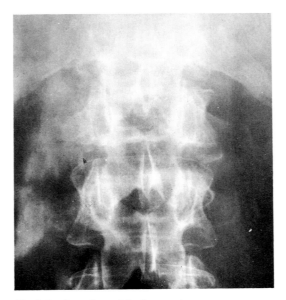

Fig. 1.4. Loss of a vertebral corner is a more common sign of vertebral disease than is loss of a pedicle.

Displaced fractures are frequently invisible on a single radiograph because the central ray was not parallel to the plane of the fracture and the plane of the fracture may be difficult to parallel radiographically. Not uncommonly, the fracture may be impossible to show on any standard radiographic study. The advent of CT scanning has shown just how often linear fractures are not demonstrated on routine radiographs. In clinical practice, one commonly fails to demonstrate longitudinal splits of bone which occur in an oblique or spiral fashion, and this most frequently in vertebral bodies and vertebral appendages. In the peripheral skeleton, such fractures tend to occur at joints where a flat articular surface (e.g. the tibia) meets a rounded articular surface (e.g. the femur), because the rounded surface acts as a wedge and splits the flat-surfaced bone longitudinally. It is unusual for these

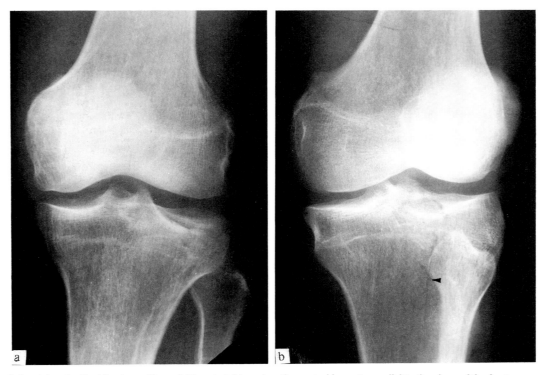

Fig. 1.5. A longitudinal fracture of bone (b) is not visible unless the central beam is parallel to the plane of the fracture.

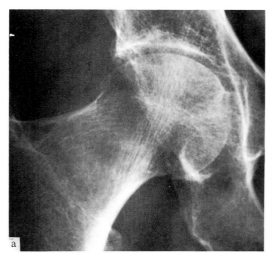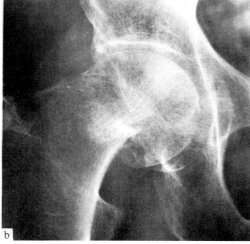

Fig. 1.6.   Fractures which are not displaced at the time of injury (a) are radiologically invisible but are no less significant in the long run (b) than are their visible counterparts.

splits to occur in either the sagittal or coronal plane and, therefore, it is unusual for the fracture to be visible on frontal or lateral radiographs. The reader will·have to decide for himself if he can diagnose an examination as normal without oblique films in the patient with a suspected fracture. Fig. 1.5 may help in this decision.

Eyes that are trained to look for fractures as black lines often miss the injury that is white. Post-traumatic increase in bone density can be due to overlap of fragments, impaction of fragments, or rotation of bone. If there is overlap or impaction the increased density will have an indistinct margin (Fig. 1.5l), whereas the rotated bone will have distinct margins (Fig. 1.7). A distinct white line may be the only sign of an important fracture such as a depression of the skull vault (Fig. 1.8).

(c)   Rotation
Although rotation is not necessarily a sign of bone discontinuity, it is most conveniently considered in this section. Rotation of a bone which is oval or rectangular in cross-section will alter its radiographic projection (Fig. 1.9). As the bone rotates its radiographic density will change, its radiographic size will change, and the clarity of its outline will change. Obviously, these changes occur in both directions but the usual triad that is considered diagnostic of rotation is decrease in size, increase in density, and increase in clarity of outline (Fig. 1.10). These changes are most obvious when two bones (e.g. vertebral bodies) are adjacent and only one is rotated. Because the radiographic projection of the rotated vertebral body is increased in anteroposterior depth there will be a step in the anterior alignment of the vertebral bodies with no similar step in the posterior alignment at the level where the rotated vertebral bodies meet the unrotated vertebral bodies.

Rotation of cortical fragments is the essential lesion of a 'ping-pong' fracture of a spherical bone such as the humeral head, and the white line of its rotation (Figs. 1.7, 1.11) will be the only sign of the presence of the injury in the absence of a tangential film. It is important to remember that frontal films taken when the central ray is not parallel to the rotated fragment will be entirely normal (Fig. 1.11a).

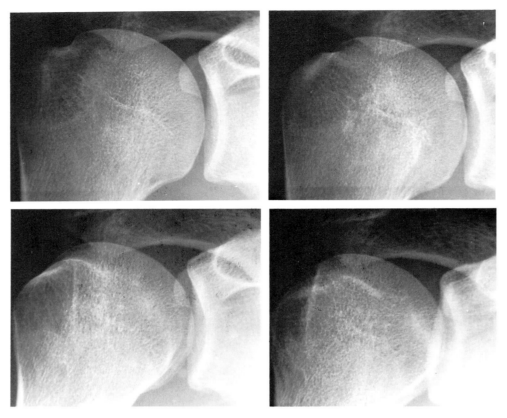

Fig. 1.7. Four views of a humeral head demonstrate that tilted cortical bone is invisible unless the incident beam is parallel to the tilted fragment.

Rotation of an angled structure will alter its radiographic projection drastically. If the rotation occurs on an axis parallel to the long axis of the structure, the radiographic projection of the angle can be increased in obtuseness but cannot be made more acute (Fig. 1.12). Conversely, if the axis of rotation is perpendicular to the long axis of the angled structure the radiographic projection can be made more acute but not more obtuse (Fig. 1.13). Clearly, a change in an angle measured on a series of radiographs can be produced by rotation, and since rotation is extremely difficult to avoid small changes should be considered to be technical rather than due to treatment or other cause.

DESTRUCTION

When bone discontinuity reaches the point where structural features are no longer visible, destruction is a more appropriate term.

(a) By infiltration

Although radiography is a two-dimensional study of gross pathology in black and white, the processes demonstrated by X-ray are not always easily translatable into gross pathological changes. For example, there is an inference that the extent of a lesion as demonstrated on a radiograph is the true extent of the lesion, but that is not necessarily so. Frequently the advancing

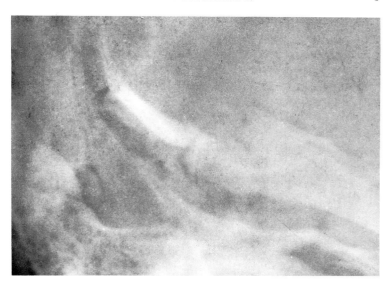

Fig. 1.8. Tilted cortical bone is sharply marginated and radio-dense. It may be the only sign of a depressed fracture of the skull.

edge of radiological bone 'infiltration' is significantly distant from the edge of the lesion, and it may not be related to the edge of the lesion at all. This is particularly true in lesions of the medullary cavity, since destruction there cannot be seen and all radiologically demonstrable changes are due to cortical damage. In osteomyelitis, a fairly small area of cortical destruction may mislead the unwary into assuming that the area of infection is equally small. Small areas of cortical destruction may be present where there is total marrow abscess. The advancing edge of bone infiltration is due to osteoporosis and it may be due to osteoporosis alone without another process being present (Fig. 1.55). It is, perhaps, more sensible to interpret 'infiltrative bone destruction' as indicating the presence of a process that the body cannot confine without inferring that it delineates the extent of the lesion.

(b) By erosion
Erosion describes disappearance of bone due to pressure from an expanding process that is trapped against the bone in a fashion that pre-

vents the expansion of the process into soft tissues. This is a reasonably accurate description of the gross pathology provided that one realizes that the extent of endosteal erosion (Fig. 1.43) or of erosion from outside (Fig. 1.20) is not an indicator of the extent of the lesion. The entire marrow cavity of a bone may be filled with an expanding process such as a chondrosarcoma with only a small area of endosteal erosion being visible.

It is a good rule of thumb that standard radiography including standard tomography cannot define the extent of a process that is destroying bone.

REPAIR

(a) Sclerosis
The pathological basis of the radiological manifestations of repair have been covered in the previous chapter, but it is worth repeating here that the radiological demonstration of repair is a sign of bone health and that sick bone will repair itself poorly and dead bone not at all.

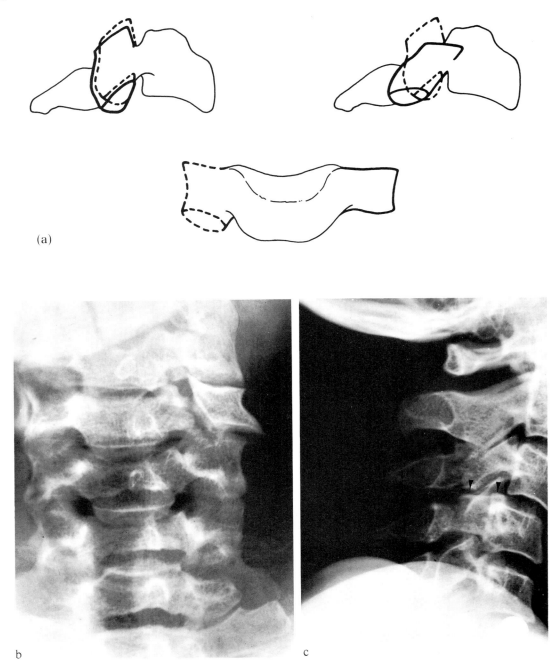

(a)

b   c

Fig. 1.9.   (a) A drawing, and (b) and (c) radiographs, demonstrating that rotated bones are smaller, more dense, and more clearly visualized than their unrotated neighbours. In practice, the visualization of a dense facet (b) alerts one to look for the horizontally lying rotated facet (c).

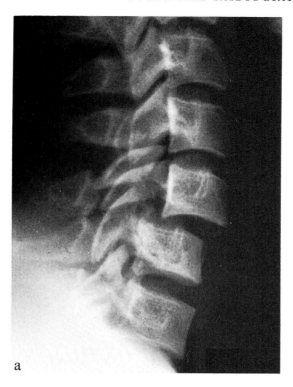

a

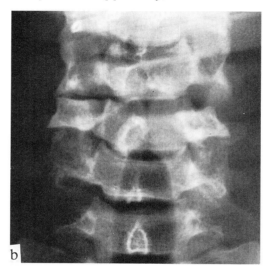

Fig. 1.10. Another example of tilted facets demonstrates that rotation can be diagnosed from a lateral film because of a difference in clarity of the outline and a difference in the anteroposterior depth of adjacent vertebral bodies. Because vertebral bodies are oval in cross-section, the rotation of one will make it appear deeper than its unrotated neighbour, frequently resulting in a step anteriorly without a step posteriorly.

b

It may be simplistic to think of bone sclerosis being an attempt by the body to replace structural strength removed by a pathological process, but it is a concept that seems to work. Once holes in bone reach a certain size, repair cannot bridge the hole and instead tends to cause sclerosis around the circumference of the previous lesion. Many examples of this can be found in daily practice, and some of the most striking are in the treated myeloma and in the treated breast carcinoma.

The stages of fracture repair and their radiological features are well known to us all, but we must remember that this is healing by secondary intention through a stage of granulation tissue (Catto 1980). Healing by primary intention has a different appearance. This type of repair is confined to the fracture or osteotomy which is internally fixed by a compression apparatus. In this circumstance, the radiological appearance may not change from the day of operation to the day of complete bone union. Perifracture osteoporosis, callus formation, and remodelling may not occur.

The commonest injury to the skeleton is physical trauma and therefore it is the commonest cause of bone repair. If only repair is seen on a radiograph, injury should be suspected as the cause; and if the repair is linear, physical trauma should be the diagnosis.

(b) Subperiosteal new bone formation
Healthy periosteum will produce bone if stimulated to do so or if physically elevated from the underlying cortical bone. In the former circumstance, the periosteal new bone tends to be solid (Edeiken *et al.* 1966) and may be serpentine, lobulated, or layered. Most authorities consider that the radiolucent layer or layers which separate the periosteal new bone from the underlying cortical bone do not contain abnormal infiltrating tissue (Volberg *et al.* 1977). The appearance

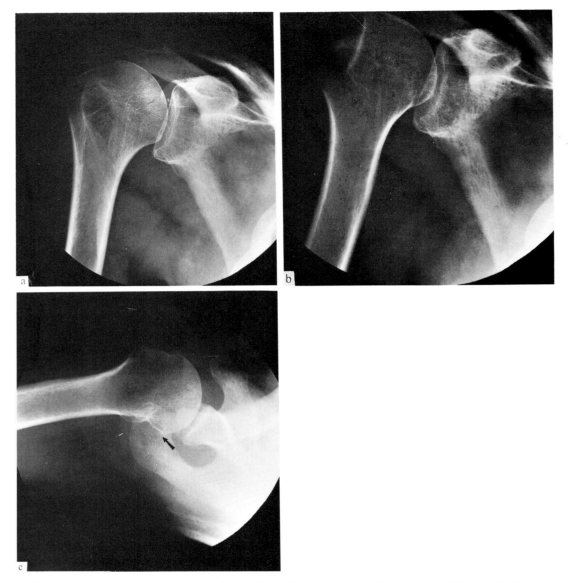

Fig. 1.11. It is important to emphasize that tilted cortical bone (b) shown by an incident beam parallel to the tilted bone (c) will be entirely invisible on a film with any other incident angulation (a).

of this type of periosteal new bone formation is therefore not a reliable indicator of the cause of the irritation. One is quite justified in concluding that layered periosteal new bone formation indicates a process which the body has not controlled, but one is not justified in diagnosing a malignant lesion.

Periosteum that is physically stripped from the underlying cortex by haemorrhage, pus, or tumour will produce new bone at a considerable distance from the cortical surface, and in this circumstance the radiolucency separating the two is filled with a combination of haemorrhage and the stripping agent. It is not surprising that

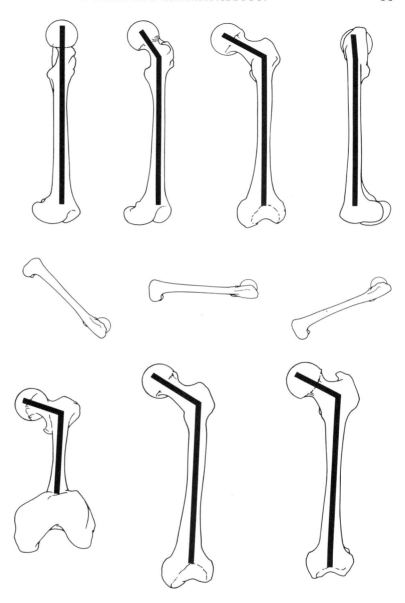

Fig. 1.12. Diagrammatic illustration of the change which occurs in the radiographic projection of an angle with rotation of the structure in the long axis. Note that the projected angle can become more obtuse but cannot become more acute than it truly is.

Fig. 1.13. A diagram demonstrates the changes which occur in the radiographic projection of an angle with rotation of the structure on an axis perpendicular to the structure. Note that the radiographic projection of the angle can be more acute but never more obtuse than the actual angle.

the periphery of the elevated periosteum is the first to re-ossify solidly, producing a 'Codman triangle'. Once again, the appearance of the Codman triangle cannot be used to justify a specific diagnosis but only to indicate that stripping has occurred. Calcification and/or ossification within the subperiosteal radiolucency may well indicate a malignant process, but if

so it is due to neo-osteogenesis rather than subperiosteal new bone formation. If this new bone formation is regular and uniform one can infer that it is occurring in an organized structure which is not likely to be a disorganized entity such as a malignant tumour.

Others have suggested that the type of periosteal reaction seen will permit differentiation of benign and malignant processes, but that is not universally accepted and it may be extremely difficult in the individual case, particularly early on when such differentiation is important (Fig. 1.2).

The radiological assessment of endosteal repair is difficult and is rarely of much practical value. It is necessary to remember that it can occur to the degree that the medullary cavity is obliterated, because that may pose problems in future interpretation.

ARCHITECTURAL DISTURBANCE

(a) *Hypertrophy*
Local overgrowth indicates an old, a chronic, or a recurrent condition. Although it is a sign of disorder it has little general application.

Where it is a specific feature of a specific disease it will be described in the chapter dealing with that disease.

(b) *Atrophy*
Bone atrophy means a decrease in the size or mass of a previously normal bone and is, therefore, the proper term to describe what is usually referred to as 'osteoporosis', 'osteopenia', 'demineralization', or other such. By far the strongest stimulus to cause atrophy in the skeleton is disuse, and this author is not sure that there is any other cause. It is impossible to maintain normal muscle mass in the absence of normal bone mass, and it is impossible to maintain normal bone mass in the absence of normal muscle mass. If this is true, one must question the practice of treating bone atrophy with a technique that does not treat muscle atrophy. Localized, generalized and periarticular osteoporosis can all be related to a decrease in muscle bulk, either generalized or localized, which should make one very cautious in interpreting bone atrophy as being part of a specific disease process or, for that matter, insisting on its presence before diagnosing a specific disease process. It is, however, an extremely important sign of bone disorder.

It has been said that generalized atrophy needs to remove at least 30% of bone mass for

it to be radiologically visible, and this probably errs on the conservative side. Precise measurements of bone density and therefore bone mass are possible, and the techniques are available, but none is in general use. In the past it has been inferred that the measuring devices were imprecise, because there was an overlap of the bone mass of patients with symptomatic bone disease with the normal population. This is not true, and the methods as described are extremely accurate. It has been my personal feeling that the vast majority of the population, and therefore the controls in all the experiments that measure bone density, have unhealthy bone. This would explain why patients with symptomatic bone disease have density measurements that overlap the normal range, and one would doubt very much that there would be an overlap of bone density in civilized patients with the healthy bones of bush natives.

The radiological diagnosis of localized bone atrophy is of much more value in routine practice. At all ages, the most active area of the long bones is the periarticular region, and disuse atrophy occurs there first, specifically around the region of the epiphyseal plate. It is irrational to expect distal bones in a limb to stay active whilst the proximal ones are disused and, in the long run, atrophy due to disuse involves all the bones distal to the lesion. Acute disuse, on the other hand, involves only the affected area for a while, and disuse atrophy is localized in the beginning.

In adults, radiologically visible bone atrophy takes about 10 days to develop and there is little use in looking for it sooner. Equally importantly, visible bone atrophy means that the process has been present for at least 10 days. Acute short-lived diseases like gout may well be over before bone atrophy develops. In the infant and young child the development of bone atrophy is much quicker but still disease may be well established before X-rays become abnormal.

Conditions which cause long-term pain are those conditions which are associated with the most severe bone atrophy and in these it may be difficult to differentiate the diseased from the normal but atrophic area. Profound bone atrophy without destruction is characterized by the preservation of the subperiosteal and subchondral cortical surfaces, giving the 'white square' so characteristic of Sudeck's atrophy. The disappearance of the subchondral or subperiosteal cortex is a radiological marker to the location of the disease in such difficult cases.

Altered growth and/or maturation are not changes that require discussion in general terms and they will be covered in the chapters covering the appropriate diseases.

Cardinal radiological signs of joint disorder

The early radiological diagnosis of joint disorder follows roughly the same path as the early clinical diagnosis in that the aim is first of all to establish that the lesion is of joint origin before deciding the type of disorder that is present.

SYNOVIAL INVOLVEMENT

(a)   Effusion
The first radiological sign of joint disorder is swelling. Obviously, soft-tissue swelling cannot be distinguished from surrounding normal soft tissues unless the swelling indents, encroaches on, or obliterates fat planes. Fortunately for radiologists, all synovial joints that have any significant range of motion are surrounded by

fat, which permits motion to occur without producing intolerable pressure changes and vacuum formation. The fat is available for radiological assessment in all joints save the shoulder and hip, and even though the radiological anatomy has only been worked out for some of the joints (e.g. the knee and elbow) they can all be assessed without great knowledge of anatomy. Subsequent chapters will cover the details of the specific areas of the body in question, and here it need only be mentioned that the perisynovial fat lies immediately superficial to the synovial capsule of a joint, often deep to the ligaments, and should be seen as a radiolucent area extending down to the capsule or occasionally to the articular cartilage. Figs. 1.14, 1.15 and 1.16 compare synovial enlargement with the normal in some less usual joints to demonstrate that it is possible to be definite about the presence of synovial abnormality.

(b)   Mass disease
The presence of synovial effusion alone does not indicate the presence of disease, and it is necessary to demonstrate synovial mass to confirm that there is a disease process as well as an effusion present. Occasionally, this mass disease can encroach on the perisynovial fat to the degree that it can be seen as lumps (Fig. 1.17) and one has no trouble in being certain that there is mass disease. Unfortunately, this is a rare observation. Synovial hypertrophy which

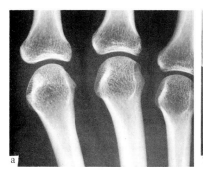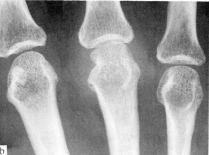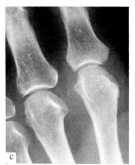

Fig. 1.14. High-resolution radiography readily permits the demonstration of synovial swelling (b and c), compared with the normal (a).

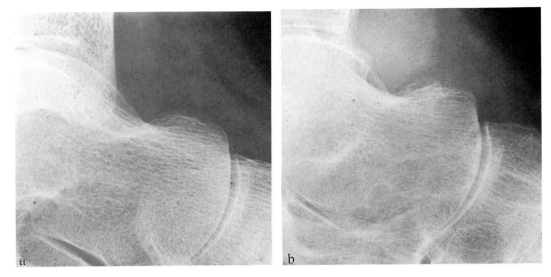

Fig. 1.15. The normal (a) versus abnormal (b) ankle joints.

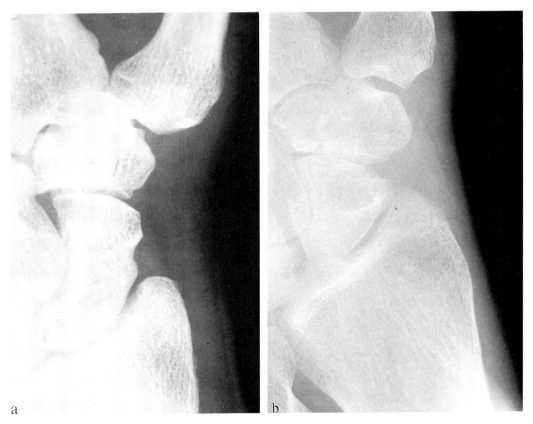

Fig. 1.16. The normal (a) versus abnormal (b) wrist joints.

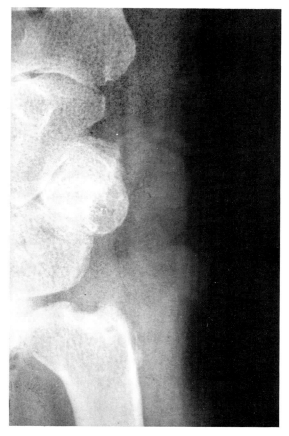

Fig. 1.17. Occasionally one can see lumpy synovium encroaching on periarticular fat which allows an unequivocal diagnosis of synovial disease rather than just synovial fluid.

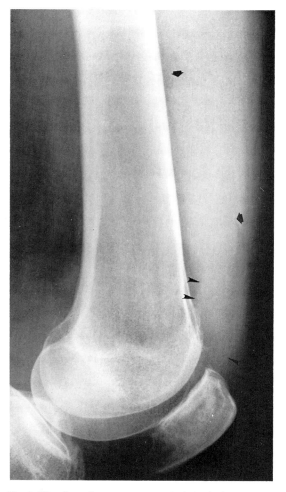

Fig. 1.18. Synovium escapes superiorly in the knee joint sparing the bones. From Butt *et al.* (1983) with permission.

does not encroach on the perisynovial fat will not be recognizable unless it causes bone change. Synovium that is not trapped by ligaments or fibrous capsule (Fig. 1.18) can expand into the soft tissues without involving the bone and can reach an enormous size with little or no bone abnormality. If, however, the synovium is trapped by the ligaments or the capsule, the expansion of the synovium occurs inwards and the bone is eroded (Fig. 1.19a). This radiological finding of early erosion does not indicate localized disease of the synovium but, rather, diffuse

disease throughout the joint visible only where the synovium is trapped. In the shoulder, for example, the erosion will be most apparent at the anatomical neck (where the synovial lining attaches), superiorly under the rotator cuff and anteriorly and posteriorly beneath the fibrous capsule, while the inferior neck is spared even though the synovium is floridly abnormal throughout (Fig. 1.19). Similarly, in the hip, the escape is inferiorly (Fig. 1.20), whereas in the knee the escape is superiorly in the suprapatellar region (Fig. 1.18). In general terms, one

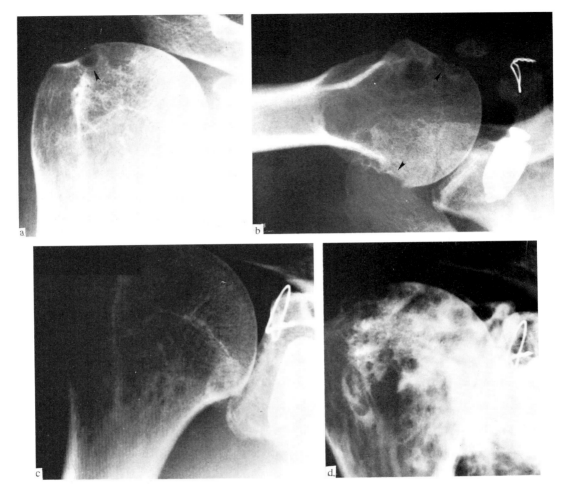

Fig. 1.19. Synovial hypertrophy causes erosion of underlying bone where the synovium is trapped by tendon insertions (a), ligament and capsular insertions (b), but spares the bone where there is room for it to expand (c), even though the synovium is diffusely involved throughout the joint (d).

should look beneath the collateral ligaments and under known tendon insertions for evidence of early synovial hypertrophy. This author has not been impressed by the necessity for an area to be bare of periosteum before an erosion can occur. If the synovium is trapped within the joint, erosion of both sides of that joint will occur.

Difficulty arises if the fibrous capsule is attached a considerable distance from the joint margins, because intracapsular erosions may well appear to be well separated from the joint

and their joint origin might not be suspected (Fig. 1.21). Equally confusing is the radiological appearance of synovium within the marrow cavity because expansion of the synovial lesion is not hindered to any great degree and a large lesion may develop with its joint origin not being suspected (Fig. 1.22a). Arthrography will often fill these 'geodes', making the origin of the lesion obvious (Fig. 1.22b). It is wise to consider the possibility of a synovial origin for any radiolucent lesion of bone which is near a joint (Fig. 1.23), even if the joint appears normal on

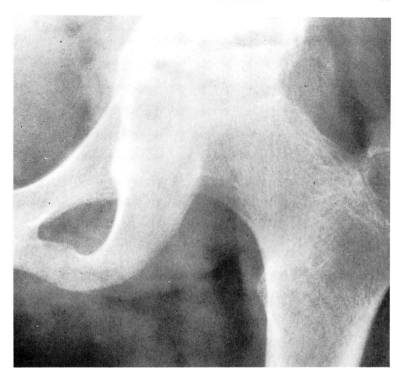

Fig. 1.20. Synovial mass disease in the hip tends to escape inferiorly without causing erosion but cannot escape superiorly where it causes bone erosion.

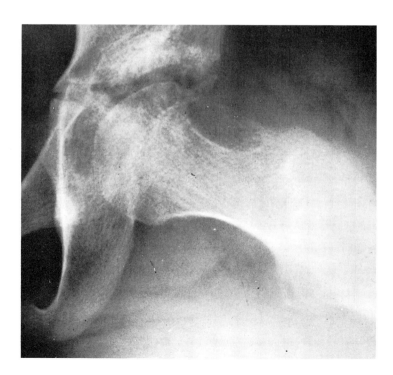

Fig. 1.21. Bone erosion caused by joint mass disease may not be suspected if the erosion is some distance from the joint as it can be in joints where the fibrous capsule inserts well away from the joint margins.

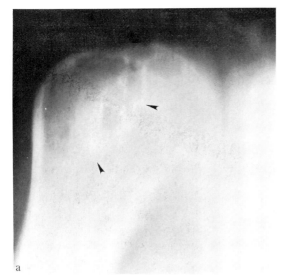

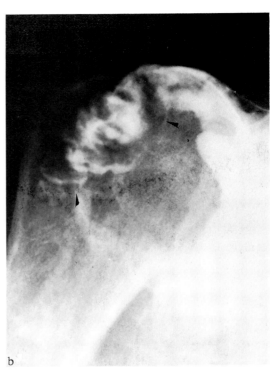

Fig. 1.22. An intra-osseous extension of synovial disease (geode) may well fool the unwary and arthrography may be necessary to demonstrate the joint origin of the lesion (b).

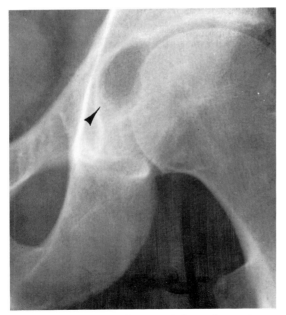

Fig. 1.23. A joint origin for any radiolucent lesion of bone near a joint must be kept in mind even though the joint appears normal.

cursory examination.

It is most important to resist the temptation to make a definitive diagnosis of the type of synovial disease on any of the observations above. A sound diagnosis of the type of joint disease cannot be made on examination of one joint only, and knowledge of the distribution of the disease is essential. The reader may well ask why it is so often done and so often got away with. Obviously, the answer is that most of the time it does not matter what the radiological diagnosis is in the patient with joint disease. When it does matter, a diagnosis made on films of a single joint will be misleading as often as it is helpful. This is particularly true early in the course of a disease.

It is possible to decide if a joint process is active or not by the presence of bone repair in the base of an erosion, especially if it can be seen that there is no soft-tissue mass accompanying the erosion. Bone repair cannot fill in holes, and all that the body can do to restore

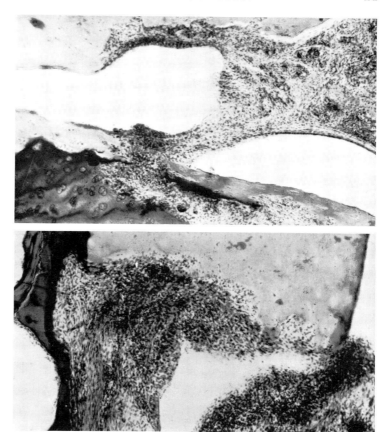

Fig. 1.24. Pannus will infiltrate beneath the articular cartilage and destroy the subchondral cortical bone as it advances. From Silberberg (1985) with permission.

strength is to reinforce the margins of the holes with sclerotic bone.

PANNUS

If the synovial expansion is caused by tumour, for instance, there may be no other radiological features of the process than those described above, but if the expansion is caused by inflammatory granulation tissue there may be more to see. The granulation tissue (pannus) has the ability to infiltrate between the layers of articular cartilage and beneath the articular cartilage, destroying the subchondral cortical bone (Fig. 1.24). This process will be seen radiologically as a localized destruction of subchondral cortical bone (Fig. 1.25), indicating that the process is localized and not generalized. Earlier, pannus will only be seen as a mass lesion at the periphery of the joint where it is trapped by the capsule, and one cannot distinguish pannus from any other joint mass at this stage (Fig. 1.26).

PROTEOLYSIS

Loss of articular cartilage will be seen as a decrease in the thickness of the 'joint space'. This narrowing can be taken to be due to proteolysis only if the change is rapid and occurs before there is extensive pannus or mechanical breakdown (Fig. 1.29). Pannus will soon interfere with the nutrition of the articular cartilage and lead to its disappearance, while mechanical breakdown causes cartilage to disappear by an unknown mechanism. If one is careful to exclude other causes of loss of joint space, the diagnosis of a proteolytic process can be made

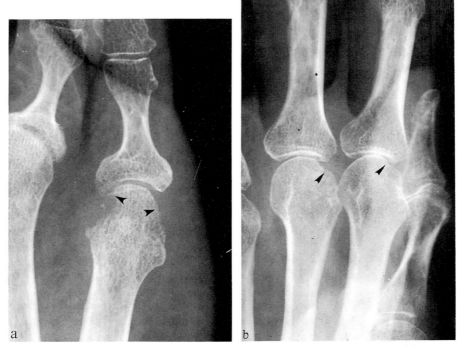

Fig. 1.25. Two radiographs demonstrate inflammatory granulation tissue (pannus) causing localized destruction of subchondral cortical bone.

which will establish unequivocally the presence of joint disease early in its course.

The definitive exclusion of proteolysis by the absence of joint narrowing could be important, as it suggests tuberculosis. One must bear in mind the possibility of proteolysis being masked by articular cartilage oedema, which has been described but which is exceedingly rare and will not persist after the onset of radiologically demonstrable pannus. Pannus without proteolysis remains the hallmark of tuberculosis, and no other diagnosis can be accepted if the disease is monarticular or pauci-articular until tuberculosis has been conclusively excluded. In this regard, a negative aspiration cannot be considered conclusive, and histological examination of the synovium must be performed.

OSTEOPOROSIS

(a) *Periarticular*
Periarticular osteoporosis is a popular sign of

arthritis and has been considered a required diagnostic sign in such conditions as rheumatoid arthritis. The periarticular regions of the long bones are the areas of the bones which are most active metabolically and are the areas which will become osteoporotic first no matter what the stimulus. Periarticular osteoporosis is, therefore, a very good sign that something is wrong but is not a very good sign that the abnormality is joint disease. For example, severe periarticular osteoporosis as seen in Fig. 1.27 can be due to disuse of bone and mislead the unwary into diagnosing the presence of polyarticular joint disease. Severe periarticular osteoporosis (Fig. 1.55) can occur in a patient without any joint disease at all and, therefore, should be interpreted with caution early in the course of a disease process. It is of considerably more value in the differential diagnosis of more advanced joint disease.

One must remember that the onset of osteoporosis will be delayed in relationship to the

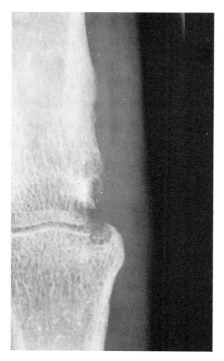

Fig. 1.26. Early bone erosion from pannus is entirely similar to bone erosion from any other synovial mass in the early stages before it is seen to infiltrate across the joint surface.

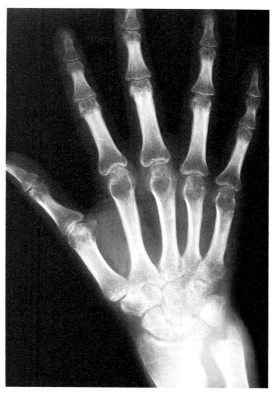

Fig. 1.27. Periarticular osteoporosis is a good sign of an abnormality in the limb but it not a good sign of joint disease. This patient with monarticular joint disease has periarticular osteoporosis of all the joints in the radiograph.

onset of the disease process, and conversely the presence of osteoporosis at the onset of a clinical complaint indicates pre-existing disease. This feature is particularly important in the diagnosis of joint abnormality in children, since virtually all initial complaints follow injury. The osteoporotic, recently injured joint is the one which was abnormal before the injury.

Disuse osteoporosis tends to involve all the bones distal to the lesion causing the osteoporosis but, again, a certain delay will occur before this will become apparent.

(b) Of subchondral cortex
The loss of subchondral cortex is a reliable early sign of joint disease. Just as preservation of subperiosteal cortical bone is the sign of bone health and its disappearance the sign of bone disease, so the preservation of subchondral cortical bone is the sign of joint health and its loss

the sign of joint disease. Even the most advanced disuse atrophy or Sudeck's atrophy will preserve subchondral cortical integrity (Fig. 1.28). On the other hand, the very earliest inflammatory arthritis will cause loss of the subchondral cortical bone (Fig. 1.29). Along with minimal joint space narrowing from proteolysis, this sign is the earliest reliable sign of joint disease.

In the small joints which are readily radiographed with high-definition techniques, it is reasonable to say that if a process has continued to the point of soft-tissue swelling and bone atrophy (Fig. 1.28), and there is no evidence of loss of subchondral cortical bone, there is no joint disease. The exclusion of joint disease, if done reliably and carefully, is the greatest con-

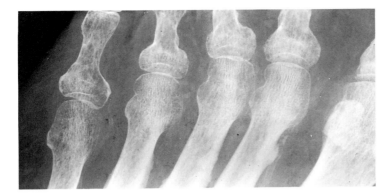

Fig. 1.28. If an infection has reached the stage of soft-tissue swelling and bone atrophy without loss of subchondral cortical integrity, the joints are not infected.

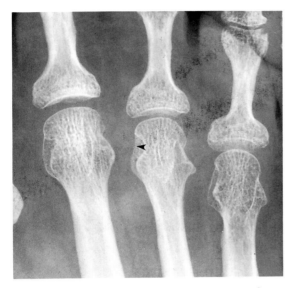

Fig. 1.29. The earliest reliable signs of the presence of inflammatory arthritis are loss of subchondral cortical integrity (arrow) and thinning of articular cartilage.

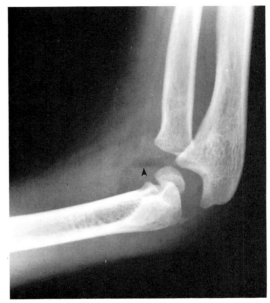

Fig. 1.30. There is no reason why a lipohaemarthrosis cannot be demonstrated with an intra-articular fracture in any joint.

tribution that radiology can make to the patient with the clinical suspicion of joint disorder.

OTHER

(a) Lipohaemarthrosis

If marrow fat is liberated into a joint it will float on blood or synovial fluid. Because marrow fat, unlike other body fat, is not encapsulated in small vesicles, it will form an interface with the fluid on which it floats and be demonstrable as a fluid level on a horizontal beam radiograph (Fig. 1.30). The appearance has been described in the shoulder and knee, but there is no reason why it should not be seen in any joint where a fracture communicates with the marrow cavity. Although a lipohaemarthrosis has been reported in the absence of fracture, the occurrence is rare and the method of excluding fracture questionable. It has not been reported in the absence of trauma and must be considered a sign of fracture if seen.

(b) Calcification

Calcification of joint structures is a part of specific disease processes and the radiography will be covered thoroughly in the sections of the book dealing with those conditions. In general, cloudy soft calcification is more likely to be symptomatic and to disappear with or just after the onset of symptoms than is hard dense calcification. The exclusion of calcification is, therefore, the most difficult in the very patient most likely to need it. It is the brave radiologist who excludes calcification on poor films.

Calcification in a gouty tophus (Fig. 1.31) is diagnostic and often must be sought in asymptomatic areas. Once again, it is worth emphasizing that an accurate diagnosis of joint disease cannot be made on films of one joint. In gout it is often more valuable to radiograph asymptomatic areas than it is to radiograph the symptomatic ones. A firm diagnosis is often possible on the standard examination when it might not even be considered in films of the symptomatic joint (Fig. 1.32).

(c) Growth disturbance

Alteration in growth, either suppression or enhancement, is a good sign of joint disorder, without being specific for any one condition. Even more, its absence is a good sign that a disorder did not start in childhood. The usual diseases associated with a growth or maturation disorder will be covered in the appropriate sections, but one is worth mentioning here because it is so commonly forgotten. By far the most potent force to influence growth is ischaemia, and often the growth disturbance is so bizarre that ischaemia is not considered in the differential possibilities.

(d) Malalignment

When severe, malalignment is not difficult to appreciate and it indicates true joint disorder. This is not true for less severe malalignment— the so-called 'subluxation'. An acute traumatic subluxation, in the sense of a little bit of dislocation, is something that this author finds hard to accept, and although it is, perhaps, possible for the supporting structures of a joint to be stretched a little and not a lot, and hence allow a slight malalignment, it is much more likely that the slightly malaligned joint is due to a spontaneously reduced dislocation. The other possibility, rarely considered, is that the 'subluxed' joint is not abnormal at all. If a normal joint is held at the extreme of its normal range of motion by a force that is external to the joint, the joint will appear subluxed. Fig. 1.33 demonstrates the author's normal (he hopes) index

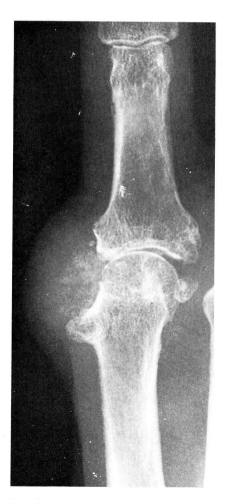

Fig. 1.31. The calcified tophus is diagnostic of gout.

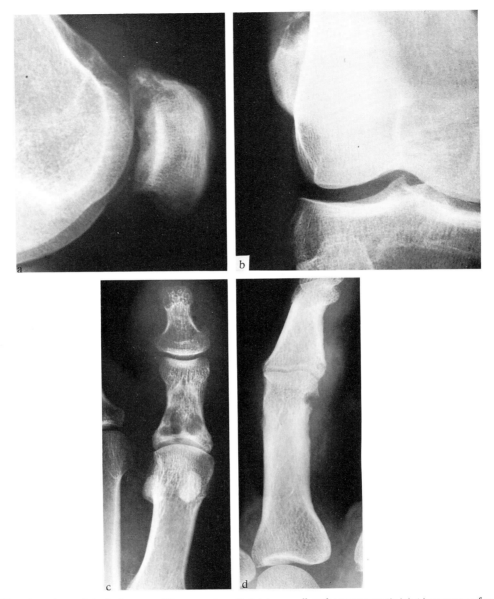

Fig. 1.32. A routine radiological survey of the asymptomatic joints as well as the symptomatic joint is necessary for a sensible diagnosis in the patient with joint disease. Few people would have considered gout in this patient if only the symptomatic knee and not the asymptomatic feet and hands had been X-rayed.

finger held at the limit of normal extension by an external force (his other index finger). Note how the MCP joint is 'subluxed'. If one were to hide this joint in the body so that the forces acting on it could not be seen, the appreciation of the cause of the appearance would not be easy. For example, a rotational subluxation of C1 on C2 (Fig. 1.34) occurred following injury, and it is tempting to call it abnormal and to infer that treatment is indicated. This C1/C2 'subluxation' is in fact rotation of C1 on C2 to compensate for a fixed rotation of the neck in

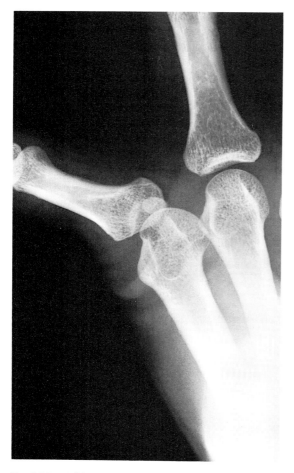

Fig. 1.33. Subluxation of the index MCP joint is due to traction on the finger. Note that this joint is not abnormal. Post-traumatic subluxation is often due to a lesion somewhere else causing a normal joint to be held in the extreme of normal motion. It is tempting to call the normal joint abnormal and to look no further.

the opposite direction. In other words, the C1/C2 subluxation is a perfectly normal motion, and if there is an abnormality in the neck it is at some other level. The author would like to see the term 'subluxation' after an acute injury reserved to describe this type of appearance because it indicates that the pathological process is somewhere else. It is unlikely that this dream will come true and one must continue to view reported subluxation with suspicion.

(e) Periostitis
Periosteal new bone formation tends to occur in those joint diseases which are vicious with severe inflammation, pain and disability. It is not surprising that it is seen in Reiter's syndrome, infection, and hypertrophic pulmonary osteoarthropathy more often than in rheumatoid arthritis. Unfortunately, it can occur in virtually any arthritis and has little differential value in the individual patient. In the past, it was said not to occur in tuberculosis, but this is not true. It must be emphasized that bacteriological diagnosis must be made bacteriologically and not radiologically.

(f) Plantar fasciitis
Plantar fasciitis can be recognized on radiographs of high quality early in its course. Why the attachment of the plantar fascia to the os calcis should become inflamed in a patient with joint disease is not known, but it is a dependable sign of joint disease and is presumed to be a sign of the rheumatoid variants and not of rheumatoid arthiritis. Early in the disease, its presence excludes rheumatoid arthritis. Although later the appearance is that of proliferation, early findings are due to loss of subperiosteal cortical integrity (Fig. 1.35a). It must be emphasized that the plantar fasciitis referred to is not a calcaneal spur, which this author considers a normal variant.

(g) Achille's bursitis
Achille's tendon bursitis is a common but non-specific finding indicating the presence of bursitis, but it is not of value in differentiating the various forms of arthritis. The author considers that Achille's bursal inflammation can be due to many causes, including local trauma, but it is a sign that must be explained (Fig. 1.35b).

The principle that underlines the radiological diagnosis of joint disorder is that the presence of joint disease can be determined from a study of the symptomatic joint but the type of joint disorder cannot. A correct diagnosis of the type of arthritis that is affecting a patient's shoulder

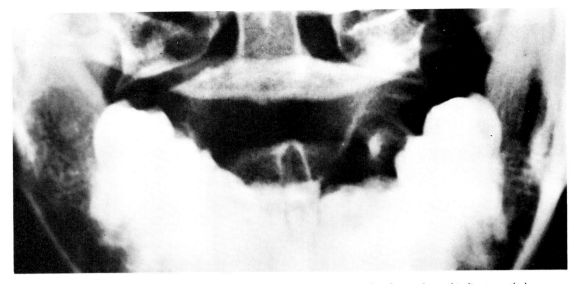

Fig. 1.34.   Rotational subluxation of C1 on C2 is a normal response to spasm of neck muscles and indicates pathology somewhere else.

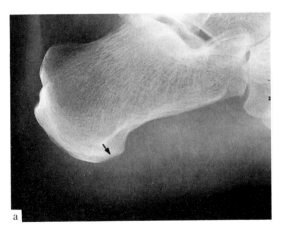

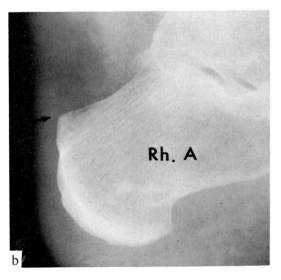

Fig. 1.35a.   The earliest sign of plantar fasciitis is loss of the subchondral cortical integrity in the area of the insertion of the plantar aponeurosis. Cf. the normal (Fig. 1.35b).

Fig. 1.35b.   Swelling of the Achilles tendon bursa shown by filling in of the normal radiolucent triangle (cf. Fig. 1.35a) behind the superior corner of the posterior surface of the os calcis. This is a non-specific sign and further findings must be looked for before a diagnosis can be written on the films.

based on radiographs of the shoulder alone is a lucky guess. It seems ludicrous to suggest to a patient with a sore shoulder that one is going to X-ray his feet, but if it is not done an early definitive diagnosis will not be possible. Conversely if high-definition radiography of the hands, wrists, feet, os calcis, and the SI joints are obtained, a definitive diagnosis of the presence and type of arthritis should be possible in the vast majority of patients.

Miscellaneous

TOMOGRAPHY

The purpose of non computer-assisted tomography is to decrease the amount of detail recorded on the radiographic film and in so doing to accentuate a plane of interest. Although it is an illusion that the tomograph increases the definition of a particular part or that there is information on a tomogram that is not present on a standard radiograph with the same projection, the illusion is valuable in clinical practice. As a radiologist, one has the obligation to demonstrate pathological processes clearly and distinctly enough that even the less experienced interpreter will make no mistake. Tomography is underused for this purpose and there should be no objection to using it to clarify a radiological observation.

Tomography is essential in certain areas of the skeleton where routine radiography cannot project overlapping structures clear of each other and a typical example is its use to demonstrate the lateral masses of the cervical spine. Only stereoscopic lateral radiography and tomography can separate the lateral masses one from the other whilst maintaining a lateral projection, and unless one or other of these techniques is routinely used, major injuries of one set of lateral masses will not be recognized (Fig. 1.36). Most of us who routinely use one technique or the other feel that the commonest bone injury of the cervical spine is a unilateral lateral mass fracture, whereas those who do not would rarely make such a diagnosis.

If a longitudinal fracture cannot be demonstrated by radiography other than in the plane of the fracture because all projections superimpose normal cortex on the fracture plane, will tomography not prevent that and demonstrate the fracture? Practical experience would suggest that the loss of definition is such that the fracture will not be visible.

It must be emphasized that tomography will not demonstrate medullary bone destruction which is invisible on standard radiographs, and it cannot be used to delineate the extent of a medullary lesion in bone.

Precise measurement of the level of the tomographic plane can be obtained with a simple device described by Samuel (1965, personal communication). An 'N' of metal placed perpendicular to the plane of the tomogram will show on the tomogram as three spots, and the proportionate distance between these can be used to calculate the precise location of the plane on a film obtained perpendicular to the 'N' (Fig. 1.37).

TRACTION PHENOMENA

(a) 'Looseness'
The unarguable radiological sign of looseness is the demonstration of displacement, and it does not matter if one is examining a joint prosthesis or a loose body. Apart from a chance radiological observation of a change in position, the demonstration of displacement requires the deliberate intervention of the radiologist, and traction is the usual method employed. It is generally accepted that the appearance of the radiolucent crescent of Legg–Perthes disease seen only in the frog-leg position is due to the traction that occurs on the femoral head in this position. If this is true, why not use traction to diagnose Legg–Perthes disease earlier and with the patient in a normal position? The suction effect of an intact articular surface on the opposing loose surface of an osteochondral fracture or osteochondritis dissecans should be sufficient to dislodge it if traction is applied to the limb. Traction under screening control can be

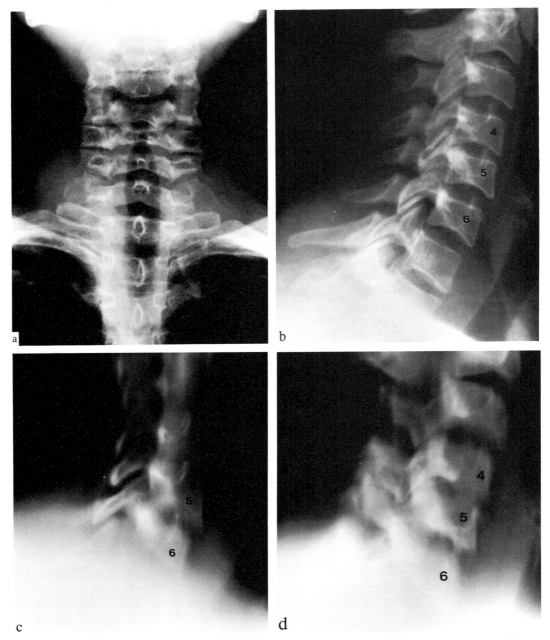

Fig. 1.36. Tomography and stereoscopy are the only radiographic techniques which will avoid superimposition of the lateral masses on a lateral film permitting the demonstration of an old fracture of the lateral mass of C5 (d) separate from the normal lateral mass of C5 on the other side (c). Although the frontal film suggests an abnormality of the lateral masses due to the rotation sign, it is not possible to confirm the abnormality on a standard lateral projection (b).

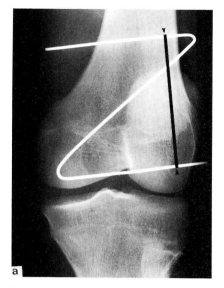
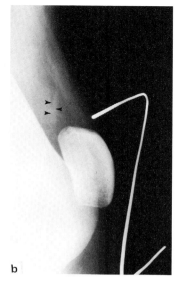
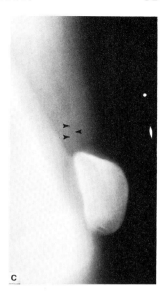

Fig. 1.37. During tomography the level of any particular section (c) can be drawn on a frontal film (a) by measuring the proportionate distance between the three metallic spots seen anterior to the patella on the tomographic section. From Butt *et al.* (1983) with permission.

very gentle, need not be painful, and is worth trying before more invasive procedures.

The author has found that most loose prostheses will move if pulled, and he feels that it is difficult to accept other signs of looseness if vigorous traction does not cause displacement.

(b) Vacuum phenomena
Martell and Poznanski (1970) describe the value of producing a vacuum defect in the hip joint by traction, since they found that this excluded the presence of an effusion in the joint. If the displacement produced by the traction was significant (greater than 1 mm), the absence of a radiologically demonstrable vacuum phenomenon indicated the presence of an effusion. The production of a vacuum phenomenon on the other side with similar traction was further evidence that the abnormal joint contained an effusion. Unfortunately, vacuum phenomena in other joints do not exclude an aspiratable effusion and this applies particularly to the shoulder and to the knee.

Spontaneously occurring vacuum phenomena have been described in normal joints, in degenerated immobile joints (e.g. symphisis pubis), and in traumatized discs. This author is hesitant to accept a vacuum phenomenon as indicative of significant disease processes.

Traction has been used to produce a vacuum phenomenon around a loose prosthesis and is an elegant way of avoiding arthrography.

Errors in diagnosis

DUE TO INADEQUATE OR INCOMPLETE EXAMINATIONS

(a) Those that are poor examinations
If one reviews errors in radiology in general, and in skeletal radiology in particular, one will find the most common cause to be reporting an incomplete or inadequate examination. If that is true, how can one get away with reporting poor films? The answer lies in the enormous

amount of medically unnecessary radiography being performed, and where there is no possibility of providing medically useful information it does not matter how bad a study is. If the reader were to review his cases in which medically useful information could have been obtained from good radiographs, he will see quite clearly that he does not get away with reporting bad ones. It is a good rule of thumb that although a positive diagnosis might be made on a bad film, one may never infer 'normal'.

(b)   Those that are considered good examinations
There is no room in a text of this sort to discuss the errors that arise from poor radiographic technique, but it may be instructive to look at some errors that have occurred during the interpretation of 'good' radiographs in order to understand some of the principles that underlie standard radiography. Traditionally, certain

studies have been accepted even though they are inadequate by definition.

Studies that are routinely single projections. Of these, the 'pelvis to show the hips' is the most common. Fig. 1.38 demonstrates that one cannot justify the diagnosis 'normal' on a single frontal film of the hips no matter how often one does so. A single frontal film of the shoulder with the humerus in external rotation is commonly performed, but this examination cannot be relied on for the diagnosis of 'normal', even in the injured patient (Fig. 1.11a). Single-view examinations for an initial diagnosis should be abandoned.

Studies that are routinely underpenetrated. Once again, the pelvis and hips are the commonest culprits. An underpenetrated pelvis film cannot be interpreted as normal (for example, Fig. 1.39a, b), since more penetration may demonstrate bilateral ischaemic necrosis of the femoral

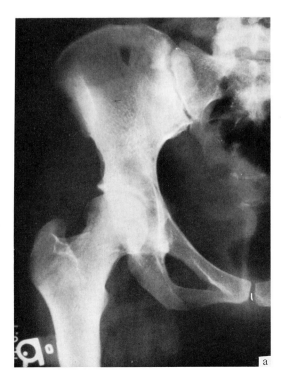

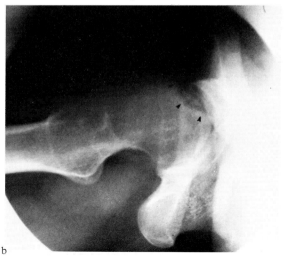

Fig. 1.38.   A frontal film alone (a) is not adequate for the initial examination of the hips.

a   b

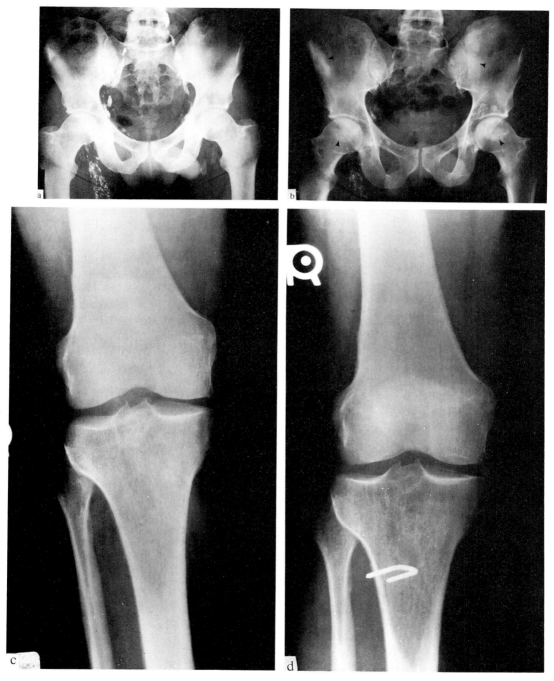

Fig. 1.39. The radiographs of two patients demonstrate the difficulty that can arise if underpenetrated films are interpreted. In both cases the salient diagnostic features were not recognized on the initial examination.

heads. Fig. 1.36(c, d) shows that the difficulty is not confined to the hip joint. It is not easy to avoid this error, but if one remembers that the radiographically 'pretty' bone film is usually underpenetrated it may help.

Studies that are routinely non-frontal or non-lateral. It has been accepted that one frontal film can demonstrate the lumbar spine even though only three of the five vertebrae are shown on it. The diagnosis 'normal' should not be made in the absence of an inclined frontal film of L5 (Fig. 1.40). In the cervical spine, one routinely accepts a frontal film which shows no vertebral bodies at all (Fig. 1.36a). What is assumed to be vertebral body on a casual glance is, in fact, lamina. Similarly, the lamina in the dorsal spine (Fig. 1.41) can simulate vertebral bodies.

Studies suffering from inertia. For some reason, recent technical advances have not filtered through to skeletal radiography. Modern generators and tubes are now sufficiently advanced that the large focal spot can be abandoned and microfocus tubes of 0·09 mm are commercially available. It is no longer necessary to use screen–film combinations that were developed for the pregnant abdomen, and the new screens provide high-definition radiography at reasonable speed. The recent advances permit exquisite bone radiography to be performed as a routine without increasing the workload or the time of the examination.

There is little point in attempting to exclude early bone disease on standard radiographic film now that processor-compatible mammographic film is available.

Buckland-Wright (1981) is opening new doors with his experimental microfocal radiography. By using a 2·5 micron focal spot he is able to demonstrate pathological changes which one would have considered microscopic, and can show these in living bone. One awaits further progress with great interest.

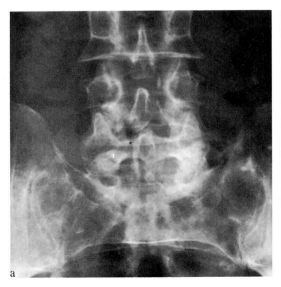 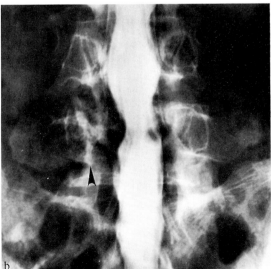

a   b

Fig. 1.40. A single frontal film of the lumbar spine is not adequate to demonstrate all the vertebrae in the lumbar spine, and lesions such as body and pedicle destruction (b) may well not be suspected unless an inclined frontal film of L5 is obtained.

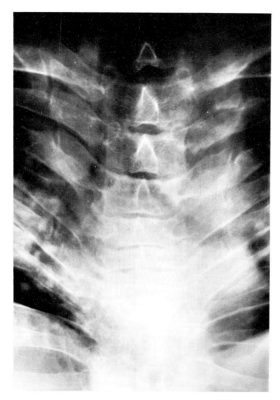

Fig. 1.41. An anteroposterior projection of a kyphotic dorsal spine shows that the laminae can simulate vertebral bodies on a frontal film. No vertebral body is visible on this film.

DUE TO ONE'S TENDENCY TO IGNORE THE FUNDAMENTAL DEFICIENCIES OF RADIOGRAPHY

(a) Its inability to demonstrate medullary bone destruction

Standard radiography, including standard tomography, is unable to demonstrate the integrity of the marrow cavity of bone; in particular it cannot demonstrate the extent of lesions which occupy this space. Lödwick (1971) has investigated this failing thoroughly and the interested reader is directed to his original work. Two examples from his text suffice to illustrate that medullary bone destruction cannot be demonstrated in the adult (Fig. 1.42). Several conclusions follow from this observation. The first is

that any small 'central' radiolucency in a bone shaft must be cortical or endocortical in location (Fig. 1.43). Secondly, the size of a medullary lesion cannot be predicted from the radiographs and a 'small' lesion may well fill the medullary cavity. Thirdly, 'trabeculation' within a lesion is much more likely to be due to residual uneroded endocortical bone between areas of erosion than it is to be due to actual bony bridges across the centre of a lesion. Fourthly, the 'advancing edge' of a tumour may not be its edge. In fact, as the edge is a zone of advancing osteoporosis, the 'tumour edge' may be neither the tumour nor its edge. (Surely this goes a long way to explain why healthy osteoporosis can mimic a destructive tumour [Fig. 1.55].) Finally, the size of a purely destructive medullary lesion will almost always be underestimated by an assessment of the cortical (the radiologically visible) involvement.

(b) Its inability to verify bone continuity

If planes of separation of bone cannot be demonstrated on radiography unless the radiographic beam is parallel to the plane of the cleavage, and if the plane of cleavage is one that does not lend itself to radiographic projection, the integrity of a bone cannot be guaranteed. The advent of CT scanning has shown us just how often apparently normal bones are fractured longitudinally. Fig. 1.44 demonstrates (with a little tongue in cheek) trabecular continuity across a joint which would be considered diagnostic of fusion but which is shown to be an overlap phenomenon alone. Although this is a trivial example, picture the process deep in the body and it becomes apparent how difficult it is to prove bone continuity or, for that matter, bone union. Radiographic examinations to establish bone union should be, therefore, attempts to demonstrate bone discontinuity. This distinction is necessary in the individual patient in order to decide the radiographic investigation to be followed. Fig. 1.45 illustrates the reasonably common difficulty of demonstrating union of a femoral neck fracture, even with the aid of tomography. If one remembers,

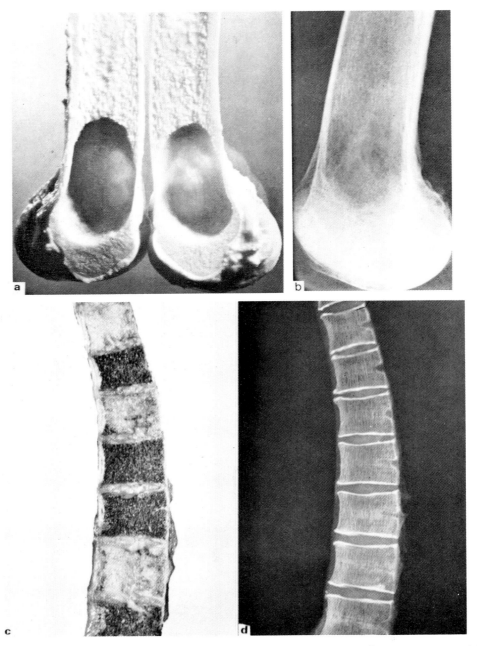

Fig. 1.42. Visibility of bone destruction. (a) Bisected distal femur with trabecular bone and inner cortex removed. Edges of hole in trabecular bone are perpendicular, but those in area of cortical destruction are sloping. (b) Radiograph of (a) after halves were fitted together and submerged in water phantom. None of the edges of bone destruction are evident, in spongy bone because relative density is small and in cortex because of lack of sharp edges. The pattern of trabecular bone is gone. (c) Section of spine involved in metastatic carcinoma. (d) Radiograph of (c). (a) and (b) from Lodwick (1964) with permission. (c) and (d) from Lodwick (1965) with permission.

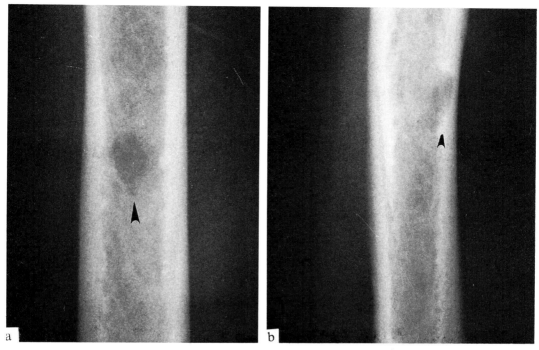

Fig. 1.43. A 'central' radiolucency is endocortical or cortical in location and a suitable oblique film (b) will demonstrate this fact.

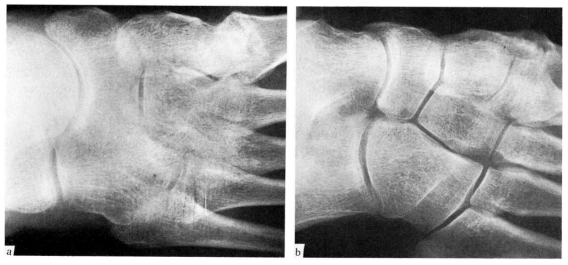

Fig. 1.44. The radiological demonstration of bone continuity even at trabecular level is not reliable. An oblique film (b) demonstrates that the tarsal 'fusion' (a) is an overlap phenomenon alone.

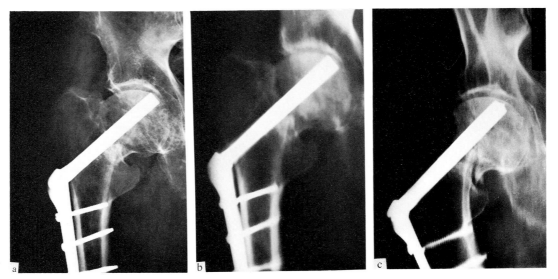

Fig. 1.45. Oblique projections are necessary to demonstrate non-union of the femoral neck. The most successful radiographic projection (c) is 30° internal rotation.

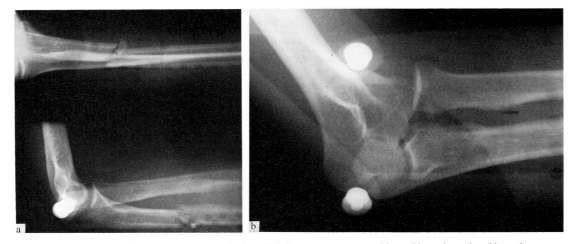

Fig. 1.46. An oblique film (b) demonstrates clearly that all dislocations are not readily visible on frontal and lateral projections. The oblique films were obtained without moving either patient or limb.

however, that one is attempting to demonstrate a fracture rather than to demonstrate union, one will realize that the X-ray beam must be parallel to the plane of the suspected fracture and be able to answer the question by rotating the femur internally.

That planes of cleavage (i.e. incomplete union) can defy radiographic demonstration is undoubtedly the explanation of the reasonably common occurrence of refracture of a radiographically and clinically solidly united femoral shaft fracture. Sufficient union occurs to resist clinical displacement, but sufficient cleavage remains causing the bone to break with weight-bearing.

(c) Its inability to record dynamic factors

There is a tendency to assume that the radiographic image is a true record of things as they are and of things as they were, rather than to appreciate that it is often only a brief glimpse of a changing process. Errors from this cause occur most commonly after injury, because one infers that the position of the bones at the time of the radiography was the position of the bones at the time of the injury. Very few bones can break without giving way afterwards, yet one rarely thinks of this 'giving way' whilst interpreting radiographs. A few seconds thought about mechanisms of injury, force lines and the resultant movement of the bones will often permit a radiological diagnosis that was not initially apparent. Fig. 1.46 illustrates an injury that can be discovered if this concept of 'giving way' is remembered. The clinical significance of an injury is not altered by the time at which an X-ray was taken, and the sequence dislocation–then X-ray–then reduction is not much different clinically from the sequence dislocation–then reduction–then X-ray. The radiological diagnosis, however, is immensely more difficult with the second sequence and the problem requires further discussion.

If there is no displacement of the fragments at the time of a fracture, the fracture will not be visible radiologically. A scaphoid fracture is the best-known example of this type of injury,

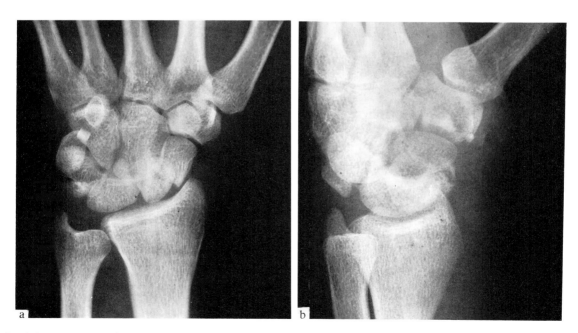

Fig. 1.47. A trans-scaphoid perilunar dislocation of the wrist causes mid-carpal rotation, preventing a lateral radiograph of both wrist and hand being obtained at the same time. The resultant oblique view (b) tends to hide the presence of the dislocation. Significant displacement of a fractured scaphoid as seen on the frontal film (a) does not occur in the absence of a mid-carpal dislocation.

but many karate injuries and the occasional subcapital fracture of the femur are other examples that must be kept in mind (Fig. 1.6). Careful perusal of the films for the earliest signs of displacement may be necessary to confirm bone injury. Most clinicians are aware of the possibility of undisplaced fractures in the above circumstances, but even they tend to err when the above kind of injury is associated with another, clinically more evident, injury. Bone scintigraphy is a useful adjunct to the diagnosis of

the undisplaced fracture and its use will be covered in a subsequent chapter.

Fractures of bones such as the scaphoid, which are usually difficult to visualize, should be viewed with suspicion if they are obviously displaced. In order for a scaphoid fracture to displace significantly (Fig. 1.47a) there must be disruption of those forces which normally resist that displacement—namely the intracarpal ligaments. A displaced fracture of the scaphoid is, therefore, a prime indicator of the presence of a

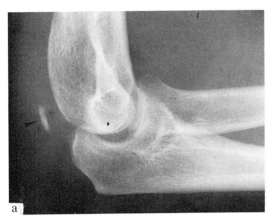

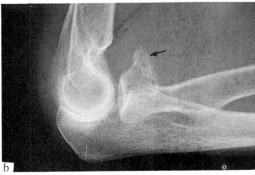

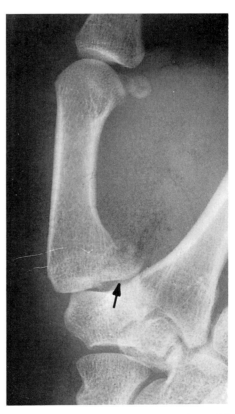

Fig. 1.48. The elbows of two patients following injury demonstrate the importance of careful assessment of 'chip' fractures. The partial avulsion of a tendon insertion (a) is relatively minor compared to the avulsion of a ligament or capsule insertion (b) because the latter indicates a spontaneously reduced dislocation.

Fig. 1.49. The displaced 'chip' fracture of the base of the metacarpal of the thumb indicates an unreduced dislocation. Note it is not the chip that is dislocated but the bone from which the chip arose.

mid-carpal fracture–dislocation. Usually, these fracture–dislocations cause rotation of the mid-carpus, which prevents lateral projections of both the wrist and the hand being obtained on the same exposure. The resultant oblique film of the carpus (Fig. 1.47b) goes a long way to hide the dislocation.

The avulsion of ligamentous, capsular, or periosteal attachments to bone is commonly seen on radiographs as chip or flake fractures. If this is the only radiological observation, one tends to consider it a minor injury. Fig. 1.48 succinctly illustrates that chip fractures may be more than they seem and that there is a distinct difference between the avulsion of a tendon insertion and of a ligament insertion. Forceful muscle contraction may avulse a tendon insertion (Fig. 1.48a) with no other injury, whereas a ligament insertion cannot be avulsed and displaced without some other injury occurring, usually a dislocation of the joint (Fig. 1.48b). In the example illustrated it is easy to infer that both elbows have injuries of similar magnitude, the one with a chip fracture posteriorly, the other with a chip fracture anteriorly. A little thought will, however, lead to the deduction that the posterior chip is due to partial avulsion of the triceps tendon insertion and therefore not of great significance, whereas the anterior chip fracture is due to avulsion of a capsule insertion and therefore indicates a spontaneously reduced dislocation of the elbow. Figs. 1.49–1.54 present a number of cases in which an occult dislocation can be recognized by the tell-tale chip fracture. Elliot *et al.* (1972) have pointed out, quite correctly, that the size of the chip is not important.

Occasionally, dynamic factors other than displacement must be considered in radiological assessment, and one of these is blood supply. Fig. 1.55a is difficult to interpret unless one appreciates that the oddly 'destroyed' bone is, in fact, normal bone responding by osteoporosis to the insult of distal ischaemia. The ischaemia protects the distal bones from radiological change. In this case, a quick look at the clinical

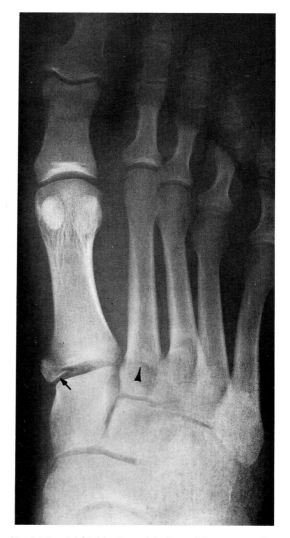

Fig. 1.50. A 'chip' fracture of the base of the metatarsal of the great toe indicates spontaneously reduced dislocation of this joint.

specimen (Fig. 1.55b) makes the diagnosis easy. Picture a similar segmental ischaemia hidden deep within the body. It is clear that the ischaemic bone will fail to respond to normal stimuli, just as the distal foot failed to respond,

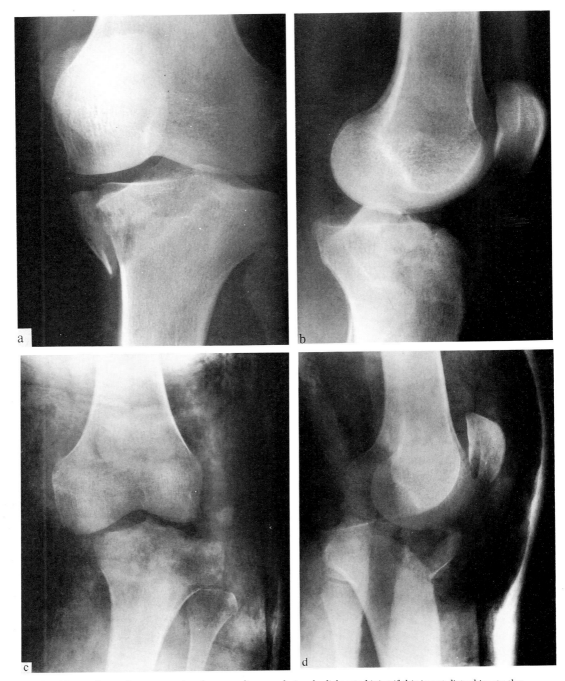

Fig. 1.51. Most radiographers are neat and may realign an obviously dislocated joint if this is not disturbing to the patient. The reasonable realignment of the knee joint should not mislead the unwary into assuming that this is less than a complete dislocation. A follow-up film 24 hours later (c, d) gives a more graphic illustration of the extent of the injury. The most important injury, i.e. that to the popliteal artery, is not visible.

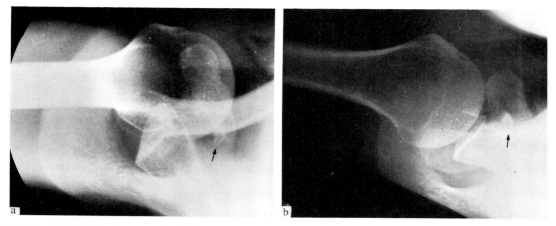

Fig. 1.52. The 'chip' fracture as a sign of dislocation is readily apparent on a film obtained before the dislocation is reduced (a), but it may not be apparent that it has the same significance if the film is obtained after reduction (b).

and the bones will not become osteoporotic. Surely this is the radiological sign of bone ischaemia.

Failure to respond to stimuli for growth or osteoporosis is a much more valuable and valid sign of bone death than are the other signs commonly found in the literature. Using this criterion, one can differentiate the infected foot with ischaemic bone from the infected foot with normal bone. It is true that dead bone in a milieu of tissue fluid will gradually become calcified and hence gradually increase in density, but the majority of the increased density shown on consecutive radiographs is due to a lack of osteoporosis rather than to an increase in bone mass. The signs of bone sclerosis and fragmentation which occur are a result of revascularization and trauma and are not, *per se*, signs of ischaemia. One would have hoped that this concept would have been accepted by now but one still reads with dismay of the surprise that researchers exhibit when infarcted bone has a normal radiological appearance. (Kernohan *et al.* 1983).

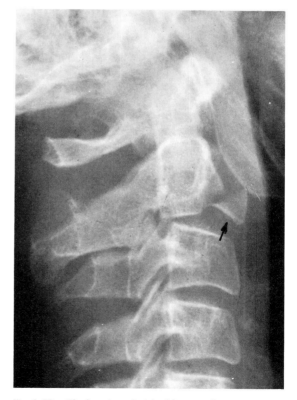

Fig. 1.53. The location of a 'chip' fracture does not alter its significance as long as it is indicative of a capsular or ligamentous avulsion.

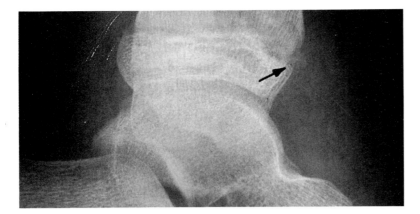

Fig. 1.54. If spontaneous reduction is close to perfect a 'chip' fracture may be the only sign that displacement has occurred and been spontaneously reduced.

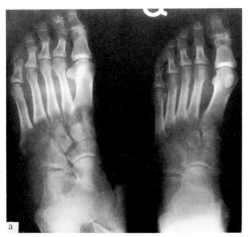

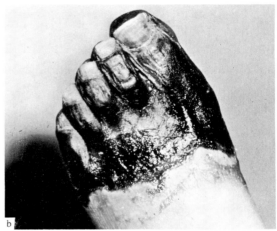

Fig. 1.55. Dead bone does not respond to normal stimulus for atrophy. 'Destroyed' bone, even with an indistinct edge, may be just normal osteoporosis.

References

ARDRAN G.M. (1957) Dose reduction in diagnostic radiology. *Brit. J. Radiol.* **30**, 436–8.

BUCKLAND-WRIGHT J.C. (1981) Microfocal radiography in the quantitative assessment of experimentally induced inflammatory arthritis in guinea pigs. *J. Pathol.* **135**(2), 127–45.

BUTT W.P., LEDERMAN H. & CHUANG S. (1983) Radiology of the suprapatellar region. *Clin. Radiol.* **34**, 522.

CATTO M. (1980) *Muir's Textbook of Pathology*, 11th Edition, pp. 87–92. London: Edward Arnold Ltd.

EDEIKEN J. (1981) General radiological approach to bone lesions. *Roentgen Diagnosis of Dieases of Bone*, 3rd Edition, pp. 8–10. Baltimore: Williams & Wilkins.

EDEIKEN J., HODES P.J. & CAPLIN L.H. (1966) New bone production and periosteal reaction. *Amer. J. Roentgenol.* **97**, 708–18.

ELLIOT J.M. JR, ROGERS L.F., WISSINGER J.P. & LEE J.F. (1972) The hangman's fracture. *Radiology* **104**, 303–7.

KERNOHAN J.G., CALVERT P.T., CATTERALL A., ALI S.Y. & SAYERS D. (1983) Experimental temporary vascular occlusion of the growing femoral head. Presented to the British Orthopaedic Association.

LODWICK G.S. (1964) *Radiol. Clin. N. Amer.* **2**, 209.

LODWICK G.S. (1965) In *Tumours of Bone and Soft Tissue* (ed. M.D. Anderson Hospital). Chicago: Yearbook Medical Publishers.

MARTEL W. & POZNANSKI A.K. (1970) The value of traction during roentgenography of the hip. *Radiology* **94**, 497–503.

SILBERBERG R. (1985) Diseases of joints. In *Anderson's Pathology*, 8th Edition (ed. Kissane J.), p. 1831. St Louis. The C.V. Mosby Co.

VOLBERG F.M., WHALEN J.P., KROOK L. & WINCHESTER P. (1977) Lamellated periosteal reaction: a radiologic and histologic investigation. *Amer. J. Roentgenol.* **128**, 85–7.

WOODS C.G. (1972) *Diagnostic Orthopaedic Pathology*, pp. 268–70. Oxford: Blackwell Scientific Publications.

Chapter 2
Contrast Medium Investigations

I. WATT

An ever-increasing spectrum of contrast medium investigations is available in the investigation and management of bone and joint disease. Once considered refined and esoteric, procedures such as arthrography are now available in most district general hospitals. The indications for individual techniques are in a constant state of flux due both to the availability of alternative imaging techniques and also to changing clinical relevance of those investigations to patient management. For example, computerized tomography may be argued now to be the best initial investigation for putative degenerative disc disease but, because it is not readily available in many centres, radiculography remains the mainstay. Low-dose Myodil/Pantopaque myelography is now totally outmoded, whereas single-contrast knee arthrography retains a place.

It is essential to remember that contrast medium investigations, indeed all radiological investigations, demonstrate anatomy and physiology and do not reveal symptoms such as pain. Hence, the correlation between the demonstration of an abnormality and its relevance in the light of a patient's symptoms often requires a quantum leap of logic fraught with difficulty. All clinicians will know that to ascribe a back pain to a bulging annulus on radiculography is a dangerous step. Furthermore nothing is achieved by undertaking time-consuming, expensive and potentially hazardous contrast medium investigations unless it is clinically relevant, for example to seek the answer to a given problem (is the medial meniscus torn?) or to evaluate a particular circumstance (how extensive is the soft-tissue extension of a bone tumour?). Arguably no radiological investigation should ever be 'routine'. Some, such as arthrography, may be requested in the knowledge of their relative accuracy, safety and availability. Others, such as discography, should be part of an agreed investigational logic. No doubt radiologists need to learn technique and interpretation and clinicians require reassurance of the value and reliability of radiological investigations. Close co-operation, particularly during the early learning stage, will be fruitful and must be encouraged.

One final rule, never undertake a contrast medium examination without adequate plain films beforehand. Osteochondritis dissecans does not need an arthrogram to diagnose, and radiculography is unnecessary to evaluate back pain if a large secondary deposit is shown on a plain film.

Since in day-to-day bone and joint radiology arthrography remains the most common contrast medium investigation to be requested, this subject will be considered under a single heading with specific reference to individual joints. Contrast medium investigations relating to the spine are grouped together into anatomical regions rather than discussed as separate techniques.

Arthrography

INTRODUCTION

Arthrography has been refined considerably since the first demonstration of its feasibility in the knee within ten years of the introduction of X-rays (1905). Almost all joints are amenable to arthrography, the knee, hip, shoulder, wrist and ankle being the most well established. Detailed descriptions of techniques are beyond the scope of this chapter but important points will be emphasized.

It may be argued that adequate double-contrast arthrography of the knee is now the benchmark against which alternative diagnostic techniques are judged. Having progressed from merely indicating the feasibility of demonstrating the soft-tissue structures of the knee in 1905 through the introduction of double-contrast techniques in 1931 to modern spot film imaging, the technique has been refined constantly and made more accurate.

Indications

The most common is internal derangement of the knee, either at the time of injury or following an unsatisfactory response to conservative management. The advent of high-quality arthrography (or arthroscopy) may make it improper to undertake exploratory arthrotomy for the latter indication. Arthrography, arguably, should be performed before any knee is opened for potential meniscal, hyaline cartilage or cruciate ligament injury, since clinical symptoms and signs are notoriously inaccurate or inappropriate. Furthermore there is an acknowledged incidence of unsuspected double meniscal lesions and the known association between ligamentous, meniscal and capsular abnormality which requires evaluation. Arthrography is also the simplest means of investigating potential joint rupture and may be used to evaluate a monarthropathy or recurrent joint symptoms of uncertain origin. In common with the hip joint the use of arthrography to assess complications following total knee replacement (*vide infra*) is increasing.

Contraindications

There are no absolute contraindications to knee arthrography. A history of a major allergic reaction to previous injections of contrast medium, particularly if 12 months or more before the study, may be taken to be a relative contraindication, and only then if there is evidence that this was of an anaphylactic rather than vasovagal nature. It is unlikely that a major allergic reaction will occur if a previous reaction was of a trivial nature such as urticaria or flushing. If necessary an air-only single-contrast arthrogram may be considered a safe alternative. Pyarthrosis has been considered a contraindication to arthrography, but the single-contrast technique may be beneficial insofar as it provides fluid for aspiration, culture and sensitivity (contrast medium being neither bactericidal nor bacteriostatic) and demonstrates sinus tracks from a joint. The potential danger of inducing an air embolus exists when a double-contrast technique is employed in a knee with acute haemarthrosis. However, this eventuality has only been reported when gas has been injected directly under pressure.

Complications may be divided into several groups. Firstly, trivial and inevitable consequences include the persistence of gas within the knee joint for some 3–4 days following the arthrogram. This may be considered unpleasant by some patients, certainly high-altitude flying is not to be recommended on the day of injection! A higher incidence of pain and discomfort occurs if a sodium-containing salt has been used rather than a meglumine salt, although histological studies have demonstrated that both are irritant. Many patients complain of transient pain and swelling, no doubt related to the positive contrast agent; this is less marked, however, when the newer generation of non-ionic, low-osmolality contrast agents are employed (for example, metrizamide or iopamidol). Accidental extravasation of either air or contrast medium degrades the images but has no other significance. It is better to re-book the patient for a further study than to press on under these circumstances.

More significant complications include transient allergic synovitis, in about 1–5% of patients, and pyarthrosis in 1/25 000. Major allergic reactions occur but are extremely rare, lesser phenomena such as urticaria occurring in 1/1000 examinations.

Choice of technique will depend on the clinical indications for the study. Most workers would accept that double-contrast arthrography is superior in the assessment of meniscal and cruciate ligament injuries. On the other hand, the single-contrast technique is considered sufficient to demonstrate the presence of a popliteal cyst or joint rupture, although it may be argued that a double-contrast technique may demonstrate the aetiology of the recurrent joint effusion which induced the joint rupture, for example an occult meniscal tear. When performed for the detection of loose bodies the choice is difficult. With a double-contrast technique frothing may obscure small bodies. A single-contrast technique may obscure them with too high a density. The author prefers a diluted single-contrast technique (of the order of 140 mg iodine/ml) with pluridirectional tomography. Delayed images may show absorption of contrast medium by cartilaginous loose bodies (Fig. 2.28b).

The knee joint should be needled using an ordinary 21-gauge venepuncture needle, aiming for the mid-part of either the medial or lateral articular facet of the patella, the choice being individual, with the needle parallel to the table top. In order to avoid the infrapatellar or suprapatellar fat pads an intra-articular location may be confirmed either by injecting a small quantity of air, and demonstrating its spread to both sides of the knee joint, or by fluoroscopic control. The latter is recommended, particularly during the learning phase. Prior to the injection of any contrast medium meticulous aspiration of joint fluid is mandatory, since this alone has the greatest influence on film quality and hence diagnostic accuracy. This is facilitated by placing a firm sandbag behind the popliteal fossa prior to aspiration. An injection of 3–4 ml of a positive contrast agent containing 280–300 mg/ml of iodine is recommended, since volumes in excess of this produce pools within joint recesses, obscuring the double-contrast effect and therefore degrading the image. 0·3 mg of

adrenaline reduces the absorption rate of contrast medium and prolongs useful screening time, particularly useful in a teaching situation. 40–50 ml of air are introduced, the quantity dependent on patient tolerance, the object being to distend the knee joint as much as posible. No advantage is gained by the filtration of air or in the injection of an alternative gas such as carbon dioxide or oxygen. Aspirated joint fluid should be sent routinely for bacteriology and microscopy: crystals if crystal arthritis is suspected and rheumatological assessment if investigation of a monarthropathy is undertaken.

Having injected contrast medium it is essential that the joint surfaces should be coated adequately, otherwise tears will be missed (Fig. 2.1a, b). This can usually be achieved by lying the patient prone and gently flexing and extending the knee several times; occasionally careful exercise is useful. An overvigorous mixing or inadequate joint aspiration may cause frothing or dilution of contrast medium, reducing the quality of image. Most commonly, arthrogram images are recorded using an overcouch intensifier system, screening the patient in the prone position. High-quality images are obtained using a low kV_p, of the order of 50–55, a short exposure time to minimize movement blur, and a small focal spot to reduce geometric unsharpness. Automatic density control is not recommended. It is important to obtain multiple images of each meniscus under direct fluoroscopic control, a minimum of eight of each meniscus since tears may be localized and discrete (Fig. 2.2a, b). In both compartments it is essential to image the extreme posterior horns of the menisci if tears are not to be overlooked. This will require turning the patient from side to side rather than simply rotating the leg. Flexion and extension are necessary to skyline the meniscus adequately. Varus and valgus stress permit joint distraction and enhance the double-contrast effect (Fig. 2.3a, b). This may be facilitated by either cross-table bands, the use of lead rubber-gloved hands or a table-top fixation device such as the Arthrostress (Picker International Ltd).

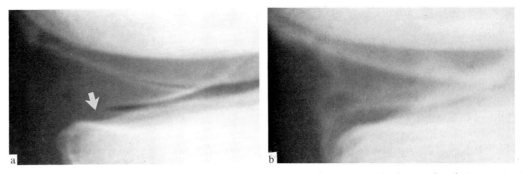

Fig. 2.1. (a) Posterior horn of medial meniscus. The whole of the joint surface is incompletely coated so that no contrast medium is present between the meniscus and the tibial plateau laterally (arrowed). (b) Following exercise coating is now complete and an extensive meniscal tear is demonstrated.

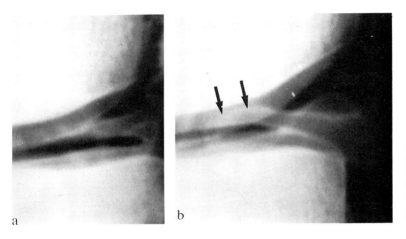

Fig. 2.2. (a) Mid-part of medial meniscus shows a blunted apex. (b) On the next image, with a few degrees of further rotation, a parrot-beak tear is shown with the fragment turned into the joint line (arrows).

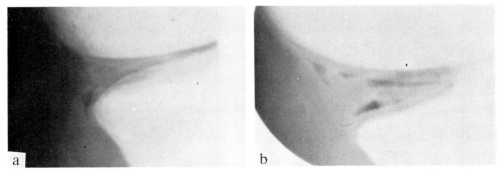

Fig. 2.3. (a) A view of the posterior horn of the medial meniscus is inadequate insofar as the meniscus has not been skylined and the joint not distracted due to inadequate valgus stress. Questionable abnormal lines of contrast medium are present within the meniscus. (b) Following correction of both of these faults a very obvious tear of the medial meniscus is demonstrated.

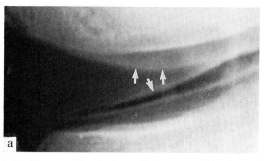 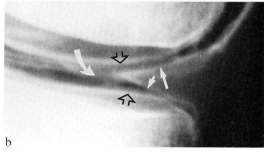

Fig. 2.4. The normal posterior medial meniscus (a) is larger than (b) the normal anterior horn of the other knee. The meniscus is outlined by contrast medium (closed arrows) as is hyaline cartilage (open arrows). Because this is a three-dimensional image the apex of the free margin can be seen extending around the joint (curved arrow).

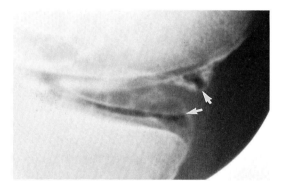

Fig. 2.5. Contrast medium frothing in joint recesses produces a soap-bubble opacification over the posterior horn of the medial meniscus. All these lines of opacity may be demonstrated to extend outside the line of the posterior horn and terminate in recesses (arrowed).

Interpretation requires experience and close mutual co-operation between radiologist and clinician. Feedback of clinical findings will facilitate this process since there is undoubtedly a learning period during which errors will be made, due mainly to the complex anatomy of the knee. One may forget that the images are three-dimensional compressed into two, and not tomograms.

In the *medial compartment* the meniscus is outlined as an isosceles triangle, larger posteriorly than anteriorly, and firmly attached to the medial collateral ligament so that the meniscus in profile does not contain either positive or negative contrast medium within its outline (Fig. 2.4a, b). However, artefacts may be projected across the meniscus, particularly those due to recesses between the meniscus and the synovium. Hence it is essential to trace all lines of contrast medium projected in the meniscus to see whether or not they can be demonstrated to extend beyond the confines of the meniscus and, for example, to terminate at a margin of a recess (Fig. 2.5). Most commonly, recesses are demonstrated inferior to the posterior horn of the medial meniscus and inferior to both horns of the lateral meniscus. In the medial compartment, however, deep recesses may be confused with incomplete tears (Fig. 2.6) and a helpful differential sign is rapid absorption of contrast medium in a tear on a delayed image (Fig. 2.10). In the *lateral compartment* more difficulty occurs since the popliteus tendon and its bursa pass through the joint line posteriorly (Figs. 2.7, 2.8). Hence contrast medium is present in the outline of the meniscus as a normal event (Fig. 2.9). Demonstration of the suspensory struts supporting the posterior horn of the medial meniscus is vital, since this represents a major potential site of trauma (Fig. 2.10). The remainder of the meniscus is attached firmly laterally. The meniscus is more uniform in size than the medial and is more extensive. The anterior horn is biconcave (Fig. 2.11). It may be obscured by recesses or synovial lines accompanying the patellar tendon or infrapatellar fat pad.

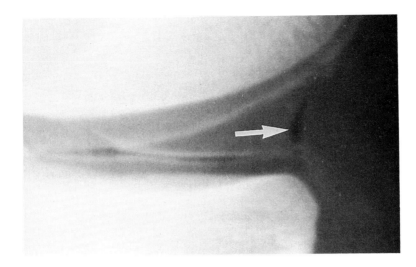

Fig. 2.6. An extensive inferior tear is shown separating the posterior horn of the medial meniscus from the joint capsule (arrow). This should not be confused with a deep recess.

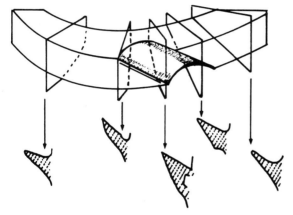

Fig. 2.7. A line drawing demonstrates the tunnel created by the popliteus tendon and its bursa passing obliquely across the posterior horn of the lateral meniscus. The meniscus viewed from behind is therefore grooved and tangential images will vary depending on the angle and position of the tunnel relative to the meniscus.

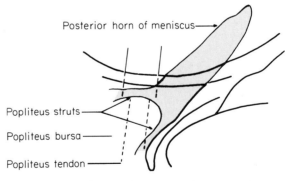

Posterior horn of meniscus—

Popliteus struts—
Popliteus bursa—
Popliteus tendon—

Fig. 2.8. A line drawing demonstrates the posterior horn of the lateral meniscus as it is most usually seen. The two attachments of the posterior horn around the popliteus tendon or struts are demonstrated.

In spite of these difficulties, the majority of meniscal tears represent a straightforward diagnostic proposition (Figs. 2.12, 2.1b, 2.2, 2.3, 2.6, 2.10, 2.13). Other meniscal abnormalities include the demonstration of cysts, which are undramatic compared with the clinical features, when usually a small horizontal tear is demon-

strated (Fig. 2.14a, b). Contrast medium is very rarely shown to extend into the clinically palpable cyst. When arthrography is undertaken in younger people the possibility of a discoid meniscus should be considered, manifest arthrographically by failure of the meniscus to taper to a point or by its excessive extent across the

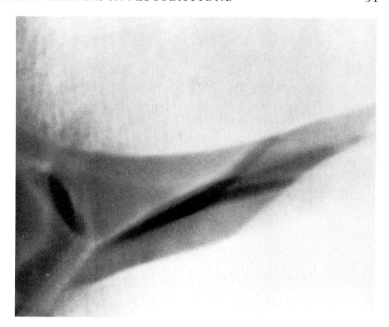

Fig. 2.9. The normal posterior horn of the lateral meniscus from a routine arthrogram. Compare this with Fig. 2.8.

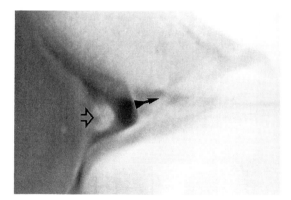

Fig. 2.10. Disruption of the popliteus struts of the posterior horn of the lateral meniscus results in a medial displacement of the meniscus (closed arrow) and an irregular nubbin representing the torn struts (open arrow). Note the absorption of contrast medium into the disrupted struts.

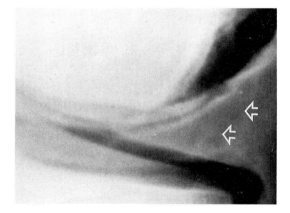

Fig. 2.11. Normal anterior horn of lateral meniscus. The small radiolucencies and their surrounding density (arrows) are a normal finding in this region. The exact anatomical cause is uncertain.

joint line (Fig. 2.15). A complete discoid meniscus may cause compartmentalization of the knee joint (Fig. 2.16a, b), a phenomenon also seen with an inferior plica. An incomplete discoid meniscus may be overlooked unless multiple images have been taken.

Pitfalls in meniscal assessment include artefacts created by recesses and by popliteal cysts overlying the posterior horn on the medial site. On occasions a small mid-part of the medial meniscus may be misinterpreted as the residuum of a tear or as a torn meniscus itself. Where the anterior horn merges into the transverse ligament the change in outline also may be misinterpreted as a tear. Pitfalls related to the lateral meniscus are largely due to the

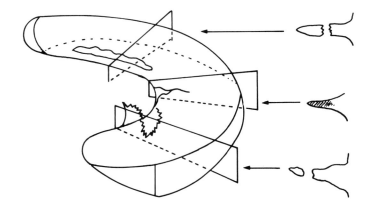

Fig. 2.12. A line drawing demonstrates the concept whereby meniscal tears are demonstrated. A bucket-handle, a radial, and a parrot-beak tear are demonstrated together with a drawing of appearances on tangentialized views. Note the absorption of contrast medium in the radial tear.

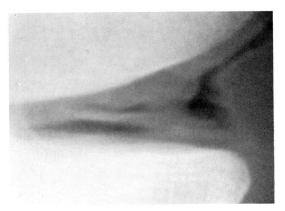

Fig. 2.13. Posterior horn of the medial meniscus is severely torn with multiple fragments. The meniscus has also been largely torn from its insertion into the medial collateral ligament.

presence of the popliteus bursa. Since naturally occurring lines of contrast medium cross the meniscal outline, the confidence with which tears are diagnosed is inherently less. Hence even in inexperienced hands accuracies of diagnosis in excess of 90% should be achieved in the medial compartment but less, about 85%, in the lateral compartment. It is important to realize that if accuracy is judged against surgical findings the latter may themselves be suspect. Posterior horn tears may be overlooked if only an anterior arthrotomy has been performed; the meniscus may be torn during its removal; the meniscectomy knife may pass through a pre-existing tear which is therefore not recognized. Other causes of confusion include the presence of chondrocalcinosis, hence

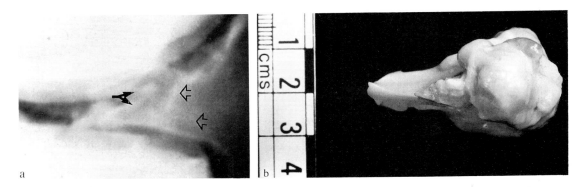

Fig. 2.14. (a) The anterior horn of the lateral meniscus demonstrates a horizontal cleavage tear (closed arrows) with some intravasation of contrast medium into the meniscus (open arrows). (b) A clinical photograph demonstrates the cystic meniscus with its torn anterior horn.

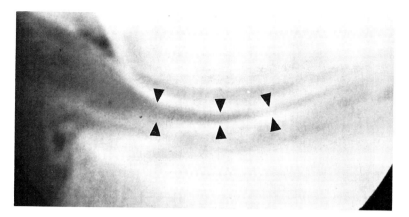

Fig. 2.15. Discoid lateral meniscus. Here a double-contrast arthrogram has not been stressed so that there is effectively a single-contrast view of a discoid meniscus extending right across the joint into the intercondylar region. Note the failure of tapering to an apex (arrowheads).

suggesting intravasated contrast medium due to tears, and, on occasions, the presence of meniscal ossicles in the posterior horns.

Following *meniscectomy* the meniscal appearances are quite different. The meniscus appears more of an equilateral shape, is less well defined, and exhibits early absorption of contrast medium. The value of arthrography lies in the detection of tears in residual horns and in assessing the quality of hyaline cartilage rather than in looking for re-tears of the regenerate meniscus, which requires considerable further trauma.

The *cruciate ligaments* are demonstrated as an intra-articular triangular structure, the anterior margin of the anterior cruciate and the posterior margin of the posterior cruciate only being demonstrated. The former is demonstrated by a straight line extending from the intercondylar notch to an insertion 7–8 mm posterior to the anterior joint line. Cruciate ligaments are demonstrated to best advantage either by a lateral film taken with the patient's knee hanging over the side of the table with anterior tibial traction, or during fluoroscopy with similar traction (Fig. 2.17a, b). On occasions lateral tomography may be necessary. In all instances it is important to apply traction in order to tense the anterior cruciate ligament and to displace the infrapatellar fat pad anteriorly, away from the anterior cruciate ligament, otherwise its outline may be obscured. There is a significant false-negative detection

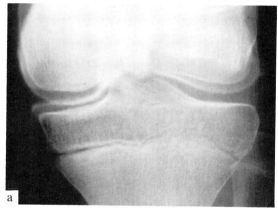

a

Fig. 2.16a. Single-contrast arthrogram demonstrates that contrast medium has coated only the upper (femoral) surface of a complete discoid lateral meniscus. Note that no contrast medium has passed between the tibial surface and the hyaline cartilage of the tibial condyle.

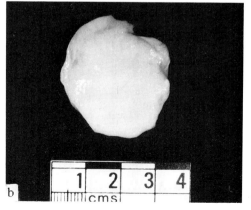

b

Fig. 2.16b The excised specimen seen from the femoral aspect.

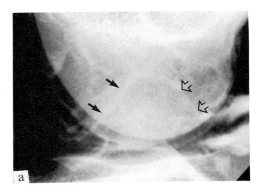

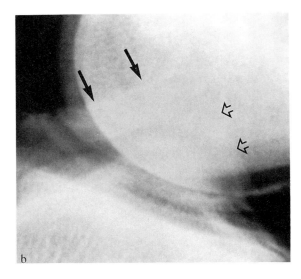

Fig. 2.17. Normal cruciate outlines demonstrated (a) by horizontal beam lateral film with tibial stress, (b) during fluoroscopy. The anterior cruciate outline is identified by closed arrows and the posterior cruciate by open arrows.

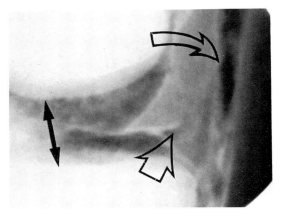

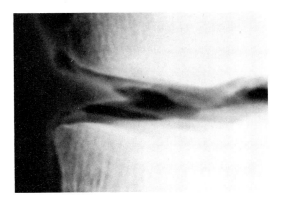

Fig. 2.18. A knee arthrogram performed on the day of acute injury. The posterior horn of the medial meniscus is extensively torn (open arrow). A capsular tear is present with extravasation of contrast medium through the medial collateral ligament (open curved arrow). The collateral instability is demonstrated by the ability to widen the joint space (closed arrow) with valgus stress. Note the slight frothing of contrast medium due to a residue of joint fluid. Nonetheless a highly diagnostic arthrogram has been achieved in the presence of an acute haemarthrosis and joint rupture.

Fig. 2.19. Acute chondral fracture. An arthrogram was performed in the belief that a medial meniscal tear had occurred. The mid-part of the medial meniscus is shown here to be normal, but immediately adjacent to it in the femoral condyle is shown a large crater due to a chondral fracture. The separate fragment is not demonstrated on this picture.

rate of tears. Hence any irregularity or bowing of the anterior cruciate outline should be regarded with suspicion as representing a partial tear with an intact synovium. Frank irregularity or collapse of outline implies unequivocally a complete tear. The presence of an inferior plica may cause a false-negative result. Com-

puterized tomography may be helpful for the assessment of the cruciate ligaments.

When arthrography is performed in *acute trauma* it is usually not possible completely to aspirate the knee joint. Nonetheless, the technique is most helpful in demonstrating capsular tears and ligamentous ruptures (Fig. 2.18). The

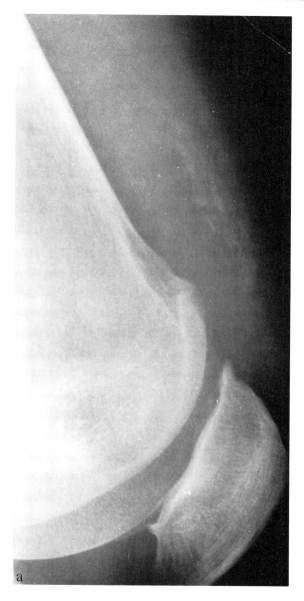

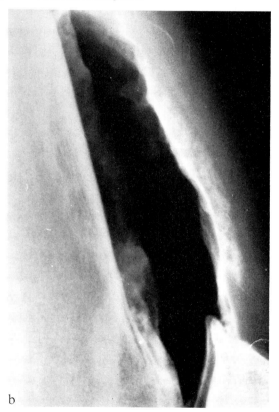

Fig. 2.20. Synovial chondromatosis. (a) A plain film reveals amorphous calcification in an enlarged suprapatellar pouch and degenerative disease of the patellofemoral joint. (b) A localized view from a double-contrast arthrogram demonstrates nodular irregularity of the whole of the synovial outline of the suprapatellar pouch confirming the diagnosis.

former may seal rapidly and not be apparent within a day or two, and the latter may only be manifest later as minor varus or valgus instability. Arthrography represents a relatively simple means of demonstrating the presence of intra-articular disease prior to the early repair of ligamentous damage. It may also distinguish

one cause of a locked knee from another (Fig. 2.19).

Synovial assessment with the double-contrast technique may demonstrate solitary lesions such as pigmented villonodular synovitis or multifocal abnormalities such as synovial chondromatosis (Fig. 2.20a, b).

Joint rupture is best detected by the single-contrast technique. Following the aspiration of joint fluid, 40–50 c.c. of a single-contrast agent are injected, usually 60% meglumine iothalamate. It is important to exercise the knee and to take further films following such exercise, since the initial film may not demonstrate joint rupture (Fig. 2.21). The diagnosis is absolute if the feathery appearance of contrast medium extending between muscle planes is demonstrated (Fig. 2.22). Joint ruptures seal rapidly within 24–48 hours.

Arthrography versus arthroscopy

In general there is little to choose between the relative accuracies of expert arthroscopy and arthrography. Arthroscopy requires general anaesthetic and is more invasive. Nonetheless, its advantages include the better demonstration of the cruciate ligaments, the anterior halves of the menisci, the synovium and hyaline cartilage, and the opportunity to biopsy. In addition, it demonstrates more clearly the subtle features of hyaline cartilage fibrillation and ulceration in early degenerative arthritis. Arthrography, on the other hand, is shown to be superior in the assessment of the posterior horns of the menisci, particularly inferior tears, the posterior joint capsule, and joint ruptures. Because of its less invasive nature it is recommended as the initial investigation of choice for internal derangement and joint rupture, whereas arthroscopy may be valuable in the assessment of chondromalacia patellae and other obscure knee joint pains or symptoms. Clearly the role of knee arthrography will be reviewed with the further extension of operative arthroscopy. At present, however, this latter remains a time-consuming technique with limited availability.

HIP ARTHROGRAPHY

Children

There are two major indications for hip arthrography: firstly in the assessment of congenital dislocation of the hip, and secondly in some patients with Perthes' disease (*see* Chapter 9).

In *congenital dislocation* the purpose of arthrography is to demonstrate any intrinsic factor

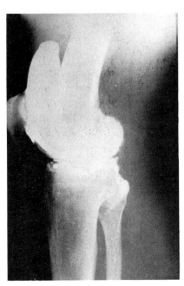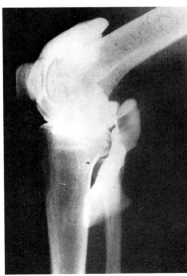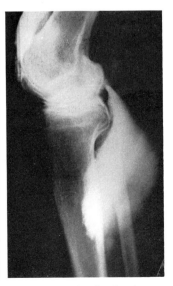

Fig. 2.21. A Baker's cyst is demonstrated on sequential images. The image on the left was taken immediately after the injection of contrast medium and no abnormality is shown. Following exercise a large lobulated popliteal cyst is demonstrated. This is shown to be much larger on the right-hand film following another period of exercise.

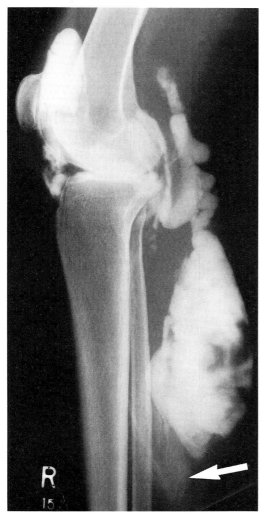

Fig. 2.22. In addition to a large lobulated Baker's cyst due to rheumatoid disease, extravasation from rupture is demonstrated into muscle planes (arrow). Note the feathery quality of the extravasation. Note also the large mass lesions in the popliteal cyst due to fibrin bodies.

which may prevent complete reduction by closed means and to evaluate those factors which will require surgical intervention should this be necessary. Those factors include, for example, inversion of the labrum, hypertrophy of the ligamentum teres, and capsular wasting.

There is no absolute contraindication to arthrography. The study, however, needs to be performed under general anaesthetic in order to prevent movement artefacts, to ensure patient co-operation, and to permit a full range of movement for radiography. Several needle approaches may be made to the hip joint, avoidance of the femoral vessels and their major branches being the objective of the approach. The needle may be inserted either anteriorly or at 45° to the midline with an anterolateral approach. Some authors prefer an inferior approach with leg abducted, the needle aimed directly to the head and parallel to the table top. A fine lumbar puncture needle (22-gauge, $2\frac{1}{2}''$) is appropriate with a short bevel aimed to enter the joint parallel to hyaline cartilage. Many experienced workers enter the joint blindly, having palpated the femoral head by movement of the hip joint. If a blind technique is used, it is useful to note that when the needle enters the joint cavity local anaesthetic may be injected freely without resistance and disconnecting the syringe will permit it to drip back out. When fluoroscopy is used the needle should be aimed to strike the femoral head in its upper, outer quadrant, thereby avoiding the non-visualized fibrous labrum and the relatively tight capsule along the femoral neck. External rotation or marked abduction during needling are to be avoided, since this tightens the capsule and makes satisfactory location of the needle more difficult. A flexible connector is useful to inject the contrast medium under fluoroscopic control.

The neonatal hip accommodates about 1 ml of a positive contrast medium; in children 1 ml per year of age is injected up to the adult volume of about 10 ml. Sodium salts should be avoided since these certainly cause synovial irritation and pain in adults. It is essential also not to use too high a density contrast medium, since soft tissue structures such as the ligamentum teres may be obscured. Sixty per cent meglumine iothalamate diluted one to one with normal saline is a good choice.

Fluoroscopic time and the number of subsequent radiographs should be minimized in view of radiation dosage and, wherever possible, gonad protection should be employed. Images may be recorded either on multiple radiographs or by video in order to demonstrate dynamic anatomy and to assess whether true reduction can be achieved and, if so, in which position. AP, AP internal/external rotation, abduction and frog-leg films are conventional. An attempt should be made in the frog-leg position or in the fully abducted, internally rotated position to obtain full reduction.

Complications are rare but significant and include the possibility of septic arthritis and avascular necrosis. There is, however, no alternative means of demonstrating the intrinsic factors which may prevent full reduction in congenital dislocation. On occasions, osteomyelitis of the pubic bones has been recorded. The femoral vessels could be damaged during an anterior approach. Finally, the risks of general anaesthetic will also need to be considered in patient selection.

In *Perthes' disease* the objectives of the study are different. To some extent they are less clear-cut in clinical terms since no uniform agreement exists on the surgical management of the disease. The study is undertaken to demonstrate whether there is flattening of the cartilage anlage, shown by pooling of contrast medium, and to demonstrate the degree of extrusion of the cartilage anlage outside the line of the labrum, particularly in the Catterall type IV hip. In the 4–8 year age group the hip accommodates 4–8 ml of contrast medium and it is preferable to inject under fluoroscopic control to avoid overdistension which may then cause extravasation and obscure anatomy. The use of a short lumbar puncture needle remains satisfactory. Many studies will require general anaesthetic.

Images are recorded as in CDH, but in addition particular care is taken with frog-leg and abduction films to demonstrate the maximum position of containment if varus rotational osteotomy is being considered.

In those rare cases where hip pain redevelops in early *adolescent life*, arthrography may be undertaken to detect labral tears, and in *adult life* arthrography may be undertaken to evaluate those rare cases where a persistent osteochondral defect is present. In these circumstances the study is designed to demonstrate whether or not this is separate and hence whether contrast medium tracks around the osteochondral fragment beneath the hyaline cartilage outline. It may be necessary to perform tomography in order to be sure this is not happening.

Adult life

In adult life the most common indication for hip arthrography is the assessment of painful total hip replacements. Loosening can often be assessed from plain films by movement of either component on push–pull film pairs, and indeed where this can be demonstrated, and there is no question of infection, arthrography may be deemed superfluous. However, minor degrees of cement separation are relatively common, particularly around the outer third of the acetabular cup and in the upper lateral femoral neck, and arthrography is necessary to demonstrate whether contrast medium extends abnormally from the joint into the interface between cement and bone (Fig. 2.23a, b). Abnormal separation between cement and metal clearly does not require arthrographic confirmation since it is easily visible on plain film. The injection of local anaesthetic during the arthrogram is an important adjunct since hip pain may be ablated by local anaesthetic, and this adds strongly to the weight of clinical suspicion that the device is the cause of the patient's symptoms.

Whilst infection may be inferred radiographically by the presence of ill-defined periosteal new bone formation or cortical resorption, arthrography presents the opportunity of aspirating joint fluid for bacteriological assessment (both aerobically and anaerobically). Scintigraphy is an important first investigation in the assessment of painful hip replacement and it may be used to select those patients in whom hip aspiration/arthrography should be undertaken, particularly when infection is being considered.

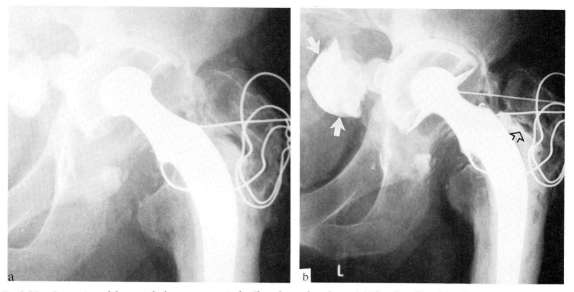

Fig 2.23. Loosening of the acetabular component of a Charnley arthroplasty. (a) The plain film. (b) Following the injection of contrast medium there is extension from the hip joint around the acetabular cement and into the pelvis, surrounding the extruded cement (closed arrows). A small quantity superomedial to the femoral neck (open arrow) is insignificant.

An anterolateral approach is recommended using a lumbar puncture needle. This, however, needs to be longer than that used in childhood, and a minimum of four inches is recommended. Some difficulty may occur in inserting a 22-gauge needle, depending on the thickness of soft tissues, and a broader needle may be required. It often feels as though an apparent mass of fibrous tissue surrounds the hip, but difficulty is seldom experienced in knowing when the hip joint is entered since the sensation of metal hitting metal is characteristic. The target is the femoral head, the needle being inserted high on the neck or on the femoral head to avoid both the acetabular cup and residual labrum/osteophyte. If no joint fluid can be aspirated, having confirmed an intra-articular position with contrast medium, saline should be injected and re-aspirated and sent for bacteriology. Again the injection of contrast medium is easier via a flexible connector so that adequate distension may be achieved under fluoroscopic control. The 'normal' hip accommodates about 8 ml of 60%

meglumine iothalamate or the equivalent. Unlike the childhood arthrogram it is preferable to use high-density contrast medium, since the detection of fine tracts of contrast medium between bone and cement is made much easier. In the normal hip the capsule is relatively tight around the acetabular cup, the femoral head and neck. Contrast medium should not enter the 'joint'. It is normal for contrast medium to track around at least one-third of the acetabular cup, particularly superolaterally, and the upper centimetre or two of the lateral femoral neck. Communication with other soft-tissue structures, including the gluteal bursa, should not occur. Routine anteroposterior, and internal and external rotation films should be supplemented by a lateral examination, preferably a true lateral shooting through the groin rather than rolled into the Lowenstein position. The study should be supplemented by a traction film, since it may be possible to demonstrate a plunger effect, moving the whole cement bulk within bone. Photographic or digital subtraction may

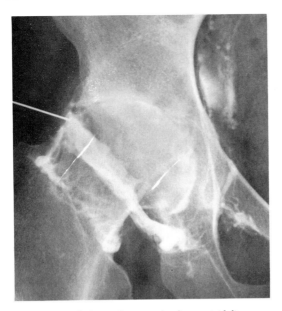

be used in order to demonstrate contrast medium tracts with greater certainty by removing the dense radio-opacity of metal. Where infection is present the extent of sinus tracts will be demonstrated and accordingly larger volumes of contrast medium may be required.

Other, less common, indications for hip arthrography include the assessment of monarthropathies, for example the distinction between pigmented villonodular synovitis and osteoarthritis or to assess the local effects of a polyarthropathy (Fig. 2.24). Arthrography may be required in the detection of loose bodies (Fig. 2.25a, b) or related abnormalities (Fig. 2.26a, b). Some workers advocate the use of a double-contrast technique, but it is possible that air bubbles may be confused with radiolucent loose bodies.

Complications are few. Apart from transient stiffness and a slight reduction in range of movement for a day or two no untoward side-effects are usually reported beyond those described above under 'knee'.

Fig. 2.24. Right hip arthrogram in rheumatoid disease. Note the markedly nodular quality of the synovial outline, virtual loss of hyaline cartilage, brisk lymphatic filling including lymph nodes in the pelvis.

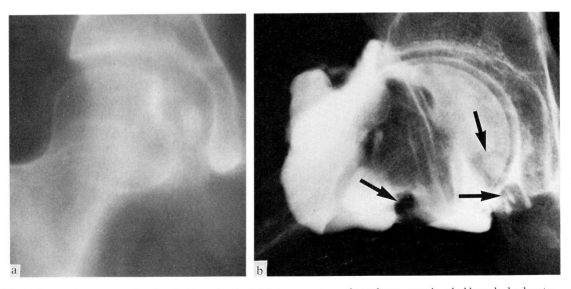

Fig. 2.25. Post-traumatic osteochondral loose bodies. (a) A tomogram reveals a solitary osteochondral loose body close to the fovea. However, an arthrogram (b) demonstrates further non-opaque loose bodies as radiolucent filling defects (arrows).

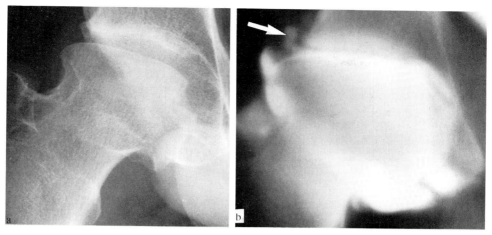

Fig. 2.26. A young adult with recently painful Perthes' disease. (a) The plain film demonstrates old Perthes' disease but little evidence of degenerative arthritis and a well-preserved joint space width. (b) A tomogram during arthrography demonstrates a fissured, torn labrum (arrow) with some overall attrition of hyaline cartilage thickness.

SHOULDER ARTHROGRAPHY

The two major indications for shoulder arthrography are in the assessment of rotator cuff injuries and the after-effects of dislocation of the shoulder joint.

Choice of technique
A single-contrast arthrogram is an accurate reproducible means of demonstrating complete tears of the rotator cuff, incomplete tears of its inferior surface (Fig. 2.27), and adhesive capsulitis, as in a frozen shoulder. In adhesive capsulitis it may be used also as a form of therapy in which progressive distension of the shoulder joint is made by further injections of contrast medium until such time as the joint ruptures. This is then followed by intensive physiotherapy and, on limited experience, is very effective!

The double-contrast method has the advantage, however, of coating disrupted tendons, and in particular facilitating the assessment of the width and extent of supraspinatus tears. In addition, there is better delineation of the glenoid labrum and clearer demonstration of the bicipital sheath and the long head of biceps. Hill–Sachs deformities may be better appreciated (Fig. 2.28a, b).

Without doubt symptoms are more frequent following shoulder arthrography than hip or knee arthrography, but are significantly less with the double-contrast technique than with the single. Experience suggests that even the newer, low-osmolality, positive contrast agents induce an appreciable morbidity. Maximal onset of symptoms, usually discomfort, occurs after the patient has left the department and may only be referred to at subsequent out-patient visits. Symptoms may last for several days, particularly when a double-contrast technique has been employed, as the resorption of residual nitrogen in the injected air is gradual.

The procedure may be undertaken under fluoroscopic control. The needle is inserted vertically, aiming just slightly lateral to the joint in order to avoid the labrum. Insertion may also be performed without the use of fluoroscopy when the landmark is the coracoid process, the needle being inserted one finger's breadth lateral to this and angulated slightly to the midline. In order to avoid the bicipital tendon sheath the arm should be externally rotated slightly to the 'thumbs up' position. Too much external rotation will tighten the joint capsule, making insertion more difficult. The ideal needle

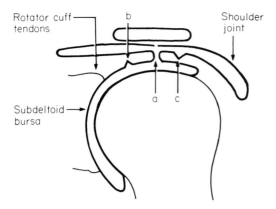

Rotator cuff
tendons

b

Shoulder
joint

Subdeltoid
bursa

a   c

Fig. 2.27. A line drawing shows the relationship between the shoulder joint and the subdeltoid bursa. Complete rupture of the supraspinatus tendon (a) permits contrast medium to extend from the shoulder joint into the subdeltoid bursa. The tear of the inferior surface is shown as a defect (b) but an abnormality of the superior surface (c) can only be demonstrated by a subdeltoid bursogram. An intrinsic abnormality affecting neither the upper nor the lower surface will not be demonstrated by any contrast medium technique.

is a 22-gauge lumbar puncture needle because of its short bevel and a 4″ needle may be necessary when the patient is particularly muscular. A flexible connector permits fluoroscopic control as contrast medium is injected, firstly confirming the intra-articular position of the needle, and secondly permitting adequate but not overdistension of the joint. When a double-contrast technique is employed 3–4 ml of a positive contrast agent such as 60% meglumine iothalamate are injected, together with 0·3 mg of adrenaline and about 10 ml of air. After gentle passive mixing anteroposterior views in internal and external rotation are recorded in the erect position, together with abduction views. Prone and supine axial films are taken to demonstrate the glenoid labrum in double contrast. Supine tomography of the inferior labrum may be performed with the patient rolled towards the injured side. Computed tomography, where available, may be a helpful adjunct. Specific views of the bicipital sheath may be taken if required.

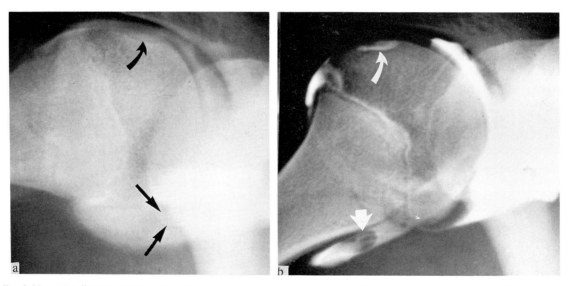

Fig. 2.28. (a) Following anterior dislocation a single-contrast arthrogram reveals a chondral fracture with a cartilaginous loose body in the bicipital tendon sheath (closed arrow) and a residual Hill–Sachs deformity in the humeral head (curved arrow). (b) A delayed image following manipulation demonstrates that the cartilaginous loose body has now absorbed contrast medium and is opaque (arrows). The Hill–Sachs defect is again demonstrated with a cartilage defect (curved arrow).

Interpretation is usually straightforward. If the rotator cuff is torn, contrast medium will extend from the shoulder joint into the subdeltoid bursa (Fig. 2.27). The extent of this tear may be judged by the degree of separation of the margins. If the inferior aspect of the rotator cuff has been torn a defect will be demonstrated. However, partial defects within the body of the rotator cuff tendons or superiorly cannot be shown by this technique and subdeltoid bursography should be performed (*vide infra*).

In the assessment of apparent dislocation the arthrogram is scrutinized for labral tears both on the prone and supine axial views and on tomograms. Computerized tomography may be particularly helpful in this respect. Recurrent dislocation is usually associated with abnormal distensibility or ballooning of the capsule anteriorly or posteriorly. In the commoner recurrent anterior dislocation there is a lack of distinction between the subcoracoid and axillary pouches. Associated osteochondral defects including Bankart and Hill–Sachs lesions may be demonstrated (Fig. 2.25). Fluoroscopic examination, with contrast medium *in situ*, may be informative, particularly in the axial projection using a mobile intensifier, when additional information about subluxation or dislocation is

forthcoming, in particular to assess the position of dislocation and the extent of instability.

Arthrography, by the single-contrast technique, may be employed immediately after an acute injury in order to demonstrate capsular rupture for surgical repair. Other less common indications include the detection of loose bodies and the assessment of synovial diseases, for example rheumatoid disease.

Subdeltoid bursography
Contrast medium may be introduced into the subdeltoid bursa (Fig. 2.29) by inserting a needle vertically under fluoroscopic control just distal to the tip of the acromion. When an area of reduced resistance is detected a test injection is made and contrast medium injected under fluoroscopic control.

Recurrent injuries to the rotator cuff are often associated with inability to distend the bursa due to multiple adhesions, but discrete tears of the upper surface of the rotator cuff may be demonstrated by a defect in the floor of the subdeltoid bursa. Impingement syndromes may be diagnosed when on abduction of the arm contrast medium pockets in the subdeltoid bursa because it cannot move freely under the acromion.

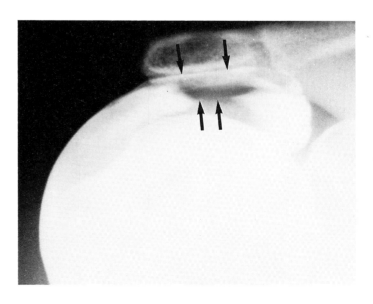

Fig. 2.29. Normal subdeltoid bursography with the upper surface of the rotator cuff demonstrated. Note the smooth outline of the subdeltoid bursa and its subacromial extension and the sharp outline of the rotator cuff.

WRIST ARTHROGRAPHY

Wrist arthrography is performed to diagnose triangular ligament tears and other traumatic abnormalities including scapholunate diastasis.
Occasionally it has a place in rheumatoid disease to demonstrate synovial mass lesions and
joint rupture into both tendon sheaths and soft
tissues.

The wrist is needled using an ordinary small
skin infiltration needle from the distal radius
angling cephalad to allow for the normal oblique articular surface. Fluoroscopy is usually
unnecessary since the needle slips easily between the radius and scaphoid but when a large
mass lesion or considerable swelling is present
it may be necessary to check position. An
intra-articular location is confirmed by ease of
injection and local anaesthetic dripping back
from the needle. The normal wrist joint accommodates between 1 and 3 ml of contrast
medium, a non-sodium salt being recommended. Larger volumes are necessary when an
extension occurs from the wrist joint, for example into tendon sheaths. Adequate filling
may be judged by the patient's sensation of fullness in the volar aspect of the wrist. Apart from
transient stiffness and some discomfort no

symptoms are usually ascribed to wrist arthrography, although it is the author's experience
that men frequently faint during the procedure!

Radiographs should be performed in the
anteroposterior and lateral projections. Radial
and ulnar deviation films are necessary when
triangular ligament rupture is sought (Fig.
2.30a, b). This diagnosis is substantiated by the
demonstration of contrast medium tracking
through the triangular ligament into the distal
radioulnar joint. The normal wrist joint probably does not communicate with the intercarpal
or intermetacarpal joints, although cadaver
studies have suggested that this may be a normal phenomenon in up to 25% of patients.
Communication with tendon sheaths is always
abnormal however. For practical purposes the
leakage of contrast medium from the wrist joint
between the carpal bones suggests scapholunate
or lunotriquetral ligamentous disruption which
may be demonstrated on localized views. Where
such injury is sought, in addition to standard
films, flexion and extension films are valuable,
together with a clenched fist film in the anteroposterior projection.

Although ganglia do not readily fill from
wrist arthrography, very delayed films may
demonstrate diffuse, faint opacification.

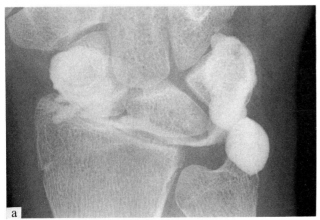
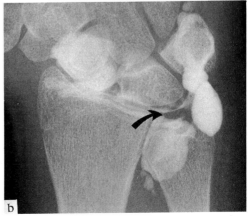

Fig. 2.30. (a) Normal wrist arthrogram. Contrast medium outlines the distal radius, the triangular ligament and the
proximal carpal row. The styloid and ulnar bursae are normal phenomena, as is the communication to the
trapeziopisiform joint. (b) Following radial and ulnar deviation contrast medium has extended through a tear of the
triangular ligament (curved arrow) to outline the distal inferior radioulnar joint.

ANKLE ARTHROGRAPHY

The use of arthrography in assessment of disorders of the ankle joint has not achieved universal acclamation. This is due, in part, to a lack of a uniform view in clinical management of acute traumatic lesions. Furthermore, variable communications between the ankle joint and other surrounding structures in normals make it difficult to define abnormal criteria.

Ankle arthrography is employed primarily after acute trauma and in chronic post-traumatic situations with persistent symptomatology. The ankle joint is needled anteriorly under fluoroscopic control since landmarks are often difficult to palpate. Approximately 8 ml of a positive contrast agent are injected, outlining an anterior and posterior recess, the articular surfaces of the talus, distal tibia and about a centimetre of the distal inferior tibiofibular synostosis. Extension of the ankle joint into the peroneal sheath occurs in about 12–14% of the normal population and into the tibial sheath in about 8% (Fig. 2.31a, b). Communication with

subtalar joints is present in about 10% of normals. However, if contrast medium extends more than a few millimetres into the inferior tibiofibular synostosis the unequivocal diagnosis of traumatic diastasis may be made, which in one-third of cases occurs in the absence of an overt fracture of the malleoli. Stress films may aid this diagnosis. Acute ligamentous injury may be diagnosed by extravasation of contrast medium from the ankle joint around the malleoli. However, it is necessary to investigate promptly since such synovial ruptures heal in a few days and thereafter only ankle stress tests, either varus or valgus, anterior or posterior, may provide indirect diagnostic signs. If contrast medium extends around the tip of the distal fibula it suggests rupture of the anterior talofibular ligament, best visualized on the external oblique view. Anterior calcaneofibular disruption results in extension into the peroneal sheath. It has been suggested that if the criterion for surgical repair is the rupture of the ankle into this sheath peroneal tenography may be a more appropriate means of making the diag-

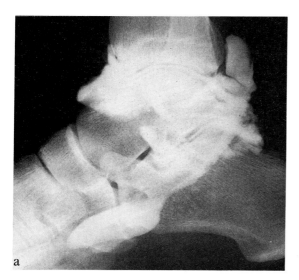

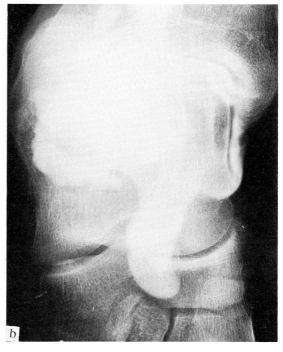

Fig. 2.31. Normal ankle arthrogram. Communication is shown between the ankle joint and the tibialis tendon sheath. This may be a normal finding. Note in the penetrated plantarflexed view a good delineation of the hyaline cartilage of the ankle joint is achieved.

nosis. Extension of contrast medium from the ankle joint around the medial malleolus indicates disruption of part or all of the deltoid ligament.

On occasions ankle arthrography may be used to demonstrate whether or not an osteochondral fragment is separated and, akin to the hip or elsewhere, tomography is a useful adjunct in order to detect discrete tracking of contrast medium around the fragment. Post-traumatic adhesive capsulitis is demonstrated by a small contracted ankle capsule with a markedly reduced range of movement and lack of distensibility. One characteristic of this diagnosis is the difficulty of placing a needle freely in the ankle joint in order to inject the contrast medium.

OTHER JOINTS

Numerous other joints are amenable to arthrography but are not often examined. Some examples are summarized.

Elbow. Double-contrast arthrography has been advocated, using gravity, to move 1 ml of 60% meglumine salt plus adrenaline and air around the elbow joint. Its use has been proposed particularly for the detection of intra-articular loose bodies. Disruption of the radial annular ligament may also be detected, together with osteochondral defects.

Interphalangeal and metacarpophalangeal joints. Arthrography has been advocated for the assessment of discrete volar plate injuries, collateral ligament avulsions and capsular ruptures (Fig. 2.32). An example in which a synovial mass lesion was evaluated is shown in Fig. 2.33.

Acromioclavicular joint. Arthrography demonstrates derangement of the articular disc and acromioclavicular ligament disruption with subluxation. Extravasation of contrast medium

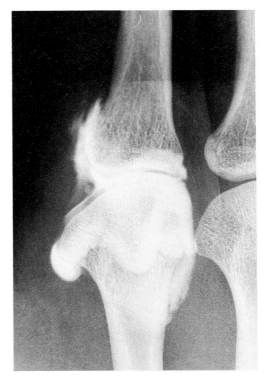

Fig. 2.32. A tear of radial collateral ligament of the index finger MCP joint. Note extravasation of contrast medium and irregularity of volar plate.

from the joint around the coracoid process permits an indirect diagnosis of disruption of the coracoacromial (if contrast medium reaches only the lateral aspect of the coracoid process) and trapezoid and conoid ligaments (if it is medial to the coracoid process).

Temperomandibular joints. The assessment of reduced range of movement, due to disruption of the articular disc, can be made from plain films. However, if local surgery is advocated, rather than condylectomy, arthrography of the inferior articular cavity demonstrates disruption of the disc or other abnormality.

Subtalar joints. Arthrography may occasionally be of use in detecting incomplete, fibrous, tarsal coalition.

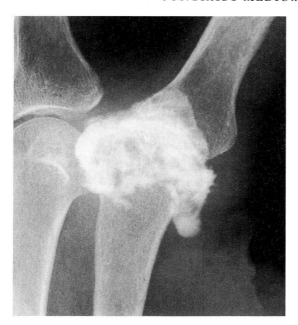

Fig. 2.33. Pigmented villonodular synovitis of the index finger MCP joint. Note the considerable synovial thickening and nodular irregularity throughout the joint.

Lumbar facet joints. The subject is discussed under 'lumbar spine investigations'. In summary, it is an uncommonly used tool in the further understanding of some patients with low back pain.

Spinal investigations

In most centres the major indication for spinal investigation is degenerative disc disease. Historically, the investigation of choice has been a myelogram using an oil-based contrast medium such as Myodil/Pantopaque. In the United Kingdom it was traditional for a small quantity of Myodil to be injected (of the order of 6–9 ml), which was then screened the whole length of the neural canal and left *in situ* after the completion of the study. In North America larger quantities were introduced and re-aspirated at the completion of the study through a variety of needles, cannulas and catheters. Today an impressive armamentarium of other investigations is available, the indications for which wax and wane. Initially the impetus for these further investigations, such as lumbar venography and epidurography, was based on known limitations of the diagnostic accuracy of Myodil myelography, in particular its inability to delineate lateral root sheath lesions. Even now, when safe water-soluble contrast medium examinations are available, an awareness remains of the unacceptability of some of the after-effects of these examinations and a requestioning of their diagnostic efficacy. For example, it has been recently suggested that radiculography has not altered the accuracy of diagnosis in patients being operated on for lumbar disc protrusions. Also, evidence is growing that modern generation computerized tomography has a high diagnostic accuracy in the anatomical demonstration of degenerative disc disease and its related abnormalities. Regrettably in the United Kingdom such data are not generally available. It is likely that the full value of CT has not yet been appreciated, neither, perhaps, have its limitations been fully delineated.

This section propounds the value, indications and limitations of spinal contrast medium techniques, including radiculography, and offers some thoughts on the suggested logic for their use in individual clinical circumstances.

LUMBAR SPINE

Degenerative disc disease provides a major challenge for radiologists to demonstrate its localization, to confirm the level and to detect whether or not there is sequestration, prolapse or mere protrusion. Furthermore, posterolateral compression from facet osteoarthritis, or pseudarthrosis from spondylolysis, must be assessed and ligamentum flavum redundancy demonstrated. Finally, acquired or developmental spinal stenosis requires evaluation. Radiculography fulfils this role.

Radiculography

The advent of safe water-soluble contrast media (for example metrizamide and iopamidol) has appreciably increased the diagnostic accuracy of myelography. Because of the inherently lower osmolality of the water-soluble agents root sheath filling is superior compared with that

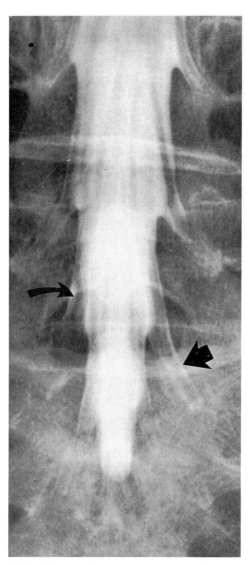

Fig. 2.34.   Metrizamide radiculogram. A fairly discrete root sheath lesion is shown. Compare the normal left S1 root (arrow) with the amputated right root sheath. Note also the displaced S1 nerve root (curved arrow).

obtained either by oil-based contrast media, such as Myodil, or by gas. Metrizamide in a 200 mg/ml dilution has an osmolality of 320 milliosmoles per litre compared with Myodil at 1570. Improved root sheath opacification means that more laterally placed root abnormalities can be regularly visualized (Fig. 2.34). Consequently, whilst little change has occurred in the accuracy of diagnosis in central disc protrusion, and indeed in intrathecal abnormalities, an appreciable improvement in the detection rate of posterolateral disc lesions has been achieved with these agents. In addition, the water-soluble agents are eliminated rapidly, whereas residual Myodil is absorbed at the rate of about 0·5 ml per year.

The water-soluble contrast media, however, have disadvantages. Whereas running Myodil to the cervical spine from lumbar puncture had little effect on contrast medium concentration, the ready miscibility of water-soluble agents has required a much more meticulous technique in moving the contrast medium, and indeed the lower specific gravity has also made it more difficult to handle. It is preferable therefore to do a separate cervical puncture if specific information is required about the cervical spine. It is no longer appropriate to obtain whole-spine views merely because the contrast medium is present in the subarachnoid space. Accordingly, the indications for radiculography or myelography should be clear in the clinician's mind when requesting a study, and the objectives should be considered by the investigating radiologist.

Whilst Myodil is an amazingly safe agent with immediate after-effects comparable only to lumbar puncture, it is associated with a significant delayed incidence of adhesive arachnoiditis, recognized of recent years, the clinical significance of which has not been fully evaluated. It is most marked when subsequent surgery has been performed or when a bloody tap occurred at the time of injection. Indeed Myodil should not be injected after a bloody tap. Adhesive arachnoiditis also occurred with meglumine iocarmate (Dimer X) now unavailable. Currently available water-soluble contrast media do not seem to have the same effect. Metrizamide is associated with a high incidence of headache (30–40%), nausea and dizziness (about 10%) and other symptoms affecting 3–5% of cases, including myoclonic spasms, fever, back pain and occasional psychomotor disturbances, including retention of urine, transient leg pain and paraesthesiae. This agent is contraindicated when an epileptiform tendency is known or when phenothiazines, monoamine oxidase inhibitors, tricyclics or antihistimine drugs have been regularly prescribed. Iopamidol seems to result in far fewer sequelae than metrizamide, dose for dose. However, some adverse reactions do occur with both agents in the 24–48 hours after injection, when patients may develop late headache with photophobia and neck stiffness, perhaps when they have been discharged home. Little is known about the aetiology of these symptoms. They are more common when contrast medium has been injected into the cervical canal, and in females. They are positively worse when the patient has been inadequately hydrated prior to the study or when hydration has been restricted thereafter. Minimizing the size of the lumbar puncture needle (a maximum of a 22-gauge needle should be used) and enforced bed rest for the first 24 hours have been shown to be beneficial, although the latter has been refuted recently. Cigarette smoking should be discouraged. Some data suggest that the incidence of side-effects reflects the concentration and hence osmolality of the contrast medium used. The late headaches, photophobia and neck stiffness are presumed to be related to continued CSF leakage due to dural tears. Epidural blood patching can be dramatically therapeutic in this circumstance.

Radiculography should never be undertaken without the benefit of adequate plain films, including flexion and extension views. If, for example, attention is paid to such features as widened interpedicular distances, posterior vertebral body scalloping and dysraphism, the incidence of unexpected intrathecal tumours will be minimized.

Radiculography is best undertaken in the pre-surgical assessment of unresponsive low back pain with a sciatic distribution, in the evaluation of spinal stenosis (either acquired or developmental) (Fig. 2.35a, b), or in putative cauda equina tumours and dysraphic anomalies (Figs. 2.36a, b and 2.37a, b). No absolute contraindications are recognized other than those indicated above. Metrizamide may be withheld in those patients with appropriate drug or epileptic history, and a large-volume Myodil study may be undertaken if other agents are unavailable. Evidence exists, however, that a water-soluble contrast medium may be safely used in a patient who has had a previous major reaction to an intravenous contrast medium, possibly because receptors in the brain differ from those in the lung.

The exact choice of contrast medium agent is individual. Metrizamide has the disadvantage of requiring reconstruction but may be made to any predetermined iodine concentration. Iopamidol, on the other hand, is ready-made but with a preordained concentration, and seems considerably less likely to induce as many side-effects. A volume of between 10 and 15 ml of either agent with 200 mg/ml of iodine is adequate for the vast majority of lumbar studies. Smaller volumes are necessary when significant spinal stenosis is present or the possibility exists of a significant space-occupying lesion. A relatively high lumbar puncture (L2–3) is best in order to avoid the majority of disc lesions and to be cephalad to the worst affected segments of spinal stenosis (usually L3–4, 4–5). Puncture at an even higher level is possible with care. Performance of lumbar puncture in the erect sitting position is often technically easier because of improved back flexion, overall ease in palpation of landmarks and the raised hydrostatic pressure of CSF enhancing the distinctive 'ping' sensed when the needle passes through the dura. A short bevelled needle is essential, and having obtained a clear tap advancement of the needle by a millimetre or two will largely avoid accidental subdural injection. If contrast material is injected too rapidly miscibility seems enhanced, possibly due to a

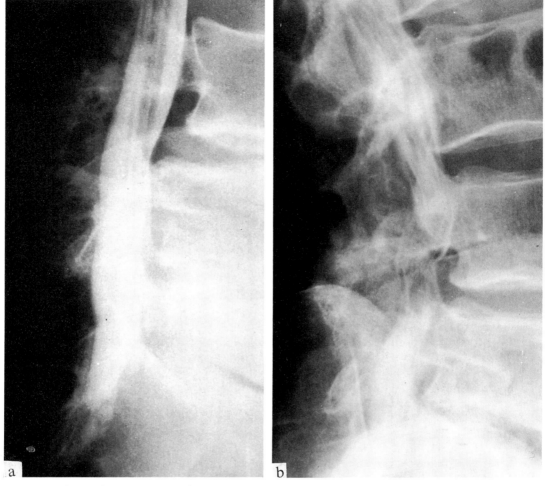

Fig. 2.35. (a) Flexion, (b) extension views during metrizamide radiculography. The dynamic nature of spinal stenosis is demonstrated with considerable narrowing, particularly at L4–5, during back extension. Note also the L4–5 discal instability.

Venturi effect, with resulting poor densities of contrast medium.

If a high-volume Myodil study is being performed a re-aspiration needle, such as the Cuatico, should be used with injection volumes of 12–18 ml. It is essential to have the needle in the midline and the patient prone during the injection in order to avoid damaging nerve roots. Consequently fluoroscopy is essential during the procedure, preferably biplanar. The site of puncture must correspond to the most dependent part of the lumbar curve. Low-volume Myodil myelography no longer has a place in clinical practice because of its inherently poor accuracy, in comparison with radiculography, and the increased incidence of adhesive arachnoiditis. Significant complications are few. Many patients experience transient pain in the back and/or radiating down the leg, reflecting their symptomatic pain, following the injection

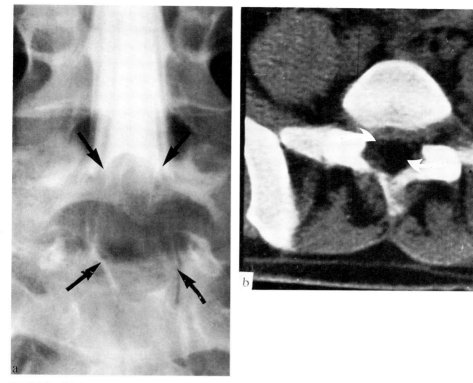

Fig. 2.36. (a) An unsuspected cauda equina tumour detected during a radiculogram for low back pain and sciatica. Note the intrinsic space-occupying lesion (arrows) with re-entrant angles and a smooth outline. (b) A CT scan at the same level demonstrates a lesion with the same attenuation coefficient as fat between muscle planes, establishing the diagnosis of a lipoma of the cauda equina.

of significant volumes of contrast medium. This is related, perhaps, to raised intrathecal pressure. Such patients almost always have an appropriate disc lesion. Severe pain during the injection is frequently associated with a space-occupying lesion causing virtual spinal block. If no lesion is demonstrated in the lumbar region it is always worthwhile examining the thoracic canal. Many also complain of transient dulling of hearing, likened to entering a tunnel in a train. Slight angulation of the needle, away from the midline, may result in pricking a nerve root, trapped in a lateral recess. Whilst uncomfortable to the patient this is not known to produce permanent sequelae. Other minor needle-related artefacts include extra- and subdural injections, and pseudodisc lesions produced by a

haematoma from the vascular annulus caused by too deep a needle position.

Radiographs must include oblique views to demonstrate, in profile, the nerve root sheaths, particularly L3–S1, and lateral views in flexion and extension. They should be exposed so that their centring point lies at the level of L4 for the L3–S1 roots and higher for the upper lumbar roots. This is essential since the diagnosis of a posterolateral disc protrusion may depend on discrete asymmetry or amputation of a root sheath (Fig. 2.34) and this may not be appreciated with inadequate images. In some centres horizontal beam decubitus films have been recommended to ensure maximal root sheath filling on the dependent side. Congenital variation may limit interpretation, particularly conjoint

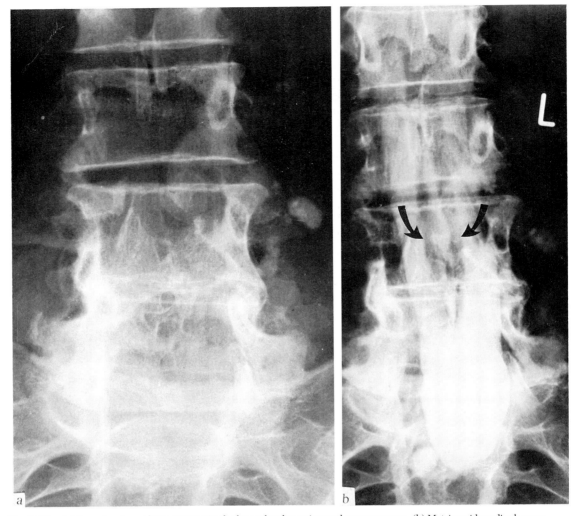

Fig. 2.37. (a) Complex dysraphism present in the lower lumbar spine and upper sacrum. (b) Metrizamide radiculogram reveals diastematomyelia with an extremely low tethered conus. The two hemicords at the conus are clearly demonstrated (arrows).

root sheaths or roots. Side-to-side comparison is then not possible since this is usually an asymmetrical phenomenon occurring in about 2% of studies, commonly involving the L5 and S1 roots (Fig. 2.38a, b). Difficulty may also occur with a high termination of the sacral sac, creating a wide space between the column of contrast medium and the back of the L5–S1 disc space. Under both of these circumstances it may be necessary to employ a second-line investiga-

tion in order to evaluate potential disc symptoms. Large arachnoid diverticula, most commonly at S1 or S2, are an incidental finding in many patients and are not known to have clinical significance, apart from a theoretical risk of flap valve obstruction and root compression. Difficulty also occurs when adhesive arachnoiditis is present because subtle root sheath abnormalities cannot be assessed or larger indentations cannot be ascribed to recurrent disc

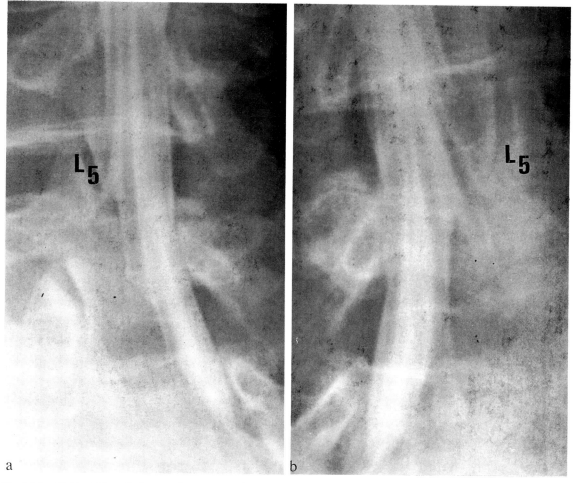

Fig. 2.38. Metrizamide radiculogram demonstrates developmental asymmetry. On the left (a) the L5 and S1 root sheathes are conjoined, on the right (b) those sheaths are separate. Side-to-side comparison is therefore not easy. The right S1 root sheath is possibly shortened (*see* Fig. 2.48).

disease with certainty (Fig. 2.39a, b). Adhesions may be seen also between nerve roots (Fig. 2.40) though their significance is uncertain.

In addition to anterolateral indentation of the column due to disc disease, attention should be paid to posterolateral indentation due to facet osteoarthritis, fibrocartilage hypertrophy and ligamentum flavum redundancy. Spinal stenosis may be appreciated, especially on the lateral film, but the dynamic nature of acquired spinal stenosis will require flexion and extension films for demonstration (Fig. 2.35a, b). These are most reliably performed by using a vertical beam with the patient flexing and extending while lying on the table; they can be conveniently recorded during fluoroscopy. If high-volume Myodil studies are being performed this may not be possible because of the in-dwelling needle.

Before completing the study it is a simple matter to examine the distal thoracic cord and conus in a water-soluble study simply by lying the patient supine and permitting the contrast medium to pool in the thoracic kyphosis. This

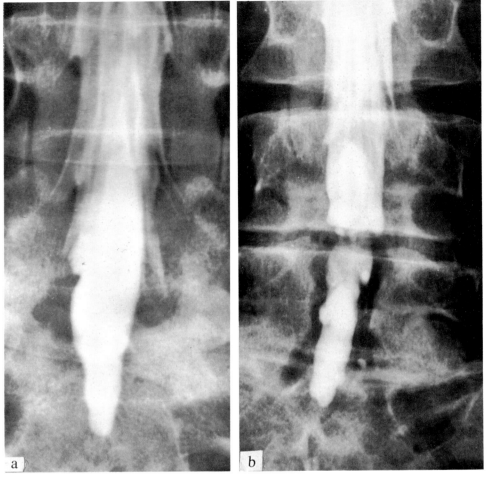

Fig. 2.39. Two examples of adhesive arachnoiditis: (a) grade 2 and (b) grade 3. Note the loss of nerve root sheath detail, wasting, irregularity of outline, and poor visualization of nerve roots, stuck by adhesions. A previous radical laminectomy has been performed in case (b).

again cannot be performed if the needle is left *in situ*, but high-volume studies should permit adequate visualization nonetheless.

Radiculography is an extremely accurate procedure in everyday practice. The vast majority of central disc protrusions are delineated and almost all posterolateral protrusions detected, so that an accuracy rate of the order of 95% should be achieved. A significant failure rate occurs with the rare, true lateral disc protrusion, or where one of the adverse factors already mentioned, for example adhesive arachnoiditis,

is present. It is important to remember that sometimes an intrathecal tumour or developmental anomaly such as neurofibromatosis is investigated in the guise of degenerative disc disease (Fig. 2.41b). On occasions disc 'indentations' are due to neoplasms or extradural abscess (Fig. 2.42a, b). A careful analysis of the radiological signs will usually lead to the correct diagnosis.

Radiculography remains the prime means of investigating spinal stenosis, either developmental or acquired. The dynamic nature can readily

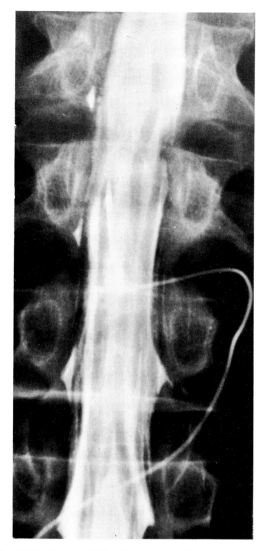

Fig. 2.40. Arachnoiditis is demonstrated between nerve roots following intrathecal chemotherapy for non-Hodgkin's lymphoma. Note the coarse quality of the fused nerve roots, and their irregular disposition.

signs, since many of the normal population have degenerative disc disease without clinical morbidity. For example, many degenerative lumbar discs have been discovered serendipitously during cervical myelography. Radiculography, indeed all contrast medium studies, falls into disrepute if patients are operated upon on the basis of X-rays alone. Nonetheless, in the majority of patients with disc-related symptoms and signs radiculography provides a highly accurate, localizing diagnostic study. Where it is undertaken in childhood, or indeed in adult life, for the assessment of dysraphism and cauda equina tumours, equally good results may be expected, although the volume of contrast medium may need to be higher. Difficulty may occur with a substantial tumour, and a clean lumbar puncture may require fluoroscopy to assist needle placement, a 'C' arm unit being most useful under these circumstances.

Discography has several major indications. Firstly, it is the only technique to demonstrate anatomical abnormality, although MRI, when available, may have a place. Anatomical normality is relevant in assessing patients for disc or spinal fusion since, for example, it is important to know that the nuclei on each side of the proposed fusion level are not already diseased. Secondly, discography is used provocatively in order to investigate low back pain syndromes, especially in patients without radicular signs or symptoms. In this situation, although anatomical abnormality may be demonstrated the test is only considered positively diagnostic if the clinical symptom complex is induced by injections into one or more disc spaces. This view is reinforced if those symptoms remit rapidly as contrast medium is absorbed. Thirdly, discography forms part of a chemonucleolysis protocol when having demonstrated an abnormal disc, in terms of both anatomy and pain responses, chymopapaine is injected (*vide infra*). Lastly, needling of the disc space is part of aspiration and/or biopsy in the diagnosis of infection and/or tumour.

be appreciated together with important signs such as nerve root redundancy.

It is important to recall that radiculography forms but one part of the evaluation of a patient with low back pain. The abnormality detected must be correlated with clinical symptoms and

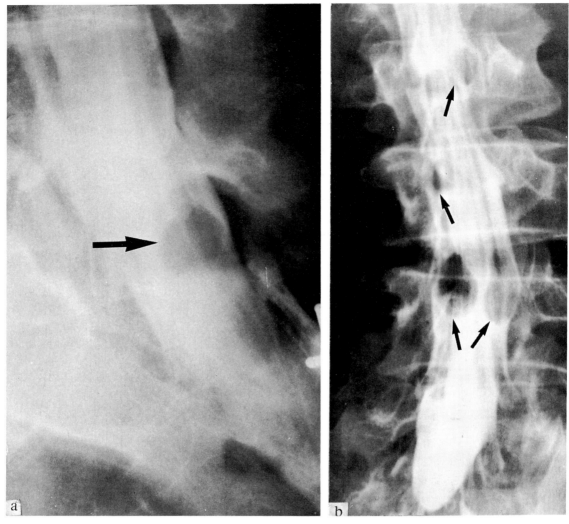

Fig. 2.41. (a) A single neurofibroma is demonstrated (arrow) involving the left S1 nerve root. (b) Multiple neurofibromata are demonstrated (arrows) in a patient with known neurofibromatosis.

Technique

There are three recommended approaches to the lumbar disc spaces. The lateral (more correctly posterolateral) approach is performed in the lateral decubitus position, with the patient lying on the left, the needle inserted some 8–10 cm from the midline and directed anteriorly from the operator at about 50–60°. The lateral placement of the needle puncture is necessary to avoid transverse processes and facet joints. A 21-gauge needle is inserted and directed to the annulus fibrosus with a track of local anaesthetic. The use of 0·5% lignocaine permits a generous volume of local anaesthetic. Once a satisfactory position has been obtained a finer 26-gauge needle is inserted through the 21-gauge needle so that the tip projects about 1 cm beyond it. It may be necessary to use biplane fluoroscopy in the learning period but with

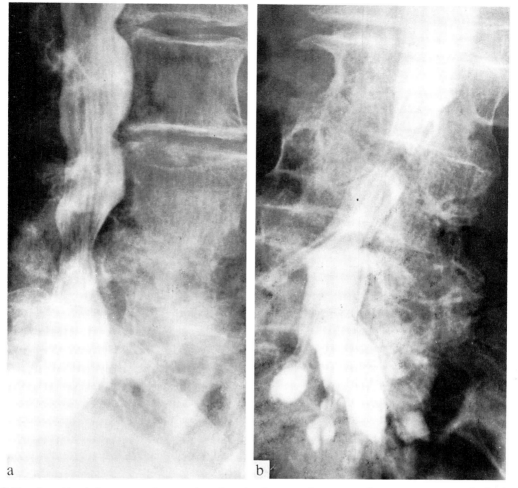

a b

Fig. 2.42. An epidural abscess secondary to tuberculous disc disease with an acquired stenosis is present at this level. Degenerative disease with disc indentation is also present more proximal to this abnormality.

experience single-plane imaging is satisfactory. Contrast medium of a non-sodium salt, for example meglumine iothalamate 60%, is injected to demonstrate the cavity in the nucleus pulposus. Since the normal nucleus (Fig. 2.43) accommodates only 1–1·5 ml of contrast medium, and injection pressure may be relatively high, a 1-ml Mantoux syringe is recommended for injection. A true intranuclear injection may be obtained more easily if side holes are drilled into the 26-gauge needle, contrast medium taking the path of least resistance. No evidence is available to know whether a true intranuclear, as compared with a perinuclear, injection is of diagnostic importance provided it is recognized as an artefactual normal (Fig. 2.46). Normal nuclei are biconcave or 'collar stud' (Fig. 2.43). It has been suggested that pressure tracings during injection not only demonstrate the true intranuclear position of injection, but also may provide information on degenerative disease.

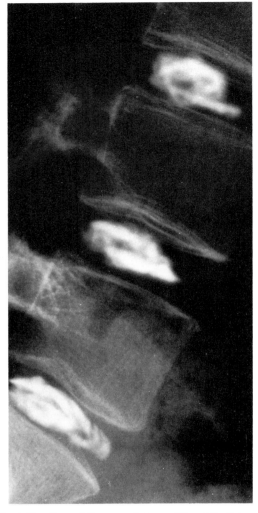

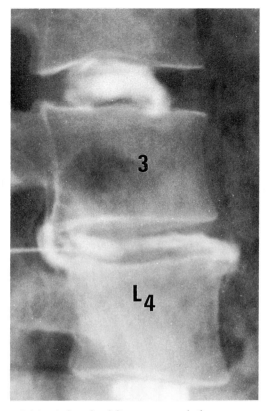

Fig. 2.43. Normal discogram between L3 and S1. Note the collar stud outline of the L3 to L5 discs and the more biconcave nature of L5–S1.

Fig. 2.44. A three-level discogram reveals three abnormalities. The L2–3 nucleus extends into a Schmorl's node in the upper end-plate of L3. This is not known to be of any direct significance. The L3–4 disc is grossly degenerated with disruption of the normal nuclear outline and leakage of contrast medium under the posterior longitudinal ligament. The needle is in position at this level. At L4–5 note the localized globular quality of the injected contrast medium. This is in a perinuclear rather than strictly intranuclear position; nonetheless it demonstrates no abnormality of the disc.

This technique is straightforward for the L3–4 and often L4–5 disc spaces. However, because of the posterior iliac crest the L5–S1 disc space requires slightly more skill, for whilst the needle puncture is virtually the same as for L4–5 it must also be directed 30° caudad. With practice it is usually possible to obtain an adequate puncture of the annulus fibrosis. Obstruction is usually caused by the transverse process of L5 or the superior facet joint at L5–S1. It is worth-while asking the patient to flex and extend the spine if the needle is just not quite in position. Very often this relatively slight movement facil-itates placement.

The posterior and posterolateral approaches cross the thecal canal. They are performed in the prone position and require biplane fluoros-copy. A 21-gauge lumbar puncture needle is inserted in the midline just below the lamina and a 26-gauge needle passed through the thecal sac and the vascular annulus into the nucleus pulposus. The posterolateral approach merely side-steps the interspinous space and requires a calculation of angle in order that the 26-gauge needle still crosses the theca in the midline. It is arguable whether a safer intraspinal contrast agent, such as iopamidol, should be used if this route is chosen, because of the potential reflux of contrast medium from the nucleus into the subarachnoid space.

Advantages and disadvantages of the technique
The lateral approach causes unequivocally more discomfort, since local anaesthetic can only be injected once the needle has passed through the lumbar muscles. Access to the lower disc spaces, particularly L5–S1, is limited by the shape of the posterior iliac crest and is, therefore, technically more difficult than either of the posterior approaches. The advantages, however, include the absence of lumbar punctures with their associated post-lumbar puncture syndromes and the avoidance of pain induced by needling the vascular annulus. Contrast medium may be injected with relative impunity since the arachnoid is intact, thus this is the route of choice if chemonucleolysis is to follow the study. The posterior approaches have disadvantages. In the true posterior approach, the needle being inserted between the spinous processes, cephalic angulation of the needle occurs and bending or manipulation of the inner needle is necessary in order to create a curve that crosses back across the thecal space to hit the midline of the disc. The posterolateral approach corrects for this, the needle crossing the theca, however, at an angle. In both approaches the slight lateral deviation of the inner needle increases the risk of pricking nerve roots trapped in lateral recesses. Passage through the vascular annulus is painful, and local anaesthetic cannot be injected. Reflux of contrast medium into the subarachnoid space can occur. Advantages include the greater probability of obtaining a true intranuclear position

than with the lateral approach and, apart from the transient painful episode when the needle passes the vascular annulus, it is common experience that patient co-operation is better with this technique.

Since discography is primarily a provocative technique it is essential to record, step by step, the patient's symptoms with an element of cross-examination. Unless clear-cut positive results are obtained (Fig. 2.45) it is dangerous to consider discography abnormal, even if anatomically so. Furthermore, pain and infirmity may be from multiple causes (Fig. 2.46a–e).

The complications of the technique are relatively few. Transthecal approaches induce post-lumbar puncture syndromes and accidental dural puncture may occur during the lateral approach. Discitis, probably of a chemical nature, occurs rarely, and even rarer is the risk of infective discitis. Transient paralytic ileus and retroperitoneal haemorrhage have also been recorded, but usually after chemonucleolysis.

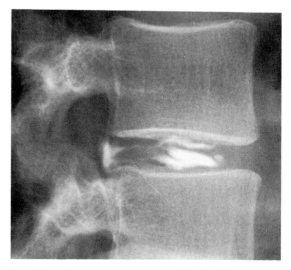

Fig. 2.45. Split annulus syndrome at L3–4 with apparently normal nucleus is shown to extend posteriorly through an annular fissure. This patient, a bank manager, experienced the sudden severe onset of low back pain without sciatica following lifting bags of silver coin. The discogram reproduced exactly his symptom complex.

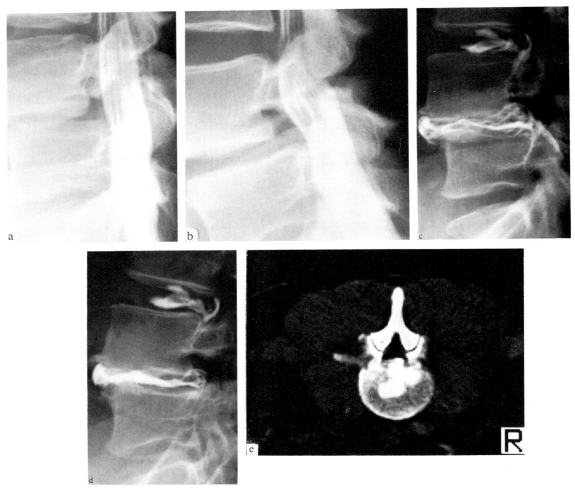

Fig. 2.46.   A young man with complex low back disease. L4–5 spondylolisthesis with bilateral spondylolytic defects is shown. Radiculography (a and b) reveals discal instability at L4–5 with dynamic spinal stenosis due to facet indentation during back extension (arrows). Discography (c and d) demonstrates a split annulus at L3–4, following which much of the symptom complex was transiently induced. The posterior extension of contrast medium is confirmed by the CT scan (e). The unstable L4–5 disc is shown to be grossly degenerate but no specific symptom was induced by injecting at this level. Consequently this patient has dynamic spinal stenosis with disc degeneration and a split annulus syndrome in addition to his known spondylolytic defect.

Chemonucleolysis

Usually, chemonucleolysis is performed in patients who are relatively young, with a short history of back pain, with radicular pain, and a failure of conservative treatment. Some workers prefer radiculography or CT to have already been performed to exclude spinal cord tumours and other intrathecal abnormalities. Following discography, by the lateral approach, and the identification of specific disc abnormality, including induced symptomatology, chymopapaine is injected in a dose of 2000–4000 units (maximum of 10 000 units) into each disc involved; no more than two discs should be injected. The injections are associated with local, transient pain. Occasional anaphylaxis is recorded. The accidental injection of chymo-papaine into the subarachnoid space induces subarachnoid haemorrhage, and consequently the posterior approach should not be used. Occasionally patients suffer paralytic ileus, but usually no more complications occur than following orthodox discography. Subsequent films will demonstrate narrowing of the injected disc with some irregularity of end-plates consistent with a chemical discitis. A few cases of transverse myelitis have occurred following chymo-papaine injection. This rare risk seems to occur only in those who have recently had some form of interference with their dura, for example epidural injections. Consequently, it is wise to postpone chymopapaine injections for 10–14 days after such an episode.

Epidural venography

Epidural venography has enjoyed a vogue based on two principles. Firstly, although venous anatomy is generally quite variable, a considerable constancy occurs with the anterior spinal veins and radicular veins (Fig. 2.47). Consequently, an abnormality such as a disc protrusion involving either an anterior bulge or a compression of the nerve root should be accompanied by appropriate venous changes. Secondly, the technique avoids subarachnoid injection and consequently may be performed on a day-case basis, avoiding all of the effects of lumbar puncture and intrathecal contrast medium. Because it demonstrates lesions along the line of root sheaths, indeed beyond them, the technique was particularly popular in countries where water-soluble contrast media were initially not available. Its use now is a second-line investigation of patients with normal or equivocal radiculograms in the presence of radicular symptoms or signs.

The study, initially performed by intraosseus injection, is now undertaken by catheterization from femoral vein puncture. Intraosseous injections, apart from being extremely painful and requiring general anaesthesia, were associated with a significant incidence of avascular bone necrosis and infection. A fine 5 French catheter

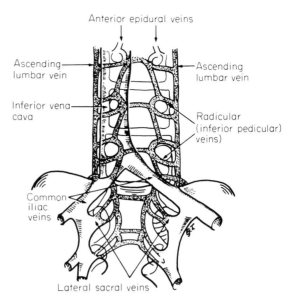

Fig. 2.47. A line drawing demonstrates the pertinent anatomy in ascending lumbar venography. The close relationship between the disc spaces and the anterior epidural veins is apparent. A constant anatomy is also found between the pedicles and the pedicular veins and therefore between the nerve roots running in relationship to the pedicles.

is preshaped with or without side holes and passed, usually from the left groin, into the left ascending lumbar vein and/or a lateral sacral vein on the contralateral side. A second catheter may be introduced so that simultaneous injections can be performed, but for ease, sequential injections are recommended. Usually the lateral lumbar vein opacifies levels craniad to L5 and the lateral sacral vein injection outlines the L5–S1 disc space. Consequently, both injections may be necessary. Between 35 and 50 ml of a non sodium-containing contrast medium, such as 60% meglumine iothalamate, are injected over a 4–5 second film run with radiographs every second. Distension and persistence of venous filling are enhanced by a compression band across the abdomen and the Valsalva technique. Visualization of veins at the lumbosacral junction is improved by a 15° craniad tilt.

Complications include those of venous catheterization and occasional vein thrombosis with persistent leg oedema, pulmonary embolus and local sepsis. In addition, pressure injection into veins may be accompanied by venous rupture, causing a self-limiting haematoma which, while requiring no special treatment, is, however, accompanied by considerable pain This is most likely to occur if a pressure injection has been made into a small vein, particularly one of the lateral sacral veins, and it may be wiser to use a hand injection at this site.

The signs which suggest disc disease relate to deformity or amputation of veins at sites where discs could indent. Hence, unilateral or bilateral obstruction of the anterior intervertebral vein at a disc space suggests a central protrusion. It may be implied also by abnormal curvature or displacement with a more discrete lesion. Posterolateral disc protrusion is suggested by displacement of a radicular vein, by delayed filling (Fig. 2.48) or complete occlusion. Less common signs include the demonstration of collateral

circulation, narrowing in calibre, or localized dilatation. The technique is unreliable when previous disc surgery has been performed or when adhesive arachnoiditis is present because in both circumstances venous anatomy is disturbed already. Nonetheless, an overall surgical correlation may be expected in some 90% of patients, a figure similar to well-chosen radiculographic investigations. Whether or not the more tedious and time-consuming examination of venography is superior to radiculography with its inherent morbidity is still a matter of debate.

Epidurography

Epidurography has enjoyed a vogue, as an alternative to radiculography, in the demonstration of both central and posterolateral disc protrusions. The advantages of the technique include the avoidance of lumbar punctures, and

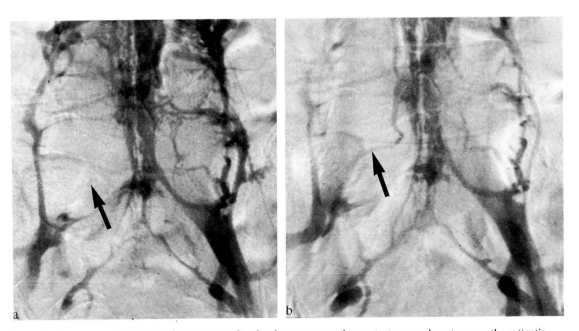

Fig. 2.48. Two consecutive images from an ascending lumbar venogram demonstrate normal anatomy on the patient's left. Delayed filling of the right inferior pedicular vein of S1 (arrow) is consistent with a posterolateral disc protrusion. This is the same patient as in Fig. 2.38 and confirms that the relatively short root sheath demonstrated on that study did represent a disc lesion.

the injection of intrathecal contrast medium, so that it may be performed as an out-patient study. By employing a catheter technique a localized study may be performed to investigate a given disc level or particular nerve root. It may also be valuable when there is a high take-off of the sacral canal. By and large demonstration of root sheaths is more extensive compared with radiculography, since the subdural space extends further than the subarachnoid space.

Two techniques are used, the dorsal interspinal approach using a Tuohy needle, or via the sacral hiatus using a catheter technique. The dorsal approach may be limited by the plica mediana dorsalis which may inhibit uniform filling of the epidural space, particularly if it is desired to look at the upper lumbar spine. The catheter technique is at its best at the L5–S1 disc space, and perhaps the L4–5 level. The use of a non-ionic or low-osmolality agent is important since subarachnoid injection of contrast medium may occur by accidental dural puncture in some 10–15% of cases. The complications of the procedure are the same as radiculography.

Abnormalities are demonstrated by mass lesions and by amputation of nerve root sheaths. False-positive results occur with fibrofatty masses of uncertain origin, as well as adhesions following arachnoiditis or previous surgery. The technique is also contraindicated in the presence of clotting or bleeding diatheses and has only limited application. Certainly it is unlikely to be of benefit where high-resolution CT is available.

Facet arthrography

It has been recognized, since the turn of the century, that some low back pain, and indeed sciatic pain, would appear to be generated from facet joint disease. The distinction, however, between this pain syndrome and those associated with degenerative disc disease has proved difficult. However, renewed interest in facet arthrography has been rekindled following reports of high success rates in the treatment of all types

of back and leg pain following transection of the nerve supply to, or resection of, facet joints. Akin to discography, the technique incorporates the concept of provocation by inducing symptoms from the injection of contrast medium into facet joints and by the amelioration of those symptoms following the injection of local anaesthetic and steroid. In addition, an anatomical demonstration of derangement of the joint may be shown by arthrography. Facet osteoarthritis is so common, however, that this is not necessarily useful information. Granted that injections into particular facet joints can be demonstrated to produce a recognizable clinical syndrome in the individual patient, it is reasonable to expect that transcutaneous facet block or radiofrequency denervation may provide permanent therapeutic results.

The facet joints are needled in the prone oblique position using a 22-gauge lumbar puncture needle inserted parallel to the vertical X-ray beam. There is usually a slight sensation of pain as the needle passes through the joint capsule. The normal joint is of small volume and hence it is essential to have a short bevel. The joint accommodates between 0·5 and 1·5 ml of a water-soluble non sodium-containing contrast medium. If the injection is associated with symptomatic pain, re-aspiration and replacement with an equivalent volume of a long-acting local anaesthetic (e.g. 0·25% bupivacaine hydrochloride) and a long-acting steroid (e.g. 40 mg of methylprednisolone acetate) provides a therapeutic trial. On occasions prolonged periods of symptomatic relief may be achieved.

The normal arthrographic appearances reveal a smooth capsular outline, oval in the frontal projection and S-shaped in the oblique projection (Fig. 2.49).

Abnormalities include hypertrophy of the synovium, with irregular or nodular filling defects, fibrocartilaginous hypertrophy and degenerative disease. Spondylolytic defects, when associated with a pseudarthrosis, may be demonstrated to communicate not only with the facet joint that is being injected, but also with the inferior facet joint of the same lamina.

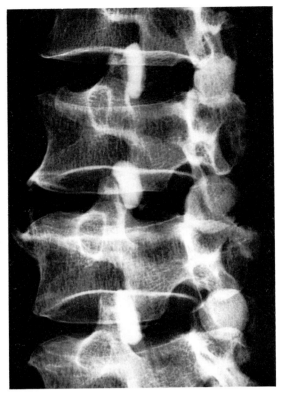

Fig. 2.49. Normal facet joints have been injected in a post-mortem specimen.

Not only may this provide information relating to the genesis of pain in spondylolysis but also the confirmation of a non-union, and therefore the necessity for operative intervention.

To summarize, the injection of contrast medium in facet joints is similar to that in discography insofar as it is a provocative investigation which may produce symptomatic pain. All induced symptoms during the study should be meticulously recorded. Furthermore, the resolution of such pain following local anaesthetic injection is relevant. The technique has, however, two disadvantages. Firstly, it may be used in those patients in whom facet joint disease is merely one part of a spectrum of causes of back pain and a partial or incomplete result may be achieved. Secondly, as a technique, it is

a painful arthrogram and carries all of the theoretical risks associated with arthrography, including septic arthritis.

Philosophy of use
Few centres have published their data on the relative merits of radiculography, epidural venography, discography and epidurography. Even those reports may have biased patient selection and it is difficult to offer a balanced approach in the use of the investigation modalities available at this time. Clearly, computerized tomography is taking, rightfully, an increasing share of first-line investigations following adequate plain-film radiography. Nonetheless, its value has not been fully ascertained and its unavailability in many parts of the world is a limiting factor. In the assessment of degenerative disc disease, particularly low back pain and sciatica, without doubt radiculography remains pre-eminent in demonstrating abnormality with a high degree of reliability. It is also relatively easy technically, if a little costly in terms of contrast medium, bed occupancy, and patient morbidity. Pharmaceutical companies continue research for contrast medium agents with lower complication rates. The use of ever-finer needles and the development of modifications of technique will almost certainly make radiculography a far more pleasant and less expensive examination.

When radiculography provides clear-cut demonstration of abnormality, and that abnormality correlates closely with clinical symptoms and signs, it is almost certainly unnecessary to proceed to any further investigations. The abnormal radiculogram which, however, does not correlate must be viewed with suspicion and appropriate further investigations undertaken. If a radiculogram is normal or produces equivocal results a second-line investigation must be undertaken. Discography or epidurography will be found to be of equally precise value in the diagnosis of disc protrusion without radicular symptoms or signs. Discography has the added advantage of being provocative and of enabling the correlation between anatomical deformity and clinical symptoms to be made, and, if chymopapaine is used, to permit therapeutic management. When radicular symptoms or signs are present epidural venography is probably the most helpful second-line investigation, because of its ability to detect more lateral disc lesions than radiculography, particularly if the involved root is above the level of L5–S1 disc.

With the increasing clarification of other low back pain syndromes there will be a concomitant reshuffling of the relative values of facet arthrography and discography. So many patients with lumbar disc disease also have facet disease, and so many 'normal' people have degenerative disc disease, that the assessment of the many variants of low back pain syndrome is fraught with difficulty, and a very close cooperation between the orthopaedic surgeon and his radiological colleagues will be necessary if the armamentarium of radiological investigation is to be used to its optimum in an individual case.

THORACIC SPINE

In orthopaedic practice the most usual indications for investigation of the thoracic spine beyond those of plain films and tomography are extradural obstruction, due to, for example, metastatic disease, trauma, meningioma, infection or a non-calcified thoracic disc. Intradural obstruction is rarer and due to such causes as ependymoma or seeded metastasis. In the younger age groups myelography has a place in the assessment of scoliosis and congenital malformations.

All three contrast agents, oil-based, water-soluble and gas, may be employed. In routine clinical practice water-soluble contrast medium is now the most useful, oil-based contrast medium being reserved for those patients in whom water-soluble agents are contraindicated, or when the whole spine is to be investigated. Gas myelography requires special apparatus, and is a complex undertaking, but is particularly valuable in the assessment of syrinx-related abnormalities.

Iopamidol or metrazamide in approximately 300 mg/ml strength is injected by the lumbar route and routine views of the lumbar canal obtained. Simply lying the patient supine and flat is adequate, in most instances, to opacify the thoracic canal fully, at least to the level of T3 or 4. Imaging in the supine projection reveals most lesions to this level (Fig. 2.50) and lateral projections may be obtained easily if the patient is turned rapidly, though carefully, on

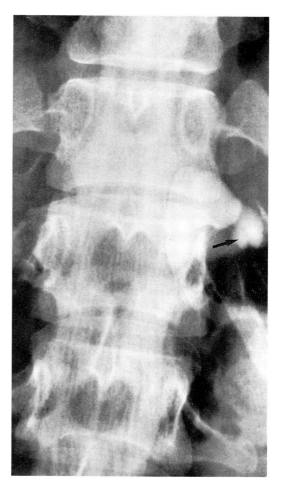

Fig. 2.50. Lateral thoracic meningocele (arrow). This was an incidental finding in a patient being investigated for low back pain and sciatica. The patient was subsequently demonstrated to have other stigmata of neurofibromatosis. The anatomy of T11–12 is clearly demonstrated.

to his side. Images higher than this may be
obtained either in the supine position or by con-
ducting the entire study prone and very carefully tipping the patient into the head-down
position. This is a difficult undertaking when a
marked thoracic kyphos is present because of
the tendency for contrast medium to be held up
at the level of the kyphos and then to flow rapidly, and dilute, once it passes this level. It is
necessary to maintain a chin-up position, extending the cervical spine, in order to prevent
contrast medium dissipating above the foramen
magnum. The supine position is thus usually
preferred for mid to lower thoracic lesions.

When the relationship between theca, canal
and vertebrae is sought, as in scoliosis or diastematomyelia, tomography is an important adjunct. It may be difficult to decide in which
plane tomography should be performed. It is
easiest to undertake this parallel to the curve of
a scoliosis and at right angles to it for the segment of spine under particular review. Early experience suggests that computerized tomography may prove helpful, but unless high-
resolution apparatus with scanning facilities
('scanogram' or 'topogram') is available the relationship between the cord and the spine will
not be visible and contrast medium must also
be injected. In complex lesions considerable limitation is caused by the partial volume effect.

When an obstructing lesion is present it is
necessary to demonstrate not only the level of
abnormality, but also its extent. Water-soluble
contrast medium is more likely to pass a significant obstruction than is an oil-based contrast
medium. Consequently, the water-soluble agent
may demonstrate both the proximal and distal
extent of an extradural mass, whereas if Myodil
is used it may be necessary to perform both
cervical and lumbar punctures.

Because water-soluble contrast medium is
readily miscible it is possible to identify normal
vascular structures such as the anterior spinal
artery (Fig. 2.51) and the artery of Adamkiewicz,
and vascular malformations may be detected
with ease.

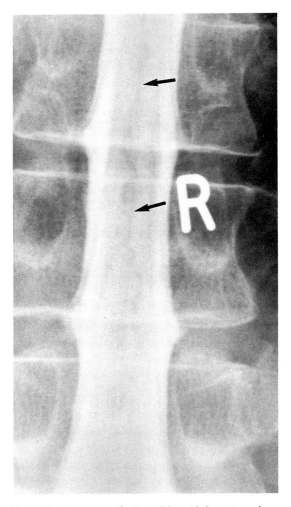

Fig. 2.51. Dense opacification of the mid-thoracic cord
following a routine iopamidol radiculogram demonstrates
clearly the anterior spinal vessels (arrows).

Further investigations, apart from spinal angiography, are very rarely necessary in the
thoracic spine. Discography is seldom performed, although a disc may be needled for the
investigation of tumour or infection. Facet joints
are extremely difficult to needle because of anatomical complexity, but costotransverse joints
are accessible for injection in some patients with
probable arthropathic pain.

CERVICAL SPINE

Major indications for the further investigation of the cervical spine include the assessment of degenerative disc disease, trauma, and the cervical spine involvement in rheumatological disorders. On occasions it is necessary to evaluate the presence of potential syrinx, tonsillar, or other space-occupying lesions of the neural canal.

Following adequate plain films, including flexion and extension images, myelography remains the single most important further investigation. Contrast medium may be injected either by lumbar puncture, and guided to the neck, or locally (Fig. 2.52a, b). Whilst Myodil may be used (Fig. 2.53), and either re-aspirated or left *in situ*, the advent of safe water-soluble contrast media, including metrizamide and iopamidol, has made local study of the cervical spine an easier proposition. Provided there are no major contraindications to the use of these agents (*see above*), the patient is laid prone with the neck extended, the patient's chin being supported by a foam pad. This may prove difficult in patients with a markedly reduced range of movement or a kyphos. The combination of a table tilt with the feet down, pillows under the chest and pads under the chin will usually produce a comfortable resting position. Patient cooperation is important, since contrast medium should be kept in the cervical spine and not be permitted to enter the basal cisterns in large quantities. Biplane fluoroscopy is desirable, but

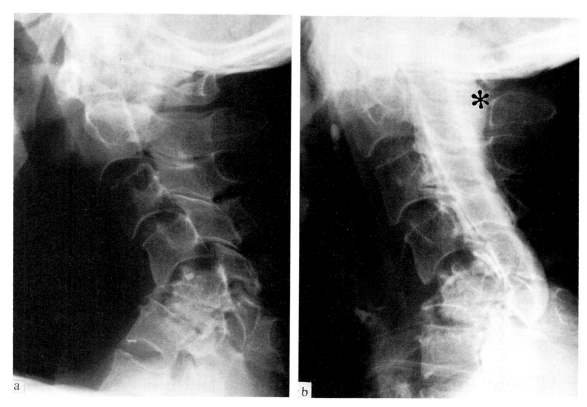

Fig. 2.52. (a) Plain film and (b) cervical myelogram in the assessment of spinal stenosis following cervical trauma. The preferred site of puncture is indicated (asterisk). A virtually complete occlusion has occurred at the C5–6 level due to both anterior indentation and laminal compression at the level of the old fracture.

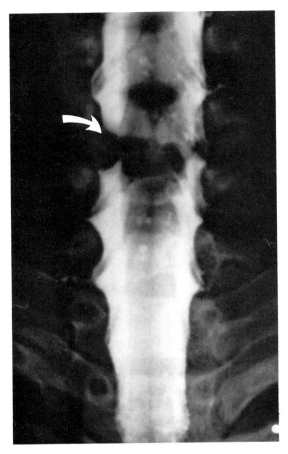

Fig. 2.53. A discrete posterolateral disc protusion is demonstrated (arrow) using a high-volume Myodil technique. No anterior disc indentation was seen on the lateral film. Note the short nerve root sheaths compared with a lumbar study.

in practice a lateral image with a 'C' arm intensifier is sufficient. A 22-gauge lumbar puncture needle is inserted just caudad and anterior to the tip of the mastoid process and is advanced parallel to the X-ray beam to strike the theca between C1 and C2 just anterior to the interlaminar line (Fig. 2.52b). Occasional checks of the position in the frontal plane are helpful but not obligatory. Usually, compared with a lumbar injection, a less clear-cut sensation is felt as the needle enters the subarachnoid space with a lumbar injection, and entry is more difficult when considerable ligamentous laxity is present, especially with rheumatoid instability syndromes. An injection of contrast medium at 300 mg/ml concentration is made under direct fluoroscopic control, using an extension tube to avoid radiation exposure to the operator. The volume injected is entirely dependent upon canal size, and freedom of flow should be judged fluoroscopically. Judicious table tilting will achieve adequate filling without overspill into the basal cisterns. The total volume (usually of the order of 8–10 ml) will be less in patients with spinal stenosis. Some workers prefer to perform lateral cervical puncture with the patient supine, the head being elevated, flexing the neck, particularly when the patient is unable to tolerate the prone position.

Radiographs are exposed in the frontal and lateral projection in order to demonstrate the cord and its relationship to the thecal canal. Attention must be paid to radiographic exposure factors in order not to overpenetrate and therefore reduce contrast. Oblique projections, rolling the patient from side to side, will demonstrate the roots. It is important to remember that root sheaths are shorter than those in the lumbar canal. In order to demonstrate the dynamic nature of spinal stenosis a flexion film may be performed, but because of the risk of increasing the volume of contrast medium running into the basal cisterns a further head tilt of the table top is prudent beforehand. Almost invariably spinal stenosis is at its worst in the neck extension position. When satisfactory cervical canal images have been recorded the patient is gradually tipped further head-up and the contrast medium imaged as it flows down the upper thoracic canal in order to detect the occasional unsuspected high thoracic disc or tumour. Contrast medium may then be left in the lumbar canal to facilitate absorption away from the brain.

In most instances this study is more than adequate to demonstrate disc lesions and to demonstrate the full extent of spinal stenosis. Complications are similar to lumbar puncture with the additional risk, however, of accidental puncture of the cord itself and vertebral arteries if the needle is directed too anteriorly. The former causes severe transient pain and hopefully no long-term effect, although transient neurological signs may occur. The puncture of a vertebral vessel is usually unassociated with permanent sequelae. When a cervical puncture is performed there is a higher incidence of headache, nausea and vomiting compared with lumbar radiculography using water-soluble agents. However, in the majority of patients the technique is tolerated well, and experience suggests that far fewer patients complain than with the extreme adverse (head-down) tilt sometimes necessary to obtain cranial flow of Myodil from the lumbar to the cervical canal.

Further investigations

The place of discography in cervical disc disease is contentious and no uniform agreement has been reached on its place. Apart from being technically more difficult, most patients find it a most uncomfortable procedure. It should probably be reserved for the preoperative evaluation of discal instability or prior to spinal fusion to confirm a symptomatic level.

An anterolateral needle approach is recommended using a short 22-gauge lumbar puncture needle. The sternomastoid muscle and the carotid sheath are displaced by deep palpation and the needle placed directly on to the anterolateral margin of the fibrous annulus. Fluoroscopic checks of position are undertaken frequently, the lateral projection being preferable. The utilization of a 'C' arm intensifier enables simple correlation in the anterior plane. When the position seems satisfactory a fine 26-gauge needle is passed through the lumbar puncture needle into the nucleus; the needle should project about half a centimetre. The normal cervical nucleus accommodates between 0·2 and 0·5 ml of contrast medium and extends more posterolaterally than the normal lumbar disc. If sodium salts are injected pain and discomfort always occur, hence 60% meglumine iothalamate or its equivalent is recommended. As in lumbar discography meticulous recording of

induced symptoms is necessary. However, it is common experience that contrast medium is frequently extravasated and spurious symptoms including heat and flushing are experienced. Accordingly, it is much more difficult than in the lumbar spine to obtain an unequivocal answer to the proposed question of 'does an injection into this disc create the symptom complex of which the patient complains?'

Complications are more frequent than in lumbar discography including the potential risk of haematoma from trauma to the cervical vessels or the thyroid gland. Discitis with or without infection also occurs, as does accidental penetration of the oesophagus. Because of these complications and the potentially equivocal results cervical discography has not achieved universal acclamation.

Trauma

In addition to meticulous attention to plain-film technique, tomography and computerized tomography, cervical myelography offers specific investigations of the cord and its roots following trauma (Fig. 2.52a, b). In particular, assessment of post-traumatic lateral meningoceles (Fig. 2.54), indicating irreversible root damage, post-traumatic syrinx formation, transection of the cord and attenuation, is relevant, with definitive prognostic significance.

Traditionally, oil-based myelography has been performed in the evaluation of these abnormalities, the injection being by lumbar puncture. Because, however, the patient is frequently paraplegic or quadriplegic or, in the case of brachial plexus avulsion injury, is in traction or otherwise incapacitated, this technique is technically difficult. It may be argued that undertaking the study is seldom urgent, except when cord compression is considered with, as yet, little neurological deficit. Accordingly, it is often better to wait until the patient's general condition is stable before pursuing cervical myelography. Lateral cervical puncture using a water-soluble contrast medium is a less difficult procedure and may be the investigation

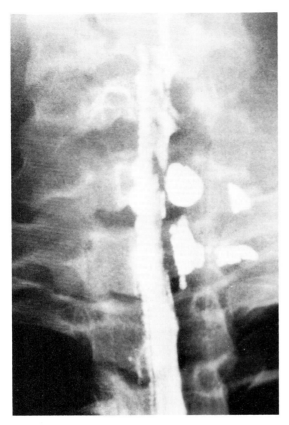

Fig. 2.54. Traumatic lateral meningoceles involving the C7 and C8 roots. The film was taken in the decubitus position using Myodil and confirms permanent nerve root avulsion at these levels.

of choice. Some evidence suggests that a gas myelogram may be a useful alternative, particularly when a syrinx is being assessed.

Rheumatoid disease and other arthropathies
The long-term sequelae of rheumatoid involvement of the cervical spine are well recognized and include atlantoaxial instability, subaxial instability and cervical discitis. Cervical myelography is therefore most frequently performed to assess cord compression and/or dynamic stenosis as a result of instability. The use of Myodil for a lumbar puncture is often an unpleasant procedure for patients with multiple painful joints and reduced mobility such as makes the simple act of turning prone a difficulty. Consequently, a cervical puncture using a water-soluble contrast medium provides a safe, reliable, accurate and relatively straightforward means of demonstrating cord compression and instability; the ease of injection and lack of necessity for tilting is appreciated both by patients and by staff.

Angiography

ARTERIOGRAPHY

Arteriography is not a common orthopaedic radiological investigation. Nonetheless it has a specific place in assessing some aspects of skeletal trauma and neoplasia.

Arteriography is best performed by a selective catheter technique, from either a femoral or axillary artery puncture with the tip of the catheter being placed as close as possible to the region of interest. Without doubt the morbidity from axillary puncture is higher, even in expert hands, than from femoral puncture. Consequently, wherever possible, a common femoral artery puncture is to be preferred. Antegrade puncture can be made in order to investigate ipsilateral lower limb abnormalities. This is often technically easier than trying to pass a catheter over the bifurcation from one leg to the other. Adequate studies of the head, neck and arm vessels can be made using preshaped commercially available catheters from the groin. Injections of contrast medium are best made by pressure pump. The choice of flow rate will depend on the size of vessel being studied and its flow under the circumstances in which it is being investigated. For example, a normal superficial femoral artery will easily accommodate 6–8 ml/s but appreciably less will be needed when the vessel is occluded following trauma. It is easier and safer to undertake arteriography in the conscious patient, but the limiting factor has been pain associated with the injection of contrast medium. The newer lower osmolality

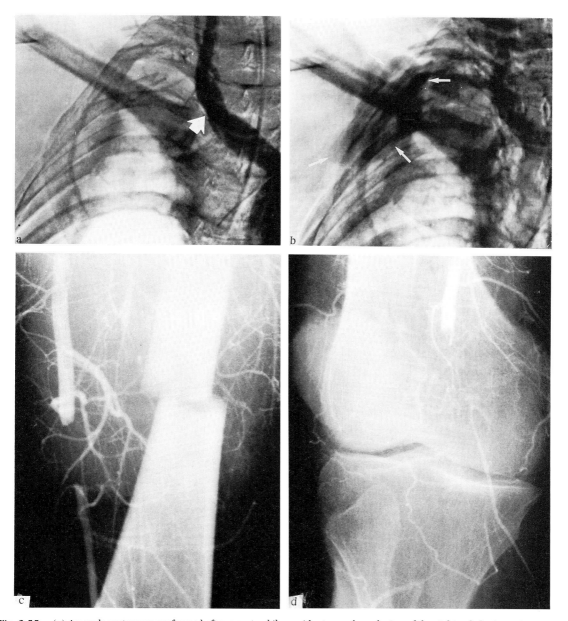

Fig. 2.55. (a) An arch aortogram performed after a motor-bike accident reveals occlusion of the right subclavian artery at its origin. The carotid artery is normal. Note multiple rib fractures. (b) A delayed image demonstrates a large false aneurysm arising from the subclavian artery (arrows). Post-traumatic occlusion of the (c) femoral and (d) popliteal arteries, both due to intimal tears. Note collateral opacification of distal vessels.

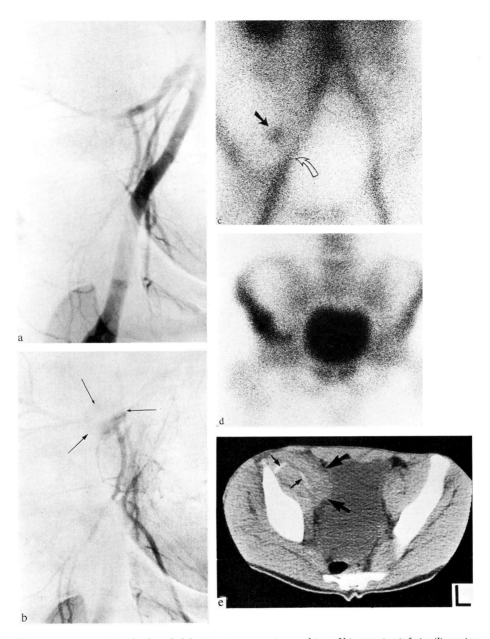

Fig. 2.56. This young man sustained a forced abduction injury causing avulsion of his anterior-inferior iliac spine. Because of persistent swelling and a falling haemoglobin a femoral arteriogram was performed. (b) On a delayed image a small false aneurysm arises from a branch of the internal iliac artery. (c) Extravasation is demonstrated on the blood pool phase of a bone scan. The extravasation (closed arrow) is in the same relationship to the iliac vessels (open arrow) as demonstrated by the angiogram. (d) The delayed phase of the bone scan shows increased activity related to the known avulsion injury. (e) A CT scan demonstrates a haematoma (large arrows) arising within the psoas which contains clot (small arrows).

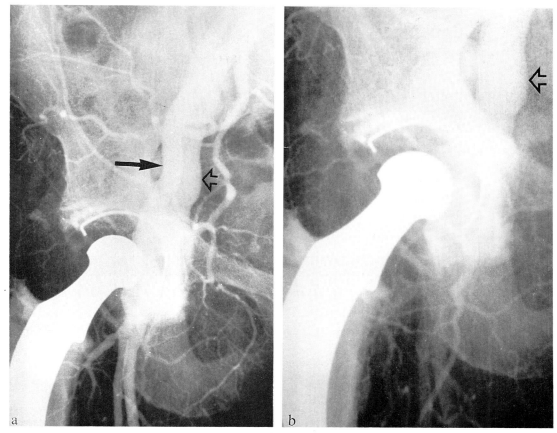

Fig. 2.57. (a) An acquired arteriovenous fistula following a Charnley arthroplasty. A femoral arteriogram demonstrates a normal external iliac artery (arrow) with early filling of the external iliac vein (open arrow). (b) A slightly later image shows extensive filling of the external iliac vein. The communication was between a branch of the profunda and the superficial femoral vein.

contrast media (metrizamide, iopamidol) are associated with considerably less discomfort, pain and flushing than the pre-existing high-osmolality agents. Although these contrast media are more expensive, they avoid the necessity of general anaesthetic and probably have less cardiovascular toxicity.

The complications of arteriography include haematoma, vessel occlusion, embolus proliferation and several other rare manifestations including dissection and arteriovenous fistula. Although significant complications are uncommon, arteriography should be undertaken only when there is a clear indication or a circumscribed objective. It is unreasonable to risk losing a limb for curiosity.

Trauma

Arteriography may be performed following injury in order to establish the degree and extent of vessel damage, for example subclavian transection or tears following motor-bike injury or femoropopliteal artery occlusion following lower limb fracture/dislocations (Fig. 2.55a–d). Some

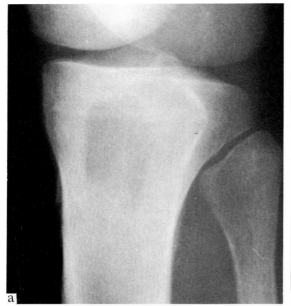

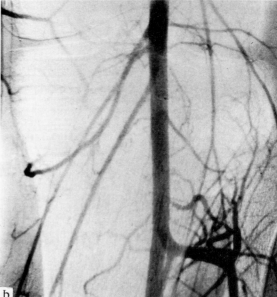

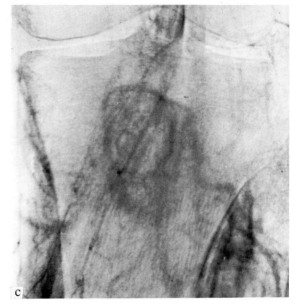

Fig. 2.58. (a) A Brodie's abcess in the proximal tibia. (b) A localized view from a popliteal arteriogram shows no abnormality of the arterial phase. (c) Delayed image shows an enhanced venous pattern with circumferential veins around the known Brodie's abcess and increased periosteal branches. This pattern of venous halo is typical of an infective bone lesion.

features on arteriography may predict the outcome of surgical reconstruction, the presence of filling defects from thrombus or intimal tears, the absence of collateral circulation, and slow drainage of contrast medium probably implying an adverse outcome. Also, a role for arteriography is rapidly developing in the manage-

ment of acute trauma, to demonstrate bleeding points (Fig. 2.56a–e) with subsequent embolization techniques to control them, particularly following pelvic fractures. This technique is highly successful, and may avoid surgery and stabilize an at-risk patient with multiple injuries.

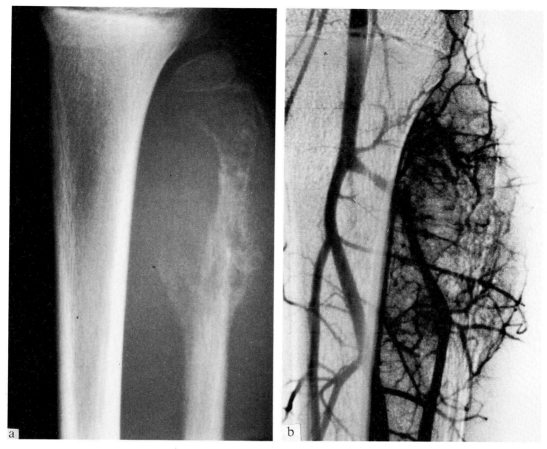

Fig. 2.59. (a) Ewing's sarcoma of the proximal fibula. (b) A femoral arteriogram shows a markedly abnormal vascular pattern. Note irregularities in calibre and size of many of the small arterial branches. Some are straight and encased, others tortuous and varying in calibre. Note also some isolated segments of abnormal vessels wandering apparently aimlessly. Note also a diffuse tumour blush.

Less commonly arteriography is necessary to assess the delayed results of an acute injury, or chronic trauma, as in the hypothenar hammer syndrome, or very rarely to demonstrate iatrogenic disease (Fig. 2.57a, b).

Neoplasm
Arteriography has three potential uses. Firstly, in the differential diagnosis of a mass lesion of bone or soft tissue. It is possible in most circumstances to distinguish between infective (Fig. 2.58a, b, c) and neoplastic conditions (Fig. 2.59a, b) on the basis of the vascular pattern, but the distinction between benign and malig-

nant is not possible if angiography is used in abstract. This is because no characteristic arteriographic feature of malignancy exists, nor does a tumour-specific angiographic pattern. Nonetheless the demonstration of encasement and pathological vessels (Fig. 2.59) is strong supportive evidence of a malignant tumour. It is more appropriate to use arteriography to distinguish between malignant tumours, for example chondroblastic osteosarcoma has a markedly abnormal vascular pattern, whereas a low-grade chondrosarcoma is essentially avascular. Arteriography may also offer prognostic information insofar as the degree of abnormal vascularity

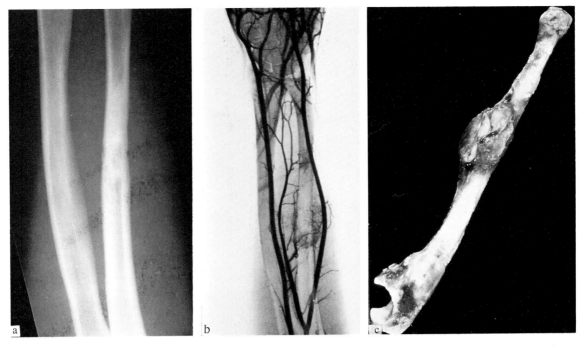

Fig. 2.60. (a) Osteosarcoma of the ulna is shown with endosteal sclerosis and bone destruction: the degree and extent of any soft tissue mass cannot be assessed. (b) A subclavian angiogram reveals an egg-sized soft-tissue mass related to the tumour. (c) This is confirmed at the excision biopsy.

may crudely reflect the aggressiveness of the tumour (for example fibrosarcoma and periosteal osteosarcoma).

The second use of arteriography is in the assessment of patients for therapy, particularly where prosthetic replacement is to be considered. Arteriography is superior to plain films in assessing both soft-tissue extensions (Fig. 2.60a, b, c) and intraosseous extension of tumour (Fig. 2.61a, b). It is probable that computerized tomography provides similar information on both soft-tissue and endosteal extent. However, it may be difficult to assess the relationship between the soft-tissue mass and great vessels on CT (Fig. 2.62a, b). It has also been suggested that bone scintigraphy offers equivalent information on the assessment of intraosseus extent of tumour, but recent evidence suggests that a bone scan overestimates tumour involvement with a larger area of photon abnormality, probably due to reactive hyperaemia (Fig. 2.63a–e). Nonetheless, the blood pool phase of a bone scan adequately demonstrates whether or not a tumour is vascular (Fig. 2.64). Arteriography has also been recommended for the selection of biopsy site, on the basis that the area of most abnormal circulation is likely to contain the most malignant features. Whilst this is undoubtedly so, it may be that the area of most tumour-specific histology is not in this region.

Thirdly, evidence is mounting to suggest that arteriography may be used in a therapeutic manner in the management of vascular benign tumours such as arteriovenous malformation, giant cell tumours and aneurysmal bone cysts. At this time the full potential and value of this technique has not been established.

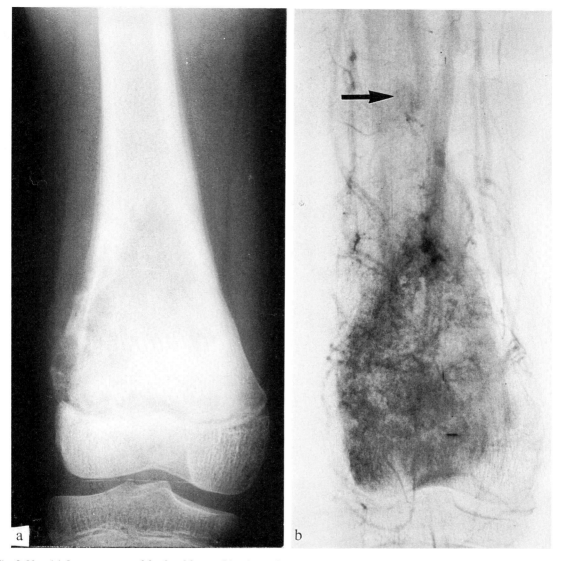

Fig. 2.61. (a) Oesteosarcoma of the distal femur. (b) A femoral arteriogram at the late stage demonstrates the intraosseous extent of the tumour. Note that the mass extends through the metaphysis to the articular surface and, in addition, a focus is shown more proximally (arrow) than may have been suspected from the plain film.

Other less frequent uses

Arteriography is the only means of demonstrating the size and extent of spinal angiomas and other arteriovenous malformations. Its use is, however, highly specialized and fraught with complications, including paraparesis.

The extent and severity of some rheumatological diseases such as scleroderma (Fig. 2.65) and other causes of Raynaud's phenomenon may be assessed using subclavian or brachial arteriography. The response of intra-arterial therapeutic agents such as reserpine or prostaglandin

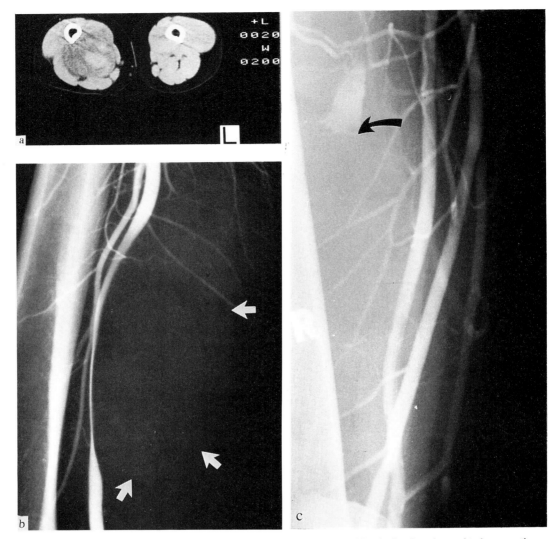

Fig. 2.62. (a) A CT demonstrates a fibrosarcoma arising in the medial aspect of the thigh. The relationship between the mass and the femoral vessels is not clear. (b) A femoral arteriogram demonstrates not only displacement of the superficial femoral artery but also obvious encasement indicating that the artery is enclosed within the tumour mass (arrows). (c) A venogram demonstrates occlusion of the superficial femoral vein within the mass lesion. Filling of the proximal part of the vein occurs by collateral circulation. The arteriogram and venogram demonstrate that both structures are encased within the tumour mass.

may be assessed also. Arteriography may be the only way of establishing a diagnosis in polyarteritis nodosa when typical small aneurysms in renal, hepatic and mesenteric arterial circulation may be demonstrated (Fig. 2.66).

Arteriography offers potential value in research to understand further such conditions as Perthes' disease and avascular necrosis of the hip in adults.

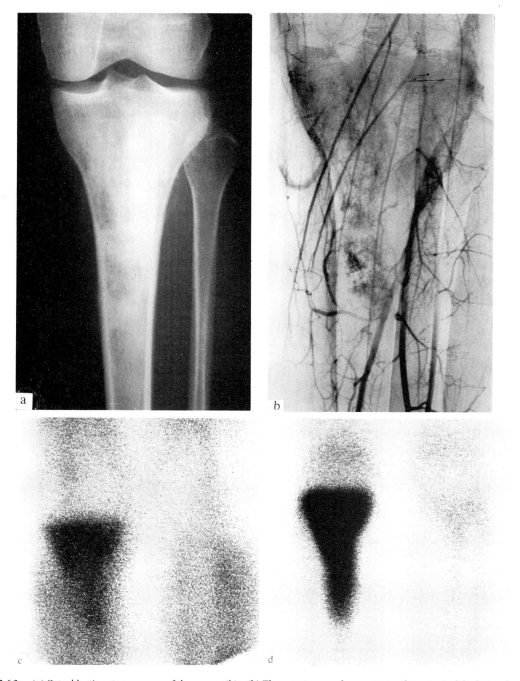

Fig. 2.63. (a) Osteoblastic osteosarcoma of the upper tibia. (b) The arteriogram demonstrates the extent of the lesion from the articular surface down to the mid-shaft. Note the abnormal vascular pattern. (c) The blood pool phase of a bone scan demonstrates much the same distribution of the tumour. (d) The size of mass lesion shown on the delayed phase is larger than on either of the previous studies. Increased activity is present also in the distal femur, probably representing disuse osteoporosis.

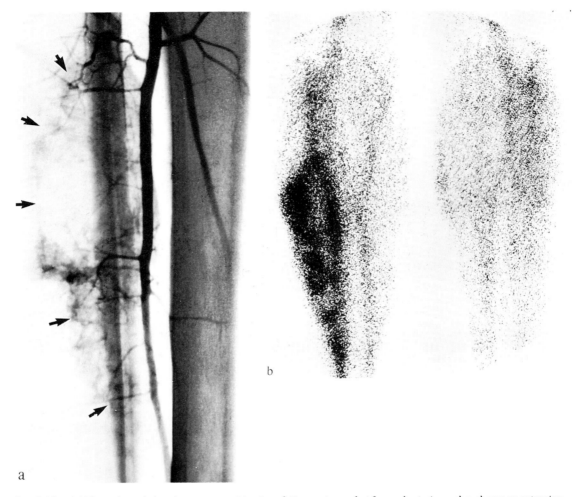

a

b

Fig. 2.64. (a) Mesenchymal chondrosarcoma arising in soft tissues, imaged at femoral arteriography, shows an extensive vascular mass (arrows). (b) The blood pool phase of a bone scan demonstrates increased activity over an area that is geographically very similar. Note that in the previous figure (2.63b, c) the blood pool phase of the bone scan mirrors the extent of abnormal vascularity not only in a bone tumour, but also, as in this case, in a soft-tissue tumour.

VENOGRAPHY

Venographic assessment of peripheral vessels is rarely required in orthopaedic practice. The most common indication is the distinction between deep venous thrombosis and joint rupture and the demonstration of deep venous thrombosis in patients with calf pain and/or pulmonary embolic disease. However, when a patient presents with calf pain and swelling and a history of joint effusion, or known knee arthropathy, it is undoubtedly preferable to perform initially a single-contrast knee arthrogram (Figs. 2.21, 2.22) or ultrasound of the popliteal fossa (Fig. 2.67), since the likely diagnosis is a popliteal cyst or joint rupture, rather than venous thrombosis. Leg venography has major disadvantages, including the potential induction of

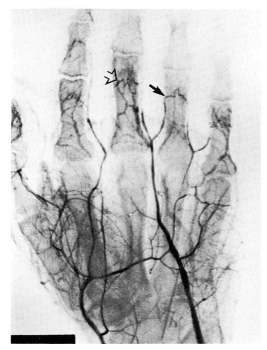

Fig. 2.65. A localized view of a brachial arteriogram in scleroderma. Note digital vessel occlusions (arrow) and anastomotic circulation between digital vessels (open arrow). Many areas of irregular calibre are present in the larger vessels.

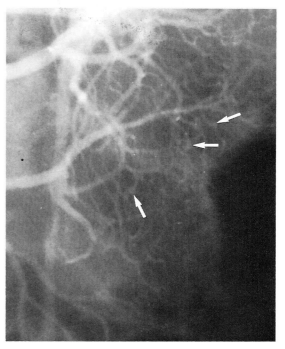

Fig. 2.66. Polyarteritis nodosa is diagnosed by the presence of small microaneurysms (arrows) in a mesenteric angiogram.

Fig. 2.67. An ultrasound scan along the posterior surface of the popliteal fossa demonstrates a transonic, liquid-filled, space-occupying lesion, subsequently confirmed to be a Baker's cyst by an arthrogram. (The patient's head is to the left, and the scale is in centimetres.) Courtesy of Dr F.G.M. Ross.

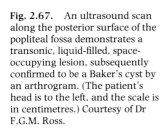
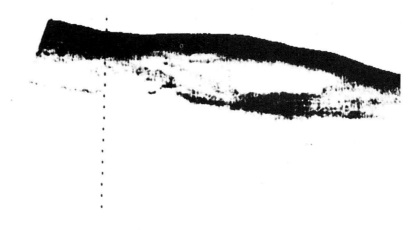

venous thrombosis by the irritant effect of the contrast medium itself. Thrombus may not be diagnosed, since totally occluded veins will not be opacified or thrombus may have formed and already dislodged into the pulmonary circulation before the study is undertaken and the venogram therefore is normal. Furthermore, the mere demonstration of thrombus does not mean that pulmonary emboli will occur. Nonetheless, leg venography is important in assessing the extent of venous thrombus, particularly craniad to the popliteal fossa, and in demonstrating its proximal extent into femoral or iliac vessels. It is possible that less invasive techniques such as isotope phlebography may provide equivalent information.

Leg venography is performed with the patient semi-erect on an X-ray table under fluoroscopic control. Having placed a tight tourniquet around the ankle a 22-gauge butterfly needle is placed in a dorsal vein of the foot, the most preferable being that adjacent to the medial aspect of the great toe MTP joint, since this drains directly into the deeper plantar arch. 50 ml of diluted contrast medium (140 mg/ml meglumine iothalamate, made by mixing 60% solution equally with saline) or similar concentrations of more expensive non-ionic agents such as metrizamide or iopamidol, are injected with fluoroscopic spot films. It is important to ensure that the proximal extent of venous thrombosis is demonstrated. It may be necessary to perform venography of the other leg in order to opacify the contralateral common iliac vein and hence show the ipsilateral level of obstruction. Very rarely, if the insertion of an inferior vena cava umbrella device is required, it may be necessary to perform intraosseous phlebography to demonstrate proximal extent. This is a painful, unpleasant procedure requiring general anaesthetic and should be reserved for exceptional circumstances.

On occasion, it will be necessary to undertake arm or leg phlebography in order to assess the extent of venous occlusion or damage to major veins as a result of previous injury prior to possible surgical reconstruction. It may be necessary also to establish the relationship between large veins and tumour masses prior to resection (Fig. 2.62c).

Tenography

Most tendon sheaths and their contents may be studied by direct needling with the injection of a positive contrast medium such as 60% meglumine iothalamate. In most instances the technique is performed in order to delineate a traumatic abnormality or to demonstrate the extent of rheumatological involvement. Naturally this is only undertaken where surgical intervention is to be influenced by its findings. The two most commonly performed are the flexor sheaths of the hand and the peroneal tendon sheath at the ankle.

Flexor tendon sheaths in the hand may be needled directly through the volar aspect of the fingers at the middle phalanx. A fine skin needle is inserted with local anaesthesia until the resistance of the periosteum is felt; a slight withdrawal and ease of injection usually indicates a satisfactory intrasheath position. This may be confirmed by injecting contrast medium under fluoroscopic control. The profunda and sublimis sheath is demonstrated and defects in, or disruptions of, the tendons are assessed. The extent of retraction and the site of the stumps may be of value in reconstruction. In addition, adhesions and tenovaginitis may be demonstrated. It may be argued, however, that since at reconstruction an incision is made at the old site of injury, and that the cut ends may be localized by manipulation of the fingers, tenography is an unnecessary study.

Abnormal findings at peroneal tenography have been suggested as the criterion for surgical repair of lateral ligament injury of the ankle, insofar as when the tear is sufficient to involve the peroneal sheath surgical reconstruction is necessary. An injection of contrast medium into the peroneal sheath is made under fluoroscopic control with a specific intention of demonstrating extravasation. There is no uniform view, however, as to whether or not surgical reconstruction of the lateral ligament of the ankle is superior to conservative management, and accordingly peroneal tenography has not received universal acclamation.

Other investigations

Although somewhat *passé* with the advent of scintigraphy and more modern investigations, sinography remains an extremely valuable technique in chronic osteomyelitis and in discharging wounds, particularly following removal of infected joint replacements. It is often easier to demonstrate sequestra by the passage of contrast medium into and around their location than to undertake tomography. Sinography is always easier with an adequate seal around the sinus tract. Preferably, a catheter should be introduced along the track. Occlusion of the ostium and an injection under a little pressure will result in superior images. Because the sinus is surrounded with the fibrous tissue and the technique is usually pain-free to the patient, the exact choice of water-soluble contrast medium is not critical.

On rare occasions numerous other techniques will be employed in the assessment of patients. Although investigations such as urethrography perhaps fall more within the province of genito-urinary surgeons, vascular studies of the brain the neurosurgeons, aortography to the thoracic surgeon (Fig. 2.68a, b), and lymphography to the radiotherapist, it is important that the orthopaedic surgeon remembers these techniques are available in the assessment of the whole patient (Fig. 2.69a, b).

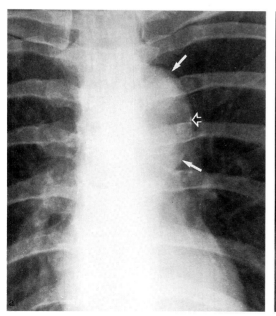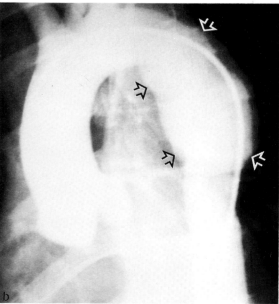

Fig. 2.68. (a) A localized view of the chest X-ray of a young woman some two years after a major road traffic accident. Note the abnormal configuration of the aortic arch (closed arrows) and the presence of calcification within the wall of the aorta (open arrow). These are the appearances of a post-traumatic aneurysm. This had been previously overlooked because attention was diverted to other significant orthopaedic lesions (this is the same patient as Fig. 2.25). (b) An arch aortogram demonstrates a post-traumatic false aneurysm (arrows).

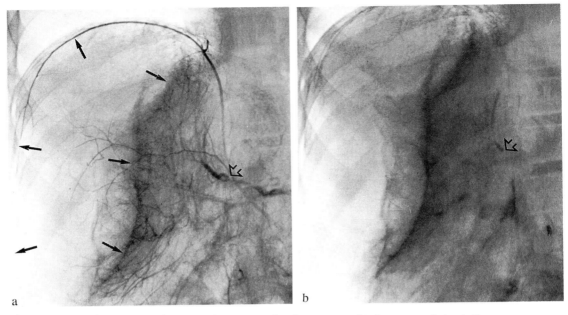

a   b

Fig. 2.69. (a) Another patient with commanding injuries elsewhere was noted to have a mass lesion in the upper abdomen and haemobilia. A mesenteric angiogram demonstrates a huge subcapsular haematoma (arrows) with partial transection of a branch of the left hepatic artery (open arrow). (b) On a slightly later image persistent filling occurs in the partially transected artery (open arrow).

Further reading

General

McCormick C. (1978) Radiology in low back pain and sciatica. An analysis of the relative efficacy of spinal venography, discography and epidurography in patients with a negative or equivocal myelogram. *Clin. Radiol.* **29**, 393–406.

Resnick O. & Niwayama G. (1981) *Diagnosis of Bone and Joint Disorders*. Section II, Radiography and related modalities in the evaluation of bone and joint disease, pp. 254–692. Philadelphia: W.B. Saunders Co.

Arthrography

Destouet J.M., Gilula L.A., Murphy W.A. & Monsees B. (1982) Lumbar facet joint injection: indication, technique, clinical correlation, preliminary results. *Radiology* **145**, 321–5.

Freiberger R.H. & Kay J.J. (1979) *Arthrography*. New York: Appleton–Century–Crofts.

Stoker D.J. (1980) *Knee Arthrography*. London: Chapman & Hall.

Epidural venography

Gargano S.P., Meyer J.S. & Sheldon J.J. (1974) Transfemoral ascending catheterization of the epidural veins in lumbar disk disease. *Radiology* **111**, 329–36.

Gershater R. & St Louis E.L. (1979) Lumbar epidural venography. *Radiology* **131**, 409–21.

Epidurography

Robertson G.H., Hatten H.T. jr & Hesselink J.H. (1979) Epidurography: selective catheter technique and review of 53 cases. *Amer. J. Roentgenol.* **132**, 787–93.

Discography and chemonucleolysis

McCulloch J.A. (1977) Chemonucleolysis. *J. Bone Jt Surg.* **59B**, 45–52.

McCulloch J.A. & Waddell G. (1978) Lateral lumbar discography. *Brit. J. Radiol.* **51**, 498–502.

Radiculography and myelography

Kieffer S.A., Binet E.F., Esquerra J.V., Hantman R.P. & Gross C.E. (1978) Contrast agents for myelography: clinical and radiological evaluation of Amipaque and Pantopaque. *Radiology* **129**, 695–703.

Skalpe I.O. & Amundsen P. (1975) Thoracic and cervical myelography with metrizamide. *Radiology* **116**, 101–6.

Chapter 3

Radionuclide Imaging of Bones and Joints
H. E. SCHÜTTE

Introduction

Despite the excellent resolution and fine shading of skeletal detail that radiography can provide, it has certain shortcomings that explain the continuing interest in other modes of diagnostic investigation of bone. For example, radiographs cannot distinguish differences in bone density before decreases in bone calcium of from 30% to 50% have occurred. Yet many diseases, in either their early or their advanced stages, involve changes of lesser magnitude. Regardless of the cause, there is a delay between the initial stimulus to destroy bone and its actual radiographic appearance. The duration of this latent period is variable, being dependent to a considerable extent on the structural characteristics of the bone being destroyed. In spongy bone of the pelvis, ribs or ends of long bones, large amounts of cancellous bone may be removed with little or no reflection of the change in the radiograph (Lodwick 1971). However, owing to the compactness of the cortex, minor alterations of the structure of cortical bone are easily discernible. The generalized loss of bone substance concurrent with ageing makes the detection of destructive changes more difficult in the elderly than in the young.

In less than 10 years, since the availability of $^{99}Tc^m$-labelled phosphate complexes, along with the advent of high-resolution, fast-imaging scintillation cameras, the evaluation of bone pathology has become revolutionary. There has been a search for better radiopharmaceuticals and imaging devices, and as the research has progressed, using a variety of different bone-

seeking radiopharmaceuticals, cumulative data have indicated that bone scans are more sensitive, but less specific, than skeletal surveys for the detection of bone disease (Mall et al. 1976, Pistenma et al. 1975, Schaffer & Pendergrass 1976, Citrin et al. 1977). A hypothetical relationship between the quality of a bone-scan image and the quality or visibility of radiographic images may be useful for the interpretation of bone scintigrams. This so-called 'evolutionary pattern', which according to Charkes (1977) accounts for over 90% of the focal lesions with reactive bone formation, can be described in terms of three phases. In the first phase the scan is abnormal (positive) but insufficient calcium has been deposited in the new bone to be detected radiographically. In the second phase the scan becomes very hot and the densities can also be seen by radiography. In the third phase the scan returns to normal (false-negative) and the radiographs become dense.

Radiopharmaceuticals used for evaluation of the skeleton

A large number of elements to some extent localize within the skeleton. The most important of these are the alkaline earths, the halogens, and the phosphate complexes. Alkaline earths include analogues of calcium, such as beryllium, magnesium, strontium, barium and radium. The factors which influence the suitability of a particular radiotracer are both biological and physical. Although radiotracers such as ^{45}Ca or ^{32}P ions may exchange for components in the hydroxyapatite and can be a measurement of changes in regional bone blood flow and new bone formation, both radionuclides decay by beta-decay, emitting beta-particles only. Therefore, the dose which can be administered to human beings for diagnostic purposes is limited.

^{85}Sr served as the routine bone-scanning agent of the 1960s, but its long physical and biological half-lives result in an unacceptably high radiation exposure to the patient (Table 3.1). $^{87}Sr^m$, also used in the past, has a much more favourable dosimetry than does ^{85}Sr, but it yields images in which the skeletal detail is obscured by high background activity. ^{18}F, a halogen capable of substituting for hydroxyl groups in the hydroxyapatite structure of bone, was introduced in the early 1970s. Despite difficulties (^{18}F can only be supplied to centres within a few hours from cyclotrons and reactor facilities), the superiority of this agent compared to ^{85}Sr and $^{87}Sr^m$, with its short half-life and energetic gamma photons, led to increasing utilization (Shirazi et al. 1974). If the $^{99}Tc^m$-labelled phosphate complexes had not been introduced in 1971 and established new standards for scintigraphic imaging of the skeleton, ^{18}F would have remained the agent of choice for radionuclide bone studies.

$^{99}Tc^m$ is an excellent radionuclide for diagnostic imaging. It decays by isomeric transition, emitting a 140 keV gamma photon, which is reasonably energetic, with a tissue half-value layer of 4 cm and there is virtually no loss in counting efficiency in sodium iodide crystals with thicknesses of 2 to $\frac{1}{2}$ inch. It can be prepared from a ^{99}Mo generator, which has physical half-life of 2.7 days and a week of useful shelf-life.

$^{99}Tc^m$ has a half-life of 6.6 hours and a favourable biological behaviour, resulting in high-quality images of the skeleton at low radiation exposures to the patient (Subramanian et al. 1975). However, as a radionuclide it has no specificity for bone by itself, and to acquire organ specificity $^{99}Tc^m$ must be linked to a specially designed carrier molecule whose biodistribution favours localization of the radioactive complex in any given organ. For example, $^{99}Tc^m$ linked to DTPA (diethylenetriaminepenta-acetic acid) will pass through the kidney like inulin, and subsequently demonstrate the kidney's function. When linked to macroaggregated albumin, it will lodge in the capillary beds of the lungs and demonstrate infarcted areas. Linked to sulphur colloid, $^{99}Tc^m$ will be phagocytosed by the reticuloendothelial cells of the liver, spleen and bone marrow. Localization in the skeleton is obtained through linkage to a phosphate complex.

THE $^9Tc^m$ PHOSPHATE COMPLEXES

The $^{99}Tc^m$ phosphate complexes are condensed phosphates or phosphonates. Phosphonates are the organic analogues of the condensed (inorganic) phosphates, containing a P–C–P rather

Table 3.1. Characteristics of suitable bone-seeking agents for scintigraphic bone studies.

Radionuclide	Half-life	Photon energy (keV)	Mean beta energy (keV)	Administered dose (mCi)	Estimated radiation dose (rad/mCi)	
					Skeleton	Red marrow
Strontium-85	64 days	514	0.014	0.1	31	11
Strontium-87m	2.8 h	388	0.082	1–5	0.15	0.5
Fluorine-18	1.9 h	511	0.28	2–5	0.18	0.4
Barium-135m	27.7 h	268	0.25	5–10	1.3	0.3
Dysprosium-157	8.0 h	326	0.02	10	0.1	0.05
Technetium-99m complexes	6 h	140	0.014	10–20	0.04	0.03

1 rad/mCi = 0.27 Gy/GBq; 1 mCi = 37 MBq

than a P–O–P linkage (i.e. the P–O–P bond of pyrophosphate and the larger chained polyphosphates; the P–C–P bond of the diphosphonates with the strong non-hydrolysable structure; and recently also the P–N–P bond of the imidodiphosphonates). Polyphosphate and pyrophosphate possess a P–O–P bond which is susceptible to enzyme degradation, compared to the non-hydrolysable diphosphonates and perhaps also the imidodiphosphonates. The degradation of pyrophosphate to shorter phosphate linkages has been documented by *in-vitro* studies, and if it does occur *in vivo* it does not seem to affect bone image quality in patients with elevated alkaline or acid phosphatase. Since diphosphonates are resistant to enzyme hydrolysis they have been used therapeutically in conditions such as Paget's disease. Recently, methylene diphosphonate (MDP) has become the tracer of choice in many institutions because of its higher skeletal uptake and faster blood clearance (Rosenthall *et al.* 1977, Fogelman *et al.* 1979a and Rudd *et al.* 1979). Studies with 24-hour whole-body retention, however, illustrate that alterations in diphosphonate molecular structure have significant effects upon specificity for bone. Different diphosphonates might be necessary for the best use in the assessment of metastatic bone disease or diffuse metabolic processes, as described by Fogelman *et al.* (1981) in normal persons. Evaluation of new bone agents should also include biodistribution studies, indicating their relative concentration in bone lesions compared to normal bone. In doing so, Subramanian *et al.* (1981) concluded that MDP is still the agent of choice for bone imaging at present time but data on the use of the recently developed $^{99}Tc^m$HDP suggest improvement of scintigraphic image quality compared to MDP (Arnt *et al.* 1985).

$^{99}Tc^m$-LABELLED SULPHUR OR ANTIMONY COLLOIDS IN BONE MARROW IMAGING

Radionuclide evaluation of bone marrow is possible with $^{99}Tc^m$-labelled sulphur or antimony colloid. The colloid particles are removed rapidly from the blood by the phagocytic cells of the reticuloendothelial system. In routine liver/spleen imaging, little activity may be seen in the bone marrow, however the relatively low quantities of tracer in the bone marrow can be demonstrated successfully by increasing exposure time and intensity of the display (Knisely 1972, Kirchner *et al.* 1981). The colloid particles of $^{99}Tc^m$–antimony colloid are much smaller than those of $^{99}Tc^m$–sulphur colloid, and Martindale *et al.* (1980) believe this might produce better marrow uptake of antimony colloids. Agents also used for bone marrow imaging are $^{111}InCl$ and ^{52}Fe (Merrick *et al.* 1975). In young children a large amount of activity is seen to be distributed along the entire length of long bones, extending into carpal and tarsal bones and phalanges. As children grow older, there is less marrow in the peripheral bones and marrow images show progressively less peripheral activity, until after the age of 20 years when an adult pattern can be observed, in which most of the radiolabelled colloid is restricted to the axial skeleton. There is, as a result of the physiological decrease of bone marrow in advancing age, a limit for the use of bone marrow imaging for avascular processes in patients of older age.

Areas where the marrow has been replaced or destroyed, for example metastases, primary tumours and bone marrow necrosis, show regionally diminished activity—'cold areas'. In contrast, cases of haemolysis, chronic blood loss and destruction of axial bone by tumour, fibrosis, etc. all promote peripheral extension of bone marrow activity, revealing pattern localizations resembling those of childhood; the only exception is that the growth plate is not seen.

GALLIUM-67

^{67}Ga is a cyclotron-produced radiopharmaceutical available as a sodium citrate complex. It did not really have clinical applications until its accumulation in lymphomatous tissue was noticed in 1969. Over the next 10 years a considerable amount of work was published on the clinical use of gallium for the localization of epithelial and lymphoreticular tumours and in the detection of acute abscesses. (Hayes 1978). It is only recently that ^{67}Ga has been used in the evaluation of skeletal disorders. (Hoffer 1980a, Taillefer *et al.* 1981, Gates 1979, Waman *et al.* 1981). It has helped in the assessment of primary tumours, osteomyelitis, eosinophilic granuloma and myeloma, all disorders known to have false-negative scans with ^{99}Tc^m phosphate complex scintigraphy.

The administered dose of ^{67}Ga ranges from 50 to 130 microcuries per kg of body weight. Almost all of this intravenous injected gallium binds to transferrin. Approximately one-third of the administered gallium is excreted by kidney and bowel in equal proportions, the bulk remaining in the liver, the skeleton and the soft tissues. The whole-body biological half-life is estimated at 20 days. Estimates of absorbed radiation dose per millicurie of administered gallium are: 0·26 rad for whole body and gonads; 0·40–0·60 rad for the bone, bone marrow and liver; and 0·90–2·00 rad for the colon. In normal tissues and in tumour the subcellular sites of localization include lysosomes and microvesicles made up of endoplasmic reticulum. In inflammatory lesions and abscesses, the localization depends to a great extent on uptake by leucocytes, but the real mechanism is not yet well understood. Accumulation of gallium in tumours is nearly complete within two hours of injection, however the very high soft-tissue background activity in bowel, liver and skeleton permits reliable images 48–72 hours after tracer administration. Interpretation of the gallium scans is advisable in combination with radiographs and other bone studies that assist in defining anatomical detail.

Mechanisms of skeletal tracer uptake

There are possibly three compartments in bone which make up the sites of radiotracer uptake. These are: the surface of bone crystals; organic components such as enzyme systems; and immature collagen. Without adequate blood supply however, no deposition would occur. Charkes (1980) has pointed out that increased blood flow through normal vessels does not proportionally add to increased tracer uptake in pathological sites. Thus the concept of 'diffusion-limited flow' has been introduced to explain the eventual fate of the tracer as it enters the extracellular space which surrounds the osteoid surface (McCarthy & Hughes 1983). Transfer to bone, however, is a slow process, controlled by diffusion laws (Hughes *et al.* 1977). In abnormal circumstances, such as fracture, infection or tumour, loss of neurogenic control may cause a hyperaemic effect by opening up normally closed capillaries by the process of 'recruitment' (Hughes *et al.* 1979).

Enzymatic systems, such as alkaline and acid phosphatase, may have a part in tracer localization. Where osteoblasts are found in abundance, active calcification and remodelling is occurring, often associated with a rise in alkaline phosphatase level. The role of immature collagen as a site for binding of radiotracers is unclear, and Sy (1981) finds it more reasonable to suggest that the surface of hydroxyapatite crystals, which is suitable for physiological processes such as chemosorbtion, is the most likely site for interactions in response to hormonal, vascular and other changes in the body. The bone crystals are slowly transformed from initial deposition of calcium and phosphate as amorphous compounds to resultant hydroxyapatite crystals. Ions, such as sodium, potassium, magnesium and carbonates, may either be absorbed in the hydration shell, or become incorporated in the crystal lattice itself. Each crystal is surrounded by a layer of hydrated ions, consisting of calcium, phosphate, hydroxyl ions and a shell of water. This layer of ions is the site of active ion interchange, while diffusion takes place between the crystal shell and the extracellular fluid. The total water content varies with age. In growing bones, water content makes up 60% of the weight, while in senile cortical bone it drops to 10%. Newly formed bone crystals are well hydrated, rather imperfect and less stable, because of the readily interchangeable ion particles. In contrast, mature crystals are less hydrated. Shell hydration is essential for diffusion to occur, and this is very likely why bone scans of the elderly lack tracer activity (Thrall *et al.* 1974, Wilson 1981, Fogelman & Bessent 1982). Another factor in relation to the relative activity concentration in normal and abnormal conditions might be the manner in which hydroxyapatite crystals are packed together. For this reason, perhaps, scans feature more tracer in trabecular and cancellous bone than in cortical bone, implementing the need for radiographic correlation.

Against this background, Sy (1981) has examined the degree of bone uptake in certain types of bone disease. In osteoporosis, there is a reduced number of crystals, which lie further apart, because the quantity of matrix is proportionally less. The crystal shell is poorly hydrated, and the internal apatite may be denser, thus resulting in less ion displacement, limited diffusion and subsequently poor activity on bone scan. In osteomalacia, there is an abundance of matrix, but this is defective and mineralizes with difficulty. The crystals, fewer in number, have a well-hydrated water shell and normal internal apatite, permitting chemosorbtion to take place. However, in severe osteomalacia, where there are few crystals, tracer deposition may be so low that overall tracer activity on the scan is not abnormally elevated. Osteitis fibrosa, whether in primary or secondary hyperparathyroidism, results from stimulation of all bone cells in response to a rise in parathormone level. Crystals are loosened, and although the shell remains well hydrated ions are easily displaceable. Some degree of remodelling occurs because of osteoblastic activity. These factors contribute to increased activity seen on the bone scan. In osteosclerosis, on the other hand, there is overmineralization, with an increased number of crystals but normal physical and chemical properties, and these factors contribute to the intense activity seen on bone scan.

In routine skeletal imaging, the injected $^{99}Tc^m$ phosphate complexes rapidly distribute throughout the extracellular fluid. Skeletal uptake of the tracer proceeds with an accumulation half-time of 15–30 minutes. Within two hours skeletal uptake is almost 50% of the administered dose (Krishnamurthy *et al.* 1976). Scanning, however, is postponed until two or four hours after tracer administration, in order to allow most of the tracer not localized in bone to be excreted in the urine, thus resulting in better images of the skeleton.

EXTRAOSSEOUS LOCALIZATIONS OF BONE TRACERS

The $^{99}Tc^m$-labelled phosphate complexes are excreted in the urine and the bowel, and some free technetium may circulate as pertechnetate ions and be excreted by gastric mucosa, the thyroid and the salivary glands. Extraskeletal sites of normal localization may subsequently include kidney, bladder, nasopharynx, breasts, etc. Incidental findings of pathological conditions of the kidneys and the bladder on bone scan have frequently been described (Maher 1975, Shah *et al.* 1981). Accumulation of tracer in breast tissue was suggested by some to be of value in the differential diagnosis of breast masses, but McDougall and Pistenma (1974) have shown that this is not the case. These bone-seeking agents may also accumulate in brain masses (Grames *et al.* 1975) and have a well-known application in the evaluation of myocardial infarction. Other pathological processes that feature focal accumulation of these agents, without radiographically evident calcifications, include inflammatory disease of muscle, healing wounds, injection sites, and malignant soft-tissue neoplasms (Ghaed *et al.* 1974, Johnson & Garvic 1980). Conditions with evident soft-tissue calcifications, such as osteosarcoma metastases to the lung, myositis ossificans, dermatomyositis, scleroderma, and diffuse intestinal pulmonary calcifications, have been reported to produce positive bone scans (Choy

& Murray 1980). Many of these sites have been the cause of problems and pitfalls in scan interpretation (Thrall *et al.* 1974).

Scintigraphic lesions observed on bone scan may show photon excess or 'hot' spots, or be photon-deficient or 'cold' spots. The mechanism of the latter is dependent on the inability of the radiotracer to be delivered to the abnormal site as a result of infarction or vascular occlusion, as in tumour or sickle cell disease. Factors that influence the detection of a photon-deficient lesion are the size of the lesion and the ability of the surrounding tissue to react on a given stimulus, and the age of the lesion at the time of the bone scan. Lytic lesions larger than 2 cm on radiographs, and without any repair manifestation, will appear as photon-deficient. Cold lesions adjacent to normal areas are usually readily apparent on the bone scan (Fig. 3.1). The indolent course of bone metastases from thyroid carcinoma, with a characteristically low rate of mineral turnover, is probably mainly responsible for the low sensitivity of bone scans in detecting skeletal involvement in these cases. Skeletal metastases from lung carcinoma and also renal carcinoma are known to be very aggressive—the bone destruction may proceed so rapidly that new bone is not yet formed when the scan is made. According to Kober *et al.* (1979) photon-deficient lesions are observed in 2·3% of all pathological bone scans. They may produce false-negative scans if the 'cold' spot is not recognized on the scan. If this possibility is suspected, the nuclear specialist may order a radiographic skeletal survey, in order to evaluate other possible photon-deficient foci of the skeleton, increasing the detection of lesions.

The degree of radionuclide uptake in bone reflects the current metabolic state of abnormal skeletal areas. In the evolution of healing lesions, such as fractures, or regression of malignant lesions after therapy, an uptake mechanism may be seen with a variable pattern of radionuclide, reflecting dynamic changes in the bone (Pabst *et al.* 1981). Subsequently one-third of all bone lesions may show some degree of photon deficiency, emphasizing the importance of serial examination for accurate interpretation of the current state. Photon-deficient areas

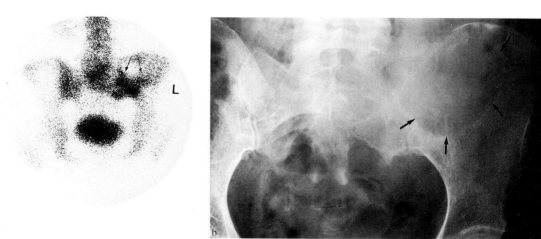

a

b

Fig. 3.1. (a) A lytic lesion (arrows) with sharp irregular border is seen in the left iliac wing, with minor sclerosis along the caudal sacroiliac joint. (b) A giant cell tumour, grade 2, was diagnosed on biopsy. On bone scan the lytic lesion is photon-deficient, but readily seen as a result of the activity in the rest of the iliac bone (arrows); obviously there is more new bone formation than expected on radiography.

may also represent artefacts (pacemakers, pocket content, etc.), post-operative deformities, and anatomical anomalies (Sy *et al.* 1975, Spencer *et al.* 1981, Tessler *et al.* 1981).

The standard bone scan consists of static images of the skeleton in both anterior and posterior projections, usually three hours after injection of the radionuclide. Because a number of disease processes may produce similar or identical images, with augmented or diminished uptake, it is often difficult to make a specific diagnosis on the basis of the static study alone. In 1975 Gilday *et al.*, and in 1976 Majd and Frankel, combined 'blood pool' and static bone images to differentiate osteomyelitis from septic arthritis and cellulitis in children. The static blood pool image was obtained immediately after injection of radiotracer and compared to the static bone image. This new acquisition was considered helpful in some cases.

Recently, flow studies have been introduced, and the static three-hour bone scan, together with the static blood pool scan and the immediate post-injection dynamic flow curve (radionuclide angiogram), is called 'three-phase scintigraphy'. This technique appears to augment the specificity of skeletal scintigraphy in patients with suspected osteomyelitis (Maurer *et al.* 1981) and to be useful in patients with reflex sympathetic dystrophy, diabetes, Legg–Perthes disease and inflammatory joint disease (Park *et al.* 1982).

The procedure is simple, the dosage of the radiotracer and the amount of radiation being similar to the conventional static bone scan. According to Maurer *et al.* (1981), three-phase images of osteomyelitis show increased blood flow, together with intense hyperaemia in the late radionuclide scan and blood pool images. Non-infectious skeletal disease is diagnosed if there is focal or diffuse abnormal skeletal uptake ranging from minimal to moderate in intensity. In soft-tissue disease the abnormal tracer uptake is seen outside bone, and septic arthritis, without associated osteomyelitis, shows symmetrical and moderate increased activity in the juxta-articular bone on both sides of the joint (Fig. 3.2).

Instrumentation

The instrument mostly used for imaging skeletal distribution of radionuclides is the scintillation or gamma camera, to which a scanning mode for displaying the whole-body distribution of the radionuclides may be added. These cameras detect the distribution of the radiopharmaceutical, by externally recording the interactions of gamma rays emitted from the body, usually with a 12-mm thick sodium iodide crystal in the camera head. The detection system involves an array of photomultiplier tubes, ranging in number from 37 to 61 in current models, which process the recorded gamma rays in the sodium iodide crystal such that each gamma ray interaction of the appropriate energy level is displayed on an XY axis, corresponding in position to its origin in the body. The resulting image may be recorded on Polaroid film, with activity displayed as a white dot, or on X-ray film, with activity displayed as black dots. With the scanning mode, the camera passes slowly over the entire body to produce a single whole-body image. The information content of this image may be limited, and individual gamma camera images (spot views) may need supplementing. The whole imaging procedure takes roughly 45 minutes. By using pinhole or converging collimators, magnification views can be generated, sometimes needed in the evaluation of small avascular areas. This magnification is not absolutely required because of improving gamma camera resolution. Recently, tomographic imaging instruments displaying multiple planes of selective activity of the body have been developed. The trend in instrumentation in nuclear medicine is probably returning to the analysis of body functions and metabolism

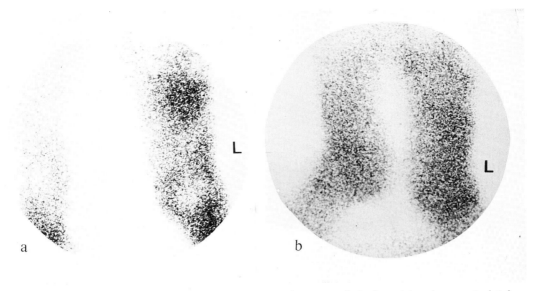

Fig. 3.2. A case of cellulitis. The blood pool image (a) shows increased tracer uptake in the metatarsal area, not related to osseous structures. On the delayed $^{99}Tc^m$ MDP scan (b) this area is normal, apart from some hyperaemia in the tarsal region.

(Budinger 1977). For detailed information on gamma camera criteria, such as sensitivity, spatial resolution, saturation performance, dead time and uniformity of resolution, see *Seminars in Nuclear Medicine*, special edition on imaging instrumentation (1977). The number of photomultipliers should not be less than 37, but the number available is not as important as the image performance of the device. Therefore spatial resolution and sensitivity should be carefully checked in order to obtain good uniformity features (Rollo 1981).

Evaluation and interpretation of bone images

To make the best use of radionuclide studies, in both the performance and the interpretation, it is necessary to have frequent consultations between the nuclear medicine staff and the referring physicians. There are various factors that may influence the quality of radionuclide bone imaging. Some are related to the patient and some are technical. When scanning is done too early after the administration of the radiotracer and the patient is not well hydrated and has not voided urine the scintigram will show too high a circulating activity. In contrast, when the study is obtained too late after tracer administration, the quality is changed accordingly by the reduced photons. When the $^{99}Tc^m$ tagging is not optimal, too many free pertechnetate ions will circulate and be found in the stomach, thyroid and salivary glands, resulting in superimposing of activities and pitfalls. Technical factors that affect image quality are reflected by the skeletal activity and the background activity ratio. Metallic or other artefacts worn by the patients during the study may absorb photons and produce photon-deficient areas, and these should be identified in time.

Patient-related factors: In renal failure, since the radiotracer is excreted by the kidneys, too much circulating activity will be present. In obese patients, the abnormal sites may be far too distant from the sodium iodide crystal to obtain adequate images and thus become a source of false-negatives. The age of the patient is important and the best detailed image is

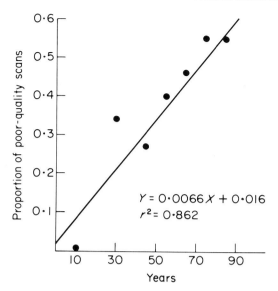

Fig. 3.3. The effect of age on the quality of bone scans. The graph shows the number of poor-quality scans plotted against age groups of patients. The linear relationship between age and the quality of images is expressed by the formula $0.0066 \times$ age $+ 0.0016$; where 0.0066 is the slope of the regression line and 0.016 a constant. From Wilson (1981) with permission.

obtained in young people, whilst in the elderly radiation activity is diffusely diminished according to the metabolic state of the skeleton. Wilson (1981) examined the effect of age on the quality of bone scans and was able to divide scan quality into five categories of image appearance. Using spine (vertebra and lumbar pedicles), soft tissue, ribs and thoracic pedicles and appendices as parameters, he found a linear relationship between age and the quality of images (Fig. 3.3). This relationship is thought to be important in determining normality in a particular age group, and should assist in the detection of skeletal involvement in diffuse metabolic or neoplastic disease.

FALSE-POSITIVE AND FALSE-NEGATIVE
SCAN RESULTS

Muroff (1981) states that an appreciation of the physiology of bone scanning agents, together with thorough clinical history and an examination of the patient, will decrease the uncertainties of bone scan interpretation. He has concluded: 'there are no false-positive scans, only inaccurate explanations for the findings'. Some of the *sources for false-positive* scans, e.g. the extraosseous activity in glands, intestines, etc., have already been discussed. There are, however, some normal anatomical variations which must be recognized if false-positive interpretation is to be avoided (Thrall *et al.* 1974, Döge *et al.* 1977, Harbert & Desai 1985). Certain parts of the skull, especially the base, when viewed tangentially may simulate pathological hotspots. For this reason suspected skull lesions must always be demonstrated '*en face*'. Three sites of shoulder uptake are usually seen, corresponding to ossification centres of the humerus, coracoid process and acromioclavicular joint. The deltoid tuberosity in the proximal third of the humerus may sometimes show increased uptake in some normal cases (Fink-Bennett & Vicuna-Rios 1980) and sometimes left- or right-handedness and excessive weight-bearing on knees show slight increased tracer uptake, which might cause diagnostic uncertainty.

Ossification centres of the sternum can, on occasion, simulate metastatic deposits. Extraskeletal uptake of radiotracer will faintly outline the heart pool, liver, kidneys and bladder, and assessment of these organs should be a part of every scan evaluation. Possible artefacts should be removed prior to scanning, especially those surface objects which attenuate activity. Also, sources of contamination, such as tracer spill, and urine, saliva, etc. containing radionuclide tracer, should be sought when there is inappropriate activity not corresponding to skeletal structures. Sometimes special supplementary views are needed to separate the superimposition of different foci of activity. Uptake increase on an anterior scan of the lower neck could be due to metastasis or cervical degenerative disease, but more often represents an artefact due to positioning related to spinal lordosis and superimposition of spine and mandible (Oppenheim & Cantez 1977). A small amount of tracer invariably extravasates at the injection site, and care should therefore be taken not to administer the radiotracer near areas of suspected abnormalities. It may be quite difficult to differentiate increased activity in solitary malignant lesions from degenerative disorders. Usually, malignant lesions are hyperaemic and therefore relatively 'hotter'. Radiographic correlation of these sites is often needed for accurate interpretation.

False-negative scans frequently result from the presence of lytic lesions or foci with little or no reparative bone formation, producing so-called photon-deficient or 'cold' lesions. Multiple myeloma is notorious in this respect, and the false-negative rate may be as high as 20–27% (Wahner *et al.* 1980, Woolfenden *et al.* 1980). When multiple myeloma is excluded, the false-negative rate is approximately 3%, and in these cases other means of diagnostic imaging are necessary to rule out skeletal disease. Bone pain should alert the clinician to the possibility of the need for radiographic correlation, when the bone scan is equivocal. (Schütte 1979).

Frankel *et al.* (1974a) observed that symmetrical skeletal involvement sometimes produced false-negative scans. In these cases bone accretion is so rapid that renal excretion becomes negative, thus producing 'superscans'. It is important to recognize the absence of kidney visualization, because superscans, by their diffuse tracer uptake, may be erroneously interpreted as normal. The linear relationship between age and image quality (Wilson 1981) is also helpful in differentiating superscans from normal scans. In patients with acute renal failure, increased soft-tissue accumulation is obvious.

LOCALIZATION AND PATTERN
RECOGNITION IN DECISION-MAKING

Since abnormalities on bone scan lack specificity, radiograms should be made of those areas which appear abnormal on scintigraphy. Localization and certain patterns of abnormalities can, however, sometimes confer some specificity. Slightly increased uptake along joint interfaces almost always reflects arthritic disorders. Metacarpophalangeal and proximal interphalangeal joints are the joints most frequently involved in rheumatoid arthritis, followed by metatarsophalangeal joints, the wrist, knees, shoulders, hips, elbows and cervical spine. Multiple focal areas of increased uptake in these areas may be a more sensitive indicator of the extent of joint involvement in early rheumatoid arthritis (Fig. 3.4). Less increased uptake in the first carpophalangeal joint may be suggestive of degenerative osteoarthritis. Blurring of the growth plates into the metaphyseal areas may represent neuroblastoma metastases in children (Murray 1980).

In patients with advanced cancer, a multifocal pattern in skull, pelvis, scapulae and long-bone diaphysis has a greater probability of representing metastatic disease compared to those in whom there is only clinical suspicion of cancer, and without clinical evidence of metastasis. According to Corcoran *et al.* (1976), 36% of the solitary lesions in cancer and noncancer patients are benign and degenerative.

The prevalence for certain parts of the body is different for malignant and non-malignant lesions, e.g. there is a 50% chance that a solitary lesion in the skull is a metastasis, whereas in the axial skeleton 80% of the solitary lesions might be malignant. In ribs this percentage is reversed, most focal bone lesions being fractures (Fogelman *et al.* 1977, Singh *et al.* 1977, Tumeh *et al.* 1985). In the extremities a solitary lesion is caused by fractures or other benign conditions in 40% of the cases.

Nearly 80% of all metastases are in the axial skeleton, 28% in the ribs and sternum, 39% in the vertebrae, 12% in the pelvis and only 10% in the skull and another 10% in the long bones (Krishnamurthy *et al.* 1977). The localization of solitary and multiple lesions in cancer and non-cancer patients is, however, not constant within each population. Rib fractures and osteoporotic vertebral compression fractures are more prevalent in older women, compared to

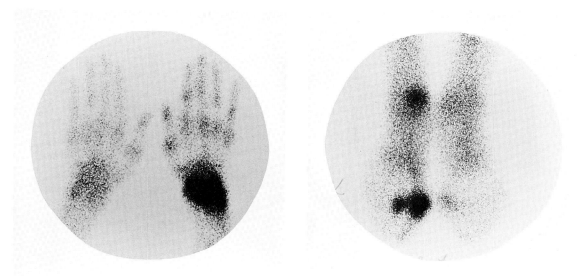

Fig. 3.4. Early rheumatoid arthritic sites are demonstrated by $^{99}Tc^m$ MDP scanning in this 34-year-old male, with normal radiographs, but with diffuse arthropathy and elevated serology.

men, and this further complicates the interpretation of bone scans in the assessment of metastatic disease in these patients. Metastases from primary tumours, such as breast and prostate, tend to spread by way of the vertebral venous plexus, and consequently are predominantly encountered in the axial skeleton, whereas metastases from lung and thyroid cancer generally enter the arterial circulation and may be encountered equally in the axial skeleton and the long bones. Knowledge of the clinical history is essential to interpret these scintigraphic images.

In general one may consider solitary and multiple scan lesions as follows:

1 It is highly probable that solitary lesions in the axial skeleton and in the long bones are of metastatic origin (venous and/or arterial spread).

2 Solitary lesions in ribs are likely to be fractures.

3 Multiple lesions in the long bones and the axial skeleton have a greater specificity for metastases (Fig. 3.5).

4 Multiple lesions in ribs alone are most likely caused by rib fractures, especially when they demonstrate a symmetrical, linear or circular pattern (Fig. 3.6).

Bone scan appearances in *metabolic bone disorders* have been recognized by Sy and Mittal (1975), Singh *et al.* (1977) and Fogelman *et al.*

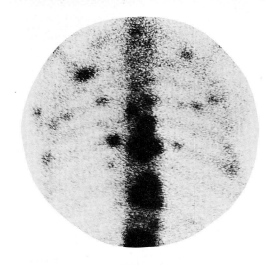

Fig. 3.5. Multiple 'hotspots' of tracer uptake in ribs and vertebral bodies are suggestive of metastases, and are very probable when the patient, like this one, is known to have prostatic cancer.

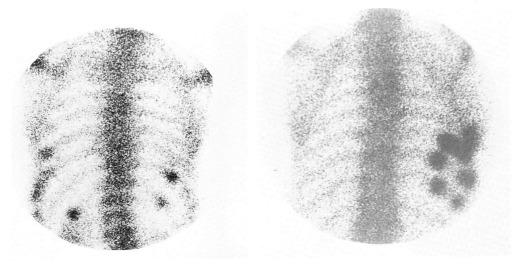

Fig. 3.6. A cluster of 'hotspots' in ribs only is characteristic of rib fractures, especially when linear, circular and symmetrical.

(1978). Fogelman (1979b) described seven metabolic features on the bone scan that are believed in general to be characteristic of metabolic bone disease. They are: increased tracer uptake in long bones, axial skeleton, and periarticular areas; prominent tracer uptake in the calvarium and mandible; the 'tie' sternum; and the faint or absent kidney images.

The patella is one of the bones to show the earliest increased activity, and when it is found outlined generalized metabolic disease must be suspected. Other causes for increased uptake in the patellae include osteoarthritis (35%), fracture, bursitis, metastasis, osteomyelitis and Paget's disease (Kipper *et al.* 1982). In osteoporosis, the features mentioned above are very poorly visualized as a result of the low bone to background ratio. In osteomalacia bone scanning has more sensitivity. The most striking bone pattern of metabolic disease is seen in renal osteodystrophy. It is thought that most of these findings are due to the effect of secondary hyperparathyroidism. Sternum uptake may be so intense, that it resembles a tie, and sometimes the ossification centres are even hotter and present themselves as a 'striped' tie.

It is important to remember that in *children* intense uptake is to be expected in the metaphyseal–epiphyseal areas of the long bones, and that this uptake diminishes with increasing age until skeletal maturation. Other areas with uptake increase are the base of the skull, the sutures, and the costochondral junctions (Murray 1980).

Finally, the scintigraphic findings of *Paget's disease* may often have a characteristic appearance. The radiotracer has a highly increased uptake and is evenly distributed throughout the affected parts of the body which are often expanded and deformed. As a rule, anatomical detail is very well visualized, e.g. in long bones the V-front can sometimes be recognized; in the pelvis a hemipelvic distribution is characteristic; in the spine one or more vertebrae may be affected; in the skull different patterns may be seen, from one spot to multiple spots, and sometimes the whole skull is highly active and grossly deformed and thickened (Shirazi *et al.* 1974, Serafini 1976, Vellenga 1981). Differentiation with metastatic disease is sometimes difficult, but generally metastatic disease presents as spotty lesions, randomly distributed, whereas

Paget's disease shows enlargement and bowing of the affected bones and there is always enhanced visibility of anatomical structures. The geography of abnormal activity is characteristic of Paget's disease on radionuclide imaging (Fig. 3.7).

SERIAL SCANNING AND QUANTITATION OF TRACER UPTAKE

In clinical bone diseases, such as acute osteomyelitis and prosthetic loosening and infection, repeat radionuclide bone studies are sometimes requested to confirm the diagnosis. Repeat studies may also be needed when a positive scan is seen without clinical evidence of disease, and should be interpreted in conjunction with radiography of the appropriate area. Serial or sequential bone scans are usually needed for the evaluation of known disease processes, as in the evaluation of maturation of ectopic bone. When the ossification reaches a plateau, tracer uptake also becomes stable and surgical therapy is more likely to be successful, with less risk of recurrence than with immature ossification (Muheim *et al.* 1973). Serial scans have been

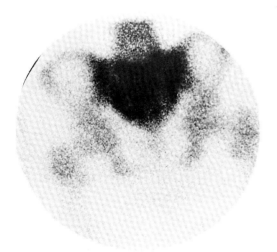

Fig. 3.7. Abnormal tracer uptake, keeping to the geography of the entire sacrum, is characteristic of Paget's disease.

performed to document the healing of fractures and bone grafts, Perthes' disease and avascular necrosis, and for the assessment of the treatment of osteomyelitis and arthritis (Rosenthall *et al.* 1982).

The most important application of serial or sequential bone studies is, however, the early detection of metastases in patients with malignant disease, in order to obtain the greatest benefit from early therapy and to assess the response to therapy. Scans taken initially and during follow-up could affect health outcomes by documenting the early presence and extent of secondary disease. The majority of publications on the progression of scan changes following metastases relate to breast cancer (Sklaroff & Sklaroff 1976, McNeil 1978, Lee 1981). Radionuclide images are usually interpreted by visual comparison with the normal contralateral, or previously unaffected, regions, rather than by quantitative measurement of activity levels from computor-processed read-outs. One might presume that the limitations resulting from this visual and quite subjective method of evaluation may be responsible for some of the misinterpretations and subsequent false-positive findings which are a feature of sequential scanning. Difficulties in identifying lesions might be produced when abnormal radionuclide uptake is only slightly higher than in the surrounding normal bone. Also, variations of exposure to the film and the amount of injected radionuclide, as well as the selection of region of interest, all have to be taken into account.

In 1974, Citrin *et al.* described a quantitative method to calculate the tumour/bone ratio by using a multichannel analyser. They developed a technique for measuring the relative activity of any region of interest by a digital profile. Such a profiling facility is normally available when the gamma camera is on line to a computer. The profile was positioned over the suspected abnormality and then over adjacent normal bone. Their technique was measured on two occasions and proved reproducible. Subsequently serial quantitative data were provided, independent of the variable exposure of the scintigrams. Since that time, many computerized techniques have been reported in benign bone disease (De Rossi *et al.* 1979), in Perthes' disease (Deutsch *et al.* 1981, LaMont *et al.* 1981), in fracture healing (Stevenson *et al.* 1974, Hughes 1980) and in sacroiliitis (Goldberg *et al.* 1978, Chalmers *et al.* 1979).

The computerized profile technique, however, has not routinely been used in daily practice. Bitran *et al.* (1980) state that serial bone scanning is a relatively crude technique for determining response to chemotherapy, since it does not reflect changes in tumour burden after successive therapy. They conclude, however, that the simple presence of stable disease on bone scan is a favourable prognostic sign, as it is associated with prolonged survival. Citrin *et al.* (1981), however, analysed serial scans during follow-up of patients with breast cancer, by using a digital model, which permitted accurate reading and measurement of skeletal abnormalities. They demonstrated significant responses on the bone scan in terms of survival length. Patients with objective responses had a median survival of 30 months. Those with stable disease had a median survival of 19 months, and those with progressive disease on the scan had a median survival of only nine months.

In cases where the effect of therapy is to be evaluated, especially when the skeleton is the only site of metastasis, it would be wise to choose one of the focal lesions as a parameter for quantitative comparison. The profile scan method could be useful to determine whether a slight difference in tracer uptake is essentially abnormal or not. One should be aware of a temporary 'flaring' of tracer uptake, due to new bone formation in the lesions, which can be recognized as a positive therapeutic effect in the first months of treatment. However, in the results of scanning reported by Alexander *et al.* (1976) the patients' response to chemotherapy could not be correlated with this flare phenomenon. Furthermore, increased tracer uptake in soft tissues, beyond the skeletal lesions (Thrall *et al.* 1975), presumably caused by regional hy-

peraemia, must be also considered as a factor which influences the profile scan.

Clinical applications of radionuclide skeletal imaging

Since the beginning of skeletal imaging in 1961, there has been an impressive growth in the number of bone scanning procedures. Charkes (1979) has listed 13 mechanisms of tracer uptake that he considers of clinical significance. This list may serve as a fine model to demonstrate the clinical applications and indications of radionuclide bone imaging (Table 3.2). Most of the mechanisms have been described on earlier pages of this chapter. In general the most frequent indications for skeletal imaging today would include:

Malignant bone disease
1   Screening for metastases.
2   Localization of metastases for diagnostic biopsies.
3   Evaluation of the extent of primary bone neoplasms.
4   Evaluation of disease modification following therapy.

Benign bone disease
1   Defining the polyostotic nature.
2   Determining whether a lesion is the cause of pain.
3   Characterizing the nature of the lesion.

Inflammatory lesions
1   To diagnose acute osteomyelitis, before the radiographic changes are evident.
2   To evaluate the nature and the extent of recurrent chronic osteomyelitis.
3   To differentiate between osteomyelitis and cellulitis.
4   To evaluate articular inflammatory disorders.

Table 3.2 Mechanisms of skeletal tracer uptake. From Charkes (1979) with permission.

Mechanism	Examples
1 Reactive bone formation	Metastases, infection, fracture, infarction
2 Malignant new bone	Osteogenic sarcoma, chondrosarcoma
3 Heterotopic new bone	Myositis ossificans, pulmonary ossification, cancer (in lymph nodes)
4 Decreased bone blood flow	Infarction
5 Increased bone blood flow, 'recruitment'	Stroke, sympathectomy, fracture, osteomyelitis, neuropathy, alpha-adrenergic drugs
6 Decreased cardiac output (increased cardiac output)	Congestive heart failure, cardiomyopathy (not detectable 1–2 h after dose)
7 Dystrophic calcification	Hypercalcaemia, uraemia (stomach, lungs, kidney, joints)
8 Blood count	Various tumours, cellulitis
9 Soft-tissue uptake	Aspergillosis, tumour, stroke, synovitis, myocardial infarction
10 Hormonal	Hyperparathyroidism, hyperthyroidism
11 Accretion	Delayed uptake (into hydroxyapatite)
12 Increased bone surface	? Mteloma (skull)
13 Destruction without reaction	Tumour, infection, infarction

Disorders of special orthopaedic interest

1 Trauma: to evaluate suspected child abuse; to evaluate the nature of fractures and non-union.

2 Prosthesis: to evaluate painful prosthesis for infection or loosening.

3 To evaluate and manage aseptic bone necrosis.

4 To evaluate bone pain.

METASTATIC AND PRIMARY MALIGNANT BONE TUMOURS

95–97% of the skeletal lesions will be demonstrated on bone scans, with the exception of multiple myeloma, the highly aggressive metastatic tumours, and the indolent thyroid metastases, incapable of producing significant reparative bone. Pistenma *et al.* (1975) described 200 patients with biopsy-proven primary cancer who had been evaluated radiographically and scintigraphically. The yields of false-negative radiographs and scans were 9·1%

and 0·4% respectively. Of the radiographs, 17% were false-negative. It is now widely accepted that the screening for metastatic bone disease should be done by bone scan. Because of their poor correlation with scan findings, normal serum calcium or alkaline phosphatase levels should not be used as criteria to decide whether or not to obtain a radionuclide bone study (Pistenma *et al.* 1975, Schaffer & Pendergrass 1976, Smalley *et al.* 1980, Lecklitner *et al.* 1981).

Bone pain is a major clinical finding in patients with bone metastases, the pain being caused by fractures, vertebral collapse and periosteal irritation. When these skeletal causes are ruled out, pain may be due to radiculopathy, perineuritis and herpes zoster, but of course this pain does not have a localized skeletal character. In prostatic cancer, Schaffer and Pendergrass (1976) found bone pain to have a sensitivity of 53·5% and a specificity of 88·0% for metastatic disease. Front *et al.* (1979) found only 50 of 155 metastatic sites to be painful.

However, it is the author's experience that the patients feel the site with the greatest periosteal irritation most of the time and consequently do not sense the other pathological areas. Schütte (1979) found in a population of patients with breast cancer that 84% (60/71) without bone pain had no metastases and normal scans, whereas 62% (55/89) with bone pain demonstrated metastatic bone disease. Bone pain is a special feature in patients with cancers that produce aggressive osteolytic metastases. In this group of cancer patients one might wait for the bone pain as an indicator of metastatic disease before ordering radionuclide bone studies. When the site of bone pain does not correlate with abnormalities on bone scan, complementary use of radiographs should be performed (Loeffler *et al.* 1975).

Primary bone tumours
Malignant primary bone tumours are always observed as areas of intense increased tracer uptake. Blood pool studies often show hyperaemia. The regional hyperaemia may sometimes obs-

cure the exact delineation of the borders of the primary tumour (Chew & Hudson 1982). With regard to the type of the primary tumour, the bone scan cannot provide diagnostic information, but Murray (1980) described some scan changes that may show characteristic patterns in order to recognize some malignant bone tumours. According to Murray, osteosarcoma usually shows a distortion of the bony outline, often irregular, and with intense tracer uptake, showing areas of absent and patchy accumulations within. Ewing's sarcoma rarely demonstrates the patchy appearance, for it presents itself with intense uptake and a smooth expansion of the skeletal outline. Chondrosarcoma also shows an intense focal uptake with deformation of the bony outline, whilst fibrosarcomas have totally varied scan patterns. Osteosarcoma metastases in the lung have been demonstrated on bone scan (Ghaed *et al.* 1974, Gilday *et al.* 1976), and according to Hoefnagel *et al.* (1981) bone scanning should be used routinely for early detection (Fig. 3.8).

According to Goldstein *et al.* (1980a, b) 2% of the children with osteosarcoma and 11% of

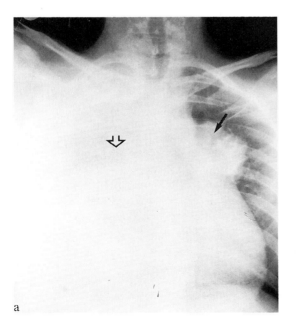

a

Fig. 3.8. There is at least one osteosarcoma metastasis visible on the radiograph (closed arrow) of the left lung (a). One may expect another faint mass (open arrow) within the fluid on the right, but the bone scan (b) demonstrates all sites of metastases to the thorax.

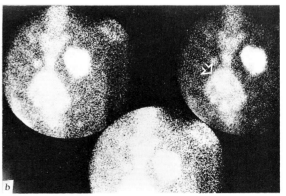

b

those with Ewing's sarcoma have bone metastases at presentation. During the follow-up, they act similarly, and about 40–45% develop metastases within the first two years. Early detection of metastatic disease and exact localization of these primary tumours seem very important now that the data indicate that treatment with chemotherapy improves survival. At presentation, all patients with osteosarcoma and Ewing's sarcoma should have a bone scan done and follow-up scans every 12 months for the first years (McNeil 1978).

Multiple myeloma

In the management of patients with multiple myeloma, bone scanning adds little. Probably as a result of insufficient new bone formation, or perhaps influenced by an osteoclast-activating factor produced by the myeloma cells, not enough detectable radionuclide is accumulated. Wahner *et al.* (1980) and Woolfenden *et al.* (1980) conclude, after comparing radiographic surveys with radionuclide studies, that radiography remains the primary method for evaluating the involvement of myeloma to the skeleton.

BENIGN BONE TUMOURS

Because benign bone tumours generally lack new bone formation and vascularity, radionuclide bone images tend to range from normal (photon-deficient) to slightly increased tracer uptake. Most of the time the pathological site is readily visualized radiographically, and all the basic features that characterize bone lesions, such as destruction, tumour expansion, periosteal reaction, margination, shape and pattern, can be distinguished with more facility. It may, however, be sometimes difficult to evaluate benign tumours, e.g. osteoid osteoma, in trabecular bone such as the spine, the femoral neck and small bones of the feet (Gilday & Ash 1976). In these instances the use of bone studies has been advocated.

Clear indications for radionuclide bone imaging for benign tumours are:

1 Establishing the multifocal nature of the entity.
2 Determining whether a benign lesion is the cause of the bone pain.
3 Characterizing the nature of the lesion.

Blood pool and three-phase radionuclide studies are considered valuable in determining the degree of hyperaemia of the lesion compared to the normal side. The nature of the lesion may be suggested when immediate post-injection flow studies do not show pooling of radiotracer, because of the relatively lesser vascularity in most benign conditions.

Osteoid osteoma

This is sometimes difficult to trace radiographically in trabecular bone, having a highly vascularized nidus, which leads to easy detection on bone scan. On post-injection dynamic studies this nidus is seen as a focus of intense activity, and the same intense activity is shown in the delayed static images (Fig. 3.9) (Gilday & Ash 1976, Mallens *et al.* 1977). As a result of the intense tracer uptake, bone scan images may be mistaken for meningioma, intracortical abscess or sclerosing osteomyelitis. In cases where the exact localization of the nidus is expected to be difficult, the radionuclide can be injected prior to the operation and the focus detected by the high uptake during the operation, using a small probe.

Benign osteoblastoma

The nidus in this aggressive benign process may sometimes be quite large, resulting in decreased tracer uptake. Depending on the localization, the tracer uptake is intense (cancellous bone) or irregular and patchy (cortical bone). Usually there is hyperaemia surrounding the lesion (Sy 1981).

Benign chondroblastoma is localized in epiphyseal ossification centres of bones, adjacent to the enchondral plate. Intense tracer uptake is caused

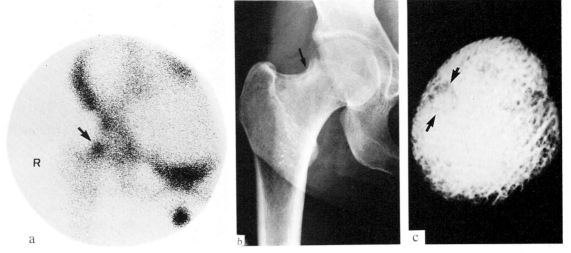

Fig. 3.9.   Increased $^{99}Tc^m$ MDP uptake in the nidus of an osteoid osteoma (a). The patient had diffuse pain in the right hip and administration of aspirin proved helpful. A faint sclerosis in the femoral neck (b) and the positive scan were indications to operate, and the nidus (c) could be extirpated.

by increased blood flow to the lesion, rather than to matrix extraction of the radionuclide (Humphry *et al.* 1980). The lesion itself is more hyperaemic than the adjacent normal bone, although increased uptake does extend to a lesser degree to the adjacent areas.

Cysts

The simple bone cysts and the aneurysmal bone cysts have no different appearance on bone scan, and have minimal to no increase of tracer uptake. Aneurysmal bone cysts, although well vascularized, have no hyperaemic component on post-injection studies. When fractured, however, cysts may show increased uptake (Gilday & Ash 1976). This feature is also described in non-ossifying fibromas and cortical defects (Greyson & Pang 1981) (Fig. 3.10).

Bone islands

These are focal areas of mature lamellar cortical bone located within trabecular bone. Most of the time they are coincidental findings on the radiographs; sometimes they change in size, this being one of the reasons for differentiation with malignant processes. The tracer uptake in bone

islands is usually normal, but sometimes increased uptake may be encountered and biopsies should be taken. Hall *et al.* (1980) believe that scintigraphic visualization is dependent on size, growth and location, but also on the sensitivity of the radionuclide tracer and the imaging device used.

Fibrous dysplasia shows increased tracer uptake along the extension of the process. Radionuclide studies are indicated to determine the polyostotic nature of the disease (Fig. 3.11).

Chondromatous benign tumours have slightly irregular, patchy increased areas of tracer uptake, and the projection outside the bony contour may suggest these lesions. After closure of the epiphyseal plates, the activity in osteochondromata usually decreases, but may flare up sometimes on malignant change.

INFECTIOUS DISEASES OF BONES AND JOINTS

Osteomyelitis and joint infection occur frequently in children and young adults. The

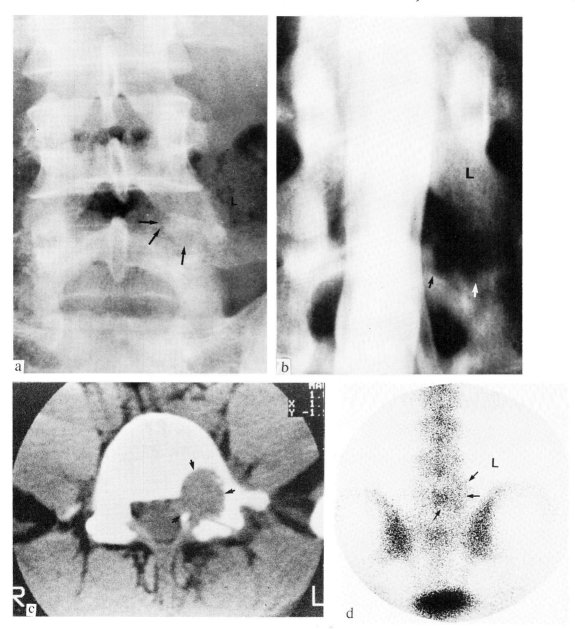

Fig. 3.10 Diagnostic limitations and possibilities are demonstrated in a 20-year-old male with aneurysmal bone cyst of L5. (a) The destruction of the vertebral body can easily be missed on the plain film. On the myelogram the lesion is better visualized tomographically (b), but on CT scan (c) the exact localization, margination and extraosseous extent is to be seen and is characteristic for a benign lesion and consistent with aneurysmal bone cyst. The bone scan (d) does not give much information, and is not conclusive without the other diagnostic images.

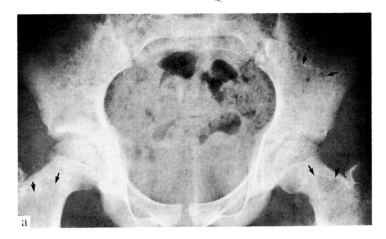

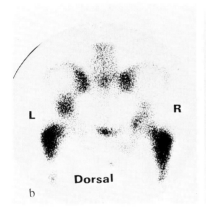

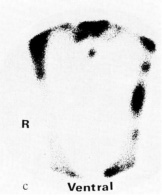

Fig. 3.11 On the radiograph of this eight-year-old girl with pubertas praecox, lytic lesions in the left iliac wing and in both trochanteric regions are seen (a). The sharp border and the ground glass appearance of the bone structure is consistent with fibrous dysplasia, and subsequently the diagnosis Albright's disease was made. The bone scan was done to determine whether other sites were present. Besides the pelvic lesions (b) lesions in the left femur were also found.

spread of the infection is usually haematogenous in these patients, whereas in adults, and diabetics, the involvement from adjacent soft-tissue infection is more frequent. Because the epiphyseal plate in infants up to one year, and in adults, does not act as a barrier to spread of infection, osteomyelitis in infants and adults frequently involves adjacent joints, unlike that in older children where the epiphyseal plate is an effective barrier.

Radiographic changes of osteomyelitis may be detected quite late after the onset of the symptoms. When the diagnosis is made by other means, e.g. radionuclide studies, and a therapeutic regimen installed, no radiographic changes may show at all (Handmaker & Leonards 1976) (Fig. 3.12). In an experimental set-

up, Norris and Watt (1981) could not demonstrate radiographic changes in rabbit tibiae at all during the first seven days. According to Nelson and Taylor (1978) the bone scan has a sensitivity of 95% and a specificity of 92% for osteomyelitis, compared with 32% and 89% respectively for radiography. Characteristically, the bone scan will demonstrate intense tracer uptake in the affected area. However, it became obvious that approximately half of the cases in children with proven osteomyelitis had scintigraphic findings that were subtle, misleading or normal (Sullivan *et al.* 1980, Ash & Gilday 1980). To differentiate between osteomyelitis and cellulitis, Gilday *et al.* (1975) and Majd and Frankel (1976) proposed the combination of bone imaging with blood pool imaging, and

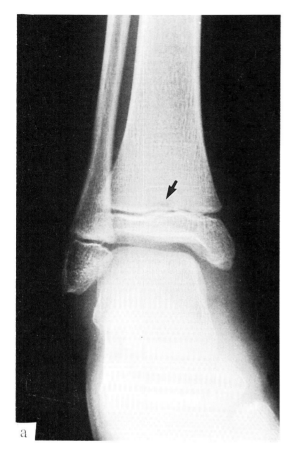

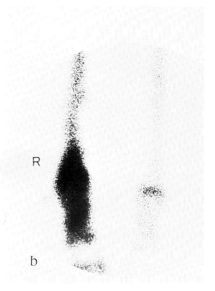

Fig. 3.12. There was some tenderness in the right lower leg for three weeks. The radiographs were normal and by the time of the scanning a small irregular lesion was seen in the metaphyseal part of the distal epiphyseal plate (a). The scan, however, is dramatically active, representing hyperaemia in acute osteomyelitis (b).

Maurer *et al.* (1981) advocated the three-phase method, starting with a dynamic angioscintigram immediately post-injection, and followed by a static blood pool scan and a delayed bone scan, to improve the chances of diagnosing osteomyelitis. Areas of cellulitis may show as 'hot' on the early images, yet show normal on the late bone scan (Fig. 3.2), whereas osteomyelitis should be associated with increased activity on the late images. Likewise, hyperaemia will be observed in septic arthritis as diffuse increased uptake in the blood pool study, persisting in delayed scans. The exact cause of the photon-deficient features in some cases of osteomyelitis is not yet known, but is probably related to thrombosis of the microcirculation of the affected area, or perhaps to compression of the vessels by pus or oedema. Norris and Watt (1981) experimented with rabbits, whose intramedullary tibial cavity was infected with *Staphylococcus aureus*. ^{99}Tc^m compound perfusion scans and 4-hour delay scans were made, as also were 24-hour ^{67}Ga scans. The perfusion scan demonstrated cold areas the first day followed by increasing activity on following days. Four-hour bone phase scans were 'cold' the first day and this persisted on the following days. The ^{67}Ga scans, however, demonstrated activity progressively from two to four days.

Differences in bone uptake in osteomyelitis might be associated with clinical circumstances, e.g. not all patients arrive early with symptoms and bone scans may consequently reflect different stages of the disease.

^{67}Ga is not dependent upon blood flow and reflects the presence of bacteria and polymorphonuclear leucocytes. Recently, many authors have advocated the use of ^{67}Ga. The ^{67}Ga scan is usually positive when ^{99}Tc^m bone scans are negative (Teates & Williamson 1977, Berkowitz & Wenzel 1980). So why not perform ^{67}Ga scans routinely on all patients suspected of having acute osteomyelitis? Handmaker (1980) answers this question as follows: 'false-negative or inconclusive scan results occur in less than 20% of patients. ^{99}Tc^m phosphate remains the best technique for screening these patients, given the low cost and radiation, and the higher spatial resolution for anatomical localization.' Hoffer and Princenthal (1981) proceed with a gallium scan when the bone scan is negative in strongly suspected osteomyelitis, or if the scan is positive but underlying chronic non-inflammatory disease is present. They never report a negative scan as having 'ruled out' osteomyelitis or joint infection. If no increased gallium uptake is observed in inflamed soft tissue, a repeat scan is done once the soft-tissue inflammatory process has been controlled with antibiotics. For follow-up studies following the process of therapy ^{67}Ga scans should be used, because the ^{99}Tc^m bone scan remains positive long after infection has resolved. Evaluation of chronic osteomyelitis may consequently have false-positive results with ^{99}Tc^m phosphate scans, however in the author's experience an intense tracer accumulation will carefully delineate the recurrent inflamed area (Fig. 3.13). In inconclusive cases ^{67}Ga scans are advocated (Alazraki *et al.* 1978).

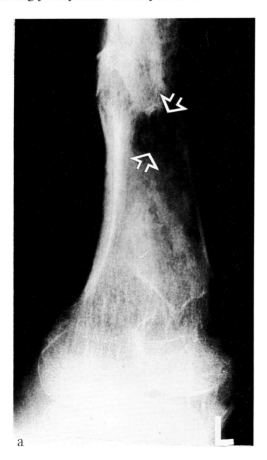

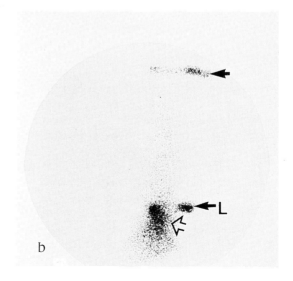

Fig. 3.13. (a) Residual sclerosis of chronic osteomyelitis of the left femur, with a lytic area (open arrow) possibly representing recurrence. (b) On the ^{99}Tc^m MDP scan the extent of the sclerosis was marked (closed arrows) and abnormal tracer uptake indeed confirms the diagnosis and the location of the recurrence.

To evaluate *inflamed joint disease*, $^{99}Tc^m$ pertechnetate and $^{99}Tc^m$ phosphate scans are utilized. Their mechanism of localization is somewhat different. The early localization of $^{99}Tc^m$ pertechnetate (TcO_4) in an inflamed joint results from increased perfusion of the inflamed synovium, a later peak occurring as a result of $^{99}Tc^m$ binding to proteins in the joint fluid. The pertechnetate study will be specific for synovitis, but false-positives have been described in concurrent cellulitis or oedema adjacent to the joints (Hoffer & Genant 1976). $^{99}Tc^m$ phosphate scans will detect osseous joint abnormalities, but may be negative in synovitis. Likewise, the phosphate scans will be positive in changes in the skeletal metabolism, localized in the periarticular regions, such as disuse osteoporosis, fractures, osteomalacia, etc., and give the misleading impression of local joint disease. In these cases $^{99}Tc^m$ pertechnetate is probably normal and more specific, although less sensitive, and in fact these non-articular conditions can be ruled out clinically and radiographically. Because of the greater sensitivity in detecting abnormal joints, and especially the central joints, such as the hips, the sacroiliac joints and the spine, joint scanning with $^{99}Tc^m$ phosphate is preferred in most institutions (*see* Table 3.2).

The role of gallium in inflammatory joint imaging has been described by Lisbona and Rosenthall (1977), Staab and McCartney (1978) and Coleman *et al.* (1982). The problem with gallium imaging remains the poor resolution with gamma camera devices, and the difficult anatomical correlation of tracer uptake, especially in infants. In septic arthritis gallium concentrates in the synovium. The same is to be seen in cellulitis. Gallium accumulation disappears during the course of therapy, and this has led to the use of this agent as a guide to therapy. Wolf *et al.* (1980) and Coleman *et al.* (1982) have described positive gallium scans in cases of rheumatoid arthritis: the consequence of these findings is that diffuse gallium and also phosphate activity is not pathognomonic of septic arthritis. Differentiation must be associated with radiographs and the clinical findings.

Rheumatoid arthritis affects the PIP and MCP joints, and intense radiotracer accumulation may be seen in active and subclinical cases. In clinically apparent cases, the bone scan can objectively document the joints involved (Shearman *et al.* 1982) (Fig. 3.14). However, the increased uptake in joints in which synovitis has clinically subsided may still be caused by persistent changes in blood flow to the subchondral bone or to reparative processes (McCarthy *et al.* 1970). In patients with persistent symptoms with absence of objective physical findings, positive bone scans suggest the presence of subclinical disease, whereas a negative scan may suggest a psychogenic component. Psoriatic arthritis, juvenile rheumatoid arthritis and sacroiliitis have all demonstrated positive scans, and the value of bone scanning in these disease processes has been reported (Weissberg *et al.* 1978).

In osteoarthritic degenerative joint disease bone imaging is always positive, reflecting the mild hyperaemia accompanying the degeneration of the joint cartilage (Desaulnier *et al.* 1974) (Fig. 4.15). In patients with osteoarthritis resulting in varus deformity of the knee, preoperative evaluation is a current application in some centres (Hoffer & Genant 1976). Medial, lateral and patellofemoral compartment involvement can be assessed, this being helpful in the choice of surgical procedures.

DISORDERS OF ORTHOPAEDIC INTEREST

Trauma

Fractures are the most common bone lesions and the proper diagnosis is nearly always made by clinical and radiographic findings. Radiographs are the most important imaging modes to establish the true nature of the fracture, e.g. the bony structure and the degree of alignment of the bones involved. However, in some parts of the skeleton, some small fractures may be hard to detect, especially when located in ribs, spine, carpus (scaphoid bone) and tarsus (Rolfe *et al.* 1981). Greenstick fractures, stress fractures and fissures may not be recognized at the

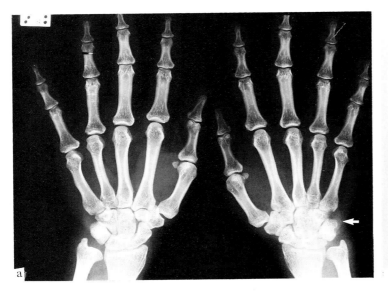

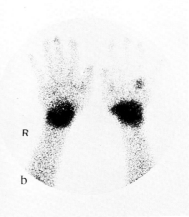

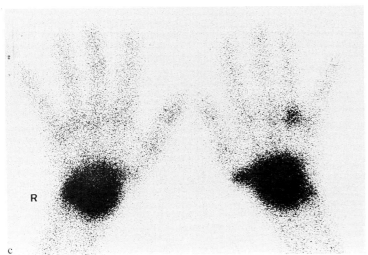

Fig. 3.14. The radiograph (a) of this patient may faintly demonstrate an erosion of the left 5th metacarpal base, suggesting rheumatoid arthritis. The $^{99}Tc^m$ MDP blood pool scan (b) and the delayed scan (c) document the joint involved.

time on radiographs and may be detected successfully by radionuclide imaging with phosphate compounds. Ganel *et al.* (1979) noted good correlation between initial radiographs showing fractures and bone scan findings in 47 patients suspected of having carpal scaphoid fractures. All 30 patients with normal bone scans failed to show evidence of scaphoid fractures.

Very important extensions to the radionuclide evaluation of fractured bone have been the evaluation of stress fractures, the battered child syndrome and delayed healing and non-union of fractures (Marty *et al.* 1976). Matin (1979) performed bone scans on 204 patients at intervals ranging from six hours to several years after traumatic fractures. He mainly examined patients with vertebral compression fractures,

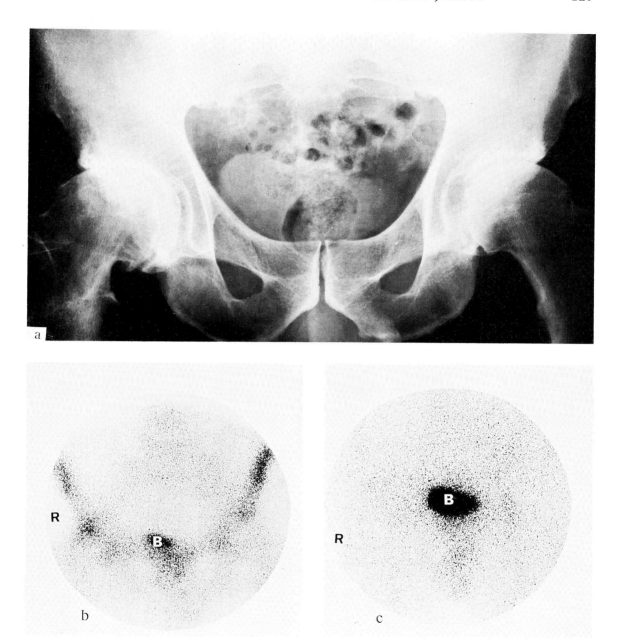

Fig. 3.15. A case of osteoarthritic joint disease (a). There is no activity seen on the post-injection radionuclide angiogram (b), ruling out excessive vascularization, such as in acute inflammatory arthritis. However, the delayed scan (c) is slightly abnormal in the right hip, due to some bone formation. B, bladder.

rib fractures and fractures of the distal extremities. The time after fracture for the bone scan to become abnormal depends upon the age of the patient and the presence of osteoporosis. Although 80% of the patients had abnormal scans within 24 hours, 95% of those under 65 years of age showed increased tracer uptake within a day after trauma at the fracture site. Thirty-seven of the 39 patients of all ages studied had positive scans within three days after trauma. Fifty-nine of the 60 studied (98%) demonstrated abnormalities at one week after injury. One was negative as a result of an impacted femoral neck fracture in osteoporotic bone.

Sequential scans performed at intervals up to 36 months after trauma showed three phases: (1) the acute stage persisting for about 3–4 weeks after trauma, characterized by a diffuse area of increased tracer uptake surrounding the fracture; the fracture line could be seen at this stage; (2) between 8 and 12 weeks after injury, a well-defined linear abnormality, with intense uptake at the fracture site is observed; (3) the healing phase is characterized by gradual diminution in intensity (evolutionary pattern, Charkes 1979) until the scan returns to normal. Some cases with increased tracer uptake in 40-year-old fractures have been described. However, by two years after trauma more than 90% of the fractures had indeed shown an uptake return to normal. Rib fractures showed the most rapid healing, with 80% normal scans in one year after injury. Vertebral compression fractures healed at a less rapid rate: 59% returned to normal in one year, 90% were normal in two years, and 97% were normal in three years. Pressure effects such as those associated with weight-bearing might be responsible for the persisting abnormal activity in fractures of the vertebral bodies, compared to fractures occurring in the rib cage.

Stress fractures
When normal or abnormal bone is subjected to repeated cyclic loading, the load being less than that which causes an acute bone fracture, stress fractures may occur. One may recognize two types of stress fracture: fatigue fractures (abnormal stress in normal bone) and insufficiency fractures (normal stress in abnormal bone). Abnormal bone has a reduced elastic resistance to stimuli, and patients with Paget's disease, rheumatoid arthritis, ankylosing spondylitis, osteomalacia, rickets, hyperparathyroidism and renal osteodystrophy may be associated with this type of stress fracture (Fig. 3.16). Fatigue fractures have been described in joggers, dancers, athletes and soldiers (Geslien *et al.* 1976, Wilcox *et al.* 1977, Meurman & Elfving 1980). Both fracture types may be encountered in patients following surgical procedures that result in altered stress or imbalance of muscular force on normal and abnormal bone, such as hip surgery and bunion surgery with subsequent arthrodesis.

The stress fracture begins as a small cortical crack, which progresses as the stimulus continues. Progression is characterized by the appearance of subcortical infarction in front of the advancing main crack in the bone. The stressed and painful bone undergoes accelerated remodelling and this produces an abnormal scan image long before radiographic findings are noted. Roub *et al.* (1979) compared radionuclide images with radiographs of 55 athletes with shin soreness and 13 asymptomatic athletes. They concluded that stress fractures are part of a continuum, rather than an isolated event like acute traumatic fractures. The bone scan is positive in stress levels of accelerated remodelling, where radiography is not sensitive.

As a result of radionuclide evaluation different sites may be found with stress fractures. Meurman *et al.* (1980) describe fractures in tarsal bones and calcanei. According to Geslien *et al.* (1976) stress fractures occur as follows: 39% in tibial plateau, 35% in calcaneum, 7·5% in metatarsal bones, and 19% in the group—femoral neck, mid-femur, distal femur or mid-tibia. The importance of early detection of stress fractures is limited to the areas of the skeleton where significant morbidity is expected, e.g. the femoral neck and tibial shaft. Here they can develop as displaced fractures and result in delayed healing.

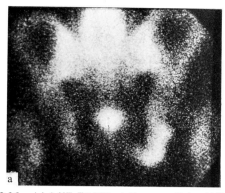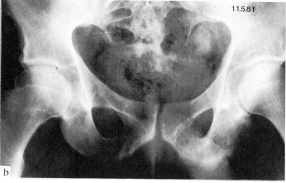

Fig. 3.16. (a) A $^{99}Tc^m$ MDP scintigram on Polaroid film of a 38-year-old male with ankylosing spondylitis. The scans show increased tracer uptake in the left ischial area. The radiograph (b) confirms a lesion, due to proliferation of new bone, considered a feature of ankylosing spondylitis, and caused by stress at points of muscle attachment.

Early recognition of child abuse

It is very important to recognize abused children in order to protect them from further harm. Concrete evidence of abuse facilitates the task of the physician to break the vicious circle of repeated attacks to the child. Lesions associated with the 'battered child syndrome' include fractures and dislocations, metaphyseal infarctions, extensive involucrum formation, metaphyseal cupping, bowing of the diaphysis and ectopic accessory epiphyseal ossification centres (De Smet *et al.* 1977). The fractures are characteristically multiple and in various stages of healing, reflecting the repeated violence. Intramedullary fat necrosis caused by traumatic pancreatitis, discharging metastatic lipase, has been reported in child abuse (Slovis *et al.* 1975). Metastatic fat necrosis produces lytic lesions in peripheral tubular bones of hands and feet that may be scintigraphically demonstrated in the early stages (Goluboff *et al.* 1978). Haase *et al.* (1980) reported on 44 children suspected of having been abused. No child with a negative scan on the day of the medical examination developed evidence of bone injury. Only skull fractures appeared to be normal on bone scan and therefore it is advisable to X-ray the skull and those parts showing focal activity on the bone scan. The bone scan may be useful to evaluate the age of different fractures. Older fractures will be less 'hot' than recent ones, and this might establish the repeated cyclic action.

Healing of fractures

Delay or arrest in the healing of a fracture is a common complication seen in orthopaedic practice. Forsted *et al.* (1978) quoted U.S. National Health Surveys for the year 1967, stating that 100 000, from the two million fractures that occur yearly in the U.S.A., go on to non-union. Factors promoting callus formation appear to be the elevation of the periosteum, the application of implants, and discontinuity in the fractured bone. The degree of callus formation, however, depends on the degree of stabilization of the fragments, their ability to obtain contact with each other and local vascularity. The distance between the fragments and the extent of the fracture line appears to be less significant (Greiff 1981). Increased risks of non-union occurring include inadequate blood supply, existing metabolic disease, poor nutritional status and, of major importance, infection.

The incidence of delayed union and non-union depends on the bone involved (Silberstein 1980). The highest incidence is found in the femur and tibia, progressively decreasing in the humerus, radius, ulna and clavicle. Greiff (1981) used $^{99}Tc^m$ polyphosphate scintimetry in experimental fractures of rabbits' tibiae, to determine the course of osteosynthetic procedures. He found that $^{99}Tc^m$ scintimetry monitors the callus formation earlier than the radiographic examinations. Hughes (1980) developed a method of quantification to measure the healing of fractures. After injecting $^{99}Tc^m$ MDP, profile scans were obtained of the fractured leg and the normal one. A pattern may be seen in different stages of healing. In healing fractures the peaks of increased tracer uptake should start on both ends of the fragments and meet in the course of some weeks. In cases of delayed union or non-union the two peaks will remain positioned on both sides of the fracture line.

McMaster and Merrick (1980) evaluated the occurrence of pseudarthrosis formation in scoliotic spine after fusion. A generalized $^{99}Tc^m$ MDP uptake, six months after the attempted fusion, correlated with solid fusion, but demonstrated one false-positive in the 71 patients. A patchy tracer uptake was considered to represent pseudarthrosis, but only six of the 12 with patchy local uptake had pseudarthrosis, and two of the 27 with a patchy generalized uptake had pseudarthrosis.

In recent years the treatment of non-united fractures with percutaneous low-grade electrical, direct-current stimulation has been shown to be effective in 60–80% of patients (Forsted *et al.* 1978). Desai *et al.* (1980) report on the role of bone scintigraphy in the evaluation of this method of treatment. Scanning appeared primarily of help in identifying those patients who may not respond to electrical stimulation of their non-united fracture. In patients with diffuse increased activity at the fracture site, there appeared to be a physiological attempt to heal the fracture, despite the longstanding non-union. In these patients with probably not enough ossified callus at the fracture site, approximately 95% responded to electrical stimulation. Increased activity at the bone-end with decreased activity at the fracture site, and finding of overall decreased activity, reflected failure of healing and inability to bridge the gap between the fragments. In the last two groups of patients no success is to be expected from electrical stimulation. Complete healing might be demonstrated by bone marrow imaging using $^{99}Tc^m$–sulphur colloid. Chafetz *et al.* (1978) demonstrated photon deficiency in areas of complete fracture healing in the ribs.

Evaluation of prosthetic implants

Replacement of hip and knee joints with prosthetic implants is now common practice. Most complications in the immediate post-operative period are related to the surgery. Following this period, the major complications are secondary to prosthetic component loosening, infection, fracture or dislocation, trochanteric complications or heterotopic bone formation. Loosening is the most frequent cause, with or without infection. This complication of hip and knee arthroplasties should be recognized as early as possible, in order to avoid progressive destruction of the bones involved compromising future surgical replacement or fusion. Radionuclide imaging has been recognized as a method for early recognition of hip and knee prosthetic loosening and infection. However, there is some disagreement over whether it is preferable to undertake arthrography, cultures of needle aspirated fluid and plain radiography. Radiographic evaluation of the painful hip is essential to rule out dislocation and fracture. Detection of prosthetic loosening is recognized by widening of the lucent zone between cement and bone or demonstration of motion between bone and prosthesis on stress films. These features, however, occur late, and the diagnosis of loosening might otherwise have been made earlier. To evaluate prosthetic loosening, many centres have added barium to the methylmethacrylate cement to make it radiopaque, and determination of prosthetic complications on plain radiographs may likewise be inexpensive and accurate (Tehranzadeh *et al.* 1981).

Arthrography has been advocated as a complementary technique in prosthetic hip and knee arthroplasty, but may have too many false-positives (Murray & Rodrigo 1975, Gelman *et al.* 1978, Tehranzadeh *et al.* 1981). Needle aspiration for cultures is considered very accurate in establishing infection and should basically be done when infection is suspected on scan or X-ray. Despite the imperfections of the bone scan in diagnosing prosthetic loosening it is probably the most reliable method for early confirmation of the diagnosis. There is some disagreement upon when the bone scan might give a worthwhile picture around the prosthesis and not show increased tracer uptake resulting from the surgery. Usually the activity is at its greatest at two months after surgery, diminishing to normal at six months. As a result bone scans done too early post-operatively might produce false-positives, and in these cases gallium studies have the same result (Williamson *et al.* 1979, Weiss *et al.* 1979). Abnormal causes of abnormal bone scans in patients with painful hip prostheses can be, according to McInerney and Hyde (1978), prosthesis removed, infection proven; prosthesis *in situ*, probably infection; protrusion of the prosthesis, Paget's disease; heterotopic bone formation, fracture in upper femoral shaft. Criteria for the distribution of tracer uptake in prosthetic loosening and infection are the following: the acetabular component is considered loose when there is marked increase of tracer uptake at the hip joint; loosening of the femoral component is diagnosed when increase of radionuclide is seen at three points i.e. medially, laterally at the intertrochanteric level, and at the distal end of the femoral component (Fig. 3.17).

Diffuse, high tracer uptake along the entire femoral and acetabular components suggests loosening combined with infection (Tehranzadeh *et al.* 1981). Because increased tracer uptake has to be compared with the contralateral side, osteoarthritis of that joint may complicate the interpretation of acetabular loosening. Weiss *et al.* (1979) state that the clue to prosthetic loosening is the focal tracer at the distal end of the femoral component, a region usually free of heterotopic bone, making evaluation easier than at the joint itself. Others claim that this distal focal spot may also be seen in normal cases. Evaluation of knee arthroplasty was reported by Gelman *et al.* (1978). Hunter *et al.* (1980) used a system of grading the scintigraphic images of femoral and tibial components and found significant differences in tracer uptake in patients with surgically proven loosening compared with those with an asymptomatic knee prosthesis. Selection of a 'normal'

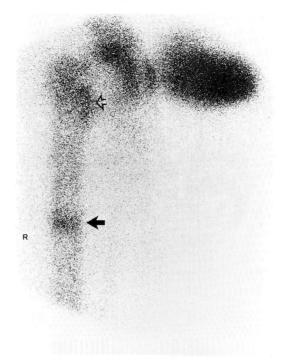

Fig. 3.17. A painful right hip after insertion of a Moore prosthesis. Tracer uptake in the lesser trochanter (open arrow) is caused by heterotopic bone, whereas the increased focal uptake in the distal end of the femoral component (closed arrow) is a clue to prosthetic loosening. Proved by operation.

level of tracer uptake for the femoral and the tibial component proved difficult. The sensitivity and specificity for the femoral component were 83% and 86% respectively. The values for the tibial component were less accurate, probably owing to the fact that the tibial prosthesis undergoes more stress and has a tendency to undergo loosening. Feith *et al.* (1976) and his associates of the University Hospital of Nijmegen, the Netherlands, advocate the use of $^{87}Sr^m$ in order to obtain better scan results. Their material is as yet quite small, however, and $^{87}Sr^m$ is not always available.

Notwithstanding that the evidence is not all that clear on the usefulness of radionuclide bone scanning as a technique for complications of orthopaedic implants, it is still advisable to proceed to bone scanning when the plain radiograph is non-diagnostic in patients with a painful hip prosthesis. When the scan is positive, one may aspirate joint fluid for cultures in order to rule out infection. On the other hand, when the $^{99}Tc^m$ MDP scan is negative or non-diagnostic, and an infection is clinically suspected, a gallium scan can be used to obtain further information.

Rövekamp *et al.* (1984) evaluated ^{111}In-labelled leucocyte scintigraphy in 32 patients after surgery of the hip. This technique gave varying results with low diagnostic accuracy of 50%. Specificity was 40% and sensitivity 70%.

AVASCULAR DISEASE, ASEPTIC NECROSIS OF BONE

Graft viability

The ability of autogenous bone grafts to reconstruct defects in the skeleton can be analysed by radiography. Enneking *et al.* (1980) found that the length of the defect did not affect the incidence of non-union, but did have an effect on the number of stress fractures in the graft. Radiographically, the grafts decrease in density during the first six months, and gradually regain their mass to become normal in two years. Stevenson *et al.* (1974) and Velasco *et al.* (1976) studied the value of $^{99}Tc^m$ phosphate bone studies in dogs and human beings respectively. In human beings, bone scans made at the end of the fourth week after graft implantation demonstrated increased uptake in the viable grafts. In cases of non-union, the graft itself remained photon-deficient. In experiments with dogs, bone scan results were seen earlier than radiographical changes suggesting graft failure.

Avascular disease in trauma of the hip

Meyers *et al.* (1977) determined the vascularity of the femoral head in patients with traumatic dislocations of the hip, femoral neck fractures, non-union of femoral neck fracture and ischaemic necrosis of the femoral head in images obtained 1–2 hours after injection of 370 MBq (10 mCi) $^{99}Tc^m$–sulphur colloid and within five days after injury in patients with fracture or dislocation of the hip. The bone scans predicted the histological findings in 95% of the cases.

Bauer *et al.* (1980) studied 34 patients with 35 fresh femoral neck fractures with $^{99}Tc^m$ MDP. Their protocol included initial radionuclide imaging accompanied by radiographs after the operation, then at 4, 8, 12, 24 and 36 months. Tetracycline was administered before the operation and biopsies taken in the femoral nail channel at operation. Major changes in normal bone scan pattern were seen shortly after fracture and nailing. Initial avascularity confirmed the fact that displaced fractures run a greater risk of femoral head necrosis than those without dislocation. The femoral head displayed a marked depression in vascular activity post-operatively in one half of the cases (Fig. 3.18).

Legg–Calvé–Perthes disease

Perthes' disease is characterized by loss of vascularity in part of the femoral ossification centre without known injury. Danigelis (1976) has observed that all children with Perthes' disease (with or without radiographic findings) have a 'cold' (photon-deficient) notch on the bone scan, involving the laterosuperior part of the femoral head, best seen on anterior frog views. The size of the cold area can be variable (Fig. 3.19). LaMont *et al.* (1981) propose a method for determining the extent of avascularity of the femoral head in suspected Perthes' disease, dividing the epiphysis into four regions, with one region in the acetabulum, and another in the trochanteric area. The values they obtained could establish the extent of the avascular insult in this disease long before such an estimate could be made on radiographs. They propose the use of the following classification: involvement of (1) the lateral third quadrant; (2) the lateral 50% of the femoral head; (3) the lateral three-quarters of the femoral head. No patients appeared to exhibit total involvement of the femoral head. This classification could be helpful for follow-up assessment. Deutsch *et al.* (1981)

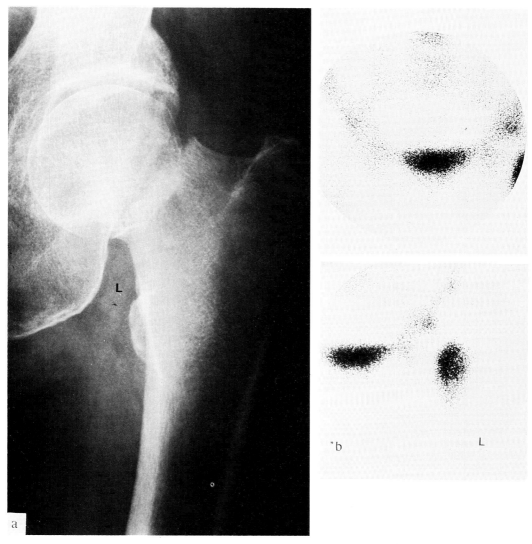

Fig. 3.18. A slightly displaced femoral neck fracture (a) with decreased tracer uptake in the left femoral head on the scan (b) due to avascularity. The fracture itself and the trochanteric area are very active due to bone formation and hyperaemia. Histologically the femoral head demonstrated areas of devitalized trabeculae.

followed 18 patients with Perthes' disease, using quantitative regional blood flow and routine delayed bone scans. Early Perthes' disease revealed a decrease in uptake in the static scan, most of the time the flow changes preceding the static images and these preceding the radiographic changes. No correlation could be made between duration of symptoms and scan changes. Serial scans in Perthes' patients showed variable patterns of flow in the same child, which may provide evidence for the concept of repeated vascular insults in these patients. In the stage of revascularization and ossification, consisting of gradual reformation of the femoral head, the scan will gradually show increase of activity, and this sometimes extends

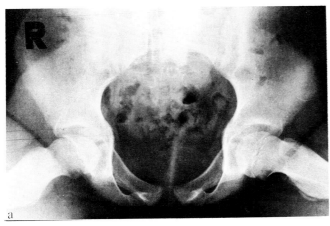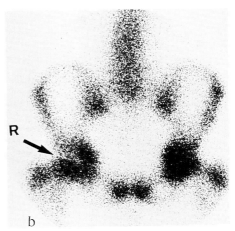

Fig. 3.19. A case of Perthes' disease. The radiograph (a) does not show abnormal changes, besides a moderate widening of the hip joint. The $^{99}Tc^m$ MDP scan (b) demonstrates the characteristic cold notch in the lateral half of the femoral head.

into the metaphysis (Fotter *et al.* 1982). The photon-deficient notch will subsequently disappear in later stages. This may complicate the interpretation of scan images in Perthes' disease. However, when revascularization has not yet reached adequate levels the flow images might be diagnostic. In this late stage radiographs will show the characteristic changes, and will mark the progressed stage of the disease. Majd (1978) reported a case of Meyer's dysplasia with normal bone scan, and subsequently excluded bilateral Perthes' disease.

Osteonecrosis is known to occur in association with lupus erythematosus, following corticosteroid treatment for immunosuppression, and in caisson disease, sickle cell disease and Gaucher disease. There is limited scintigraphic experience. Osteonecrosis of the femoral head in corticosteroid treatment has early positive radionuclide images, but in the knee smaller lesions might produce false-negative results. In comparing the relative values of radiography and scintigraphy in experimental bone necrosis produced by infarcts in rabbits, Gregg and Walder (1980) found histological evidence that areas with extensive necrosis and reactive reparative processes were only radiographically visible in a small number of cases. In contrast to the ra-

diographic findings, abnormalities were detected on bone scan as early as three weeks after damage, and once present these 'hotspots' persisted for at least three months. In a study of old lesions of caisson disease, done in a group of persons 10 years after stopping work in a high-pressure environment, normal radiographs with abnormal scans, abnormal radiographs and abnormal scans, and abnormal radiographs with normal scans were all seen. Gregg and Walder assume that lack of obvious changes on the radiographs does not mean that the process has stopped; and that early bone scanning may have a value in the early recognition of sarcomatous development of old bone infarcts, as has been reported in the lower femoral shaft.

Miscellaneous

LOW BACK PAIN

For early detection of destructive lesions of the spine, the value of radiography is limited, because of the latent period between the onset of the symptoms and any detectable changes. The value of radionuclide bone studies has been described for patients with a variety of spinal disorders. Recent investigators have shown its usefulness in the diagnosis of osteoid osteoma (Gilday & Ash 1976, Mallens *et al.* 1977) and rheumatoid arthritis and its variants (Weissberg *et al.* 1978), but according to Weissberg abnormal joints were seen with greater frequency on scanning than on radiographs—with the exception of the spine. Radionuclide bone images of the sacroiliac joints may be useful in distinguishing abnormal joints by the high tracer uptake in these joints. However, qualitative interpretation of the SI joints is considered not sensitive enough, and consequently some institutions have advocated quantitative sacroiliac scintigraphy (q.s.s.), using a computerized profile technique, in which the tracer uptake in the sacroiliac joints is compared to the sacral activity (Goldberg *et al.* 1978, Chalmers *et al.* 1979, Schütte & Park 1983).

EVALUATION OF BONE PAIN

In patients without previous known disease, radiographs should be made to evaluate the nature of the painful site(s). In almost all cases benign and degenerative disorders will be diagnosed with more precision on radiographs, and it should be remembered that in older patients one-third of the positive bone scans are caused by tracer uptake in degenerative foci. When radiographs are found to be negative or inconclusive, bone scintigraphy may be indicated.

The author has examined 70 patients with bone pain and without known malignant disease. In only one patient were metastatic lesions responsible for the bone pain. In 40 patients the bone scans were negative and no skeletal lesions were discovered on follow-up in the painful region for one year at least. In the other 29 patients with positive scans, the causes of the pain were as follows: 12 osteoporotic fractures, 7 benign conditions, and 10 Paget's disease. All these conditions were radiographically evident (Schütte 1979).

Majd (1978) examined 82 children with focal or generalized skeletal pain of obscure origin. Clinical, routine radiographic and laboratory findings were normal or equivocal. All patients with underlying diseases and with signs of acute infections were excluded. Fifty-five cases had normal scans, whereas 27 had positive scans, listed as follows: traumatic 8, inflammatory 8, neoplastic 9, benign 4, malignant 5 and Perthes' disease 2.

SOFT-TISSUE DISORDERS IMAGED BY BONE-SEEKING RADIONUCLIDES (*See also* p. 109.)

Radionuclide bone seekers for skeletal imaging are taken up by a variety of soft-tissue abnormalities. Increased vascularity, capillary permeability, cellular calcium metabolism, immature collagen and binding of $^{99}Tc^m$-labelled phosphates to phosphatase enzymes are factors to explain the localization of these bone seekers in soft-tissue lesions. The uptake to the calcified foci is perhaps similar to that absorption which occurs onto the hydroxyapatite crystals in bone when soft-tissue lesions are partly calcified.

Pearlman (1977) reported radionuclide bone studies in liposarcoma, including dynamic flow studies and static images, and found that the distribution of the radiotracer is more or less proportional to regional blood flow. The information he obtained with these studies was qualitatively similar to an angiographic study. He stresses the need of prior knowledge of location and size of feeder vessels to avoid bleeding at operation. In 60% of the cases of neuroblastoma the primary tumour may show uptake, and uptake is sometimes also seen in hepatic metastases (Smith *et al.* 1980).

At the University of Florida radionuclide bone scanning is included in the preoperative radiological staging of soft-tissue masses. Chew *et al.* (1981) have experience with some 240 patients with soft-tissue masses, and report on 113 patients for whom complete material was available. Only 29 of the 113 scans were negative, one being a soft-tissue chondrosarcoma and the remaining 28 being benign disorders. The 84 abnormal scans showed intense uptake in areas of radiographically evident calcification, but apart from this relationship no correlation was found between intensity of tracer uptake and the histogenesis, size or vascularity of the tumour. When angiograms were available, hypervascularity was present in most of the lesions which demonstrated radionuclide hyperconcentration. They report having seen five patterns of tracer abnormality, which are summarized here very briefly:

1   Isolated soft tissue hyperconcentration; within soft tissue itself.

2   Hyperconcentration in soft tissue and adjacent bone; this always indicates involvement of the bone by the soft-tissue tumour. The tumours were practically the same as seen in the first pattern. In some benign cases there was some periosteal bone formation adjacent to the soft-tissue lesion.

3   Hyperconcentration in soft tissue contiguous with normal bone; the uptake in bone is not increased, but the uptake of the soft-tissue lesion appears to be contiguous with that of the adjacent bone on available views. All lesions with this pattern were malignant.

4   Unlocalizable hyperconcentration; uptake not localizable to soft tissue or to bone.

5   Extended uptake; in bones of the lesion-bearing limb.

AMPUTATION LEVEL SELECTION

Selection of an amputation level to remove diseased, infected or gangrenous portions of extremities is made most of the time on clinical criteria. Other criteria such as angiographic patterns, skin temperature and temperature gradients all lack quantitative measurements. As a result, when primary healing of the wound is not achieved, progressively higher amputations have to be carried out, or alternatively the surgeon has to decide upon high—above the knee—levels to provide healing.

Moore *et al.* (1981) have used xenon (^{133}Xe) clearance to select the most distal amputation level that allows sufficient blood flow for healing. The condition of the patient was carefully

evaluated with respect to the extent of the pathological process. The most distal amputation level was identified and marked for xenon flow measurements, and skin blood flow was initially determined on the anterior midline of the leg. If the flow rate was less than 2·4 ml/min/100 mg tissue, the measurement was repeated at the next anatomical amputation level. The examination was performed with the patient in supine position; 0·05 ml of xenon (^{133}Xe) in sodium chloride was injected intracutaneously near the marked point. A total of 100–500 mCi was injected with a tuberculin syringe and a 26 gauge needle. After injection, the xenon activity was monitored for 10 minutes at four frames per minute by a gamma camera interfaced to a computer. The slope constant for xenon washout was calculated, and this value provided the perfusion rate. Their data demonstrated that the criterion for amputation of minimum flow of 2·4 ml/min/100 mg of tissue is applicable not only at the 'below-knee' level, but also at other amputation levels.

Conclusion

Radionuclide scintigraphic imaging with ^{99}Tc^{m} phosphate complexes (MDP) is a very sensitive screening method for detecting skeletal abnormality associated with bone turnover. It is a very convenient and non-invasive way of drawing attention to some lesions that might otherwise be overlooked on radiographs. This modality is therefore the first examination of choice when malignant or metastatic disease is suspected. Lesions that are relatively blind to radiography can be picked up scintigraphically. Skeletal lesions resulting from trauma, arthritis, infection and neoplasm may be demonstrated before radiographs become abnormal, especially when there is a high index of clinical suspicion. Further, radionuclide bone studies can be conclusive when radiographs are positive and the clinical presentation is equivocal, or both radiography and clinical history are equivocal. In acute osteomyelitis, especially in children, and in prosthetic implant infection, and also in rapidly destructive bone metastases, false-negative bone scans can occur. Radiogallium scintigraphy is advocated in these cases as a second line of approach. However, gallium is somewhat capricious, and although there is a high sensitivity to infectious processes there is a variable and unpredictable sensitivity to non-septic inflammatory conditions as well as increased bone metabolism (Rosenthall *et al.* 1982). The lesion/background ratio is low and poor imaging resolution may be a further source of diagnostic confusion. Serial follow-up studies can document the process of therapy, but Tc bone studies may remain positive long after the pathological process has resolved. Positive scans of $^{99}Tc^m$ MDP are not specific, and knowledge of the uptake mechanisms, the clinical context of the patient, and the distinction of scan patterns may be necessary to establish an accurate diagnosis.

References

ADAMS F.G. & SHIRLEY A.W. (1983) Factors influencing bone scan quality. *Europ. J. nucl. Med.* 8, 436–9.

ALAZRAKI N. (1981) Bone imaging by radionuclide techniques. In *Diagnosis of Bone and Joint Disorders* (eds. Resnick D. & Niwayama G.), p. 670. Philadelphia: Saunders.

ALAZRAKI N.P., FIERER J. & RESNICK D. (1978) The role of gallium and bone scanning in monitoring response to therapy in chronic osteomyelitis. *J. nucl. Med.* 19, 696.

ALEXANDER J.L., GILLESPIE P.J. & EDELSTYN G. (1976) Serial bone scanning using technetium-99m diphosphonate in patients undergoing cyclic combination chemotherapy for advanced breast cancer. *Clin. nucl. Med.* 1, 13–17.

ARNT J.W., PAUWELS E.K.J., CAMPS J.A.J. & HEIDEMA J. (1985) Clinical differences between bone-seeking agents. *Europ. J. nucl. Med.* 11, 330.

ASH J.M. & GILDAY D.L. (1980) Futility of bone scanning in neonatal osteomyelitis. *J. nucl. Med.* 21, 417–20.

BAUER G., WEBER D.A., CEDER L., DARTE L., EGUND N., HANSSON L.I. & STRÖMQVIST B. (1980) Dynamics of technetium-99m methylene diphosphonate imaging of the femoral head after hip fracture. *Clin Orthop.* 152, 85–92.

BERKOWITZ I.D. & WENZEL W. (1980) 'Normal' technetium bone scans in patients with acute osteomyelitis. *Amer. J. Dis. Child.* 134, 828–30.

BITRAN J.D., BEKERMAN C. & DESSER R.K. (1980) The predictive value of serial bone scans in assessing response to chemotherapy in advanced breast cancer. *Cancer* 45, 1562–8.

BUDINGER T. (1977) Instrumentation trends in nuclear medicine. *Semin. nucl. Med.* 7, 285–97.

CHAFETZ N., SLIVKA J., TAYLOR A., ALAZRAKI N.P., RESNICK D. & GOERGEN T. (1978) Decreased $^{99}Tc^m$–sulfur colloid activity in healed rib fractures. *Radiology* 126, 735–6.

CHALMERS I.M., LENTLE B.C., PERCY J.S. & RUSSELL A.S. (1979) Sacro-iliitis detected by bone scanning: a clinical, radiological and scintigraphic follow-up study. *Ann. rheum. Dis.* 38, 112–17.

CHARKES N.D. (1979) Mechanisms of skeletal tracer uptake. *J. nucl. Med.* 20, 794–5.

CHARKES N.D. (1980) Skeletal blood flow: implications for bone-scan interpretation. *J. nucl. Med.* 21, 91–8.

CHEW F.S. & HUDSON T.M. (1982) Radionuclide bone scanning of osteosarcoma: falsely extended uptake patterns. *Amer. J. Roentgenol.* 139, 49–54.

CHEW F.S., HUDSON T.M. & ENNEKING W.F. (1981) Radionuclide imaging of soft tissue neoplasms. *Semin. nucl. Med.* 11, 266–76.

CHOY D. & MURRAY I.P.C. (1980) Metastatic visceral calcification identified by bone scanning. *Skeletal Radiol.* 5, 151–9.

CITRIN D.L., BESSENT R.G., TUOHY J.B. & GREIG W.R. (1974) Quantitative bone scanning: a method for assessing response of bone metastases to treatment. *Lancet* 1, 1132–3.

CITRIN D.L., BESSENT R.G. & GREIG W.R. (1977) A comparison of the sensitivity and accuracy of the $^{99}Tc^m$-phosphate bone scan and skeletal radiograph in the diagnosis of bone metastases. *Clin. Radiol.* 28, 107–17.

CITRIN D.L., HOUGEN C., ZWEIBEL W., SCHLISE S., PRUITT B., ERSCHLER W., DAVIS T.E., HARBERG J. & COHEN A.I. (1981) The use of serial bone scans in assessing response of bone metastases to systemic treatment. *Cancer* 47, 680–5.

COLEMAN R.E., SAMUELSON C.O., BAIM S., CHRISTIAN P.E. & WARD J.R. (1982) Imaging with $^{99}Tc^m$-MDP and ^{67}Ga citrate in patients with rheumatoid arthritis and suspected septic arthritis. *J. nucl. Med.* 23, 479–82.

CORCORAN R.J., THRALL J.H., KYLE R.W., KAMINSKY R.J. & JOHNSON M.C. (1976) Solitary abnormalities in bone scans of patients with extraosseous malignancies. *Radiology* 121, 663.

DANIGELIS J.A. (1976) Pinhole imaging in Legg–Perthes disease: further observations. *Semin. nucl. Med.* 5, 69–82.

DE ROSSI G., FOCACCI C. & CATINO A. (1979) The particular usefulness of radioisotope methods in some benign bone diseases. *Europ. J. nucl. Med.* 4, 203–6.

DESAI A., ALAVI A., DALINKA M.K., BRIGHTON C. & ESTERHAI J. (1980) Role of bone scintigraphy in the evaluation and treatment of non-united fractures: concise communication. *J. nucl. Med.* 21, 931–4.

DESAULWIERS S.M., FUKS A., HAWKINS D., LACOURCIERE J. & ROSENTHALL L. (1974) Radiotechnetium polyphosphate joint imaging. *J. nucl. Med.* 15, 417–23.

DE SMET A.A., KUHNS L.R., KAUFMAN R.A. & HOLT J.F. (1977) Bony sclerosis and the battered child. *Skeletal Radiol.* 2. 39–41.

DEUTSCH S.D., GANDSMAN E.J. & SPRARAGEN S.C. (1981) Quantitative regional blood-flow analysis and its clinical application during routine bone scanning. *J. Bone Jt Surg.* 63A, 295–305.

DÖGE H., JOHANNSEN B.A. & HENNIG K. (1977) Fehler möglichkeiten bei der Interpretation der knochen szintigramme mit $^{99}Tc^m$–diphosphonat. *Roefo. Fortschr. Röntgenstr.* 126, 251–7.

ENNEKING W.F., EADY J.L. & BURCHARDT H. (1980) Autogenous cortical bone grafts in the reconstruction of segmental skeletal defects. *J. Bone Jt Surg.* 62A, 1039–58.

FEITH R., SLOOFF T.J.J.H., KAZEM I. & VAN RENS TH.J.G. (1976) Strontium-87m bone scanning for the evaluation of total hip replacement. *J. Bone Jt Surg.* **58B**, 79–83.

FIHN S.D., LARSON F.H., NELP W.B., RUDD T.G. & GERBER F.H. (1984) Should single phase radionuclide imaging be used in suspected osteomyelitis? *J. nucl. Med.* **25**, 2080–8.

FINK-BENNET D. & VICUNA-RIOS J. (1980) The deltoid tuberosity—a potential pitfall (the 'delta-sign') in bone scan interpretation: concise communication. *J. nucl. Med.* **21**, 211–12.

FOGELMAN I. & BESSENT R. (1982) Age related alterations in skeletal metabolism—24 hr whole body retention of diphosphonate in 250 normal subjects: concise communication. *J. nucl. Med.* **23**, 296–300.

FOGELMAN I., MCKILLOP J.H., GREIG W.R. & BOYLE I.T. (1977) Pseudo-fractures of the ribs detected by bone scanning. *J. nucl. Med.* **18**, 1236.

FOGELMAN I., MCKILLOP J.H., BESSENT R.G., BOYLE C.T., TURNER J.G. & GREIG W. (1978) The role of bone scanning in osteomalacia. *J. nucl. Med.* **19**, 245.

FOGELMAN I., CITRIN D.L. & MCKILLOP J.H. (1979a) A clinical comparison of $^{99}Tc^m$ HEDP and $^{99}THc^m$ MDP in the detection of bone metastases: concise communication. *J. nucl. Med.* **20**, 98–101.

FOGELMAN I., CITRIN D.L., TURNER J.G., HAY I.D., BESSENT R.G. & BOYLE I.T. (1979b) Semi-quantitative interpretation of the bone scan in metabolic bone disease. *Europ. J. nucl. Med.* **4**, 287–9.

FOGELMAN I., PEARSON D.W., BESSENT R.G., TOFE A.J. & FRANCIS M.D. (1981) A comparison of skeletal uptakes of three diphosphonates by whole-body retention: concise communication. *J. nucl. Med.* **22**, 880–3.

FORSTED D.L., DALINKA M.K., MITCHELL E., BRIGHTON C.T. & ALAVI A. (1978) Radiologic evaluation of the treatment of non-union of fractures by electrical stimulation. *Radiology* **128**, 629–34.

FOTTER R., LAMMER J. & RITTER G. (1982) Szintigraphische 5-Jahre-Studie bei Kindern mit M. Perthes. *Roefo. Fortschr. Röntgenstr.* **137**, 141–6.

FRANKEL R.S., JOHNSON K.W. & MABRY J.J. (1974a) 'Normal' bone radionuclide image with diffuse skeletal lymphoma. *Radiology* **111**, 365–6.

FRANKEL R.S. (1974b) Clinical correlation of gallium-67, and skeletal whole body radionuclide studies with radiography in Ewing sarcoma. *Radiology* **110**, 597.

FRONT D., SCHNECK S.D., FRANKEL A. & ROBINSON E. (1979) Bone metastases and bone pain in breast cancer, are they closely associated? *J. Amer. med. Ass.* **242**, 1747–8.

GANEL A., ENGEL J., OSTER Z. & FARINE I. (1979) Bone scanning in assessment of fractures of the scaphoid. *J. Hand Surg.* **4**, 540–3.

GATES G.F. (1979) The gallium 'bone scan' in acute leukemia. *J. nucl. Med.* **20**, 854–6.

GELFAND M.J., STRIFE J.L. & KEREIAKES J.G. (1981) Radionuclide bone imaging in spondylolysis of the lumbar spine in children. *Radiology* **140**, 191–5.

GELMAN M.I., COLEMAN R.E., STEVENS P.M. & DAVEY B.W. (1978) Radiography, radionuclide imaging and arthrography in the evaluation of total hip and knee replacement. *Radiology* **128**, 677–82.

GESLIEN G.E., THRALL J.H., ESPINOSA J.L. & OLDER R.A.

(1976) Early detection of stress fractures using $^{99}Tc^m$-polyphosphate. *Radiology* **121**, 683–7.

GHAED N., THRALL J.J., PINSKY S.M. & JOHNSON M.C. (1974) Detection of extraosseous metastases from osteosarcoma with $^{99}Tc^m$-polyphosphate bone scanning. *Radiology* **112**, 373–5.

GILDAY D.L. & ASH J.M. (1976) Benign bone tumors. *Semin. nucl. Med.* **6**, 33–46.

GILDAY D.L., PAUL D.J. & PATERSON J. (1975) Diagnosis of osteomyelitis in children by combined blood pool and bone imaging. *Radiology* **117**, 331–5.

GILDAY D.L., ASH J.H. & REILLY B.J. (1976) Radionuclide skeletal survey for paediatric neoplasms. *Radiology* **123**, 399.

GOLDBERG R.P., GENANT H.K., SHIMSHAK R. & SHAMES D. (1978) Applications and limitations of quantitative sacroiliac joint scintigraphy. *Radiology* **128**, 683–6.

GOLDSTEIN H., MCNEIL B.J., ZUFALL E. & TREVES S. (1980a) Is there still a place for bone scanning in Ewing's sarcoma? *J. nucl. Med.* **21**, 10–12.

GOLDSTEIN H., MCNEIL B.J., ZUFALL E., JAFFE N. & TREVES S. (1980b) Changing indications for bone scintigraphy in patients with osteosarcoma. *Radiology* **135**, 177–80.

GOLUBOFF N., CRAM R., RAMGOTHA B., SINGH A. & WILKINSON G.W. (1978) Polyarthritis and bone lesions complicating traumatic pancreatitis in two children. *CMA Journal* **118**, 924–8.

GRAMES G.M., JANSEN C., CARLSEN E.N. & DAVIDSON T.R. (1975) The abnormal bone scan in intra-cranial lesions. *Radiology* **115**, 129–34.

GREGG P.J. & WALDER D.N. (1980) Scintigraphy versus radiography in the early diagnosis of experimental bone necrosis. *J Bone Jt Surg.* **62B**, 214–21.

GREGG P.J. & WALDER D.N. (1981) A study of old lesions of caisson disease of bone by radiography and bone scintigraphy. *J. Bone Jt Surg.* **63B**, 132–7.

GREIFF J. (1981) Bone healing in rabbits after compression osteosynthesis, studied by $^{99}Tc^m$ (Sn) polyphosphate scintimetry and autoradiography. *J. nucl. Med.* **22**, 693–8.

GREYSON N.D. & PANG S. (1981) The variable bone scan appearance of non-osteogenic fibroma of bone. *Clin. nucl. Med.* **6**, 242–5.

HAASE G.M., ORTIZ V.N., SFAKIANAKIS G.N. & MORSE T.S. (1980) The value of radionuclide bone scanning in the early recognition of deliberate child abuse. *J. Trauma* **20**, 873–5.

HALL F.M., GOLDBERG R.P., DAVIES J.A.K. & FAINSINGER M.H. (1980) Scintigraphic assessment of bone islands. *Radiology* **135**, 737–42.

HANDMAKER H. (1980) Acute hematogenous osteomyelitis: has the bone scan betrayed us? *Radiology* **135**, 787–9.

HANDMAKER H. & LEONARDS R. (1976) The bone scan in inflammatory osseous disease. *Semin. nucl. Med.* **6**, 75–105.

HARBERT J. & DESAI R. (1985) Small calvarial bone scan foci—normal variations. *J. nucl. Med.* **26**, 1144–8.

HAYES R.L. (1978) The medical use of gallium radionuclides: a brief history with some comments. *Semin. nucl. Med.* **8**, 183–91.

HOEFNAGEL C.A., BRUNING P.F., COHEN P., MARCUSE H.R. & VAN DER SCHOOT J.B. (1981) Detection of lung metastases from osteosarcoma by scintigraphy using $^{99}Tc^m$-methylene diphosphonate. *Diagn. Imaging* **50**, 277–84.

HOFFER P.B. (1980a) Status of gallium-67 in tumor detection. *J. nucl. Med.* 21, 394–8.

HOFFER P.B. (1980b) Gallium and infection. *J. nucl. Med.* 21, 484–8.

HOFFER P.B. & GENANT H.K. (1976) Radionuclide joint imaging. *Semin. nucl. Med.* 6, 121–37.

HOFFER P.B. & PRINCENTHAL R. (1981) Scintigraphy in inflammatory osseous disease. In *Bone Scintigraphy* (eds. Pauwels E.K.J., Schütte H.E. & Taconis W.K.), pp. 53–8. The Hague: Martinus Nijhoff.

HORTOBAGYI G.N., LIBSHITZ H.I. & SEABOLD J.E. (1984) Osseous metastases of breast cancer: clinical, biochemical, radiographical and scintigraphical evaluation of response to therapy. *Skeletal Radiol.* 10, 137–46.

HUGHES S.P.F. (1980) Radionuclides in orthopaedic surgery. *J. Bone Jt Surg.* 62B, 141–50.

HUGHES S.P.F., DAVIES D.R., BASSINGTHWAIHTE J.B., KNOX F. & KELLY P.J. (1977) Bone extraction and blood clearance of diphosphonate in the dog. *Amer. J. Physiol.* 232, H341.

HUGHES S.P.F., LEMON G., DAVIES D.R., BASSINGTHWAITE J.B. & KELLY P.J. (1979) Extraction of minerals after experimental fracture of the tibia in dogs. *J. Bone Jt Surg.* 61A, 852–66.

HUMPHRY A., GILDAY D.L. & BROWN R.G. (1980) Bone scintigraphy in chondroblastoma. *Radiology* 137, 497–9.

HUNTER J.C., HATTNER R.S., MURRAY W.R. & GENANT H.K. (1980) Loosening of the total knee arthroplasty: detection by radionuclide bone scanning. *Amer J. Roentgenol.* 135, 131–6.

JOHNSON R.J. & GARVIC N. (1980) Case report 121. Synovial sarcoma. *Skeletal Radiol.* 5, 185–7.

KIPPER M.S., ALAZRAKI N.P. & FEIGLIN D.H. (1982) The 'hot' patella. *Clin. nucl. Med.* 7, 28–32.

KIRCHNER P.T. & SIMON K.A. (1981) Radio isotope evaluation of skeletal disease. *J. Bone Jt Surg.* 4, 673–81.

KNISELEY R.M. (1972) Marrow studies with radiocolloids. *Semin. nucl. Med.* 2, 71–86.

KOBER B., HERMANN H.J. & WETZEL C. (1979) 'Cold spots' in bone scintigraphy. *Roefo. Fortschr. Rontgenstr.* 131, 545–9.

KRISHNAMURTHY G.T., TUBIS M., HISS J. *et al.* (1977) Distribution pattern of metastatic bone disease: a need for total body skeletal image. *J. Amer. med. Ass.* 237, 2504.

KRISHNAMURTHY G.T., HUEBOTTER R.J., TUBIS M. & BLAHD W.H. (1976) Pharmacokinetics of current skeletal-seeking radiopharmaceuticals. *Amer. J. Roentgenol.* 126, 293–301.

LAMONT R.L., MUZ J., HEILBRONNER D. & BOUWHUIS J.A. (1981) Quantitative assessment of femoral head involvement in Legg–Calvé–Perthes' disease. *J. Bone Jt Surg.* 63A, 746–52.

LECKLITNER M.L., ROSEN P.R. & NUZYNOWITZ M.L. (1981) Nuclear medicine in the diagnosis and treatment of cancer. *Semin. Family Med.* 2, 279–88.

LEE YEU-TSU N. (1981) Bone scanning in patients with early breast carcinoma: should it be a routine staging procedure? *Cancer* 47, 486–95.

LISBONA R. & ROSENTHALL L. (1977) Radionuclide imaging of septic joints and their differentiation from periarticular osteomyelitis and cellulitis in pediatrics. *Clin. nucl. Med.* 2, 337–43.

LODWICK G.S. (1971) *The Bones and Joints.* Chicago: Year Book Medical Publishers.

LOEFFLER R.K., DISIMONE R.N. & HOWLAND W.J. (1975) Limitations of bone scanning in clinical oncology. *J. Amer. med. Ass.* 234, 1228–32.

LOPEZ-MAJANO V. & MISKEW D.B.W. (1980) Sacro-iliac joint disease in drug abusers. The role of bone scintigraphy. *Europ. J. nucl. Med.* 5, 459–63.

McCARTHY I.D. & HUGHES S.P.F. (1983) The role of skeletal blood flow in determining the uptake of $^{99}Tc^m$ methylene diphosphonate. *Calcif. Tiss. Int.* 35, 508–11.

McCARTHY D.J., POLCYN R.E. & COLLINS P.A. (1970) $^{99}Tc^m$ technetium scintiphotography in arthritis. II Non-specificity and chemical and roentgenographic correlations in rheumatoid arthritis. *Arthr. and Rheum.* 13, 21–32.

McDOUGALL I.R. & PISTENMA D.A. (1974) Concentration of $^{99}Tc^m$ diphosphonate in breast tissue. *Radiology* 112, 655–7.

McINERNEY D.P. & HYDE I.D. (1978) Technetium $^{99}Tc^m$ pyrophosphate scanning in the assessment of the painful hip prosthesis. *Clin. Radiol.* 29, 513–17.

McMASTER J. & MERRICK M.V. (1980) Scintigraphic assessment of the scoliotic spine after fusion. *J. Bone Jt Surg.* 62B, 65–72.

McNEIL B.J. (1978) Rationale for the use of bone scans in selected metastatic and primary tumors. *Semin. nucl. Med.* 8, 336.

McNEIL B.J. & POLAK J.F. (1981) An update on the rationale for the use of bone scans in selected metastatic and primary bone tumors. In *Bone Scintigraphy* (eds. Pauwels E.K.J., Schütte H.E. & Taconis W.K.), pp. 187–207. The Hague: Martinus Nijhoff.

MAHER F.T. (1975) Evaluation of renal and urinary tract abnormalities noted on scintiscans: a retrospective study of 1711 radioisotope skeletal surveys. *Mayo Clin. Proc.* 50, 370.

MAJD M. (1978) Bone scintigraphy in children with obscure skeletal pain. *Ann. Radiol.* 22, 85–95.

MAJD M. & FRANKEL R.S. (1976) Radionuclide imaging in skeletal inflammatory and ischemic disease in children. *Amer. J. Roentgenol.* 126, 832–41.

MALL J.C., BEKERMAN C., HOFFER P.B. & GOTTSCHALK A. (1976) A unified radiological approach to the detection of skeletal metastases. *Radiology* 118, 323–8.

MALLENS W.M.C., PAUWELS E.K.J. & TETTEROO Q.F. (1977) Bone scintigraphy as a guide to the diagnosis of osteoid osteoma. *Radiol. clin.* 46, 300–6.

MARTINDALE A.A., PAPADIMITRION J.M. & TURNER J.M. (1980) Technetium-99m antimony colloid for bone marrow imaging. *J. nucl. Med.* 21, 1035–41.

MARTY R., DENNEY J.D., McKAMEY M.R. & ROWLEY M.J. (1976) Bone trauma and related benign disease: assessment by bone scanning. *Semin. nucl. Med.* 6, 107–20.

MATIN PH. (1979) The appearance of bone scans following fractures, including immediate and long-term studies. *J. nucl. Med.* 20, 1227–31.

MAURER A.H., CHEN D.C.P., CAMARGO E.E., WONG D.F., WAGNER H.N. & ALDERSON P.O. (1981) Utility of three-phase skeletal scintigraphy in suspected osteomyelitis: concise communication. *J. nucl. Med.* 22, 941–9.

MERRICK M.V., GORDON-SMITH E.C. & LAVENDER J.P. (1975) A comparison of ^{111}indium with ^{52}Fe and $^{99}Tc^m$ sulfur colloid for bone marrow scanning. *J. nucl. Med.* 16, 66–8.

MERTEN D.F., RADKOWSKY M.A. & LEONIDAS J.C. (1983) The abused child: a radiological reappraisal. *Radiology* **146**, 377–81.

MEURMAN K.D.A. & ELFVING S. (1980) Stress fractures in soldiers: multifocal bone disorders, comparative radiologic and scintigraphic study. *Radiology* **134**, 483–7.

MEYERS M.H., TELFER N. & MOORE T.M. (1977) Determination of vascularity of the femoral head with technetium-99m–sulfur colloid: diagnostic and prognostic significance. *J. Bone Jt Surg.* **59A**, 658–64.

MOORE W.S., HENRY R.E., MALONE J.M., DAKY M.J., PATTON D. & CHILDERS S.J. (1981) Prospective use of xenon-133 clearance for amputation level selection. *Arch. Surg.* **116**, 86–8.

MUHEIM G., DONATH A. & ROSSIER A.B. (1973) Serial scintigrams in the course of ectopic bone formation in paraplegic patients. *Amer. J. Roentgenol.* **118**, 865–9.

MUROFF L.R. (1981) Optimizing the performance and interpretation of bone scans. *Clin. nucl. Med.* **10S**, 68–76.

MURRAY I.P.C. (1980) Bone scanning in the child and young adult (parts 1 and 2). *Skeletal Radiol.* **5**, 1–14 and 65–78.

MURRAY W.R. & RODRIGO J.J. (1975) Arthrography for the assessment of pain after total hip replacement. *J. Bone Jt Surg.* **57A**, 1060–5.

NELSON H.T. & TAYLOR A. (1978) Bone scanning in the diagnosis of osteomyelitis. *J. nucl. Med.* **19**, 696.

NIELSEN P.T., HEDEBOE J. & THOMMESEN P. (1983) Bone scintigraphy in the evaluation of fracture of the carpal scaphoid bone. *Acta orthop. scand.* **54**, 303–6.

NORRIS S.H. & WATT L. (1981) Radionuclide uptake during the evolution of experimental acute osteomyelitis. *Brit. J. Radiol.* **54**, 207–11.

OPPENHEIM B.E. & CANTEZ S. (1977) What causes lower neck uptake in bone scans? *Radiology* **124**, 749–52.

PABST H.W., LANGHAMMER H., SCHMID L. & SINTERMANN R. (1981) Skelettszintigraphische Verlaufs- und Therapiekontrolle beim Prostata karzinompatienten. *Roefo. Fortschr. Rontgenstr.* **135**, 44–9.

PARK W.M., SPENCER D.G., McCALL I.W., WARD D.J., BUCHANAN W.W. & STEPHENS W.H. (1981) The detection of spinal pseudarthrosis in ankylosing spondylitis. *Brit. J. Radiol.* **54**, 467–72.

PARK H.N., WHEAT J., SIDDIQUI A.R., BURT R.N., ROBB J.A., RANSBURG R.C. & KERNEK C.B. (1982) Scintigraphic evaluation of diabetic osteomyelitis. *J. nucl. Med.* **23**, 569–73.

PAUWELS E.K.H., HESLINGA J.M. & ZWAVELING A. (1982) Value of pre-treatment and follow-up skeletal scintigraphy in operable breast cancer. *Clin. Oncol.* **8**, 25–32.

PEARLMAN A.W. (1977) Pre-operative evaluation of liposarcoma by nuclear imaging. *Clin. nucl. Med.* **2**, 47–51.

PISTENMA D.A., McDOUGALL I.R. & KRISS J.P. (1975) Screening for bone metastases, are only scans necessary? *J. Amer. med. Ass.* **231**, 46–50.

RESNICK D., WILLIAMSON S. & ALAZRAKI N. (1981) Focal spinal abnormalities on bone scans in ankylosing spondylitis: a clue to the presence of fractures or pseudoarthrosis. *Clin. nucl. Med.* **6**, 213–17.

ROLFE E.B., GARVIE N.W., KHAN M.A. & ACKERY D.M. (1981) Isotope bone imaging in suspected scaphoid trauma. *Brit. J. Radiol.* **54**, 762–7.

ROLLO F.O. (1981) An intelligent approach to the selection of imaging equipment. *Clin. nucl. Med.* **105**, 16–18.

ROSENTHALL L., ARZOUMANIAN A. & LISBONA R. (1977) A longitudinal comparison of the kinetics of ^{99}Tc^m-MDP and ^{99}Tc^m-HEDP in humans. *Clin. nucl. Med.* **2**, 232–4.

ROSENTHALL L., KLOIBER R., DAMTEW B. & AL-MAJID H. (1982) Sequential use of radiophosphate and radiogallium imaging in the differential diagnosis of bone, joint and soft tissue infection: quantitative analysis. *Diagn. Imaging* **51**, 249–58.

ROUB L.W., GUMERMAN L.W., HANLEY E.N., WILLIAMS CLARK M., GOODMAN M. & HERBERT D.L. (1979) Bone stress: radionuclide imaging perspective. *Radiology* **132**, 431–8.

RÖVEKAMP M.H., VAN ROYEN E.A., REINDERS FOLMER S.C.C. & RAAYMAKERS E.L.F.B. (1984) Indium-111 labelled leucocyte scintigraphy after hip surgery. In *Blood Cells in Nuclear Medicine, Part I* (eds. Hardeman D & Najean). The Hague: Martinus Nijhoff.

RUDD T.G., ALLEN D.R. & SMITH F.O. (1979) Technetium-99^m-labelled methylene diphosphonate—biological and clinical comparisons. *J. nucl. Med.* **8**, 821–6.

SCHAFFER D.L. & PENDERGRASS H.P. (1976) Comparison of enzyme, radiographic and radionuclide methods of detecting bone metastases from carcinoma of the prostate. *Radiology* **121**, 431–4.

SCHAUWECKER D.S., PARK HEE-MYUNG, MOCK B.H., BURT R.W., KERNICK C.B., RUOFF R.W., SINN H.J. & WELLMAN H.N. (1984) Evaluation of complicating osteomyelitis with ^{99}Tc^m MDP, ^{111}In granulocytes and ^{67}Ga citrate. *J. nucl. Med.* **25**, 849–53.

SCHÜTTE H.E. (1979) The influence of bone pain on the results of bone scans. *Cancer* **44**, 2039–43.

SCHÜTTE H.E. (1981) A radiological approach to metastatic bone disease. In *Bone Scintigraphy* (eds. Pauwels E.K.J., Schütte H.E. & Taconis W.K.). The Hague: Martinus Nijhoff.

SCHÜTTE H.E. & PARK W.M. (1983) The diagnostic value of bone scintigraphy in patients with low back pain. *Skeletal Radiol.* **10**, 1–4.

SERAFINI A.N. (1976) Paget's disease of bone. *Semin. nucl. Med.* **6**, 47–58.

SHAFER R.B. & REINKE D.B. (1977) Contribution of the bone scan, serum acid and alkaline phosphatase, and the radiographic bone survey to the management of newly diagnosed carcinoma of the prostate. *Clin. nucl. Med.* **2**, 200–3.

SHAH P.J., SHREEVE W.W. & NARAYAMA MURTHY B. (1981) Iatrogenic rupture of urinary bladder: incidental finding on bone scan. *J. nucl. Med.* **22**, 564–5.

SHEARMAN J., ESDAILE J., HAWKINS D. & ROSENTHALL L. (1982) Predictive value of radionuclide joint scintigrams. *Arthr. and Rheum.* **25**, 83–6.

SHIRAZI P.H., RAYUDU G.V.S. & FORDHAM E.W. (1974a) ^{18}F bone scanning: review of indications and results of 1500 scans. *Radiology* **112**, 361–8.

SHIRAZI P.H., RAYUDU G.V.S. & FORDHAM E.W. (1974b) Bone scanning in evaluation of Paget's disease of bone. *Crit. clin. Radiol. nucl. Med.* **5**, 523.

SILBERSTEIN E.B. (1980) Nuclear orthopedics. *J. nucl. Med.* **21**, 997–9.

SILBERSTEIN E.B., SAENGER E.L., TOFE A.J., ALEXANDER G.W. & PARK HEE-MYUNG (1973) Imaging of bone metastases with $^{99}Tc^m$-Sn-EHDP (diphosphonate), ^{18}F, and skeletal radiography. *Radiology* 107, 551–5.

SINGH B.N., KESALA B.A., MEHTA S.P. & QUINN J.L. (1977) Osteomalacia on bone scan simulating skeletal metastases. *Clin. nucl. Med.* 2, 181.

SKLAROFF R.B. & SKLAROFF D.M. (1976) Bone metastases from breast cancer at the time of radical mastectomy as detected by bone scan: eight-year follow-up. *Cancer* 38, 107–11.

SLOVIS T.L., BERDON W.E., HALLER J.O., BAKER D.H. & ROSEN L. (1975) Pancreatitis and the battered child syndrome. *Amer. J. Roentgenol.* 125, 456.

SMALLEY R.V., MALMUD L.S. & RITCHIE W.G.M. (1980) Pre-operative scanning: evaluation for metastatic disease in carcinoma of the breast, lung, colon, bladder, and prostate. *Semin. Oncol.* 7, 358–69.

SMITH F.W., GILDAY D.L., ASH J.M. & REID R.H. (1980) Primary neuroblastoma uptake of $^{99}Tc^m$ methylene disphosphonate. *Radiology* 137, 501–4.

SPENCER R.P., SZIKLAS J.J., ROSENBERG R., JAE-HWI YOO & WEIDNER F.A. (1981) Hemivertebral 'disappearance' on bone scan. *J. nucl. Med.* 22, 454–6.

STAAB E.B. & McCARTNEY W.H. (1978) Role of gallium 67 in inflammatory disease. *Semin. nucl. Med.* 8, 219–34.

STEVENSON J.S., BRIGHT R.W., DUNSON G.L. & NELSON F.R. (1974) Technetium-99m phosphate bone imaging: a method for assessing bone graft healing. *Radiology* 110, 391.

STY J.R. & STARSHAK R.J. (1983) The role of bone scintigraphy in the evaluation of the suspected abused child. *Radiology* 146, 369–75.

SUBRAMANIAN G., McAFEE J.G., BLAIR R.J. & THOMAS F.D. (1975) An evaluation of $^{99}Tc^m$-labelled phosphate compounds and bone imaging agents. In *Radiopharmaceuticals* (eds. Subramanian G., Rhodes B.A., Cooper J.F. & Sodd V.J.), pp. 319–28. New York: Society of Nuclear Medicine.

SUBRAMANIAN G., McAFEE J.G., THOMAS F.D., FELD T., ZAPF-LONGO C. & PALLADINO E. (1981) Localization of new $^{99}Tc^m$-labelled diphosphonates in experimental bone lesions. Paper presented at the 19th international annual meeting of the Society of Nuclear Medicine Europe in Berne.

SULLIVAN P.C., ROSENFIELD N.S., OGDEN I. & GOTTSCHALK A. (1980) Problems in the scintigraphic detection of osteomyelitis in children. *Radiology* 135, 731–6.

SY W.M. (1981) *Gamma Images in Benign and Metabolic Bone Disease.* Boca Raton: CRC Press.

SY W.M. & MITTAL A.K. (1975) Bone scan in chronic dialysis patients with evidence of secondary hyperparathyroidism and renal osteodystrophy. *Brit. J. Radiol.* 48, 878–84.

SY W.M., WESTRING D.W. & WEINBERGER G. (1975) 'Cold' lesions of bone imaging. *J. nucl. Med.* 16, 1013.

TAILLEFER R., LEVASSEUR A. & ROBILLARD R. (1981) Ga-67 imaging in eosinophilic granuloma. *Clin. nucl. Med.* 6, 270–1.

TEATES C.D. & WILLIAMSON R.J. (1977) 'Hot and cold' bone lesions in acute osteomyelitis. *Amer. J. Roentgenol.* 129, 517–18.

TEHRANZADEH J., SCHNEIDER R. & FREIBERGER R.H. (1981)

Radiological evaluation of painful total hip replacement. *Radiology* 141, 355–62.

TESSLER F., LANDER P. & LISBONA R. (1981) Congenital absence of a pedicle with photon deficiency on bone scan. *Clin. nucl. Med.* 10, 498–9.

THOMAS S.R., GELFAND M.J., KEREIAKES J.G. *et al.* (1978) Dose to the metaphyseal growth complexes in children undergoing $^{99}Tc^m$-EHDP. *Radiology* 126, 193–5.

THRALL J.H., GHAED N., GESLIEN G.E., PINSKY S.M. & JOHNSON M.C. (1974) Pitfalls in $^{99}Tc^m$ polyphosphate skeletal imaging. *Amer. J. Roentgenol.* 121, 739–47.

THRALL J.H., GESLIEN G.E., CORCORAN R.J. & JOHNSON M.C. (1975) Abnormal radionuclide deposition pattern adjacent to focal skeletal lesions. *Radiology* 155, 659–60.

TUMEH A.A., BEADLE G. & KAPLAN W.D. (1985) Clinical significance of solitary rib lesions in patients with extra-skeletal malignancy. *J. nucl. Med.* 26, 1140–3.

VELASCO J.G., VEGA A. & LEISOREK A. (1976) The early detection of free bone graft viability with $^{99}Tc^m$: a preliminary report. *Brit. J. plast. Surg.* 29, 344.

VELLENGA C.J.L.R. (1981) Paget's disease. In *Bone Scintigraphy* (eds. Pauwels E.K.J., Schütte H.E. & Taconis W.K.). The Hague: Martinus Nijhoff.

WAHNER H.W., KYLE R.D. & BEABOUT J.W. (1980) Scintigraphic evaluation of the skeleton in multiple myeloma. *Mayo Clin. Proc.* 55, 739–46.

WAMAN A.D., SIEMSEN J.K., LEVINE A.M., HOLDORF D., SUZUKI R., SINGER F.R. & BATEMAN J. (1981) Radiographic and radionuclide imaging in multiple myeloma. Role of gallium scintigraphy. *J. nucl. Med.* 22, 232–6.

WEISS P.E., MALL J.C., HOFFER P.J., MURRAY W.R., RODRIGO J.J. & GENANT H.K. (1979) $^{99}Tc^m$-methylene diphosphonate bone imaging in evaluation of total hip prosthesis. *Radiology* 133, 727–30.

WEISSBERG D.L., RESNICK D., TAYLOR A., BECKER M. & AL-AZRAKI N. (1978) Rheumatoid arthritis and its variants: analysis of scintiphotographic, radiographic and clinical examinations. *Amer. J. Roentgenol.* 131, 665–73.

WILCOX J.R., MONIOT A.L. & GREEN J.P. (1977) Bone scanning in the evaluation of exercise-related stress injuries. *Radiology* 123, 699–703.

WILLIAMSON R.J., McLAUGHLIN R.E., GWO-JAW WANG, MILLER C.W., TEATES C.D. & BRAY S.T. (1979) Radionuclide bone imaging as a means of differentiating loosening and infection in patients with painful total hip prosthesis. *Radiology* 133, 723–6.

WILSON M.A. (1981) The effect of age on the quality of bone scans using technetium-99m pyrophosphate. *Radiology* 139, 703–5.

WINTER W.A., VERAART B.E.E.M.J. & VERDEGAAL W.P. (1981) Bone scintigraphy in patients with juvenile kyphosis (M. Scheuermann). *Diagn. Imaging* 50, 186–96.

WOLF J.A., TUOMANEN E.I. & GREENBERG I.D. (1980) Radionuclide joint imaging: acute rheumatic fever simulating septic arthritis. *Pediatrics* 63, 339–41.

WOOLFENDEN J.M., PITT M.J., DURIE B.G.M. & MOON T.E. (1980) Comparison of bone scintigraphy and radiography in multiple myeloma. *Radiology* 134, 723–8.

Chapter 4
Computed Tomography of the Musculoskeletal System

H. K. GENANT

Introduction

Impacting across many disciplines, computed tomography (CT) is undoubtedly one of the foremost advances in medical technology today. The rapid development of instrumentation since the introduction of the first scanner less than a decade ago has been discussed (Alfidi *et al.* 1975, Ambrose 1973, Baker *et al.* 1974 and Boyd *et al.* 1977), and today more than 2000 body scanners are in operation worldwide. This chapter summarizes some of the applications of the remarkable technology of CT for the orthopaedic surgeon.

Technology

The origins of CT have been shown to date back many years (Cormack 1963, Kuhl & Edwards 1968, Oldendorf 1961 and Radon 1917) and

Hounsfield has described the development of the first clinically useful brain scanner in 1970 (Hounsfield 1973). The essential components of the CT system are a scanning gantry, X-ray generator, data-processing system, viewing console, and archival storage system. Fig. 4.1 schematically shows image computation and presentation common to all CT scanners as described by Alfidi *et al.* (1975).

The cross-sectional slice, typically 0·2–1·0 cm thick, is divided into numerous small, identical elements of volume. McCullough (1975), Phelps *et al.* (1975) and Rosenfeld *et al.* (1979) have shown how an X-ray attenuation value is determined for each tissue, based on the density and atomic number of the elements within it. These computed values are expressed as CT numbers (or Hounsfield numbers) generally on a scale of -1000 for air, zero for water and $+1000$ for dense bone (Fig. 4.2). For display, the reconstructed slice is regarded as a two-

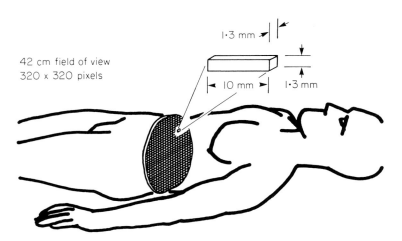

42 cm field of view
320 x 320 pixels

1·3 mm

10 mm

1·3 mm

Fig. 4.1. Schematic representation of image computation and presentation by a typical computed tomography scanner.

dimensional matrix of picture elements (pixels) and represented on a video monitor with varying shades of grey to indicate the CT numbers, the range of which can be chosen by adjusting the width of the window and its level on the monitor. Thus the quantifying and displaying of small differences in tissue density is the unique capability of CT.

Boyd *et al.* (1977), Brooks and DiChiro (1975) and Gordon *et al.* (1970) have reviewed the chronological development of commercial scanners (Fig. 4.3). First-generation brain scanners utilize an X-ray source with a tightly collimated pencil beam focused on a single sodium iodide detector on a gantry that can move transversely and also rotate. The gantry moves laterally (translation) and the beam traverses a narrow path across the subject's head while multiple readings of X-ray intensities are made. At the completion of the first transverse pass, the gantry rotates through a small angle, usually 1°, and the process is repeated through 180°, obtaining and processing a total of several hundred thousand measurements to produce a single cross-sectional image of the head. These scanners are extremely slow, requiring 5–10 minutes per scan image, and are no longer in use.

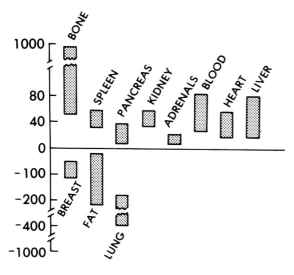

Fig. 4.2. CT number ranges for various tissues.

Second-generation scanners are capable of imaging the body as well as the head and, by using a narrow fan-beam and multiple detectors rather than single ones, have shortened scanning time to 5–20 seconds. The same translate–rotate motion of the gantry is used, but multiple readings are obtained simultaneously and large increments of rotation are employed.

Third-generation scanners are now in wide use. With a broad fan-beam that exposes the entire body with one pulse and a continuous 360° rotatory motion of the gantry, these eliminate the complex translate–rotate motion of earlier models. The fan-beam is focused on a large array of detectors—as many as 600—thus shortening the time for one complete scan to 2–10 seconds, with image reconstruction requiring 10–60 seconds. Fourth-generation scanners utilize a similar rotatory fan-beam but the detection configuration is a stationary ring—these models are also widely available.

TECHNICAL ADVANCES AFFECTING MUSCULOSKELETAL CT

As new technical advances arise and diagnostic CT procedures are upgraded, this imaging modality is becoming more important in assessing musculoskeletal disorders, replacing many conventional techniques as well as invasive or time-consuming procedures. The advantages of CT over conventional radiography have been shown: capability for three-dimensional imaging, excellent contrast resolution, accurate measurement of tissue attenuation coefficient, non-invasive nature and, in many instances, reduced radiation exposure to the patient (Genant *et al.* 1981)—these make CT a powerful tool in the assessment of the musculoskeletal system.

Several scanners currently being marketed have the capability for submillimetre resolving power for high-contrast objects such as bone. Coupled with the use of thin sections (1–3 mm), this means that high-quality images of fine bony structures can readily be obtained. The excellent contrast resolution of CT is approximately 0·3 per cent for most of the newer scanners. This

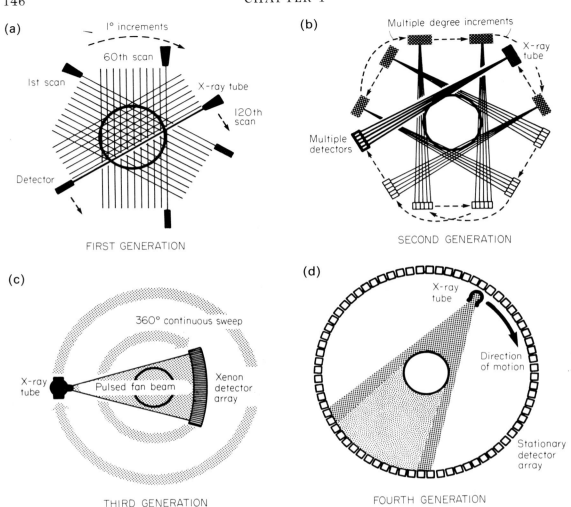

Fig. 4.3. First (a), second (b), third (c) and fourth (d) generation scanners (adapted from General Electric Co. 1976).

has long been recognized as superior to conventional films and is obtained at a radiation dose of 1–3 rads—substantially lower than with older CT models.

The average scanning time of less than five seconds for the newer systems eliminates most of the motion artefacts of older machines. In addition, rapid-sequence scanning in the dynamic mode greatly facilitates the performance of these systems—30–40 contiguous scans are generated in 5–10 minutes. Brown *et al.* (1982) and Reese *et al.* (1981) have shown how dynamic scanning obtains back-to-back scans at

relatively low milliamperage with a 1- to 2-second interscan delay for table incrementation, and Glenn *et al.* (1979) have shown how thereby, for high bone detail, 1- to 3-mm thick contiguous stacked scans provide not only excellent axial images, but also the basis for high-quality sagittal, coronal or multiplanar reformations. Thus CT has supplanted conventional polytomography for delineating subtle structural changes in anatomically complex regions of the skeleton.

In addition, variable algorithms to reconstruct original projection data are now widely available to optimize high-contrast resolving power, low-contrast detectability or other parameters—their particular usefulness for imaging bony structures has been discussed (Genant *et al.* 1981). The use of extended scales (− 1000 to + 3000 HU) permits visualization of the entire range of densities in bone. Computed radiographic localization systems are also widely offered and greatly facilitate studies in musculoskeletal disease (Fig. 4.4). Further, the two-dimensional projection radiograph indexed to the table location can be used to specify precise scanning location and gantry angulation. The best external localization systems provide an accuracy of 0·5–1·0 mm in the table location, so that the limiting factor becomes subject motion between the time the axial scans are done and the time the computed radiograph is obtained.

Thus the combination of projection computed radiography, high-resolution scanning, dynamic rapid-sequence scanning, thin-section capability and multiplanar reformation has created an exciting array of possibilities for CT imaging of the musculoskeletal system.

CLINICAL APPLICATIONS OF MUSCULOSKELETAL CT

A broad experience has been gained in the clinical applications of CT for musculoskeletal diagnoses over the past decade. The major musculoskeletal applications considered in this chapter are assessment of trauma, infection, neoplasms, low back pain syndromes, metabolic bone disease, and miscellaneous disorders—the author's own experience and a review of the literature provide the basis of discussion.

Musculoskeletal neoplasms

The localization of *primary bone tumours* by cross-sectional display (Fig. 4.5), determination of the intramedullary and extraosseous extent of the tumour (Figs. 4.6 & 4.7) and definition of the relationship between tumour and vital structure with CT scanning have been discussed (Genant *et al.* 1981, Wilson *et al.* 1978, Hardy *et al.* 1980, Berger & Kuhn 1978, De Santos *et al.* 1978, Destouet *et al.* 1979, and Schumacher

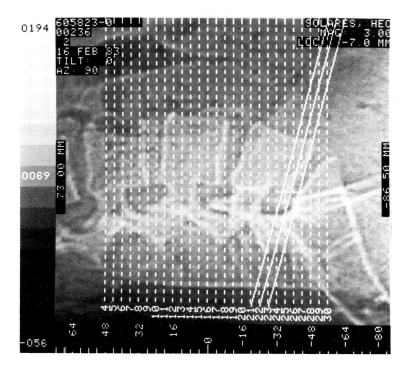

Fig. 4.4. Lateral scout view of the lumbar spine demonstrating a protocol in which 5-mm thick sections are obtained at 3-mm intervals through the neural foramen and intervertebral discs. The gantry is angled selectively to obtain true axial views.

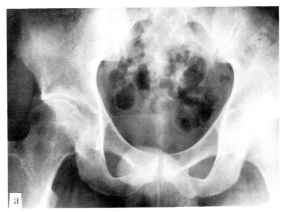

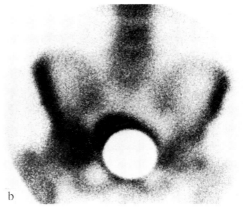

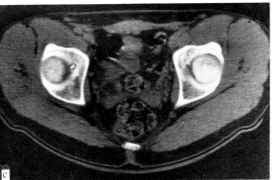

Fig. 4.5. Periarticular demineralization on a conventional radiograph (a) and increased radionuclide uptake in the acetabulum on a bone scan (b). CT scan (c) identifies the nidus of an osteoid osteoma and defines its position in the acetabulum, thereby facilitating surgical resection.

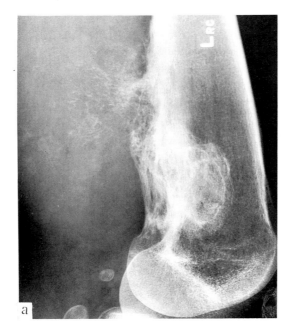

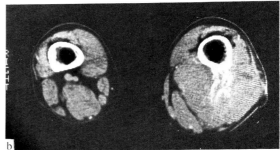

Fig. 4.6. (a) Lateral magnification radiograph of the left knee demonstrates a blastic sclerotic process involving the distal femoral metaphysis associated with aggressive periosteal reaction and a large soft-tissue mass. (b) CT scan defines the borders of the large soft-tissue component and was also useful in defining the intraosseous extent of involvement in this osteosarcoma.

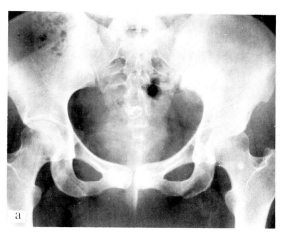

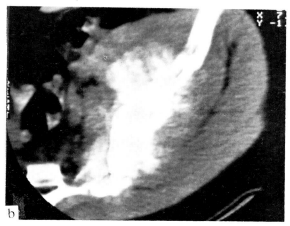

Fig. 4.7.   (a) A conventional radiograph of the pelvis of a young adult reveals mixed sclerosis and destruction of the left ilium. (b) CT scans reveal osteoblastic activity with destruction of the ilium accompanied by a large soft-tissue mass, suggesting osteosarcoma. In this case, the CT study yielded important diagnostic, prognostic and therapeutic information.

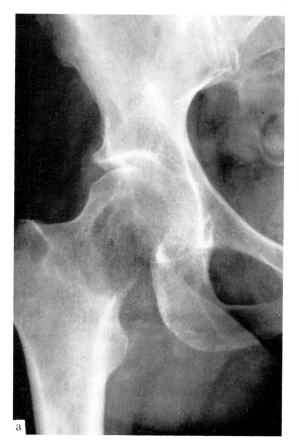

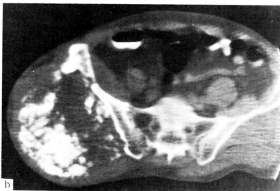

Fig. 4.8.   (a) Conventional radiograph demonstrates a lytic destructive process involving the medial aspect of the femoral head and neck. (b) CT scans demonstrate the intraosseous rather than intra-articular nature of this process and show several foci of dystrophic calcification and a mass lesion that is principally isodense with muscle. A fibrosarcoma was proved at biopsy.

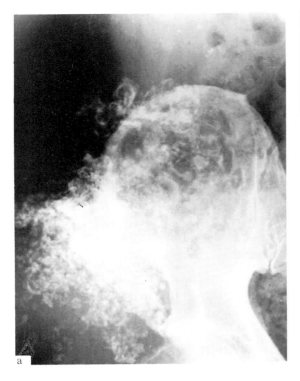

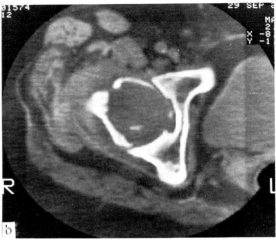

Fig. 4.9. (a) A densely calcified cartilaginous mass in the region of the right buttock. (b) The CT scan accurately defines the extent of this chondrosarcoma and reveals erosion of the ilium. A soft-tissue mass beyond the calcified portion of the mass is invading the inner pelvic wall.

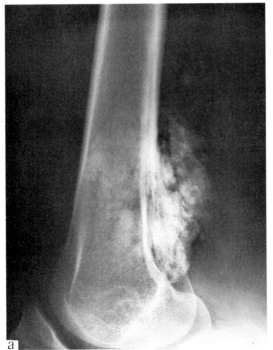

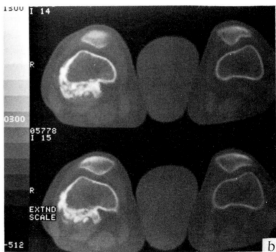

Fig. 4.10. (a) A lateral radiograph demonstrates a large ossifying mass encircling the posterior cortex of the distal femur. (b) CT scans demonstrate the intimate relationship of the ossifying mass to the underlying cortex as well as the sparing of the medullary space, supporting a diagnosis of parosteal sarcoma and bearing prognostic significance.

et al. 1978). Such assessment may have diagnostic or prognostic significance, i.e. differentiating a solid lesion from a cystic lesion, demonstrating tumour invasion beyond the cortical confines (Fig. 4.8) or revealing a soft-tissue mass outside the ossified or calcified portions of a tumour, thereby suggesting malignancy (Fig. 4.9). Of greater importance are the therapeutic implications of CT. For example, in the preoperative assessment of exophytic bony masses, CT may help to define the base of the lesion and its relationship to underlying bone (Figs. 4.10 & 4.11), indicate whether enough bone will remain after resection to preserve structural integrity, and identify vascular structures and possible vessel entrapment within the tumour. Finally, CT assessment may be important in evaluating benign but locally aggressive neoplasms to define tumour borders when the surgeon is considering an allograft or a custom prosthesis.

The superiority of CT in assessing *soft-tissue tumours* has been well established (Genant *et al.* 1981, Wilson *et al.* 1978, Berger & Kuhn 1978, Genant *et al.* 1980, Hunter *et al.* 1979 and Termote *et al.* 1980)—it not only determines the location and extent of the process but often provides a specific diagnosis (Fig. 4.12). Hunter *et al.* (1979) have shown how, for example, a sharply marginated, homogeneous, low-density mass with a CT number comparable to that of subcutaneous fat is diagnostic of lipoma (Figs.

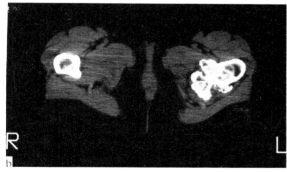

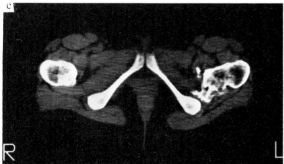

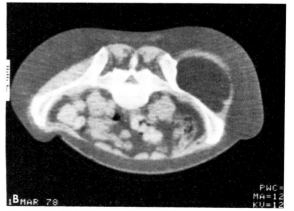

Fig. 4.11. (a) A conventional radiograph demonstrates a deforming osteochondroma involving the proximal femur. (b) and (c) CT scans demonstrate the exact relationship of the stalk of the osteochondroma to the shaft of the femur, the proximity of the calcified cap to the ischium, and the absence of a significant soft-tissue mass, suggesting benignancy.

Fig. 4.12. Gluteal mass with a density comparable to subcutaneous fat, characteristic of a benign lipoma.

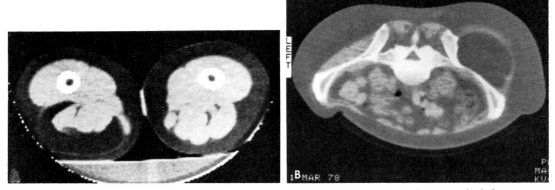

Fig. 4.13. CT reveals sharply marginated, homogeneous, low-density, soft-tissue masses of posterior thigh diagnostic of lipoma.

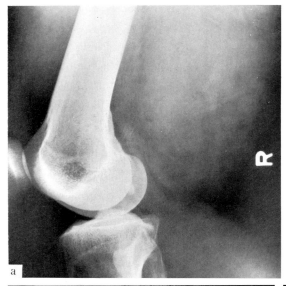

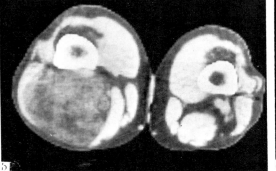

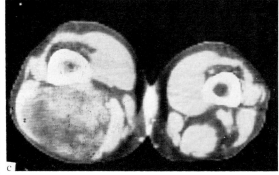

Fig. 4.14. (a) A radiograph demonstrates a bulky mass with areas of low density in the right popiteal fossa. (b) A CT scan (without contrast) reveals a large, inhomogeneous mass of overall low density located between the semimembranosus and semitendinosus muscles. (c) Following intravenous contrast, areas of higher density corresponding to vascular elements are noted within the mass.

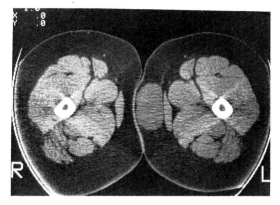

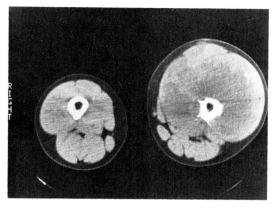

Fig. 4.15. CT scan through the proximal thighs demonstrates a well-defined, smoothly marginated, homogeneous, soft-tissue mass with a density slightly lower than that of adjacent muscle but well above that of subcutaneous fat. Precise localization by CT was helpful in planning surgical excision for this fibrous histiocytoma.

Fig. 4.16. CT scan shows a multilobulated, mixed-density soft-tissue mass with underlying bone involvement. The proximal borders of the tumour were identified in other planes, facilitating surgical planning for this malignant fibrous hystiocytoma.

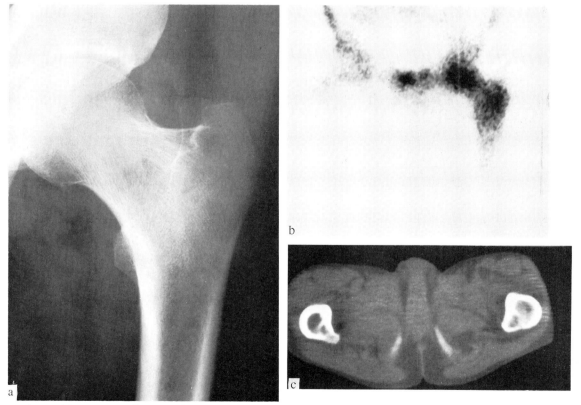

Fig. 4.17. (a) A patient with suspected metastatic disease has a normal conventional radiograph of the femur but focally increased activity on bone scan (b) in the proximal femur. (c) CT scan shows ipsilateral increased density of the medullary canal, strongly supporting a diagnosis of a metastatic focus.

4.12 & 4.13), whereas a poorly marginated, in-homogeneous mass or a mass that contains fat as well as higher density regions that enhance with contrast indicates a liposarcoma (Fig. 4.14), and how CT is largely replacing arterio-graphy for defining the boundaries of soft-tissue masses and determining their vascularity. Even lesions that are isodense with muscle (such as desmoid tumours) can be demonstrated if they are surrounded by fat (Fig. 4.15) or produce sufficient anatomic displacement (Fig. 4.16).

Locally recurrent neoplasms are best evaluated by CT scanning. When a tumour cannot be completely resected, or when local recurrence of an aggressive tumour is likely, a baseline post-operative study may be performed. CT can then be used to identify and serially assess recurrent disease.

Finally, the use of CT to evaluate *skeletal metastases* has been demonstrated (Genant *et al.* 1981, Wilson *et al.* 1978 and Helms *et al.* 1981). Although radionuclide bone scanning remains the most sensitive screening procedure, CT can be used to document the presence of suspected metastases and to evaluate the med-ullary and extraosseous extent of metastases. A suspected early metastatic focus that cannot be demonstrated by conventional radiography may be confirmed by CT demonstration of subtle osseous destruction or focal increased med-ullary density (Fig. 4.17). Such findings have been shown to be nearly diagnostic of metastases (Helms *et al.* 1981)—they may indicate the need for or the extent of radiation therapy.

Musculoskeletal trauma and infection

The role of CT in evaluating *fractures or dislo-cations* has been discussed (Genant *et al.* 1981, Brant-Zawadski *et al.* 1981, Naidach *et al.* 1979, Lange & Alter Jr 1980, Lasda *et al.* 1978

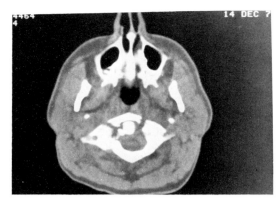

Fig. 4.18. Axial representation optimally displays a Jefferson fracture of C2.

and Wilson *et al.* 1978)—it is particularly im-portant in anatomically complex regions such as the spine (Figs. 4.18 & 4.19), sacrum, pelvis, hip (Fig. 4.20), shoulder and sternum. The cross-sectional display may optimally demon-strate the spatial relationships of fractures, the need for or the adequacy of reduction (Fig. 4.21) and the nature of associated soft-tissue injuries. It has been shown (Genant *et al.* 1981, Naidach *et al.* 1979 and Post *et al.* 1978) that as CT procedures become faster and more ac-cessible to the clinician this manner of studying complicated fractures may largely replace con-ventional tomography, which is more time-con-suming, more difficult to perform, and results in higher radiation exposure.

The diagnostic usefulness of CT in some cases of *infection* involving osseous or articular struc-tures by revealing subtle bony destruction, al-teration in medullary density or the presence of abscess formation (Figs. 4.22 & 4.23) has been discussed (Genant *et al.* 1981, Wilson *et al.* 1978, Kuhn & Berger 1979, McLeod *et al.* 1978). Hardy *et al.* (1980) have shown that it may have therapeutic value by suggesting the need for surgical drainage and debridement and by providing localization for CT-guided needle aspiration (Fig. 4.24).

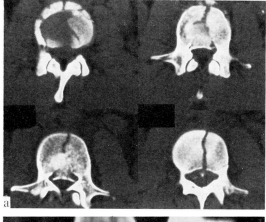

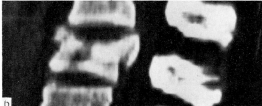

Fig. 4.19. Axial view (a), sagittal reformation (b), and coronal reformation (c) of a burst fracture of a lumbar vertebral body compromising the neural canal and accompanied by a fracture of the lamina.

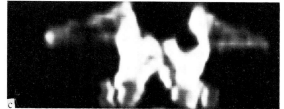

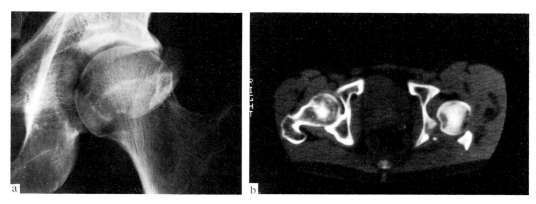

Fig. 4.20. (a) An anteroposterior radiograph of the left hip shows a fracture–dislocation with at least one and possibly more fracture fragments. (b) CT scan through the hip reveals the position of the fracture fragments and the incomplete reduction (Courtesy of Dr John S. Wilson).

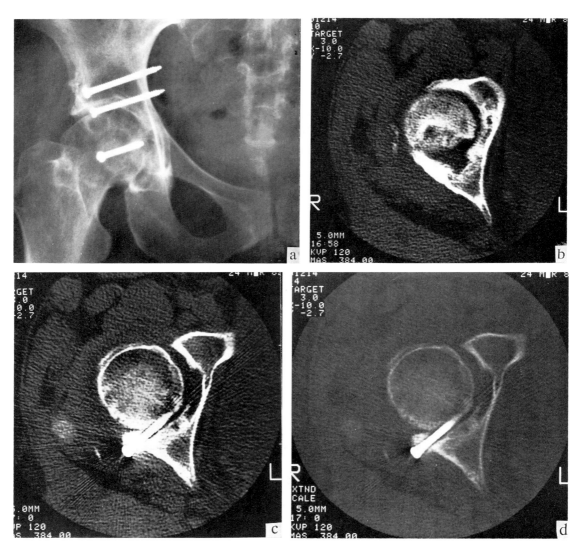

Fig. 4.21. (a) A conventional radiograph demonstrates abnormal right hip, three months following open reduction and internal fixation of acetabular fracture. (b) and (c) CT images demonstrate osseous and articular destruction resulting from screw extending into hip joint. (d) CT image using extended grey scale.

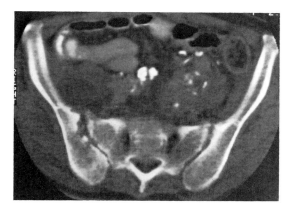

Fig. 4.22. CT clearly demonstrates pyogenic infection causing irregular destruction of the subchondral cortex of the right sacroiliac joint, focal lysis of the ilium, and a large presacral iliopsoas abscess.

Low back pain syndrome

As has been shown (Genant *et al.* 1981, Genant *et al.* 1980, Burton *et al.* 1979, Carrera *et al.* 1980, Hammerschlag *et al.* 1976, Glenn *et al.* 1979, Meyer *et al.* 1979, Ullich *et al.* 1980, Lee *et al.* 1978, Genant *et al.* 1982 and Haughton & Williams 1982), the potential of CT for evaluating the lumbar spine in patients with low back pain syndromes is just beginning to be realized. Only in the past several years have scanners with high spatial and density resolution combined with scout view localization (Fig. 4.4) become widely available.

The evaluation of the status of *lumbar intervertebral discs* and their relationship to the thecal sac in patients with low back pain syndrome is made possible by the presence of epidural fat in the spinal canal at the disc levels. Additionally, the annulus and nucleus pulposus are slightly more dense than the thecal sac—thus the interface between disc and sac can be distinguished in most cases. The normal configuration of the posterior aspect of the intervertebral disc at the L4–5 level (Fig. 4.25) is a slight upward concavity which flattens with increasing age (beyond 40 years), as Meyer *et al.* have shown (1979). In older patients a minor diffuse annular bulge producing slight downward convexity is common and has no clinical significance unless there is concomitant obliteration of epidural fat. At the L5–S1 level (Fig. 4.26), the posterior aspect of the intervertebral disc normally has a convex configuration. Epidural fat is abundant, however, and the thecal sac is not impinged upon.

Two patterns of discogenic impingement may be observed. The first, which represents a broad annular bulge, is characterized by a smooth, curvilinear convexity that impinges upon the thecal sac and obliterates epidural fat (Fig. 4.27). This appearance reflects broad discogenic degeneration without herniation of the nucleus pulposus. The second pattern, which is characterized by a discrete nodular or lumpy protrusion of the disc on the thecal sac or nerve root

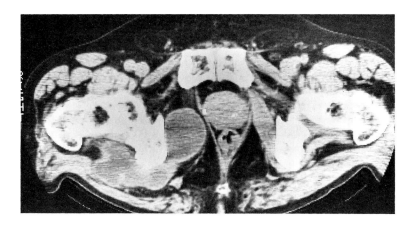

Fig. 4.23. Enlarged iliopsoas bursa due to chronic tuberculous infection.

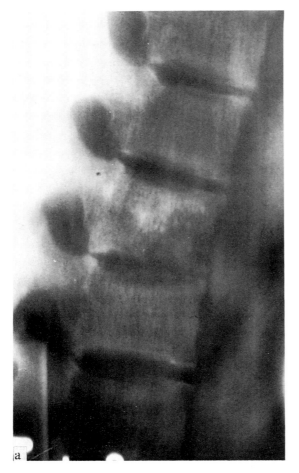

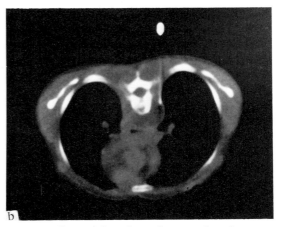

Fig. 4.24. Chronic tuberculous infection on lateral radiograph (a) with abscess formation and CT-guided aspiration (b).

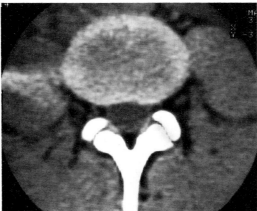

Fig. 4.25. A normal intervertebral disc at L4–5. The disc is slightly concave or flat and does not impinge upon the thecal sac and L4 nerve roots.

accompanied by focal obliteration of epidural fat (Fig. 4.28), corresponds to a herniated nucleus pulposus or annular tear, with or without a free fragment. The differentiation between these two patterns of encroachment may have therapeutic significance but cannot always be made.

The evaluation of the patency of the *neural foramina* requires a series of contiguous or overlapping scans beginning at the level of the inferior surface of the pedicle and extending caudad through the disc. Generally, the nerve roots are well outlined by epidural fat adjacent to the inner, inferior aspect of the pedicle. In sections immediately caudad, the neural foramina generally become smaller, ending at the level of the superior articular facet or pedicle of

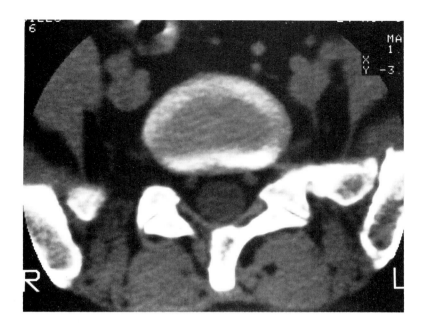

Fig. 4.26. A normal intervertebral disc at L5–S1. The disc is flat or slightly convex and does not encroach upon the thecal sac or the S1 nerve roots.

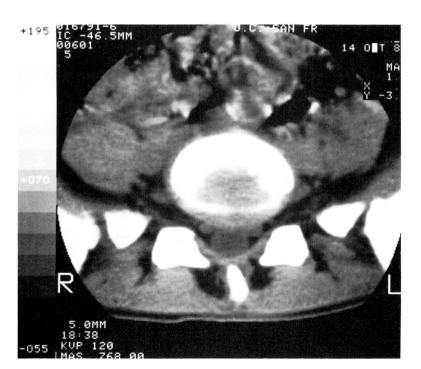

Fig. 4.27. An abnormal L5–S1 disc with a moderate, broad-based discogenic bulge that obliterates epidural fat and impinges upon the thecal sac and S1 nerve roots.

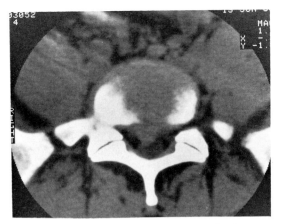

Fig. 4.28. Focal disc protrusion at the L5–S1 level indicating herniated nucleus pulposus or localized annular tear.

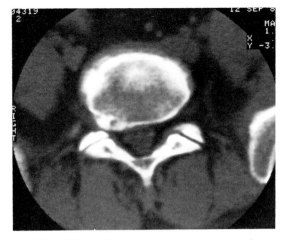

Fig. 4.29. CT scan demonstrates encroachment on the right neural foramen by osteophytic overgrowth extending from the vertebral margin.

the adjacent vertebra. A narrowed neural foramen at the level of the end-plate and disc does not by itself indicate significant nerve root compression, as the root has generally exited the foramen cephalad to the disc; the entire series of consecutive scans must be evaluated to determine significant foraminal encroachment (Fig. 4.29). Occasionally a laterally bulging or herniating disc may encroach upon the existing nerve root peripherally in the neural foramen (Fig. 4.30)—this is often undetected by myelography but is readily depicted by CT. It has been shown how sagittal and oblique reformation sometimes provide additional useful information in the evaluation of osseous neural foraminal encroachment (Genant *et al.* 1981 and Glenn *et al.* 1979).

Also, the importance of the application of CT in the evaluation of low back pain syndromes caused by *spinal stenosis* and acquired disorders that compromise the spinal cord and nerve roots has been discussed (Genant *et al.* 1981, Post *et al.* 1978, Hammerschlag 1976, Glenn *et al.* 1979, Meyer *et al.* 1979, Ullich *et al.* 1980, Lee *et al.* 1978, Genant *et al.* 1982, Haughton & Williams 1982, Coin *et al.* 1977, Roub & Drayer 1979 and Sheldon *et al.* 1977). In spinal stenosis, the cross-sectional display of CT per-

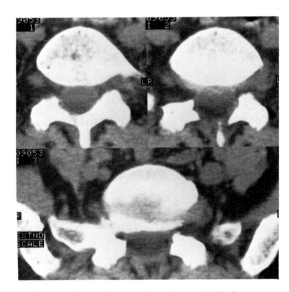

Fig. 4.30. A laterally protruding disc at L5–S1 that encroaches upon the exiting L5 nerve root.

mits precise definition of the critically important transverse configuration and size of the canal. Although measurements of the anteroposterior, transverse and cross-sectional area of the lumbar spinal canal by CT have been described (Ullich *et al.* 1980), the application and interpretation of such measurements is often difficult.

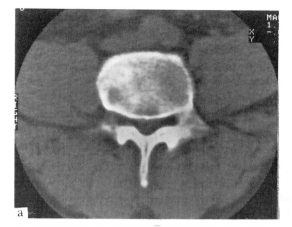

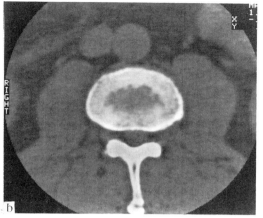

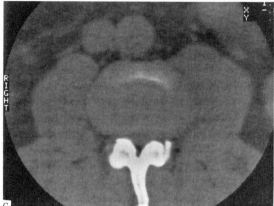

Fig. 4.31. A small central osseous canal (a) and (b) combined with broad disc degeneration (c) results in spinal stenosis.

In practice, it is generally more reliable to use the configuration and appearance of the spinal canal to assess the presence and severity of spinal stenosis qualitatively (Fig. 4.31). For example, if a relatively small osseous spinal canal and total obliteration of epidural fat at the level of the pedicle and lamina are demonstrated, osseous spinal stenosis is present. Epidural fat is usually preserved at these levels, except after laminectomy or discectomy, when fibrosis occurs. Additionally, when spinal stenosis is due to hypertrophy or the superior articular facets the spinal canal may have a compressed or trefoil configuration associated with encroachment on the lateral recesses and the nerve root (Fig. 4.32). Here again, the configuration of the

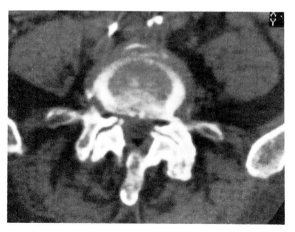

Fig. 4.32. Hypertrophy of superior articular facets results in marked lateral spinal stenosis.

spinal canal and obliteration of epidural fat are of greater importance than the absolute linear measurements.

Preliminary evaluations have been shown to suggest that CT examination of the lumbar spine is highly accurate (Genant *et al.* 1982 and Haughton & Williams 1982), and studies comparing the sensitivity and specificity of CT with those of myelography, epidural venography, and surgical exploration are beginning to appear. One can speculate that CT will assume an important role as a non-invasive screening procedure in low back syndromes. When the findings are clearly normal, conservative management can be used. When the findings are grossly abnormal and consistent with clinical data, further diagnostic procedures may be obviated. When the CT findings are equivocal or inconsistent with clinical observations, additional invasive diagnostic procedures including metrizamide-enhanced CT (Fig. 4.33) may be indicated before surgical exploration.

QUANTITATIVE BONE MINERAL ANALYSIS USING CT

It has been shown (Genant *et al.* 1981, Genant *et al.* 1982, Bradley *et al.* 1978, Cann & Genant 1980, Genant & Boyd 1977, Orphanoudakis *et al.* 1977, Pullan & Roberts 1978 and Ruegsegger *et al.* 1976) that the capability of CT to display a cross-sectional image of bone in terms of the actual attenuation coefficient for each point in it provides the potential for quantitative bone mineral analysis in metabolic bone diseases. Perhaps the most important site for application of CT mineral measurement is the spine (Fig. 4.34), where the first clinical signs of bone loss occur (i.e. vertebral fracture). Direct measurement of the metabolically active trabecular bone at this site provides a sensitive indicator of the skeletal response to metabolic stimuli. Normative data (Fig. 4.35) and clinical results are currently being generated (Genant *et al.* 1981). With the large number of whole-body

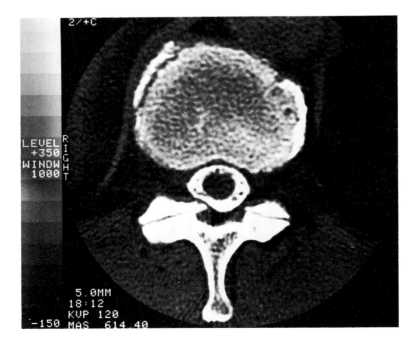

Fig. 4.33. High-resolution CT scan after intrathecal metrizamide injection demonstrates cord and roots as well as osteophytosis of right apophyseal joint.

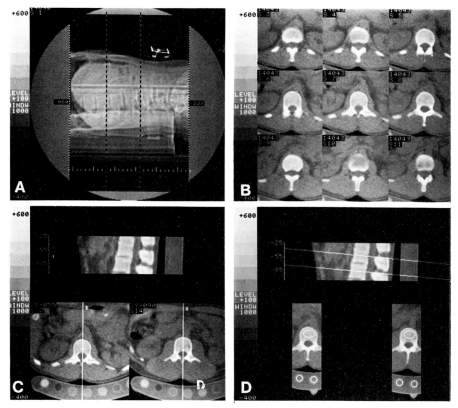

Fig. 4.34. A lateral computed radiograph (scout view) provides gross localization to upper lumbar spine (top left). A series of contiguous 5-mm thick axial sections are obtained (top right). Using advanced computer software, a sagittal reformatted image (bottom left) is generated. From the sagittal view, the midplanes of the L1 and L2 vertebral bodies are defined (bottom right), and a new, 1-cm thick synthesized image is generated in the axial plane, centred at the midplane and corrected for angulation. An oval region of interest in the synthesized images is used to determine vertebral mineral content, and a circular region of interest is used to quantify the calibration solutions.

CT scanners available, the widespread use of vertebral mineral measurements is now possible.

MISCELLANEOUS DISORDERS

The potential applications of CT for assessing the musculoskeletal system currently being investigated have been shown to include preoperative assessment of the adequacy of bone stock for total joint arthroplasty (Genant *et al.* 1981 and Genant *et al.* 1980), non-invasive evaluation of tears of the cruciate ligaments (Fig. 4.36) (Chafetz *et al.* 1981 and Pavlov *et al.* 1979), determination of patellofemoral tracking abnor-

malities (Delgado-Martins 1979), definition of the adequacy of post-cast reduction in congenital hip dysplasia (Genant *et al.* 1981 and Padovani *et al.* 1979), measurement of femoral anteversion (Hernandez *et al.* 1981), and detection of early sacroiliitis in the seronegative spondyloarthropathies (Genant *et al.* 1982 and Carrera *et al.* 1981).

CONCLUSION

The applications of CT for musculoskeletal diagnosis are increasing in number and importance. With proper use of existing systems and upgrading of diagnostic procedures, it can replace

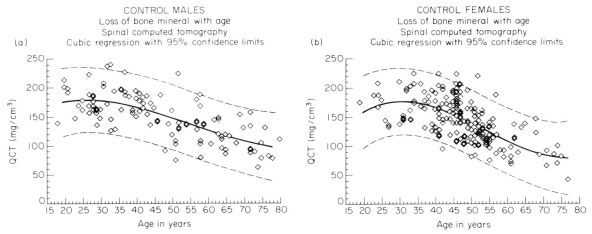

Fig. 4.35. (a) Normal male values for vertebral cancellous mineral content by QCT. (b) Normal female values for vertebral cancellous mineral content by QCT.

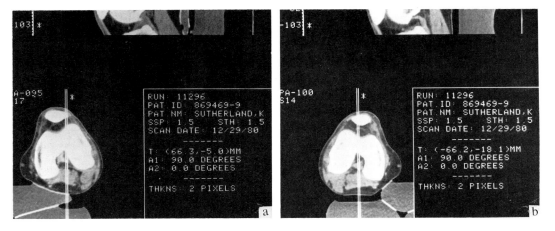

Fig. 4.36. The cruciate ligaments can be evaluated on sagittal images (top) reformatted from contiguous 1·5-mm axial sections. (a) Normal anterior and posterior cruciate ligaments. (b) A torn anterior cruciate ligament and a normal posterior cruciate ligament.

many conventional techniques and invasive procedures for skeletal imaging, as it has done for neuroradiography. The advantages of CT over conventional radiography—its three-dimensional imaging capabilities, excellent contrast resolution, accurate measurement of tissue attenuation coefficients, non-invasive character, and, in most instances, reduced radiation exposure to the patient—make it a valuable tool in musculoskeletal diagnosis.

References

ALFIDI R.J., MACINTYRE W.J., MEANY T.F., CHERNACK E.S., JANICKI P., TARA R. & LEVIN H. (1975) Experimental studies to determine application of computer assisted tomography (CAT) scanning to the human body. *Amer. J. Radiol.* **124**, 199–207.

AMBROSE J. (1973) Computerized transverse axial scanning (tomography). Part II. Clinical application *Brit. J. Radiol.* **46**, 1023–47.

BAKER H.L. JR, CAMPBELL J.K., HOUSER O.W., REESE D.F., SHEEDY P.F., HOLMAN C.B. & KURLAND R.L. (1974) Computer assisted tomography of the head. An early evaluation. *Mayo Clin. Proc.* **49**, 17–27.

BERGER P.E. & KUHN J.P. (1978) CT of tumors of the musculoskeletal system in children. Clinical applications. *Radiology* **127**, 171–5.

BOYD D.P., MOSS A. & KOROBKIN M.T. (1977) Engineering status of computerized tomography. *Opt. Eng.* **16**, 37.

BRADLEY J.G., HUANG H.K. & LEDLEY R.S. (1978) Evaluation of calcium concentration in bones from CT scans. *Radiology* **128**, 103–7.

BRANT-ZAWADSKI M., MILLER E.M. & FEDERLE M.P. (1981) Computed tomography in evaluation of spine trauma. *Amer. J. Radiol.* **136**, 369–76.

BROOKS R.A. & DICHIRO G. (1975) Theory of image reconstruction in computed tomography. *Radiology* **117**, 561–72.

BROWN B.M., BRANT-ZAWADSKI M. & CANN C.E. (1982) Dynamic CT scanning of spinal column trauma. *Amer. J. N. Radiol.* **3**, 561–5.

BURTON C.V., HEITHOFF K.B., KIRKALDY-WILLIS W. & RAY C.D. (1979) Computed tomographic scanning and the lumbar spine. Part II. Clinical considerations. *Spine* **4**, 356–68.

CANN C.E. & GENANT H.K. (1980) Precise measurement of vertebral mineral content using CT. *J. Comput. assist. Tomogr.* **4**, 493–500.

CARRERA G.F., HAUGHTON V.M., ASBJORN S. & WILLIAMS A.L. (1980) CT of lumbar facet joints. *Radiology* **134**, 145–8.

CARRERA G.F., FOLEY W.D., KOZIN F., RYAN L. & LAWSON T.L. (1981) CT of sacroiliitis. *Amer. J. Radiol.* **136**, 41–6.

CHAFETZ N.I., MARKS A.S., HELMS C.A., CANN C.E., GLICK J.M. & GENANT H.K. (1981) CT of the menisci and cruciate ligaments (abstract). Association of University Radiologists 29th Annual Meeting, New Orleans, Louisiana. *Invest. Radiol.* **15**, 366.

COIN C.G., CHAN Y.S., KERANEN V. & PENNINK M. (1977) Computed assisted myelography in disc disease. *J. Comput. assist. Tomogr.* **1**, 398–404.

CORMACK A.M. (1963) Representation of a function by its line integrals, with some radiological applications. *J. appl. Phys.* **34**, 2722–7.

DELGADO-MARTINS H. (1979) A study of the position of the patella using CT. *J. Bone Jt Surg.* **61B**, 443–4.

DE SANTOS L.A., GOLDSTEIN H.M., MURRAY J.A. & WALLACE S. (1978) Computed tomography in the evaluation of the musculoskeletal neoplasms. *Radiology* **128**, 89–94.

DESTOUET J.M., GILULA L.A. & MURPHY W.A. (1979) CT of long bone osteosarcoma. *Radiology* **131**, 439–45.

GENANT H.K. & BOYD D.P. (1977) Quantitative bone mineral analysis using dual energy CT. *Invest. Radiol.* **12**, 545–51.

GENANT H.K., WILSON J.S., BOVILL E.G. JR., BRUNELLE F.O., MURRAY W.R. & RODRIGO J.J. (1980) CT of the musculoskeletal system. *J. Bone Jt Surg.* **62A**, 1088–2001.

GENANT H.K., CANN C.E., CHAFETZ N.I. & HELMS C.A. (1981) Advances in CT of the musculoskeletal system. *Radiol. Clin. N. Amer.* **19**, 645–74.

GENANT H.K., CHAFETZ N.I. & HELMS C.A. (eds.) (1982) *CT of the Lumbar Spine: Diagnostic and Therapeutic Implications for the Radiologist, Orthopedist and Neurosurgeon*. University of California Printing Department.

GENERAL ELECTRIC CO. (1976) *Introduction of CT*. Milwaukee: General Electric Medical Systems Division.

GLENN W.V., RHODES M.L., ALTSCHULER E.M., WILTSE L.L., LOSTANEK C. & KUO Y.M. (1979) Multiplanar display computerized body tomography applications in the lumbar spine. *Spine* **4**, 282–352.

GORDON R., HERMAN G.T. & JOHNSON S.A. (1970) Image reconstruction from projections. *Sci. Amer.* **29**, 471–81.

HAMMERSCHLAG S.B., WOLPERT S.M. & CARTER B.L. (1976) Computed tomography of the spinal canal. *Radiology* **121**, 361–7.

HARDY D.C., MURPHY W.A. & GILULA L.A. (1980) CT in planning subcutaneous bone biopsy. *Radiology* **134**, 447–50.

HAUGHTON V.M. & WILLIAMS A.L. (1982) CT of the spine. St Louis: The C. V. Mosby Co.

HELMS C.A., CANN C.E., BRUNELLE F.O., CHAFETZ N.I., GILULA L.A. & GENANT H.K. (1981) Detection of bone marrow metastasis using CT. *Radiology* **140**, 745–50.

HERNANDEZ R.J., TACHDJIAN M.O., POZNANSKI A.K. & DIAS L.S. (1981) CT determination of femoral torsion. *Amer. J. Radiol.* **137**, 97–201.

HOUNSFIELD G.N. (1973) Computerized transverse axial scanning (tomography). Part I. Description of system. *Brit. J. Radiol.* **46**, 1016–22.

HUNTER J.C., JOHNSTON W.H. & GENANT H.K. (1979) CT evaluation of fatty tumors of the somatic soft-tissues: clinical utility and radiographic pathologic correlation. *Skeletal Radiol.* **4**, 79–91.

KUHL D.E. & EDWARDS R.Q. (1968) Reorganizing data from transverse section scans of the brain using digital processing. *Radiology* **91**, 975–83.

KUHN J.P. & BERGER P.E. (1979) CT diagnosis of osteomyelitis. *Radiology* **130**, 503–6.

LANGE T.A. & ALTER A.J. JR (1980) Evaluation of complex acetabular fractures by CT. *J. Comput. assist. Tomogr.* **4**, 849–52.

LASDA N.A., LEVINSOHN E.M., YUAN H.A. & BUNNELL W.P. (1978) CT in disorders of the hip. *J. Bone Jt Surg.* **60A**, 1099–2002.

LEE S.C.P., KAZAM E. & NEWMAN A.D. (1978) CT of the spine and spinal cord. *Radiology* **129**, 95–102.

McCULLOUGH E.C. (1975) Photon attenuation in CT. *Med. Phys.* **2**, 307–20.

McLEOD R.A., STEPHENS D.H., BEABOUT J.W., SHEEDY P.F. II & HATTERY R.R. (1978) CT of the skeletal system. *Semin. Roentgenol.* **13**, 235–47.

MEYER G.A., HAUGHTON V.M. & WILLIAMS A.L. (1979) Diagnosis of herniated lumbar disc with CT. *New Engl. J. Med.* **301**, 1166–7.

NAIDACH T.P., PUDLOWSKI R.M., MORAN C.J., GILULA L.A., MURPHY W. & NAIDICH J.B. (1979) CT of spinal fractures. *Advanc. Neurol.* **22**, 207.

OLDENDORF W.H. (1961) Isolated flaying spot detection of radiodensity discontinuities displaying the internal structural pattern of a complex object. *IRE Trans. bio-med. Electron. Eng.* **8**, 68–72.

ORPHANOUDAKIS S., JENSEN P.S. & RASMUSSEN H. (1977) Bone mineral analysis using single-energy computed tomography. *Invest. Radiol.* **14**, 122–30.

PADOVANI J., FAURE F., DEVRED P., JACQUEMIER M. & SARRAT P. (1979) Use and advantages of tomodensitometry in testing congenital luxations of the hip. *Ann. Radiol.* **22**, 88–93.

Pavlov H., Hirschy J.C. & Torg J.S. (1979) CT of the cruciate ligaments. *Radiology* **132**, 389–93.

Phelps M.E., Hoffman E.J. & Ter-Pogossian M.D. (1975) Attenuation coefficients of various body tissues, fluids and lesions at photon energies of 18 to 136 keV. *Radiology* **117**, 573–83.

Post M.J.D., Gargano F.P., Vining D.Q. & Rosomoff H.L. (1978) A comparison of radiographic methods of diagnosing constrictive lesions of the spinal canal. *J. Neurosurg.* **48**, 360–8.

Pullan B.R. & Robert T.E. (1978) Bone mineral measurements using an EMI scanner and standard methods. A comparative study. *Brit. J. Radiol.* **61**, 24–8.

Radon J. (1917) On the determination of functions from their integrals along certain manifolds. Abhandl. Berichte K. Saechsische gesellsch der Wissensch., Leipzig, *Math.-phys. klasse* **69**, 262–77.

Reese D.F., McCullough E.C. & Balcer H.L. jr (1981) Dynamic sequential scanning with table incrementation. *Radiology* **140**, 719–22.

Rosenfeld D., Abols Y. & Genant H.K. (1979) Analysis of multiple energy computed tomography techniques for the measurement of bone mineral content. *Proceedings of the Fourth International Conference of Bone Measurement.* Washington: U.S. Government Printing Office.

Roub L.W. & Drayer B.P. (1979) Spinal CT: limitations and applications. *Amer. J. Radiol.* **133**, 267–73.

Ruegsegger P., Elsasser U., Anliker M., Gnehm H., Kind H. & Prader A. (1976) Quantification of bone mineralization using CT. *Radiology* **21**, 93–7.

Schumacher T.M., Genant H.K., Korobkin M.T. & Bovill E.G. jr (1978) CT: its use in space-occupying lesions of the musculoskeletal system. *J. Bone Jt Surg.* **60A**, 600–7.

Sheldon J.J., Sersland R. & Leborgne J. (1977) CT of the lower lumbar vertebral column. *Radiology* **124**, 113–18.

Termote J.L., Baert A., Crolla D., Palmers Y. & Bulcke J.A. (1980) CT of the normal and pathologic muscular systems. *Radiology* **137**, 439–44.

Ullich C.G., Binet E.F., Sanecki M.G. & Kieffer S.A. (1980) Quantitative assessment of the lumbar spinal canal by CT. *Radiology* **134**, 137–43.

Wilson J.S., Korobkin M.T., Genant H.K. & Bovill E.G. jr (1978) CT of the musculoskeletal disorders. *Amer. J. Radiol.* **131**, 55–61.

Chapter 5
Other Advanced Imaging Techniques

W. M. PARK

Magnification radiography

In order to identify subtle changes in bone or joint morphology it is necessary to obtain the best quality radiographic image. High-resolution techniques have to be employed so that the sharpest possible detail can be obtained.

Optical enlargement can be obtained with the use of a magnifying glass and conventional film. This method is limited unless fine-grain industrial films such as Crystalex are used. The resultant image may be viewed with either a hand magnifying lens or an optical projector for group viewing.

Clinical studies with this technique are not new. In the early 1950s Fletcher and Rowley reported their experience with fine-grain films and photographic enlargement in the study of peripheral skeletal abnormalities. Following this, further reports appeared about the use of industrial films and optical magnification in rheumatoid arthritis. More recently, Meema et al. (1972), Weiss (1972), Genant et al. (1975, a, b, 1976, 1977), Mall et al. (1973, 1974) and Jensen and Kliger (1977) have reported extensive experience with this technique in various metabolic and arthritic disorders. Thus the clinical importance of the optical magnification technique appears established for selected skeletal examinations.

Direct radiographic magnification for skeletal radiography has received less attention than has optical magnification. Only with the recent development of X-ray tubes having small focal spots (100–150 microns) and adequate output for clinical examination has this technique become available. Clinical experience with direct radiographic magnification of the skeleton has been reported by Gordon et al. (1973), Sundaram et al. (1979), Ishigaki (1973), Doi et al. (1975) and Genant et al. (1975a, b, 1976, 1977).

Experience with magnification radiographic techniques shows that it is most valuable in studying thin-section tissue slices where detailed correlation with histological appearances is necessary. The clinical applications are in the detection of early arthropathy, joint erosion, bone destruction and hairline fractures. The bone detail thus obtained is superior to that seen with good-quality conventional radiography.

Conventional tomography

Certain structures such as the vertebral column, sternum, ribs and sella turcica may be difficult to evaluate accurately by conventional X-ray techniques in the body, because of surrounding tissue. Similarly, certain articulations may not be adequately visualized during radiography, necessitating the application of tomography. This is particularly true for the sternoclavicular, temporomandibular, sacroiliac, costovertebral, apophyseal, atlanto-occipital, atlantoaxial, subtalar and intertarsal articulations. Tomographic evaluation of joint disorders can be accomplished in several ways. Preliminary films must be taken prior to tomography and should be available during the procedure. These radiographs must also be available when the tomograms are being interpreted.

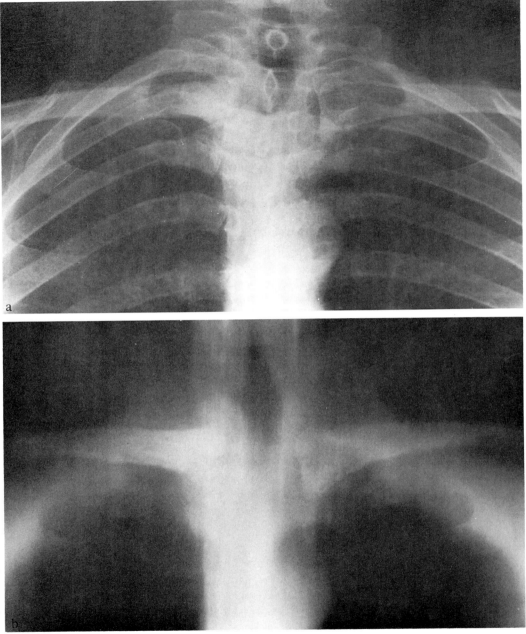

Fig. 5.1. Plain radiograph (a) and tomograph (b) of right sternoclavicular joint. A little sclerosis is seen at the medial end of the right clavicle. The extent of the lesion is better appreciated on tomography.

The optimal type of radiographic tube motion and correct thickness and spacing of the tomographic sections will vary. Fine structures such as the pituitary fossa or middle ear are best demonstrated on 1-mm slices using a circular, elliptical or hypocycloidal movement. In general, spinal and sacroiliac detail are sufficiently well seen on 1-cm or ½-cm slices using a linear movement (Fig. 5.1).

Xeroradiography

Xeroradiography is an electrostatic imaging system that utilizes selenium as a photoconductor. It is a radiographic application of the xerographic process first discovered by Carlson in 1937. This was initially applied as a photographic recording medium. McMaster and Schaffert in 1950 first used the selenium plate with X-rays for the non-destructive testing of metal castings. Initial medical application was undertaken in the early 1950s by Roach and Hilleboe who explored this system as a means of providing diagnostic X-ray facilities during civilian disaster.

In the past decade considerable investigation has been directed by Wolfe (1968, 1969) at the medical application of xeroradiography. Wolfe has written extensively on it as an imaging system for mammography, and has supported its use in other areas of diagnostic radiography. These applications include skeletal trauma, metabolic bone disease, musculoskeletal neoplasms and arthritis.

Very briefly, the image is produced by an electrostatic method which does not require silver in the film process. One of the unique features is the phenomenom of edge enhancement. There is a broad latitude in exposure factors which results in improved sharpness of the final image and is referred to as increased spatial resolution. The radiation exposure required for xeroradiography is relatively high compared to that needed for conventional screen-films radiography but is lower than for non-screen industrial film. Typical skin doses of 0·3–2·0 rads are needed for musculoskeletal application,

which generally limits the use of xeroradiography to the thinner parts of the body.

Clinical applications of xeroradiography include the demonstration of soft-tissue lesions around joints, such as Baker's cysts (Fig. 5.2) and gouty tophi. Non-opaque foreign bodies—cotton, wood, plastic, etc.—are demonstrable by xeroradiographic techniques, and it is particularly helpful in the detection of these following blast trauma. The upper and mediastinal airways, which may be difficult to see because of overlapping structures, are also well demonstrated.

Digital radiography

The success of computer-assisted tomography (CAT scanning) has illustrated the value of digitized radiographic information. The principle of

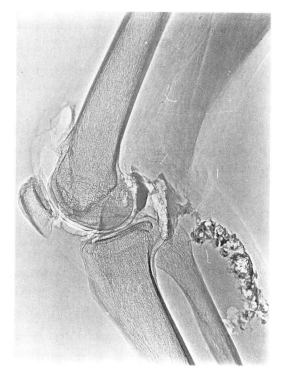

Fig. 5.2. Xeroradiography of knee following arthrography. The ruptured Baker's cyst is well demonstrated. The bone and soft-tissue detail are well seen in the one image. (Courtesy of Dr H. Harty.)

digitizing the information present in a projected X-ray image has now been further extended into conventional radiography and fluoroscopy. The transformation is performed by an analogue–digital converter. In digital form, information can be processed and manipulated at extremely high speed by a computer. The manipulation of the data can increase contrast sensitivity by the elimination of scatter, and the quantative treatment of the data allows reconstruction of the image in different modes to enhance varied features. Quantitative information also makes it possible to achieve tissue characterization.

With the development of very high-resolution television and digital fluoroscopy units it is now possible to perform angiographic examinations, both arterial and venous, following intravenous injection of contrast, rendering the angiogram effectively non-invasive. Where optimum detail is required, catheter studies using digital vascular imaging may still be necessary, but these are done using smaller doses of contrast, and the catheter need not be as selectively placed, thus making the examination much safer.

Computerized images are accumulated and stored electronically and subtracted from a preinjection image. Final images are usually presented in this subtracted form. Digital angiography has rapidly become an established technique and is already in routine use where equipment is available. While the detail is not yet as good as that obtained by conventional arteriography it, in many instances, is sufficiently diagnostic to plan treatment. It can also be used as a screening examination and allows patient selection for the more invasive tests. With digital equipment many angiograms can be carried out as an out-patient procedure. As arterial pictures can be achieved via an intravenous injection, arterial pictures can be obtained in situations previously impossible or extremely hazardous. The main clinical application of digital vascular imaging is in the detection of cerebral, peripheral and coronary arterial disease.

As yet it has not had a direct impact on orthopaedic practice but is of great value in the investigation of associated arterial disease.

Emission tomography

Routine radionuclide studies performed with a gamma camera have an inherent limitation, projection of a three-dimensional object onto a two-dimensional display. The third dimension, depth, is usually obtained by complementary views at different angles. Activity from overlying or underlying structures can obscure the region of interest. Emission tomography overcomes these difficulties by producing images of the distribution of activity within structures, analagous to computerized tomography. This also allows visualization of smaller lesions. Apart from the anatomical information, functional information about cellular activity is also obtained, as measurements of blood flow, oxygen utilization and glucose metabolism in normal and diseased tissue can be obtained with certain radiopharmaceuticals. Emission tomography can be performed in two ways. In the first method, ECAT scanning, pharmaceuticals labelled with the more conventional radioisotopes are used and images are obtained by rotating the gamma camera around the patient, the data being analysed by computer techniques. In the second method, positron emission tomography (PET), specialized expensive equipment is required with access to cyclotron-produced isotopes. The technique is still limited to a few centres.

The clinical application of ECAT scanning is now well established in the brain, liver and heart, and its greater sensitivity in the detection of lesions is proven. Its role in other areas of the body is not yet established (Fig. 5.3).

Radionuclide emission tomography, although an old concept, still has not achieved widespread acceptance because of the high cost of equipment necessary to provide most of the capabilities required. Future developments of radiopharmaceuticals, and the outcome of detailed

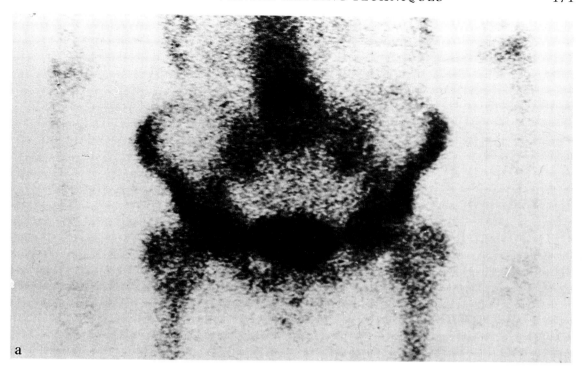

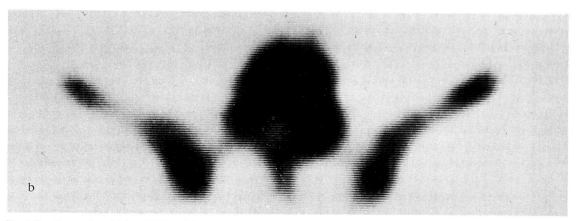

Fig. 5.3. Conventional (a) and ESCAT (b) image of spine. (a) Hot L5 is seen on the routine scan at L5; this is due to metastasis. (b) ESCAT scan at L5 level demonstrates the distribution of abnormal activity in the vertebral body. (Courtesy of Dr I. Watt.)

current clinical trials in many laboratories, should provide valuable information to determine the cost–benefit relationship for radionuclide tomography as a routine diagnostic procedure.

Ultrasound

The role of ultrasound as a non-invasive diagnostic modality is well established. The basic principle of ultrasound is that tissues of different structures have different reflective properties.

Fluid is transonic, air totally reflective. Images are obtained by electronically converting the reflected echoes and reconstructing images of the tissues through which the sound echoes have passed. Early images were only present in graph form—A scanning. Nowadays most scanners in clinical use are of the real-time type. There is no radiation with ultrasound, and as far as is known it is a totally harmless form of investigation at levels used in diagnostic procedures. It is used extensively in organ imaging in heart, liver, kidney and pelvic pathology.

In the neonate and young child the anterior fontanelle, as long as it remains patent, provides a window to the brain. Routine scanning to detect intraventricular or intracerebral haemorrhage is the norm in premature nurseries. Ultrasound cranial scanning is also the routine method for the assessment of hydrocephalus while the fontanelle remains open.

Doppler ultrasound techniques now play a major role in the detection of arterial disease in the carotid, iliac and femoral vessels and have been used with some success in the detection of venous thrombosis.

The role of ultrasound in orthopaedics is more limited, as bone is impervious to ultrasound. Ultrasound has been used in the detection of CDH, and in the assessment of spinal dysraphism and the tethered cord, in the assessment of soft-tissue lesions, bursae and Baker's cysts. Its other role in orthopaedics is the indirect one of assessing metastatic lesions in the liver and kidney and the detection of abscess cavities (Fig. 5.4).

Interventional radiography

Successful diagnosis by biopsy by needle puncture and aspiration was described by Martin and Ellis in 1930. Intermittent reports followed, detailing clinical experience with improved biopsy needle design, improved histopathological diagnosis by cytology and improved radiol-

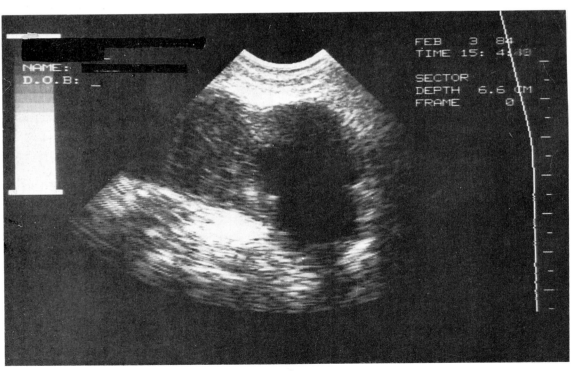

Fig. 5.4   Ultrasound of abscess cavity distal to the shaft of prosthesis.

ogical techniques. The last decade has seen the firm establishment of the technique as an alternative to open biopsy. Its advantage lies in the lessened morbidity, and shortened hospital stay compared with open biopsy, and definitive treatment can be started sooner. The procedure is done under fluoroscopic control under local or general anaesthesia, as is clinically indicated. A variety of biopsy needles may be used, and include the Craig, Jamshedi, Ackerman, Johnson and Tru-cut needles. Biopsy material is sent for cytological examination and bacterial culture where appropriate. The most frequent indications are for needle biopsy diagnosis of a lytic bone deposit where the primary is unknown, or the confirmation that a lesion is metastatic when the primary is known. It is also extensively used to confirm suspected infection, with the aspiration of material for bacteriological diagnosis. Contraindications are few but the procedure has a reported complications rate of 0·2%, some of which are serious. The serious complications are death, paraplegia and meningitis. Less serious complications are pneumothorax and transient paraplegia and paresis. The decision to carry out the biopsy must only be taken after consideration of other less invasive techniques which might yield diagnosis. Close liaison with the pathology and bacteriology departments is essential prior to starting the procedure, so that aspirated and biopsied material is properly processed. The optimum site for biopsy must be chosen. CT and radionuclide studies may aid this decision and the biopsy may need to be under CT control.

Thermography

Infrared thermography provides information about surface temperature distribution. By using microwave frequencies it is possible to penetrate deeper into the subcutaneous tissues, permitting detection of their thermal patterns. The possibility of using thermography for clinical diagnosis was first described in 1974 by Barrett and Myers, Edrich and Hardee, and Enander and Larson. Since then papers describing

the use of thermography for the detection of breast, bone and thyroid cancer have been published. The surface temperature over tumours is greater than that of surrounding tissues. The major role of thermography in orthopaedics is in assessing joint inflammation and the response to treatment of anti-inflammatory drugs. Inflamed joints will have a higher surface temperature than surrounding tissues and this is detected by microwave thermography (Fig. 5.5). The technique provides an objective assessment of the degree of inflammation and helps to eliminate subjectivity when assessing the efficiency of an anti-inflammatory drug.

The technique has failed to gain widespread acceptance in spite of its non-invasive properties, and is not routinely available in most departments. The neoplastic diseases can be detected more reliably by other techniques. While

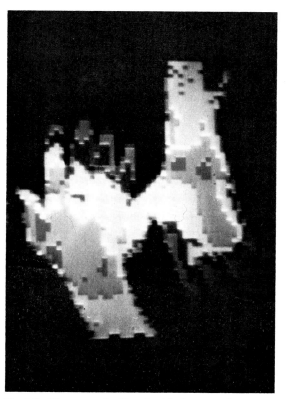

Fig. 5.5 Thermograph of hands with rheumatoid arthritis. There is marked increase in temperature in the affected hand (Courtesy of Dr I. Watt.)

it is an excellent method of assessing temperature variations over joints, the technical requirement of a stable environment in the room in which the examination is done is not easy to maintain. Variation in room temperature interferes with reliability and reproducibility. This, combined with the highly specialized application, has not led to widespread use.

References

Magnification radiography

BOOKSTEIN J.J. & VOEGLI E. (1971) A critical analysis of magnification radiography. *Lab. Invest. Radiol.* **98**, 23–30.
DOI K., GENANT H.K. & ROSSMAN K. (1975) Effect of film graininess and geometric unsharpness on image quality in fine detail skeletal radiology. *Invest. Radiol.* **10**, 160–72.
FLETCHER D.E. & ROWLEY K.A. (1951) Radiographic enlargements in diagnostic radiology. *Brit. J. Radiol.* **24**, 598–604.
GENANT H.K., KOZIN F., BERMAN C. *et al.* (1975a) The reflex sympathetic dystrophy syndrome. A comprehensive analysis using fine detail radiography, photo absorptiometry and bone and joint scintigraphy. *Radiology* **117**, 21–32.
GENANT H.K., DOI K. & MALL J.C. (1975b) Optical versus radiographic magnification for fine detail skeletal radiography. *Invest. Radiol.* **10**, 160–72.
GENANT H.K., DOI K. & MALL J.C. (1976) Comparison of non-screen techniques (medical versus industrial film) for fine detail skeletal radiology. *Invest. Radiol.* **11**, 486–500.
GENANT H.K., DOI K. & MALL J.C. (1977) Direct radiographic magnification for skeletal radiology. An assessment of image quality. *Radiology* **123**, 47–55.
GORDON S.L., GREER R.B. & WEIDNER W.A. (1973) Magnification Roentgenographic technic in orthopaedics. *Clin. Orthop.* **91**, 169–73.
ISHIGAKI T. (1973) First metatarsal phalangeal joint of gout macroroentgenographic examination in six times magnification. *Nippon Acta Radiol.* **33**, 839–54.
JENSEN P.S. & KLIGER A.F. (1977) Early radiographic manifestation of secondary hyperparathyroidism associated with chronic renal disease. *Radiology* **125**, 645–52.
MALL J.C., GENANT H.K. & ROSSMAN K. (1973) Improved optical magnification for fine detail radiography. *Radiology* **108**, 707–8.
MALL J.C., GENANT H.K., SILCOX D.C. *et al.* (1974) The efficacy of fine detail radiography in the evaluation of patients with rheumatoid arthritis. *Radiology* **112**, 37–42.
MEEMA H.E., RABINOVICH S., MEEMA S. *et al.* (1972) Improved radiological diagnosis of azotemic osteodystrophy. *Radiology* **102**, 1–10.
MILNE E. (1971) The role and performance of minute focal spots in roentgenology with special reference to magnification. *CRC crit. Rev. radiol. Sci.* **2**, 269–310.
SUNDARAM M., SHIELDS J., BRODEUR A., POLING E.R. (1979)

Versatile ceiling tube mount for direct magnification radiography. *Amer. J. Radiol.* **132**, 4–81.
WEISS A. (1972) A technique for demonstrating fine detail in bones of the hands. *Clin. Radiol.* **23**, 185–7.

Xeroradiography

BAO-SHAN JING, VILLANEUVA R. & DODD G.D. (1977) A new medical technique in the evaluation of prosthetic fitting. *Radiology* **122**, 534–5.
ENGELSTADT B.L., FRIEDMAN E.M. & MURPHY W.A. (1981) Diagnosis of joint effusion on lateral and axial projections of the knee. *Invest. Radiol.* **16**, 188–92.
KALLISHER L. (1975) Xeroradiography in lymph node disease. *Radiology* **115**, 67–71.
KRAMAN B. (1979) Transvenous xeroarteriography: non-invasive method for demonstrating peripheral arteries. *Amer. J. Roentgenol.* **133**, 245–50.
MARSHALL K.A., SADOWSKY N.L. & SIGMAN D. (1978) Xeroradiography in the diagnosis of facial fractures. *Plast. reconstr. Surg.* **62**, 207–11.
NESSI R. & DE YOLDI G.C. (1978) Xeroradiography of bone tumors. *Skeletal Radiol.* **2**, 143–50.
OTTO R., POULIADIS G.P. & KUMPE D.A. (1976) The evaluation of pathological alteration in juxta osseous soft tissue by xeroradiography. *Radiology* **120**, 297–302.
PAULUS D.D. (1980) Xeroradiography—an depth review. *CRC crit. Rev. diagn. Imaging.* **12**, 309–84.
PETERS N.D. *et al.* (1978) Xeroradiography in evaluation of cervical spine injuries. Technical note. *J. Neurosurg.* **49**, 620–1.
ROSENFIELD N.S. *et al.* (1978) Xeroradiography in the evaluation of acquired airway abnormalities in children. *Amer. J. Dis. Child.* **132**, 1177–80.
SCOTT J.R. & KRAMER S.A. (1978) Pediatric tracheostomy. Radiographic features of difficult decannilation. *Amer. J. Roentgenol.* **130**, 893–8.
SMITH F.W. & JUNOR B.J.R. (1977) Xeroradiography of the hands in patients with renal osteodystrophy. *Brit. J. Radiol.* **50**, 261–3.
THOMSON D.H., STANSEY C.R. & MILLER T. (1978) Xeroradiographic detection of foreign bodies. *Laryngoscope* **88**, 254–9.

Digital radiography

CRUMMY G.B., STREGHORST M.F., TURSKI P.A. *et al.* (1982) Digital subtraction angiography: current status and use of intra-arterial injection. *Radiology* **145**, 303–9.
GUTHANEN D.F. & MILLER D.C. (1983) Digital subtraction angiography in aortic dissection. *Amer. J. Roentgenol.* **141**, 157–61.
GUTHANEN D.F., WEXLER l., ENZMANN D.R. *et al.* (1983) Evaluation of peripheral vascular disease using digital subtraction angiography. *Radiology* **147**, 393–9
MISTRETTA C.A., CRUMMY A.B. & STUORTHER C.M. (1981) Digital angiography—a perspective. *Radiology* **139**, 273–7.
RIEDERER S.J. & KRUGER P.A. (1983) Intravenous digital subtraction. A summary of recent developments. *Radiology* **147**, 633–9.
WOOD G.W., LUKIN R.R., TOMSILK T.A. *et al.* (1983) Digital subtraction angiography with intravenous injection. As-

sessment of 1000 carotid bifurcations. *Amer. J. Roentgenol.* **140**, 855.

ROSEN R.J., ROVEN S.J., TAYLOR R.F. *et al.* (1983) Evaluation of aorto-iliac occlusive disease by intravenous digital subtraction angiography. *Radiology* **148**, 7–9.

Emission tomography

ACKERMAN R.H. (1982) Clinical application of positron emission tomography (PET). *Radiol. Clin. N. Amer.* **20**, 9–14.

BURDINE J.A., MURPHY P.H. & DEPREY E.G. (1979) Routine computed tomography of the body using routine radiopharmaceuticals. Clinical applications. *J. nucl. Med.* **20**, 108–14.

COWAN R.J. & WATSON N.E. (1980) Special characteristics and potential of single proton emission computed tomography in the brain. *Semin. nucl. Med.* **10**, 335–45.

DECHIRO G., DELAPAZ R.L., BROOKS K.A. *et al.* (1982) Glucose utilization of cerebral gliomas measured by F18 fluorodeoxy glucose and positron emission tomography. *Neurology* **32**, 1323–9.

GRONEMEYER S.A., BROWNELL G.L., ELMALEH D.R. & ATHANASOULIS C.A. (1980) Transverse section imaging of soft tissue tumors and peripheral vascular disease. *Semin. nucl. Med.* **10**, 392–9.

KHAN O., ELL P.J., JARRITT P.H. *et al.* (1981) Comparison between emission and transmission computed tomography of the liver. *Brit. med. J.* **283**, 1212–14.

PHELPS M.E. (1977) Emission computed tomography. *Semin nucl. Med.* **7**, 337–65.

PHELPS M.E., HOFFMAN E.J., COLEMAN R.E. *et al.* (1976) Tomographic images of blood pool and perfusion in brain and heart. *J. nucl. Med.* **17**, 603–12.

SCHELBERT H.R., HENZE E. & PHELPS M.E. (1980) Emission tomography of the heart. *Semin. nucl. Med.* **10**, 355–73.

WOLFE A.P. (1981) Special characteristics and potential for radiopharmaceuticals for positron emission tomography. *Semin. nucl. Med.* **11**, 2–12.

Thermography

ARONEN H.J., SUARENTA H.T. & TAAVITSAINEN M.J. (1981) Thermography in deep venous thrombosis of the leg. *Amer. J. Roentgenol.* **137**, 1179–83.

BARRETT A.H. & MYERS P.C. (1975a) Microwave thermography, a method of detecting subsurface thermal patterns thermography. In *Proceedings of the First European Congress, Amsterdam, 1974. Bibl. radiol.* **6**, 45–56.

BARRETT A.H. & MYERS P.C. (1975b) Subcutaneous temperature: a method of non-invasive sensing. *Science* **190**, 669.

BARRETT A.H., MYERS P.C. & SADOWSKY N.L. (1977) Detection of breast cancer by microwave radiometry. *Radiol. Sci.* **12**, 167–71.

BINDER A. *et al.* (1983) A clinical and thermographic study of lateral epicondylitis. *Brit. J. Rheumatol.* **22**, 77–81.

DI PIETRO S. *et al.* (1982) Critical evaluation of the use of thermography in the investigation of scintigraphically cold thyroid nodules. *Invest. Radiol.* **17**, 607–9.

EDRICH J. & HARDEE P.C. (1974) Microwave radiometric detection and location of breast cancer. *Proc. I.E.E.E.* **62**, 1391.

ELDRICH J. & SMYTH C.J. (1977) Millimetre wave thermograph as subcutaneous indicator of joint inflammation. In *Proceedings of the Seventh European Microwave Conference, Copenhagen, 1977.* 713.

ENANDER B. & LARSON G. (1974) Microwave radiometric measurements of the temperature inside the body. *Electron Lett.* **10**, 317.

GRENNAN D.M. *et al.* (1982) Infra-red thermography in the assessment of sacroiliac inflammation. *Rheumatol. Rehabil.* **21**, 81–7.

LEROY Y. (1982) Microwave radiometry and thermography: present and prospective. In *Biomedical Thermology*, pp. 485–99. New York: Alan R. Liss.

RAJ A.P., ASKE C. *et al.* (1981) Thermography in the assessment of peripheral joint inflammation—a reevaluation. *Rheumatol. Rehabil.* **20**, 81–7.

STERNS E.E. *et al.* (1982) Thermography in breast diagnosis. *Cancer* **15**, 323–5.

Ultrasound

BABCOCK D.S. & BOKYUNG K. HAN (1981) The accuracy of high resolution real time ultrasonography of the head in infancy. *Radiology* **139**, 665–77.

BARNES R.W. (1981) Ultrasound techniques for evaluation of lower extremity venous disease. *Semin. Ultra.* **2**, 276.

BERNARDINO M.E., THOMAS J.L., MAKLAD M.F. (1982) Hepatic sonography. Technical considerations, present applications and possible future. *Radiology* **42**, 249–52.

GRAF R. (1980) Diagnosis of congenital hip joint dislocation by ultrasonic compound scanning. *Arch. orthop. traumat. Surg.* **97**, 117–33.

GRAMIAK R. & NANDA N.C. (1979) New techniques in cardiac imaging with ultrasound: state of the art. *Radiology* **133**, 669–77.

HOLM H.H., ALS O. & GAMMELRAARD J. (1979) Percutaneous aspiration and biopsy procedures under ultrasound visualisation. *Clin. diagn. Ultra.* **1**, 137.

KAUFMAN S.L., BARTH K.H., KADIR S. *et al.* (1982) Hemodynamic measurements in the evaluation and follow up of transluminal angioplasty of the iliac and femoral arteries. *Radiology* **142**, 329–36.

NOVICK G., GHELMIN B. & SCHNEIDER M. (1983) Sonography of the neonatal and infant hip. *Amer. J. Roentgenol.* **141**, 639.

RUBIN J.M. & DOHRMANN G.J. (1983) Intra-operative sonography of the spine. *Radiology* **146**, 173–7.

SLASKY B.S., LENKEY J.L., SKOLNICK M.L. *et al.* (1982) Sonography of soft tissues of extremities and trunk. *Semin. Ultra.* **3**, 288.

TURNIPSEED W.D., SACKETT J.F., STROTHEN C.M. *et al.* (1982) Comparison of standard cerebral anteriography, with non-invasive Doppler imaging and intravenous angiography. *Radiology* **145**, 582–3.

Needle aspiration biopsy

GRIFFITHS H.J. (1979) Interventional radiology: musculoskeletal system. *Radiol Clin. N. Amer.* **17**, 475–84.

HAAGA J.R. (1979) New techniques for CT guided biopsies. *Amer. J. Roentgenol.* **133**, 633–41.

HARDY D.C., MURPHY W.A. & GILULA L.A. (1980) Computed tomography in planning of percutaneous bone biopsy. *Radiology* **137**, 447–50.

LALLI A.F. (1970) Roentgen guided aspiration biopsies of skeletal lesions. *J. Canad. Ass. Radiol.* **21**, 71–3.

LEGGE D., ENNIS J.T. & DEMPSEY J. (1978) Percutaneous needle biopsy in the management of solitary lesions of bone. *Clin. Radiol.* **29**, 497–500.

MARTIN H.E. & ELLIS E.B. (1930) Biopsy by needle puncture and aspiration. *Ann. Surg.* **92**, 169–81.

MAZET R. & COZEN L. (1952) The diagnostic value of vertebral body needle biopsy. *Ann. Surg.* **135**, 245–52.

MURPHY W.A., DESTOUET J.M. & GILLULA L.A. (1981) Percutaneous skeletal biopsy 1981: a procedure for radiologists. Results review and recommendations. *Radiology* **139**, 545–9.

TEHRANZADEH J., FREIBERGER R.H. & GHELMAN B. (1983) Closed needle biopsy: review of 120 cases. *Amer. J. Roentgenol.* **140**, 113–15.

VAN SONNENBERG, FERRUCI J.T., MUELLER P., WITTENBERG J. & SIMEONE J. (1982) Percutaneous drainage of abscess and fluid collections. Techniques, results and applications. *Radiology* **142**, 1–11.

Chapter 6
Bone and Joint Measurement

E. HIGGINBOTTOM & G.A. EVANS

The upper limb

THE SHOULDER

Acromiohumeral distance (Fig. 6.1, Weiner & McNab 1970)

Degenerative changes and rupture of the rotator cuff overlying the humeral head can sometimes be recognized by proximal migration of the humeral head. A standard anteroposterior radiograph of the shoulder is taken with the arm at the side in neutral rotation. The interval between the humeral head and the inferior portion of the acromion has a normal range of 7–14 mm. Narrowing to 5 mm or less is abnormal, and was found in 44% of 59 patients with a proven rotator cuff rupture.

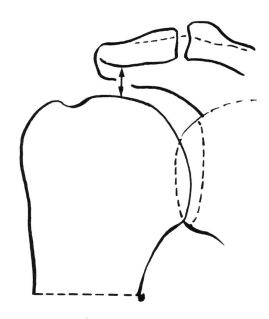

Acromiohumeral interval

Fig. 6.1.

THE ELBOW

1 Carrying angle (Keats *et al.* 1976)

The normal elbow has a slight valgus alignment known as the carrying angle. This may be affected by fractures, especially a supracondylar fracture during childhood.

The measurement may be made radiographically in an anteroposterior projection with the elbow extended fully and the two humeral epicondyles equidistant from the film. Lines are drawn along the long axes of the humerus and ulna, and a transverse line is drawn tangential to the humeral articular surface as shown in Fig. 6.2. The normal ranges of the bony alignment are as in Table 6.1.

Table 6.1.

	Male	Female
Carrying angle	2–26° (11°)	2–22° (13°)
Humeral angle	77–95°	72–91°
Ulnar angle	74–99°	72–93°

2 Baumann's angle (Fig. 6.3, Baumann 1929, Jones 1977)

This measurement allows assessment of the reduction of a displaced supracondylar fracture of the humerus. The anteroposterior projection should be taken with the fracture held reduced. If the fracture has been treated by closed reduction, and the position maintained by flexion of the elbow in a collar and cuff, it is important to take a 'shoot-through' projection of distal humerus. Extension of the elbow in these circumstances will allow the fracture to displace. Both elbows are radiographed.

Baumann's angle is formed by a line drawn along the lower border of the lateral humeral metaphysis and a line drawn at right angles to

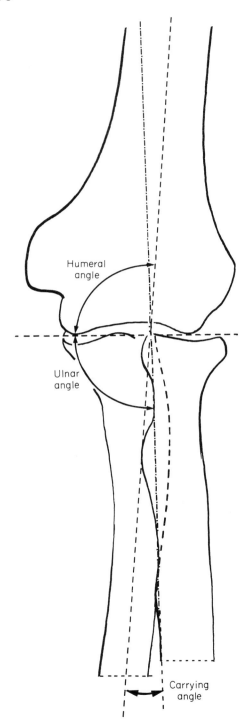

Humeral
angle

Ulnar
angle

Carrying
angle

Fig. 6.2.

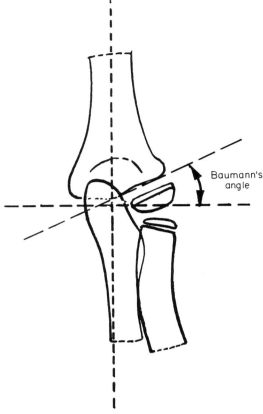

Baumann's
angle

Fig. 6.3.

the long axis of the humerus. Unfortunately, the bony detail is sometimes difficult to define, especially when the projection is taken by the 'shoot-through' technique. The objective of treatment is to achieve a reduction with the Baumann's angle symmetrical. An increase in the angle indicates cubitus varus, and a decrease indicates cubitus valgus.

3   Radial head alignment (Fig. 6.4, Storen 1959)

The relationship between the radius and the humerus is difficult to determine in young children where epiphyseal ossification centres have not yet appeared, because of the distance between the distal end of the humerus and the proximal end of the radius. This makes the diagnosis of dislocation of the radial head difficult.

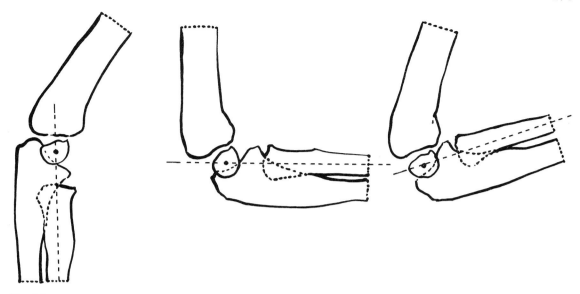

Fig. 6.4.

The projection of choice is a lateral view of the elbow with the joint flexed. A line extending along the mid-axis of the radius should pass through the centre of the capitellum in all positions of elbow flexion.

THE WRIST AND HAND

1 Articular inclination (Keats *et al.* 1966)
The normal alignment of the distal radius and ulna may be disturbed by fractures or by skeletal dysplasias such as dyschondrosteosis (Madelung deformity) and diaphyseal aclasis.

On a standard *anteroposterior projection* the angle measured is formed by the longitudinal axis of the radius and a line passing tangentially from the tip of the radial styloid process through the base of the ulnar styloid process. The proximal ulnar angle is usually less than a right angle (average 83°), and the normal range for males is 72–93°, for females 73–95° (Fig. 6.5a).

On the standard lateral projection the angle measured is formed by the longitudinal axis of the radius and a line drawn tangentially across the most distal points of the radial articular surface. The proximal ventral angle formed is usually less than a right angle (average 85°),

and the normal range for males is 79–93° and for females 80–94° (Fig. 6.5b).

2 Carpal angle (Fig. 6.6, Harper *et al.* 1974)
On an anteroposterior projection of the wrist, taken with the hand in a neutral position, the carpal angle is formed by two tangents. The first tangential line touches the proximal contour of the scaphoid and lunate and the second line touches the triquetrum and lunate. The obtuse angle formed has considerable deviation with age, sex and race, ranging from 110° to 150°. The angle is slightly greater in the black than the white population. On average the angle is also greater in girls than boys, but there is no appreciable sex difference in adults.

3 Flexion and extension ranges (Fig. 6.7, Brumfield *et al.* 1966)
Overall flexion and extension of the hand on the forearm represents the combined ranges of motion at the radiocarpal, intercarpal and carpometacarpal joints. The total range and relative contribution by the different elements can be affected by congenital abnormalities such as intercarpal fusions, and by ligamentous and joint injuries.

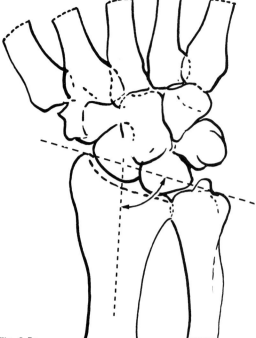

Fig. 6.5a.

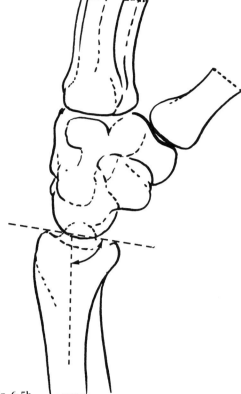

Fig. 6.5b.

On a true lateral of the wrist and hand taken in full flexion and extension the following lines are drawn:

(a) The longitudinal axes of the radius and second metacarpal bone.

(b) The transverse axis of the lunate as a line tangential to its intercarpal surface. A perpendicular to this line is then constructed.

Table 6.2 gives the average values for the combined ranges of flexion and extension.

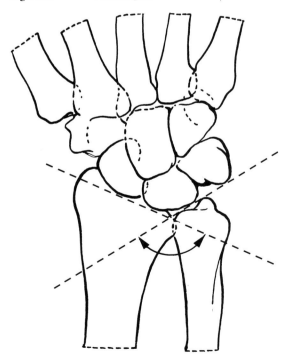

Fig. 6.6.

Table 6.2.

Combined extension and flexion	Males	Females
Total range (angles 1 + 4)	151°	156°
Radiocarpal (angles 2 + 5)	60°	65°
Intercarpal (angles 3 + 6)	77°	82°

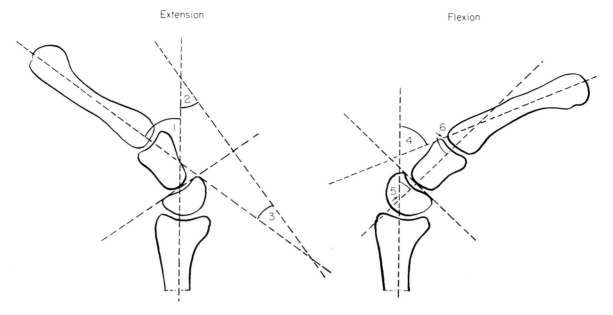

Extension   Flexion

Fig. 6.7.

4 *Carpal instability* (Fig. 6.8, Linscheid *et al.* 1972)

Traumatic rupture of the intercarpal ligaments may produce instability of the carpus, the pattern of which can be identified and quantified on a routine lateral radiograph of the wrist held in the neutral position. In the normal hand the longitudinal axes of the radius, lunate, capitate, and third metacarpal are collinear. The scapholunate angle formed by the longitudinal axes of the scaphoid and lunate averages 46° (range 30–60°).

Carpal instability can be divided in two main types: dorsal and palmar. In the commoner dorsal variety the lunate is dorsiflexed and displaced ventrally with respect to the longitudinal axes of the radius and the capitate, which are no longer collinear. This is usually associated with rotational displacement of the scaphoid so that its axis is almost perpendicular to the radius, and the scapholunate angle is increased. In the palmar variety of instability there is palmar flexion of the lunate relative to the long axes of radius and capitate, and there may be

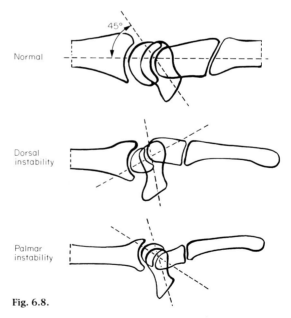

Fig. 6.8.

additional dorsal subluxation of the lunate on the radius. The scaphoid often appears foreshortened but there is no increase of the scapholunate angle.

5 *Metacarpal length* (Fig. 6.9, Garn *et al.*
1972)
Metacarpal and phalangeal length may be
measured, and when compared with the standard measurements for an age range from two
years to adult life it is possible to construct a
pattern profile for the evaluation of skeletal malformations. Measurements are made on a posteroanterior projection of the hand, with a tube
distance of 36 inches. The whole length of the
bone is measured, including epiphyses, with the
exception of the 'hook' at the base of the third
metacarpal, which is excluded.

6 *Metacarpal index* (Joseph & Meadow 1969,
Parish 1966)
The ratio of metacarpal length to minimum
width may be abnormal and allow confirmation
of congenital abnormalities. In Marfan's
syndrome the metacarpal index is above the
normal range, and it is below normal in Morquio's disease. Measurements are made on a
posteroanterior projection of the hand, with a
tube distance of 30 inches. The metacarpal
index is calculated by measuring the axial
length and minimal width of the second, third,
fourth and fifth metacarpals. The sum of the
lengths is divided by the sum of the widths (Fig.
6.9).
   The metacarpal index during infancy increases slowly with growth. Marfan's syndrome
has an index of 7 or greater.

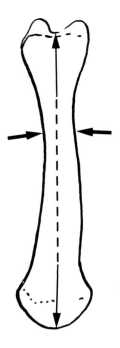

Fig. 6.9.

Table 6.3. Normal indices.

Age (months)	6	12	18	24	Adult
Male	5·23	5·2	5·28	5·4	6·86 (5·9–8·1)
Female	5·6	5·75	5·82	5·84	7·6 (6·3–8·9)

7 *Skeletal maturation* (Pyle *et al.* 1971)
It is essential to assess skeletal growth and bone
age when planning the correction of leg-length
discrepancy by growth-arrest techniques such
as epiphyseodesis and growth-plate stapling.
   In order to improve the accuracy of the timing of these procedures the bone age should be

assessed on several occasions. For this reason
the methods of assessing skeletal development
which require extensive exposure of the body
are not applicable because of the large cumulative radiation doses. The bone age is therefore
assessed on repeated hand radiographs according to the technique described by Greulich and
Pyle (1959) or Tanner *et al.* (1975). The
patient's film is compared with the published
standard radiographs of the same sex. The standard radiograph which appears to resemble the
patient's film most closely designates the bone
age or stage of skeletal maturation. The specific
radiographic technique and method of assessment are described fully by Greulich and Pyle
(1959) and Tanner *et al.* (1975) respectively.

The lower limb

THE HIP JOINT

Most measurements of the hip joint relate to
comparisons between normal and abnormal
values, and between one side and the other. In

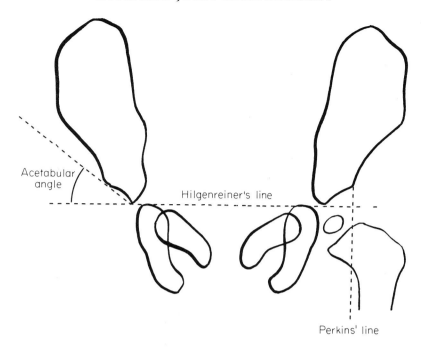

Fig. 6.10.

the neonate and the infant most of the important structures such as the acetabular rim and femoral head are radiolucent. The assessment of available landmarks, with the drawing of lines and measurement of angles, determines the relationship between the unseen femoral head and the visible part of the acetabulum. The objective is to identify lateral or proximal displacement of the femur in relation to the acetabulum, and to assess the ossific development of the acetabulum, and femoral head and neck.

1   Acetabular angle (Fig. 6.10, Hilgenreiner 1925)
This is a method of assessing the ossification and development of the acetabulum during the first months and years of life. The angle is increased in acetabular dysplasia, which is usually secondary to dislocation or subluxation of the femoral head.

The patient lies supine and an anteroposterior projection of the pelvis is obtained, with the central ray perpendicular to the film and centred to a point 2·5 cm above the symphysis pubis. The usual tube–film distance is 100 cm. It is essential that there is no pelvic rotation or asymmetry.

A horizontal line is drawn through the triradiate cartilages at the upper ossific margins (Hilgenreiner's line). Oblique lines are drawn from these latter points to the lateral acetabular margins, thus forming the acetabular angles. The normal measurements in the white population are shown in Table 6.4. Single measurements are unsatisfactory in assessing or predicting acetabular development. There may also be considerable interobserver variation of the measurement.

Table 6.4.

	Female	Male
At birth	28·8 ± 4·8°	26·4 ± 4·4°
Age 6 months	23·2 ± 4·0°	20·3 ± 3·7°
Age 12 months	21·2 ± 3·8°	19·8 ± 3·6°

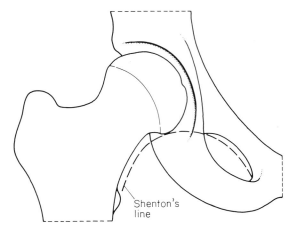

Fig. 6.11.

2   Perkins' (Ombredanne) line (Perkins 1928, Bertol *et al.* 1982)

This allows assessment of the relationship between the femoral metaphysis, or at a later stage the ossified femoral head, and the acetabulum. The position of the patient and the radiographic projection is as for (1) with the legs held together in neutral rotation.

A vertical line is drawn down from the lateral margin of the acetabulum, perpendicular to Hilgenreiner's line. The centre of ossification of the femoral head lies below the horizontal line and medial to the vertical line. In cases of dislocation it will be above and lateral to these lines. Reduction of the vertical distance from the acetabular margin to the femoral metaphysis measures cephalad displacement of the femur. Prior to ossification of the femoral head, the distance between the medial metaphysis and nearest point on the ossified ischium may be measured and should be less than 5 mm (Fig. 6.10).

3   Shenton's line (Fig. 6.11, Shenton 1911)

This is an assessment of proximal migration of the femoral head and neck in relation to the pelvis.

The patient lies or stands with the legs together and in neutral rotation. A routine anteroposterior projection of the pelvis or hip is obtained centred 2·5 cm superior to the pubic symphysis.

In the normal hip Shenton's line is an even arc of continuous contour between the superior border of the obturator foramen and the inferior margin of the femoral neck. In the dislocated or subluxated hip the line is broken as the femoral neck is displaced proximally. The line may be slightly interrupted if the radiograph is taken when the normal hip is held in external rotation and adduction.

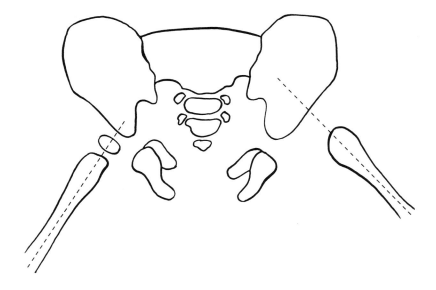

Fig. 6.12.

4 *Von Rosen projection* (Fig. 6.12, Andren &
Von Rosen 1958)

This radiographic projection is taken in order to
demonstrate irreducible dislocation of the femoral head during infancy, prior to ossification
of the capital femoral epiphysis. The patient lies
supine with the hips abducted not less than
45° and internally rotated. An anteroposterior
radiographic projection is taken, centred 5 cm
above the symphysis pubis and at a standard
distance of 100 cm.

A longitudinal line is drawn proximally along
the femoral shaft. In a normal hip its medial
continuation passes within the acetabulum or
through the corner of the acetabular roof, and
crosses the spine at the L4 vertebra. In a dislocated hip the line lies higher, crossing the
anterior superior iliac spine and passing above
the L3 vertebra. A reducible dislocation of the
hip may be overlooked by this technique, as the
femoral head may enter the acetabulum in abduction and internal rotation.

5 *Centre–edge angle of Wiberg* (Fig. 6.13,
Wiberg 1939, Tonnis 1976)

This technique assesses the relationship of the

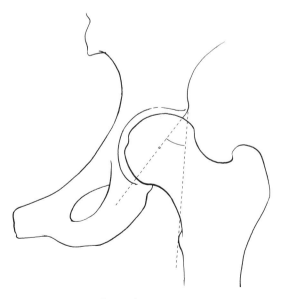

Fig. 6.13.   Centre–edge angle.

femoral head to the acetabulum and is a
measure of acetabular cover. Measurements are
abnormal in acetabular dysplasia, with or without subluxation of the femoral head.

On the routine anterior–posterior projection
of the pelvis, centred 2·5 cm above the pubic
symphysis, an angle is formed between Perkins'
line and a line drawn from the most lateral
ossified margin of the acetabulum to the centre
of the ossified nucleus of the femoral head. The
technique is of relevance in the age range 5–20
years. The measurement is considered abnormal
if less than the following angle:

Age range:	5–8 years	19°
	9–12 years	25°
	13–20 years	26–30°

As a single measurement this appears to give
the best indication as to the long-term prognosis
of the joint.

6 *The teardrop distance* (Fig. 6.14, Eyring *et al.*
1965)

This measures lateralization of the ossified
femoral head from the medial wall of the
acetabulum, which may occur as the earliest
radiological sign of Perthes' disease.

Routine anteroposterior projection with the
central ray perpendicular to the plane of the
film, centred over the mid-pelvis and a tube–
film distance of 100 cm. Positioning does not
alter the measurement provided the hip is not
rotated internally or externally more than 30°,
flexed more than 30° or abducted more than 15°.

The teardrop shadow becomes visible when
the infant is a few months old. It consists of
three lines formed by the floor of the acetabulum, the inner wall of the lesser pelvis, and a
short connecting curved line that corresponds
to the cortex of the acetabular notch. Measurement is made from the lateral margin of the
teardrop to the medial border of the proximal
femoral metaphysis, and is independent of the
child's age. Asymmetry greater than 2 mm or a
teardrop distance of more than 11 mm is abnormal.

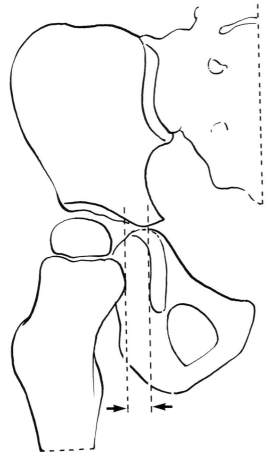

Fig. 6.14.

7   *Sharp's acetabular angle* (Fig. 6.15, Sharp 1961, Johnson *et al.* 1979)

This allows measurement of the acetabular inclination following closure of the triradiate cartilage, and assesses acetabular development in the older child and adult.

Routine anteroposterior projection of the pelvis, centred 5 cm above the pubic symphysis, ensuring the absence of pelvic rotation or asymmetry.

A baseline is drawn connecting the inferior margins of the pelvic teardrops. An angle is formed between this line and a further line connecting the inferior teardrop and the lateral margin of the same acetabulum. Normal values are as follows:

Age range:		
	Less than 3 years	$47° \pm 3$
	3–10 years	$45° \pm 2$
	10–14 years	$43° \pm 2$
	14–18 years	$41° \pm 3$
	Adults	$35° \pm 3$

8   *Articulotrochanteric distance* (Fig. 6.16, Edgren 1965, Langenskiold & Salenivs 1967)

This is an indirect measure of the femoral neck length. It is used to assess the disturbance of proximal femoral growth which may occur following Perthes' disease or as a complication of the treatment of congenital hip dislocation.

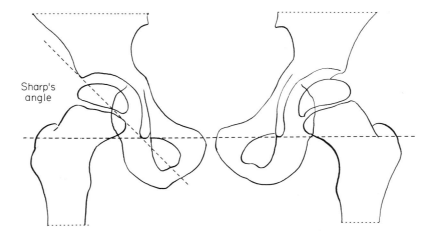

Sharp's angle

Fig. 6.15.

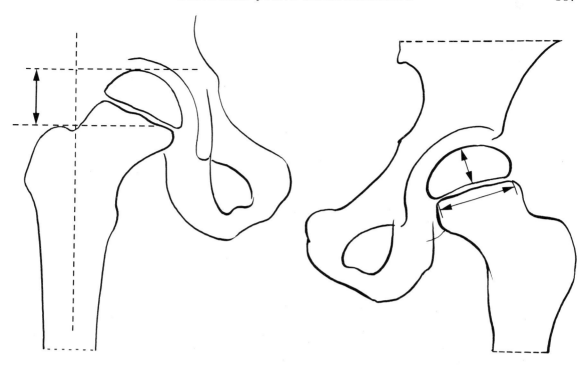

Fig. 6.16. Fig. 6.17.

Routine anteroposterior projection of the pelvis and proximal femurs, ensuring that the hips are in neutral rotation.

The distance is measured from the top of the greater trochanter to the level of the articular surface on the top of the femoral head along a line parallel to the long axis of the femoral shaft. A comparison is made with the opposite hip. The normal range for children between 5 and 13 years of age is 16 ± 3.6 mm for boys and 23 ± 4.5 mm for girls. This distance is decreased by severe damage to the proximal femoral growth plate and the greater trochanter may grow above the level of the femoral head.

9 Epiphyseal quotient (Fig. 6.17, Eyre-Brook 1936, Heyman & Herndon 1950)

This is an indirect measure of the sphericity of the femoral head which is used as part of the assessment of treatment in children with Perthes' disease. It is one of several femoral head, neck, and acetabular quotients that have been described. Measurements are made on a routine anteroposterior projection of the pelvis and hips. The maximum height of the epiphysis, as a line perpendicular to the growth plate, is divided by its widest diameter to give the epiphyseal index. The normal index, expressed as a percentage, is between 45 and 55 under seven years of age and between 35 and 45 over seven years of age. The epiphyseal quotient is the ratio of one epiphyseal index divided by that for the opposite normal hip, and the normal result should be close to 1·0. Sphericity of the head can be measured directly using the circle template described by Mose (1964).

10 Detection of minor epiphyseal displacement

The purpose of this technique is to detect minor degrees of displacement which may occur in adolescent children with slipping of the capital femoral epiphysis. On a standard anteroposterior radiograph of the femoral head a straight

(a)   ANTEROPOSTERIOR   (b)   LATERAL

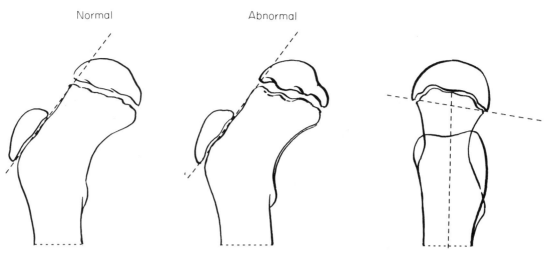

Fig. 6.18.

line is drawn up the superior border of the femoral neck. The line normally crosses the outer
portion of the epiphysis which bulges laterally
beyond this plane. If the line is tangential, or
lateral, to the head, this indicates displacement
of the epiphysis (Fig. 6.18a)

A more definitive measurement can be taken
on a lateral projection of the femoral head and
neck. A line is drawn along the axis of the neck
and should bisect the base of the epiphysis at
the midpoint. A line drawn across the base of
the epiphysis normally forms an angle of 85–90°
with the axis of the neck. This angle decreases
when the epiphysis slips posteriorly and can
serve as a measure of the displacement (Fig.
6.18b).

*11 Measurement of anteversion of the femoral
neck* (Fig. 6.19, Billing 1954)
There are many radiographic methods for measuring anteversion which are being superseded
by other techniques which utilize ultrasound,
computerized axial tomography and nuclear
magnetic resonance. Two basic radiographic
systems have been described. The first attempts
a direct measurement, and the other is an indirect measurement from anteroposterior and

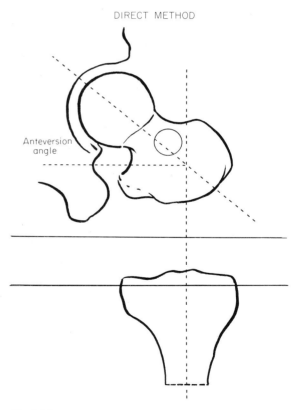

Fig. 6.19.

lateral radiographs, using a trigonometric calculation to obtain the angle of anteversion.

The direct method of Budin and Chandler (1957). The patient is seated on the X-ray table with the grid cassette placed vertically behind him. The knee is flexed to 90° over the edge of the table with the lower leg suspended vertically. The central ray passes along the length of the femur. The proximal tibia must be shown on the film. As this is a high kilovoltage technique gonadal protection is essential and repetition should be avoided. It is probable that this method should be used only on thin children under six years of age.

The measurement technique is based on the fact that there is a direct relationship between the longitudinal axis of the flexed tibia and the coronal (bicondylar) plane, which is perpendicular to it. The axis of the femoral head and neck can be drawn on the film. Thus the actual angle which the femoral neck makes with the coronal plane is directly recorded on the film.

Age-related normal angles of anteversion with this technique are as shown in Table 6.5.

Indirect method of Magilligan. This method is advantageous in the respect that both radiographic projections are standard ones and there is no need for additional exposure to radiation. Both films are taken with the patient lying supine with the femurs parallel to the table top, the knees flexed 90° and the lower legs suspended vertically over the end of the table. An anteroposterior film is obtained and the neck–shaft angle (α) measured. A lateral film is then taken with a horizontal beam, and the cassette placed lateral and parallel to the femoral neck by placing it at the same angle to the femoral shaft as the angle α. The neck–shaft angle (β) on the lateral film is then measured. The precise position of the lines for the measurement of angulation is probably the source of greatest inaccuracy. Determination of the true angle of anteversion is derived from the trigonometric relationship between the two measured angles and can be obtained from tables published by Magilligan (1956).

THE KNEE

1 Coronal plane (Fig. 6.20, Keats *et al.* 1966)
In the anteroposterior radiographic projection of the knee the centre point is 1 cm below the

Table 6.5.

Age (years)	Anteversion angle
0–1	30°–50°
1–2	30°
3–5	25°
6–12	20°
12–15	17°
16–20	11°
20	8°

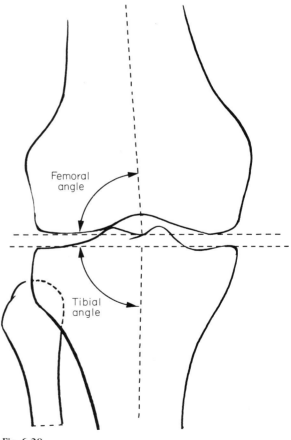

Fig. 6.20.

patella. The patella is centralized over the femur, and a number of patients require slight external rotation of the limb to achieve this.

The femoral angle (Table 6.6) is formed by a line drawn along the shaft of the femur and a line drawn tangentially along the inferior aspect of the femoral condyles. The femoral angle, which overlies the lateral condyle, is less than a right angle.

The tibial angle (Table 6.6) is formed by a line drawn along the tibial shaft and a line drawn tangentially to the tibial plateau. The tibial angle overlies the lateral tibial condyle.

Table 6.6. Femoral and tibial angles: normal values.

	Femoral angle	Tibial angle
Male	75–85°	85–100°
Female	75–85°	87–98°

2   Sagittal plane

Patellar position (Fig. 6.21, Insall & Salvati 1971). The relationship of the patella and femur can be assessed on the lateral projection of the knee. Proximal displacement of the patella is called patella alta, and this predisposes to lateral subluxation from the condylar groove of the femur.

The knee should be in a true lateral position with the femoral condyles superimposed, and the joint semiflexed. The central X-ray should be projected through the joint space, perpendicular to the plane of the film.

The height of the patella is measured from its proximal posterior border to the distal pole. The length of the patellar tendon is measured from its proximal posterior attachment, immediately above the apex of the patella, to the notch on the proximal margin of the tibial tubercle. These two measurements are approximately equal and the normal variation does not exceed 20%. There is a statistically significant increase of tendon length in patients with clinically demonstrable lateral subluxation of the patella.

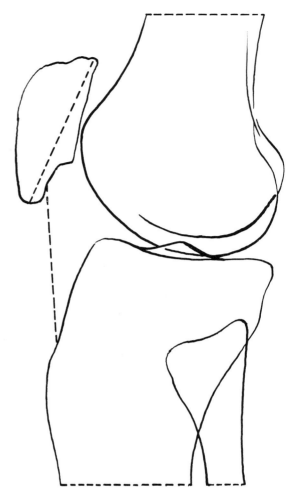

Fig. 6.21.

Tibial plateau angle (Fig. 6.22, Moore *et al.* 1974). The extent of tibial condylar depression and displacement following injury can be measured on a lateral projection of the knee and proximal tibia. A line is drawn along the anterior cortex of the tibia and it is bisected by a second line drawn along the tibial plateau. A further line is drawn from this point perpendicular to the anterior cortical line. The angle created by this perpendicular and the line along the plateau is called the tibial plateau angle.

The normal angle varies between 7° and 22° with a mean of 14° and a standard deviation of $\pm 3 \cdot 6°$.

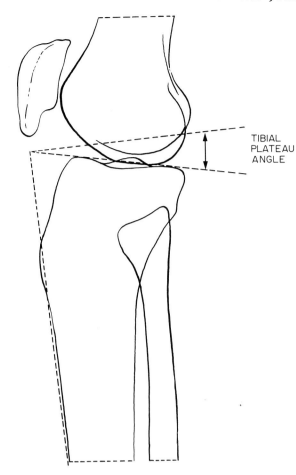

Fig. 6.22.

and the knee supported over the end of the table in 45° flexion. The quadriceps muscle should be relaxed. The tube is angled distally at 30° from the horizontal femur, and the film cassette is placed 30 cm below the knee, resting on the shins and perpendicular to the X-ray beam.

In Fig. 6.23 the highest points in the medial (B) and lateral (C) condyles and the lowest point of the intercondylar sulcus (A) are joined to form the sulcus angle (BAC). This angle is bisected (AO). A line is also drawn from the lowest point of the articular ridge of the patella (D) to the intercondylar sulcus. The angle DAO is described as the *congruence angle*. All values medial to the reference line AO are designated as minus, and those lateral as plus. The average congruence angle is −6°, with a standard deviation of 11°. Any angle greater than +6° is regarded as abnormal, irrespective of age, sex, side and patella alta. The sulcus angle is also flatter in the symptomatic knees with lateral patellar subluxation.

Laurin's projection (Fig. 6.24, Laurin *et al.* 1979). The patient lies supine with the hip semiflexed and the knee supported in 20 degrees of flexion. The tube is directed in a cephalad

3 Axial views

The normal relationship of the anterior surface of the femur and the patella has been defined using axial radiographs. Such projections may demonstrate abnormal lateral displacement of the patella in children or adolescents presenting with pain and a mechanical derangement of the joint. Most patients with recurrent subluxation or dislocation of the patella do not have lateral displacement of the patella on the routine anteroposterior and classic skyline radiographs.

Merchant's projection (Merchant *et al.* 1974). The patient lies supine with the hips extended

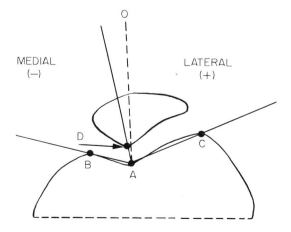

Fig. 6.23.

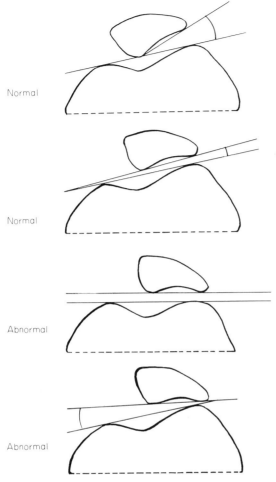

Normal

Normal

Abnormal

Abnormal

Fig. 6.24.

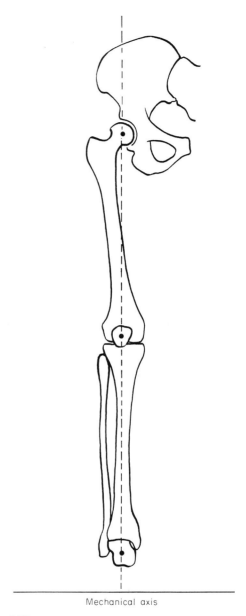

Mechanical axis

Fig. 6.25.

direction so that the beam is almost parallel to the anterior border of the tibia and passing through the patellofemoral joint. The cassette is held immediately proximal to the knee and positioned perpendicular to the beam.

A line is drawn to connect the anterior aspects of the femoral condyles and a second line drawn along the lateral facet of the patella. Normally the angle formed by these two lines opens laterally. In patients with subluxation of the patella these lines are parallel or the angle opens medially.

4   Long leg film (Fig. 6.25)

The purpose of this radiograph is to demonstrate the mechanical alignment of the hips, knees and ankles on the same anteroposterior projection while the patient is weight-bearing.

Normally the mechanical axis passing from the centre of the femoral head to the talus passes through the centre of the knee. The axis will be displaced inside the knee with genu varum deformity, and outside the knee with valgus deformity. The technique allows preoperative quantification of the deformity, and verification of the post-operative correction.

The patient stands erect with the patellae directed forwards and the tube centred on the knees. A long film is required to include the hips, knees and ankles on the same projection, and the whole film is exposed.

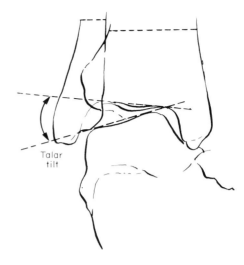

THE ANKLE AND FOOT

1 Stress views of the ankle (Fig. 6.26)

Stress inversion and anterior draw radiographs (Lindstrand & Mortensson 1977, Landeros *et al.* 1968) demonstrate instability of the talus within the ankle mortise due to rupture of the lateral ligament of the ankle. In order to obtain a clear view of the mortise and talar tilt (Leonard 1949, Rubin & Witten 1960, Lauren *et al.* 1968), the anteroposterior radiograph is taken with the leg internally rotated 10–20° so that the central ray is perpendicular to the transmalleolar plane. Inversion stress is applied slowly and progressively by the protected hands of the examiner holding the heel and distal tibia. Sudden inversion will cause peroneal muscle spasm and pain which will reduce or prevent the demonstration of instability. This test is more reliable when performed under general or spinal anaesthesia. The lateral radiograph should be taken in the transmalleolar axis. Anterior displacement of the talus may be demonstrated by resting the heel on a wooden block and pushing posteriorly on the tibia immediately above the ankle.

The interpretation of the stress inversion radiograph is difficult, as up to 25° of tilt has been recorded in uninjured ankles, and there may also be a normal asymmetry of 19°. However, the asymmetry of tilt is usually less than 10° in uninjured ankles. In general, talar tilt that

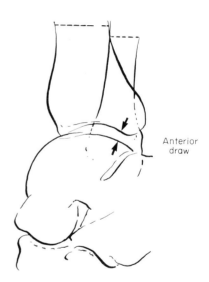

Fig. 6.26.

occurs only when the foot is plantarflexed is due to rupture of the anterior talofibular ligament, and a tilt that is present with the foot both plantarflexed and plantigrade indicates additional rupture of the calcaneofibular ligament. The anterior draw test is positive when the talus displaces forward in the ankle mortise, and indicates rupture of the anterior talofibular ligament. More than 3 mm of displacement is regarded as abnormal.

2   The calcaneum

The normal shape of the calcaneum may be disturbed by a crush fracture.

To demonstrate Boehler's angle (Boehler 1931) the ankle must be in the radiographic lateral position with both malleoli superimposed, and the central ray directed to the medial malleolus at 100 cm distance. Care must be taken not to overrotate the ankle joint.

The angle is made up by lines drawn tangentially to the anterior and posterior elements of the superior surface of the calcaneum. The normal range is between 28° and 40° but the average is between 30° and 35°. Less than 28° is abnormal (Fig. 6.27).

For a full assessment of fractures of the calcaneum the axial projection and Anthonson's oblique (Anthonson 1943) are required. The weight-bearing position of the heel, in relation to varus or valgus deformity, can be demonstrated and quantified according to the technique described by Cobey (1976).

3   The talocalcaneal angles and forefoot alignment (Simons 1978, Templeton 1965)

The talus and calcaneum are ossified at birth but the navicular bone cannot be demonstrated

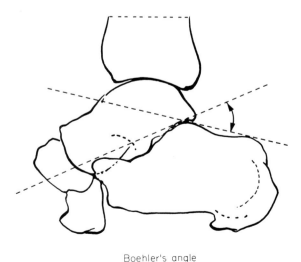

Boehler's angle

Fig. 6.27.

radiographically until the third or fourth year. Abnormal relationships of the hindfoot and forefoot, including talonavicular subluxation or dislocation, can be inferred from the assessment of anteroposterior and lateral radiographs of the foot when it is weight-bearing or alternatively, in a small infant, held in dorsiflexion. Such radiographs assist with the diagnosis, and with the assessment of the severity of deformity, and the effectiveness of surgical correction in congenital deformities such as club foot and vertical talus.

On the *anteroposterior projection* the lines drawn along the long axes of the ossific nuclei of the talus and calcaneum converge posteriorly to form a talocalcaneal angle, which in infants and young children measures 20–40°, and in children over five years of age measures less, 15–30°. This angle is decreased with a varus deformity of the hind foot and increased with a valgus deformity. The forward extension of the talar axial line passes either along the first metatarsal shaft, or inside the shafts by a maximum of 20° (talometatarsal angle). If the talar line passes outside the first metatarsal shaft this indicates medial deviation of the forefoot. The forward extension of the calcaneal axis usually falls along the fourth metatarsal (Fig. 6.28a).

On the *lateral projection* the lines drawn along the ossific nuclei of the talus and calcaneum converge anteriorly to form a talocalcaneal angle of 35–55° on maximum dorsiflexion of the foot during infancy, and 25–50° on a weight-bearing radiograph in an older child. Reduction of this angle indicates equinovarus deformity of the hind foot. During infancy forward extension of the talar axial line passes inferior to the first metatarsal bone, but at five years of age or older it passes along the metatarsal shaft (Fig. 6.28b).

In a child with congenital equinovarus deformity of the foot the talocalcaneal angle is reduced on both radiographic projections and the axis of the first metatarsal is displaced inwards and downwards in relation to the talar axis, indicating an additional equinovarus deformity of the forefoot (Fig. 6.29).

NORMAL FOOT

(a)   Anteroposterior

Anteroposterior

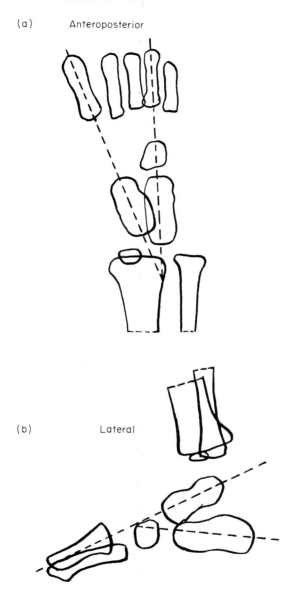

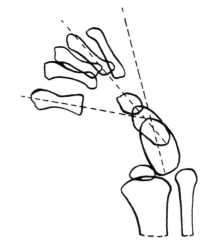

Lateral

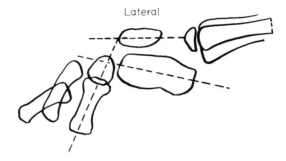

(b)   Lateral

Talipes equinovarus

Fig. 6.29.

Fig. 6.28.

In a child with metatarsus adductus the talocalcaneal angles are normal as there is no hindfoot deformity. However, on the anteroposterior projection the axis of the first metatarsal is displaced inwards in relation to the talar axis, indicating forefoot adductus. In addition the axes of the metatarsals tend to converge posteriorly, whereas in a normal foot they are very nearly parallel (Fig. 6.30).

A simple cavus deformity of the foot is due to equinus of the forefoot in relation to the hindfoot. The axis of the first metatarsal is inclined below the talar axial line. In addition the angle formed by a line drawn tangential to the inferior border of the calcaneum and a line along the axis of the fifth metatarsal is more acute than the normal range of 150–175° (weight-bearing) (Fig. 6.31).

Metatarsus adductus

Anteroposterior

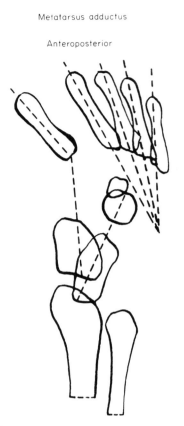

Fig. 6.30.

Lateral

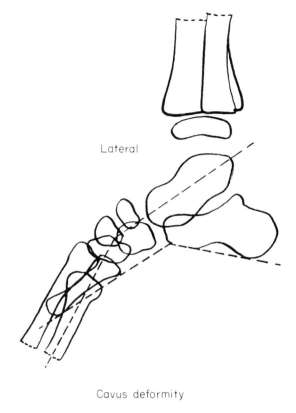

Cavus deformity

Fig. 6.31.

Leg length measurement (Tachdjian 1972)
Children may be born with a discrepancy of leg length which increases with growth, or, alternatively, damage to one of the femoral or tibial growth plates during childhood may cause a progressive discrepancy. Radiographic measurement of the leg lengths allows accurate assessment of the severity, site and rate of progression of the discrepancy. This in turn facilitates the selection and timing of corrective procedures.

The technique utilizes three separate radiographic exposures with the beam sequentially centred directly over the hip, the knee and the ankle of the patient, who is lying supine. The distance between the major joint surfaces is calibrated by means of a centimetre rule placed on the same surface as that upon which the patient is lying. This allows measurement of the total

leg length discrepancy and the proportions in the femur and tibia.

There are two possible sources of inaccuracy. Firstly, the technique does not take into account any asymmetry of the pelvis or feet. Secondly, if the patient moves between any of the exposures the examination is invalidated.

The spine

As a general principle the radiation dose for the patient should be kept to a minimum by the following techniques:

(a) Protection of the gonads if this does not obscure relevant detail.
(b) Fast film/screen combination.
(c) Adequate filtration upon the X-ray tube.
(d) Adequate collimation/narrow diaphragm.

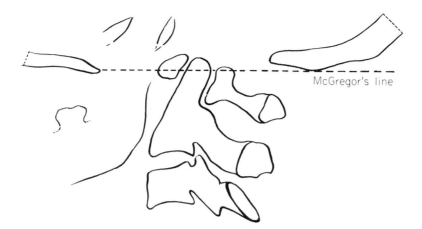

McGregor's line

Fig. 6.32.

(e) Special dose-reducing techniques where applicable.

(f) Clearly defined protocols for different clinical presentations.

1 Basilar invagination of the skull by C1 vertebra (Bull *et al*. 1955, Hinck & Hopkins 1960)
The cervical spine may invaginate into the base of the skull as a congenital anomaly, or secondary to generalized weakening of the skeleton, as in osteogenesis imperfecta, osteomalacia, hyperparathyroidism and Paget's disease. This abnormal relationship can be determined radiographically by the following techniques.

McGregor's line (McGregor 1948, Fig. 6.32) is drawn on a lateral projection which is centred to C2 vertebra, with a tube distance of 72 inches. A line drawn from the posterior edge of the hard palate to the most caudal part of the occiput normally passes just above the tip of the odontoid peg, the mean position of the tip relative to this line being 0.39 ± 3.02 mm. The odontoid is displaced superiorly in the presence of basilar invagination.

2 Atlas–odontoid distance (Fig. 6.33, Locke *et al*. 1966, Hinck & Hopkins 1960)
Some forward shift (up to 2 mm) of a vertebral body on its caudal neighbour is normal if it occurs evenly throughout the neck. In children,

more pronounced shift of one vertebra on another is seen in a quarter of cases. Following injury, this displacement is not abnormal unless accompanied by physical signs of restricted neck movement. However, marked atlantoaxial displacement may occur without pain as the result of skeletal dysplasias such as Morquio's disease and spondyloepiphyseal dysplasia congenita.

A lateral projection of the neck is centred on the thyroid cartilage, with the head and neck

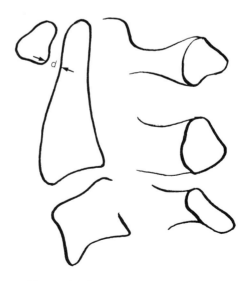

Diagnosis of atlantoaxial subluxation

Fig. 6.33.

held in a neutral position and a tube distance of 72 inches. The distance between the postero-inferior margin of the anterior arch of the atlas and the anterior surface of the odontoid process is measured. The maximum atlas–odontoid displacement found in a normal child is 5 mm, with a mean distance of 2 mm. In 95% of normal adults the measurement is between 2 and 4 mm with the head held neutral, and on forward flexion the range measures 1·8–3 mm.

3 Anterior displacement of C2 vertebra (Fig. 6.34, Swischuk 1977)

Differentiating pseudodislocation of the cervical spine from true fracture–dislocation of C2 on C3 is often difficult in children. In the presence of anterior displacement of the C2 vertebral body it has been noted that the alignment of the posterior arches and spinous processes of the upper three cervical vertebrae is distinctly different in cases with physiological and with pathological displacement.

On a true lateral projection of the cervical spine a line is drawn through the anterior cortex of the posterior arches of the C1 and C3 vertebrae. If this line touches or comes within 1 mm of the front of the same point on the C2 vertebra it is normal. If the line misses the C2 arch by 2 mm or more it is highly suggestive of a fracture–dislocation through the C2 vertebra. A false-positive interpretation may occur if the C2 vertebra is angulated forwards by muscle spasm without anterior displacement of the body.

4 Measurements for cervical instability below C2 vertebra

Augustus White III *et al.* (1975) in a series of cadaveric experiments measured the physiological limits of intervertebral displacement and angulation in the cervical spine. They found that:

(a) Instability is present if there is more than 2·7 mm horizontal displacement of one vertebral body relative to the one immediately inferior, when measured with mechanical gauges. A correction was made for X-ray magnification, and it is claimed that acute forward displacement of 3·5 mm or more on a standard lateral radiograph of the neck indicates the spine is unstable.

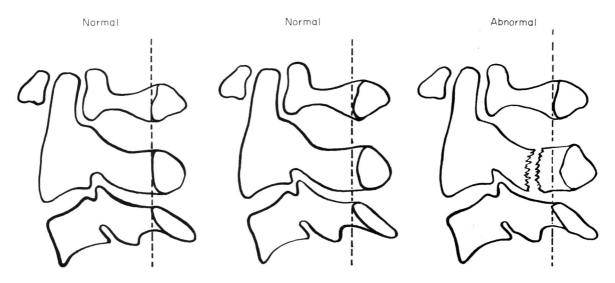

Normal   Normal   Abnormal

No displacement   1 mm displacement   2 mm or more displacement

Fig. 6.34.

(b) The upper limit of physiological angular displacement of adjacent vertebrae was an 11° difference compared with the adjacent cervical segments. Lines are drawn along the inferior vertebral end-plates on a lateral radiograph and the angles formed at each spinal segment are measured. The measurement is not affected by X-ray magnification.

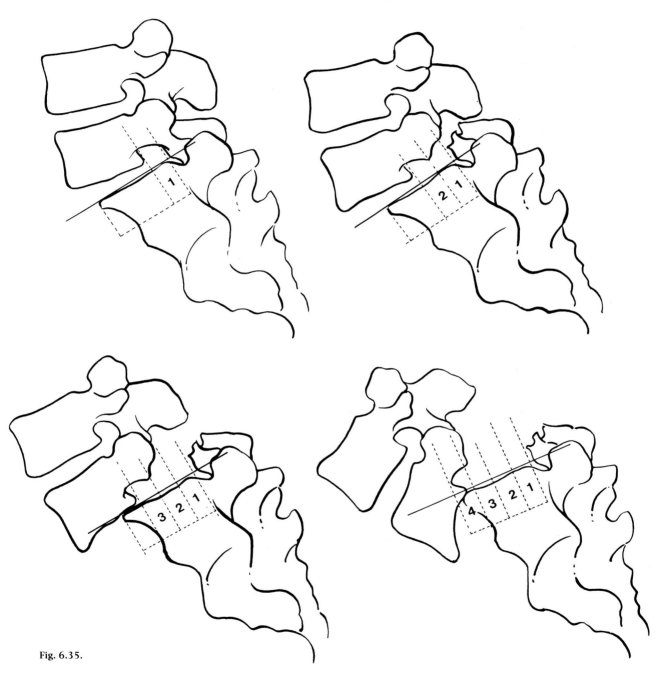

Fig. 6.35.

5   *Spinal instability in spondylolisthesis*

There are several techniques for assessing the severity of vertebral displacement, which when measured on a series of X-rays of the same patient will quantitate the progression of displacement. A true lateral radiograph of the lumbosacral junction is obtained with a focus/film distance of not less than 100 cm.

Meyerding's classification (Meyerding 1932) is based on the relationship between the superior surface of the sacrum and the posteroinferior corner of the body of the fifth lumbar vertebra. The superior surface of the sacrum is divided into four quarters, as shown in Fig. 6.35, and the position of the fifth lumbar vertebra graded accordingly.

Garland and Thomas (1946) have described a technique for assessing early or minor displacement. A line is drawn proximally from the anterior margin of the superior surface of the sacrum, perpendicular to the sacral end-plate. The anteroinferior corner of the fifth lumbar vertebral body is normally 1–8 mm behind this line (Fig. 6.36).

O'Brien (personal communication) describes a method which is particularly suitable for patients with severe displacement or spondyloptosis, where there has been remodelling of the anterosuperior margin of the sacrum. An angle is measured by drawing lines along the superior borders of fifth lumbar and second sacral vertebrae. This technique demonstrates a lordotic angle in the normal spine, and severe displacement represents a kyphotic deformity (Fig. 6.37).

6   *Assessment of scoliosis*

After clinical examination a number of children will be referred for radiographic assessment. The following technique is suggested so that the radiation dose is kept to a minimum, especially in the radiosensitive area of the

(a)   (b)

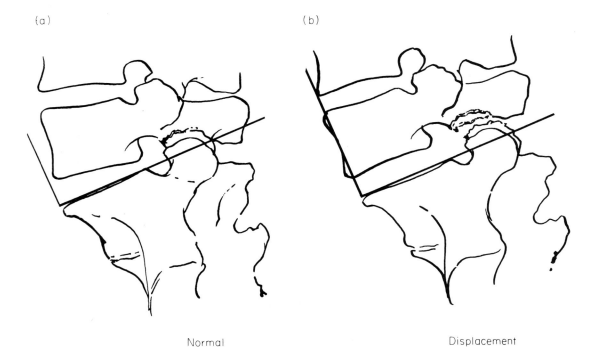

Normal   Displacement

Fig. 6.36.

female breast. The radiograph is taken with the patient erect in the posteroanterior position. An air gap technique is used with a minimum air gap of 22 cm between cassette and sternum and a tube/focus/film distance of at least 3 m, and preferably 3·5 m. The size of cassette is dependent upon age and height of the patient, but it may be necessary to use cassettes up to 95 cm in length. At these tube/film distances field coverage is not a problem.

A full 'scoliosis series' will consist of the following projections:

1 Anteroposterior projection whole spine erect.
2 Lateral projection whole spine erect.
3 Anteroposterior projections whole spine erect, one with left lateral flexion and the other with right lateral flexion.
4 Posteroanterior projection of the chest for rib cage deformity.
5 Coned lateral projection L5/S1 region supine.
6 Hand to include wrist joint for bone age assessment.

One of the projections should include the iliac crests for the assessment of skeletal maturity. Sequential radiographic assessment will usually require the erect anteroposterior projection alone.

(a) *Angular deformity.* Scoliosis is a curvature in the coronal plane of the spine. The Scoliosis Research Society recommends measurement of the deformity by the technique described by Cobb (1948). Two lines are drawn along the superior and inferior end-plates respectively of the upper and lower vertebrae which tilt maximally towards the concavity of the curve (end vertebrae). Alternative anatomical landmarks may be used, such as the superior or inferior borders of the pedicles, if the end-plates are indistinct. These lines form the Cobb angle. It may be necessary to construct perpendiculars to these lines for technical reasons in order to measure lesser angles on the radiograph (Fig. 6.38).

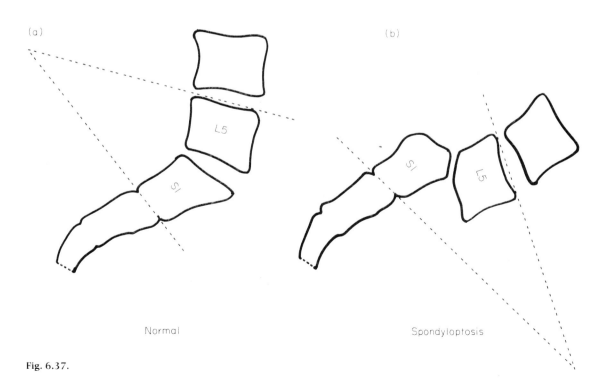

(a)   Normal

(b)   Spondyloptosis

Fig. 6.37.

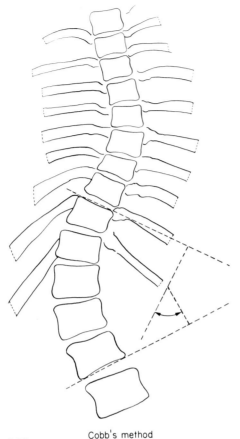

Fig. 6.38.   Cobb's method

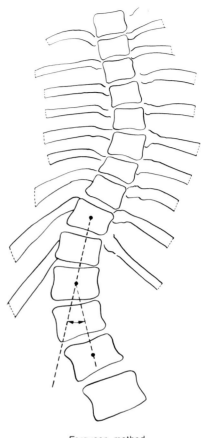

Fig. 6.39.   Ferguson method

Stagnara *et al.* (1977) have indicated that as the Cobb angle increases the accuracy of the measurement decreases, because scoliosis is associated with rotational deformity of the vertebrae. They have suggested that if the patient is screened and rotated so that the central ray passes perpendicular to the anterior surface of the mid-vertebra of the curve, and the patient is then radiographed in this oblique position, the new measurement reflects the deformity more accurately. This technique may also provide better definition of congenital abnormalities and diastematomyelia.

The measurement technique described by Ferguson (1949) is more accurate than Cobb's method for angles of less than 50°. The end vertebrae and the vertebra at the apex of the curve

are identified. The apical vertebra has the most rotation and the most deviation from the vertical axis of the patient. Lines are drawn through the centres of these vertebral bodies as shown in Fig. 6.39, and the inferior angle formed is the recorded deformity.

(b) *Rotational deformity.* Vertebral rotation can be assessed by the method described by Nash and Moe (1969). In the normal vertebra there is symmetry between the pedicles and the lateral borders of the body on the anteroposterior radiograph. As rotation occurs the pedicle on the convex side of the curve appears to move further from the lateral edge of the vertebra towards the midline. The rotational deformity has been graded as shown in Fig. 6.40. The interval

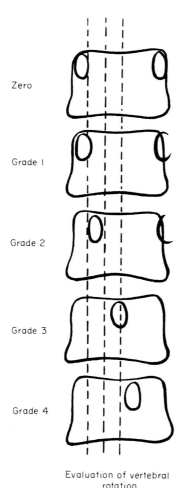

Zero

Grade 1

Grade 2

Grade 3

Grade 4

Evaluation of vertebral
rotation

Fig. 6.40.

from the lateral edge of the vertebra to the mid-line is divided into three, and there is a fourth grade beyond the midpoint.

(c) *Skeletal maturity.* Fusion of the vertebral ring apophyses coincides with complete cessation of spinal growth, which has significance in relation to the prognosis and treatment of spinal deformities. Other techniques for assessing skeletal development are the evaluation of bone age on a radiograph of the left hand, and the grading of ossification of the iliac crests as described by Risser (1958). Normally ossification of the iliac epiphysis starts at the anterior spine and progresses posteriorly to the posterior superior iliac spine. Once complete ossification has occurred, fusion of the epiphysis with the ilium takes place. Risser divided the iliac crest into four quarters, and graded the ossification from 1 to 4 as it reaches these quadrants. Finally, Risser 5 + indicates fusion of the epiphysis, which correlates with the cessation of growth (Fig. 6.41).

7   The rib–vertebral angle (Mehta) (Fig. 6.42)
The majority of cases of infantile idiopathic scoliosis resolve spontaneously. Mehta (1972) has described a radiographic technique which identifies the progressive curves at an early stage with approximately 80% accuracy. On an anteroposterior radiograph of the spine the relationship is defined between the apical vertebra of the curve and its adjacent ribs. The rib–vertebral angle is formed by a line drawn along

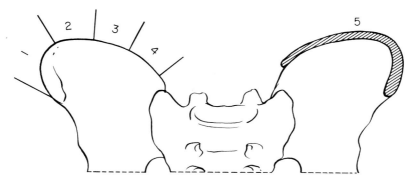

Fig. 6.41.   Ossification of iliac epiphysis

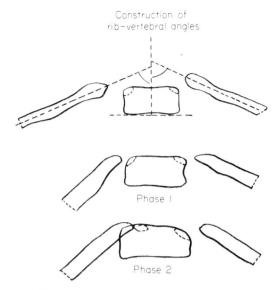

Construction of
rib—vertebral angles

Phase 1

Phase 2

Fig. 6.42.

the mid-neck and midpoint of the head of the rib to the perpendicular drawn from the vertebral end-plate. The difference in the measured angles on the right and left sides is recorded. The relationship of the rib head on the convex side to vertebral body is also noted. The features are interpreted as follows:

Phase 1. The heads of the ribs do not overlap the vertebral body. A rib–vertebral angle difference of 20° or more indicates a potentially progressive curve. A more accurate prognosis can be made after three months. If the difference remains unchanged or has decreased, it indicates a resolving scoliosis.

Phase 2. The head of the rib on the convex side overlaps the vertebral body, indicating considerable rotational deformity. None of these curves resolved spontaneously.

8   Assessment of kyphosis and lordosis (Moe *et al.* 1978)

The most frequent indication for the sequential radiographic assessment of kyphosis is Scheuermann's disease of the spine. The standard projection is a lateral 2-m standing film of the spine with the arms held parallel to the floor and the hands resting on a support. Additional projections include a supine hyperextension view to assess flexibility of the kyphosis, and in the 20–30% of cases with a mild scoliosis a true lateral of the deformity, as opposed to a lateral of the patient, may be obtained. The degree of kyphosis and lordosis is then measured by marking the end-plates of the vertebrae which are maximally tilted into the curves, as for the Cobb measurement in scoliosis. The superior border of the sacrum is considered to be the end vertebra for the measurement of lumbar lordosis. Unfortunately, the normal ranges of lumbar lordosis are unknown, and it is considered that in a growing child a thoracic kyphosis greater than 40° is abnormal.

References

ANDREN L. & VON ROSEN S. (1958) The diagnosis of dislocation of the hip in newborns and the primary results of immediate treatment. *Acta radiol.* **49**, 89–95.

ANTHONSON W. (1943) *Acta radiol.* **24**, 306.

BAUMANN E. (1929) Bruns' Beiträge zur Klinischen. *Chirurgie* **146**, 48.

BERTOL P., MACNICOL M.F. & MITCHELL G.P. (1982) Radiographic features of neonatal congenital dislocation of the hip. *J. Bone Jt Surg.* **64B**, 176–9.

BILLING L. (1954) Roentgen examination of proximal femur end in children and adolescents. *Acta Radiol. suppl.* **110**.

BOEHLER L. (1931) Diagnosis, pathology and treatment of fractures of the os calcis. *J. Bone Jt Surg.* **13**, 75–89.

BRUMFIELD R.H., NICHEL V.L. & NICKEL E. (1968) Joint motion in wrist flexion and extension. *Sth. Med. J.* **59**, 909–10.

BUDIN E. & CHANDLER E. (1957) *Radiology* **69**, 209.

BULL J.W.D., NIXON W.L.B & PRATT R.T.C. (1955) Radiological criteria and familial occurrence of primary basilar impression. *Brain* **78**, 229–47.

CAFFEY J. (1956) Contradiction of congenital dysplasia–predislocation hypothesis of congenital dislocation of hip through study of normal variation in acetabular angles at successive periods in infancy. *Pediatrics* **17**, 632–40.

COBB J.R. (1948) Outline for the study of scoliosis. *American Academy of Orthopaedic Surgeons Instructional Course Lectures* **5**, 261–75.

COBEY J.C. (1976) Posterior roentgenogram of the foot. *Clinical Orthopaedics and related Research* **118**, 202–7.

EDGREN W. (1965) Coxa plana. *Acta orthop. scand. suppl.* **84**.

EYRE-BROOK A.L. (1936) Osteochondritis deformans coxae juvenilis or Perthes' disease: the results of treatment by traction in recumbency. *Brit. J. Surg.* **24**, 166–82.

EYRING E.J., BJORNSON D.R. & PETERSON C.A. (1965) Early diagnostic and prognostic signs in Legg–Calvé–Perthes' disease. *Amer. J. Roentgenol.* **93**, 382–7.

FERGUSON A.B. (1949) *Roentgen Diagnosis of the Extremities and Spine*, 2nd Edition. New York: Hoeber.

GARLAND L.H. & THOMAS S.F. (1946) Spondylolisthesis: criteria for more accurate diagnosis of true anterior slip of involved vertebral segment. *Amer. J. Roentgenol.* **55**, 275–91.

GARN S.M., HERTZOG K.P., POZNANSKI A.K. & NAGY J.M. (1972) Metacarpophalangeal length in the evaluation of skeletal malformation. *Radiology* **105**, 375–81.

GREULICH W.W. & PYLE S.I. (1959) *Radiographic Atlas of Skeletal Development of the Hand and Wrist*, 2nd Edition. Stanford: Stanford University Press.

HARPER H.A.S. (1974) *Invest. Radiol.* **9**, 217.

HEYMAN C.H. & HERNDON C.H. (1950) Legg–Perthes' disease. A method for the measurement of the roentgenographic result. *J. Bone Jt Surg.* **32A**, 767–78.

HILGENREINER H. (1925) *Med. Klin.* **21**, 1385, 1425.

HINCK V.C. & HOPKINS C.E. (1960) Measurement of the atlanto-odontal interval in the adult. *Amer. J. Roentgenol.* **84**, 945–51.

INSALL J. & SALVATI E. (1971) Patella position in the normal knee joint. *Radiology* **101**, 101–4.

JOHNSON R.M., CARY J.M., OZONOFF M.B. & KELSEY J.L. (1979) Sharp's acetabular angle in children from two to fourteen years of age. In *Pediatric Orthopaedic Radiology* (ed. Ozonoff M.B.), p. 117. Philadelphia: Saunders.

JONES D. (1977) Transcondylar fractures of the humerus in children: definition of an acceptable reduction. *Proc. roy. Soc. Med.* **70**, 624–31.

JOSEPH M.C. & MEADOW S.R. (1969) The metacarpal index of infants. *Arch. Dis. Childh.* **44**, 515–16.

KEATS T.E., TEESLINK R. & DIAMOND A.E. (1966) Normal axial relationships of the major joints. *Radiology* **87**, 904–7.

LANDEROS O., FROST H.M. & HIGGINS C.C. (1968) Post-traumatic anterior ankle instability. *Clinical Orthopaedics and related Research* **56**, 169–78.

LANGENSKIÖLD A. & SALENIUS P. (1967) Epiphyseodesis of the greater trochanter. *Acta orthop. scand.* **38**, 199–219.

LAURIN C.A., OUELLET R. & ST-JACQUES R. (1968) Talar and subtalar tilt: an experimental investigation. *Canad. J. Surg.* **11**, 270–9.

LAURIN C.A., DUSSAULT R. & LEVESQUE M.D. (1979) The tangential X-ray investigation of the patellofemoral joint. *Clinical Orthopaedics and related Research* **144**, 16–26.

LEONARD M.H. (1949) Injuries of the lateral ligaments of the ankle: a clinical and experimental study. *J. Bone Jt Surg.* **31A**, 373–7.

LINDSTRAND A. & MORTENSSON W. (1977) Anterior instability in the ankle joint following acute lateral sprain. *Acta radiol. Diagn.* **18**, 529–39.

LINSCHEID R.L., DOBYNS J.H., BEABOUT J.W. & BRYAN R.S. (1972) Traumatic instability of the wrist: diagnosis, classification and pathomechanics. *J. Bone Jt Surg.* **54A**, 1612–32.

LOCKE G.R., GARDNER J.I. & VAN EPPS E.F. (1966) Atlas–dens interval (ADI) in children: a survey based on 200 normal cervical spines. *Amer. J. Roentgenol.* **97**, 135–40.

McGREGOR M. (1948) Significance of certain measurements of skull in diagnosis of basilar impression. *Brit. J. Radiol.* **21**, 171–81.

MAGILLIGAN D.J. (1956) Calculation of the angle of anteversion by means of horizontal lateral roentgenography. *J. Bone Jt Surg.* **38A**, 1231–46.

MEHTA M.H. (1972) The rib–vertebra angle is the early diagnosis between resolving and progressive infantile scoliosis. *J. Bone Jt Surg.* **54B**, 230–43.

MERCHANT A.C., MERCER R.L., JACOBSEN R.H. & COOL C.R. (1974) Roentgenographic analysis of patello-femoral congruence. *J. Bone Jt Surg.* **56A**, 1391–6.

MEYERDING H.W. (1932) Spondylolisthesis. *Surg. Gynec. Obstet.* **54**, 371.

MOE J.H., WINTER R.B., BRADFORD D.S. & LONSTEIN J.E. (1978) *Scoliosis and Other Spinal Deformities*. Philadelphia: Saunders.

MOORE T.M. & HARVEY J.P. (1974) Roentgenographic measurement of tibial-plateau depression due to fracture. *J. Bone Jt Surg.* **56A**, 155–60.

MOSE K. (1964) *Legg–Calve–Perthes' Disease. A Comparison betwee Three Methods of Conservative Treatment*. Copenhagen: Universitetsforlaget.

NASH C.L. & MOE J.H. (1969) A study of vertebral rotation. *J. Bone Jt Surg.* **51A**, 223–9.

PARISH J.G. (1966) Radiographic measurements of the skeletal structure of the normal hand. *Brit. J. Radiol.* **39**, 52–62.

PERKINS G. (1928) *Lancet* **1**, 648.

PYLE S.I., WATERHOUSE A.M. & GREULICH W.W. (1971) *A Radiographic Standard of Reference for the Growing Hand and Wrist*. Cleveland: Case Western Reserve University Press.

RISSER J.C. (1958) The iliac apophysis: an invaluable sign in the management of scoliosis. *J. Bone Jt Surg.* **11**, 111–119.

RUBIN G. & WITTEN M. (1960) The talar tilt angle and the fibular collateral ligaments: A method for the determination of talar tilt. *J. Bone Jt Surg.* **42A**, 311–26.

SHARP I.K. (1961) Acetabular dysplasia: the acetabular angle. *J. Bone Jt Surg.* **43B**, 268–72.

SHENTON E.W.A. (1911) *Diseases in Bone*. London: MacMillan.

SIMONS G.W. (1978) Analytical radiography and the progressive approach in talipes equino-varus. *Orthop. Clin. N. Amer.* **9**, 187–206.

STAGNARA P., COUNOD J. & CAMPO-PAYSAA A. (1977) Arthrodeses dans le traitement des cyphoses et des cyphoscolioses. *Int. Orthop.* **1**, 199–214.

STOREN G. (1959) *Acta chir. scand.* **116**, 144.

SWISCHUK L.E. (1977) Anterior displacement of C2 in children: physiologic or pathologic? *Radiology* **122**, 759–63.

TACHDJIAN M.O. (1972) *Pediatric Orthopedics* Vol. 2, 1486–9. Philadelphia: Saunders.

TANNER J.M., WHITEHOUSE R.H. & MARSHALL W.A. (1975) *Assessment of Skeletal Maturity and Prediction of Adult Height: TW2 Method*. New York: Academic Press.

TEMPLETON A.W., McALISTER W.H. & ZIM I.D. (1965) Standardization of terminology and evaluation of osseous relationships in congenitally abnormal feet. *Amer. J. Roentgenol.* **93**, 374–81.

TONNIS D. (1976) Normal values of the hip joint for the evaluation of X-rays in children and adults. *Clinical Orthopaedics and related Research* **119**, 39–47.

WEINER D.S. & MacNAB I. (1970) Superior migration of the humeral head: a radiological aid in the diagnosis of tears of the rotator cuff. *J. Bone Jt Surg.* **52B**, 524–7.

WHITE A.A., JOHNSON R.M., PANJABI M.M. & SOUTHWICK W.O. (1975) Biomechanical analysis of clinical stability in the cervical spine. *Clinical Orthopaedics and related Research* **109**, 85–96.

WIBERG G.G. (1939) Studies on dysplastic acetabular and congenital subluxation of the hip joint with special reference to the complication of osteoarthritis. *Acta chir. scand. suppl.* **58**.

SECTION II
PRACTICAL CLINICAL PROBLEMS

Chapter 7
Skeletal Trauma in the Adult

B. JONES & P. M. ROZING

In a busy radiology department traumatology forms a considerable part of the radiological workload. X-rays are vital for the diagnosis of a fracture when all that may be seen externally is swelling due to haematoma formation. The film will show the location of the fracture and any complications which may require immediate operative intervention. Following diagnosis and treatment, follow-up films are essential to monitor healing and the continuing good position of the bones. It is the pile of trauma films that is often left to the trainee radiologist to report. This task may be tedious as about 90% are normal and any fractures are obvious. However, it is the information obtained from these vast amounts of trauma films that gives the radiologist the most valuable groundwork in his understanding of the principles of film-reading. He develops his powers of observation and a method of analysis that will remain with him for the rest of his career as a radiologist.

The principles of radiographic examination in the emergency patient require special consideration in those who are severely traumatized. Most commonly, today, these cases are the result of a car crash or a factory accident. These patients require very swift evaluation and treatment if they are to survive. To operate successfully this system requires teamwork. Radiodiagnostically the authors have modified a system advocated by Kingma in Groningen. Basically it involves a system of timed repeat X-rays of the chest and abdomen interspersed with other pictures of the skeleton. Rapid changes, possibly fatal, in the chest and abdomen can be more closely followed and a decision to operate more optimally timed. Typically, the patient arrives in the X-ray room with a team of doctors and nurses in attendance. An anaesthetist maintains an airway with an endotracheal tube, and the casualty doctor sets up an intravenous infusion to maintain blood pressure, and is usually trying to assess the injuries by the time the radiologist arrives. During the day a qualified radiologist supervises the series of X-rays, beginning with a lateral neck film and followed by supine chest and abdomen films. Frequently, because of splenic or liver rupture or gastrointestinal laceration, these are sent quickly to the operating room. Speed is essential and the maximum information concerning the patient's injuries should be ascertained. Following the first abdominal film an intravenous excretion urography is performed as a routine. One or two subsequent large abdominal films are then sufficient to ascertain if there are two functioning kidneys and any surgically correctable renal damage. Two further chest X-rays at 15 and 30 minute intervals are made to evaluate mediastinal widening and development of pleural fluid or pneumothorax. In between these radiographs the rest of the patient's injuries such as skull and limbs are X-rayed.

It is thus possible, with teamwork and the minimum of confusion, to complete the radiodiagnostic work-up within half-an-hour, thereby presenting a patient for immediate surgery or intensive care in a resuscitated state and with considerable knowledge of his injuries. This, of course, works very well with the one severe case, but should there be several then the radiologist has to be prepared to commandeer more X-ray rooms and personnel, if need be interrupting the organized programme of the day in order to assess these severely injured

patients quickly. It is unfortunate if a patient
should die on the way to a modern well-
equipped casualty unit, but it is a tragedy if the
patient dies within the unit because of lack of
organization or too much delay.

When considering fractures to long bones in
the adult it is important to remember how the
bones differ from those of the child. Most bones
will tend to break at their weakest point. In
children this is often the epiphyseal plate. In the
adult it is the area that takes the greatest strain
in the healthy bone, such as femoral neck, distal
tibia, distal radius, and subcapital area of the
humerus. But often, as shall be seen later with
regard to sports injuries, the bones are very
strong and the traumatic energy is preferen-
tially dispersed in the form of dislocations or
ligament ruptures.

In older people the form of the injury will be
affected by any pathology that the bone may
have, such as osteoporosis, infiltrations, metastases or old osteomyelitis. Infiltrative bone marrow diseases have a special predilection for
pathological fracture.

It is important for the orthopaedic surgeon to
know the stand or position of the fracture and
this should be noted by the radiologist. Is the
fracture angulated? If so, which way, dorsal or
ventral, etc., overlapping, partial apposition, distraction, or rotated?

A basic rule of fracture radiology is always to
take views in two planes at right angles. This is
to show not only the presence of fractures but
also the degree of dislocation, which can be misleading if only one projection is taken. Often
just repeating a picture with the X-ray tube
moved slightly off-centre can show a difficult-
to-see fracture line. All fracture lines will run in
the plane of the greatest weakness.

If the X-ray beam strikes the fracture end-on
it will be seen, but if the plane runs obliquely
then the absorption of the beam becomes diffuse
and no sharp fracture will be seen (Fig. 7.1).
This is why not all of the fracture is seen in a
spiral shaft fracture (Fig. 7.2) and traction may
be required to separate the fragments (Fig. 7.3).
Also the oblique fracture can cause problems

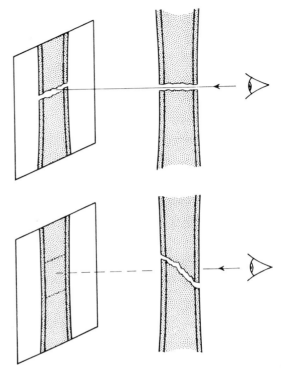

Fig. 7.1. Schematic representation of how an oblique
fracture may be missed if only one view is made.

(Fig. 7.4). Sometimes delaying a repeat picture
for several days may allow resorption of a fracture line due to hyperaemia, or the formation of
a thin periosteal reaction due to subperiostal
bleeding may be seen.

However, it has been shown that on isotope
scans fractures appearing as hotspots may be
seen as early as 24 hours, and certainly within
three days (Figs. 7.5, 7.6 and 7.7). A negative
scan after this time is sufficient to exclude a
fracture. Comparison views of adjacent limbs
are of more practical use in children. However,
slightly oblique or rotated views can often show
an elusive fracture (Fig. 7.8). Sometimes it can
be said that the answer to a radiological problem lies in the next film taken! It is difficult to
detect fractures in certain areas, such as in the
sacrum (Fig. 7.9), upper thoracic spine and
talus. If in doubt it is possible to proceed to
immediate tomography, linear being often quite
adequate in most cases.

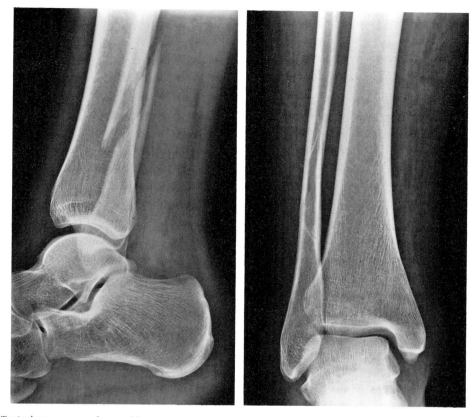

Fig. 7.2. Typical appearance of a spiral fracture, in this case occurring in the fibula.

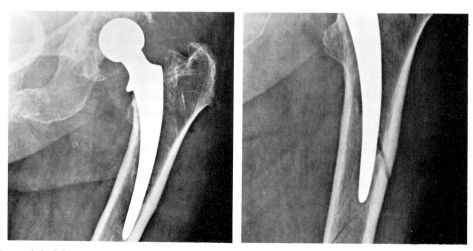

Fig. 7.3. Femoral shaft fracture not seen on initial films (left) but there was a strong clinical suspicion. Fracture (right) was then demonstrated by repeating the picture with slight traction of the leg. The prosthesis was coincidental.

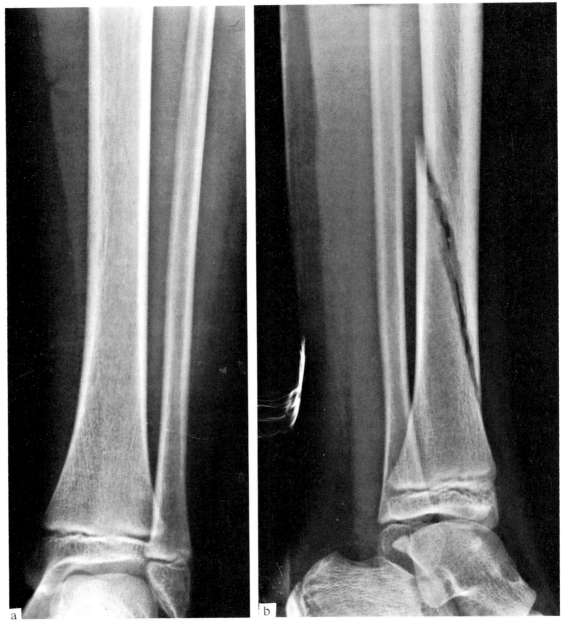

Fig. 7.4.   Oblique-running tibial shaft fracture only seen on lateral film (b) emphasizing the basic importance of taking more than one view.

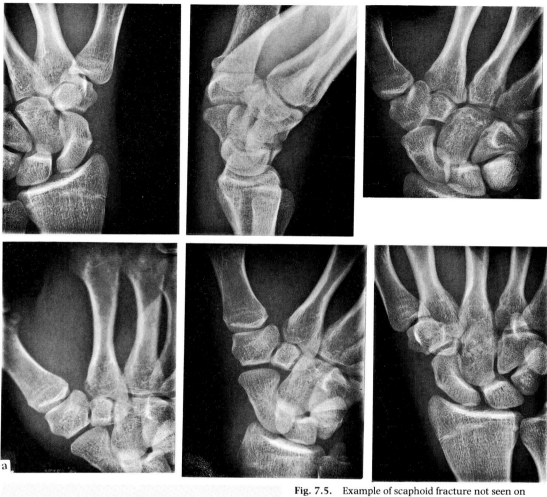

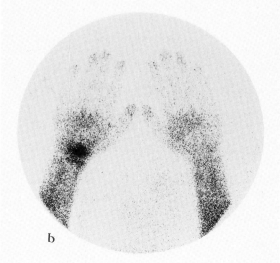

Fig. 7.5. Example of scaphoid fracture not seen on conventional views (a) but treated as fracture following positive isotope scan (b). Healing fracture subsequently shown later on conventional X-rays. Isotope scans of fractures can be positive as early as 24 hours after the trauma. This method precludes the need for delaying repeat films for 10 days or so before a definite diagnosis can be made.

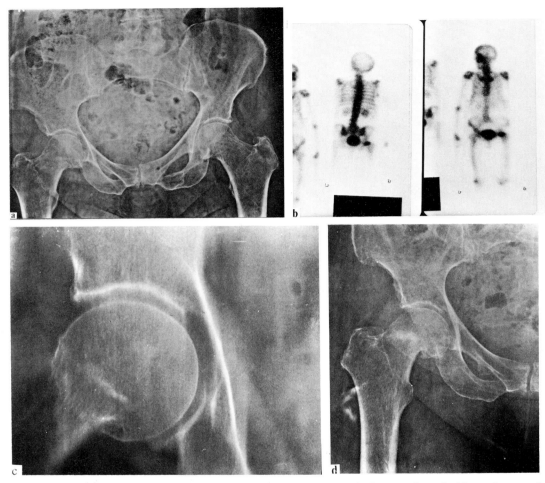

Fig. 7.6. Elderly lady fell at home. Initial pelvis film (a) showed vague sclerotic shadow in right neck of femur. Because of clinical suspicion of a fracture an isotope scan was performed (b) showing hotspot over right femoral neck. A tomogram (c) shows more clearly the sclerosis due to impacted trabeculae. Following conservative treatment (d) notice the inferior dislocation of femoral head and more obvious sclerosis.

A further basic principle of trauma radiology is to radiograph the joints on both sides of any fracture. This is especially important for paired bones such as radius and ulna or tibia and fibula. It is possible that a fracture of one bone may affect its partner some distance away from the site of injury. Thus a femoral shaft fracture may be associated with a hip dislocation or, more commonly, this can be exemplified by the Galeazzi and Monteggia fractures.

A Monteggia fracture–dislocation (Fig. 7.10) involves a fracture of the middle or proximal third of the ulna associated with dislocation of the radial head. There are various types depending on whether the radial head dislocates anteriorly, posteriorly or laterally. There is a rare fourth type where there is also a fracture of the radius just distal to the bicipital tuberosity.

A Galeazzi fracture is a fracture of the distal third of the radius accompanied by dorsal dislocation of the ulna. By definition there must be

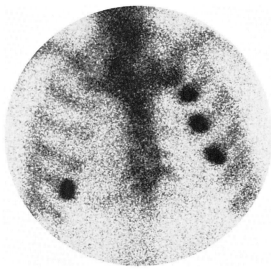

Fig. 7.7. Fractures of ribs a coincidental finding on a bone scan for another reason. The typical row of hotspots differentiates them from metastases.

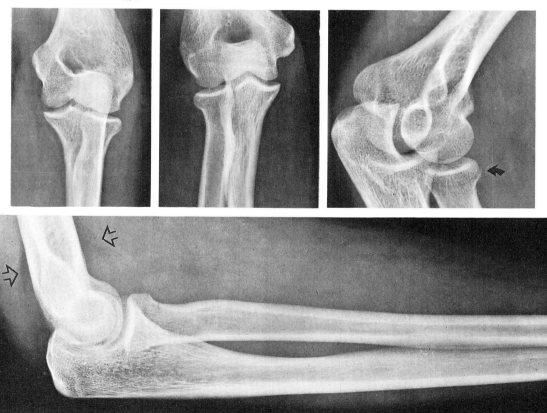

Fig. 7.8. Radial head fracture difficult to see without extra views (closed arrow). Notice positive fat pad signs anterior and posterior (open arrows) to the humerus.

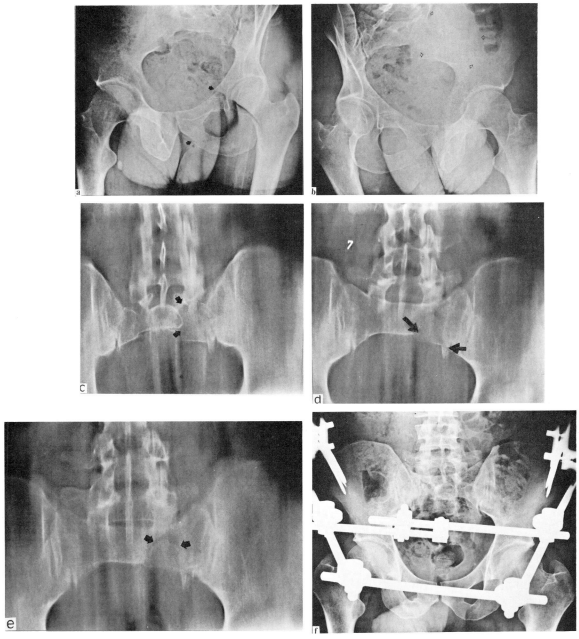

Fig. 7.9. Fracture of left sacral ala only clearly seen by tomography. Initial standard series of AP and two obliques shows fractures of the left superior and inferior pubic rami (a, closed arrows). Notice density difference caused by haematoma formation in front of the sacral fracture (b, open arrows). Linear tomography (c–e) was performed directly after the plain films showing the sacrum fracture (arrows). This extra knowledge allowed the surgeon strongly to suspect pelvic instability and he introduced pelvic ring stabilization rods with a good result (f).

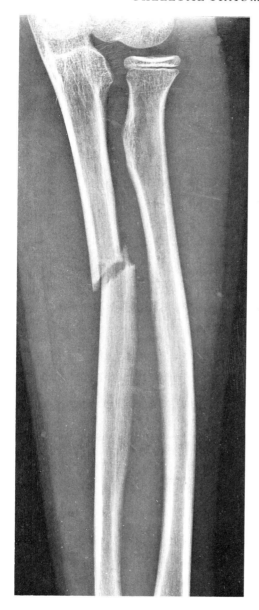

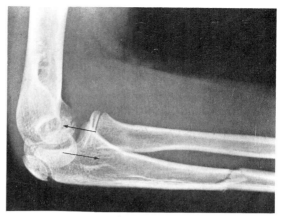

Fig. 7.10. A Monteggia fracture–dislocation in the forearm of a 14-year-old boy who was kicked whilst playing football. Although having pressure pain over the radial head the dislocation was missed. A proximal third ulnar fracture with anterior dislocation of the radial head (Monteggia type I) occurs in about 5% of such cases. A line drawn through the length of the radius does not pass through the capitulum (arrows).

tearing of the triangular fibrocartilage of the distal radioulnar joint. There may be an associated avulsion fracture of the styloid process or fracture of the ulnar head. Injury is usually due to a direct blow on the dorsum of the wrist or to a fall. It is said to be more common than the Monteggia fracture (Fig. 7.11).

Fracture–dislocations of joints are important to diagnose because of the greater risk of complications involving the articular joint surfaces. The radiologist should always mention if a fracture line enters a joint. In a dislocation there has been complete disassociation of both joint surfaces (Figs. 7.12, 7.13). It is not surprising,

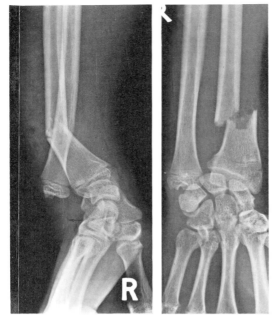

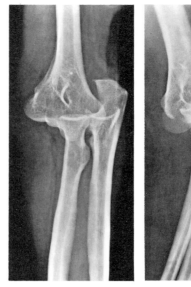

Fig. 7.13. Anterior humeral dislocation of the elbow. The patient fell onto elbow whilst in a very drunken state.

Fig. 7.11. A Galeazzi fracture–dislocation in a 19-year-old male following a fall from moped presented with wrist pain, swelling and ventral angulation of distal radius. Note that the carpal bones retain a normal radiocarpal relationship and the avulsed fragment of the styloid process (arrow). The injury was treated by closed reduction under anaesthesia followed by six weeks in plaster. There was an excellent functional end result.

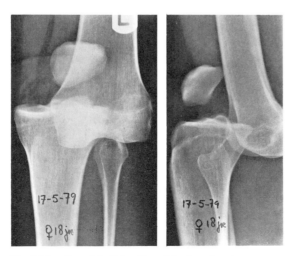

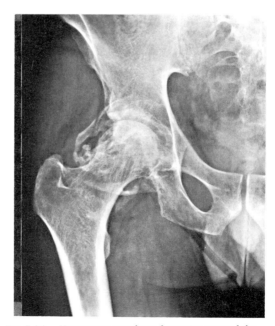

Fig. 7.12. Complete dislocation of the knee in a teenager occurred during friendly fighting. Subsequently reduction was performed and there were no further complications on follow-up.

Fig. 7.14. Heterotopic new bone formation around the hip joint following reduction of a posterior dislocation of the femur. The patient lay in a coma for a period of time after the accident.

therefore, that subsequent osteoarthritis might ensue. Calcification in and around the joint capsule may result in limited joint movement. Indeed early passive joint movement following surgical reconstruction of the joint is advised, to prevent stiffness and heterotopic new bone formation (Fig. 7.14). Signs of intra-articular fracture include fat/blood fluid level in the joint (Fig. 7.15), elevated fat pads indicating an effusion into the joint (Fig. 7.8), and a fracture line entering a joint (Fig. 7.16). Air in the joint space indicates an open joint injury.

Shoulder

A trauma to the shoulder joint can result in a dislocation or a fracture. Owing to its high mobility and insufficient bony encapsulation the shoulder joint is commonly dislocated. A dislocation is most frequently seen in the second and third decade. The bone is strong and withstands the powerful force so the capsule and ligaments give way. Later in life the bone breaks.

DISLOCATION OF THE GLENOHUMERAL JOINT

In a dislocation of the glenohumeral joint the humeral head can be dislocated anteriorly, posteriorly, inferiorly and superiorly. There are also very rare subclavicular and transthoracic types. Most common is the anterior and posterior dislocation. There are different types of anterior dislocation. The most common type is the subcoracoid dislocation (Fig. 7.17) and the second most common is the subglenoid dislocation (Fig. 7.18). The cause is commonly a violent episode. After a dislocation the glenohumeral joint will be damaged. The anterior capsule ruptures or is detached from the inferior glenoid with labrum and periosteum. The subscapularis muscle and

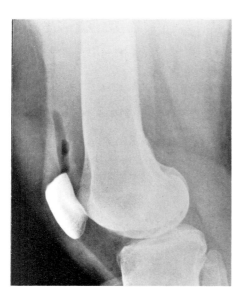

Fig. 7.15. Fat–blood meniscus in the suprapatellar pouch in a patient with intra-articular tibial plateau fracture.

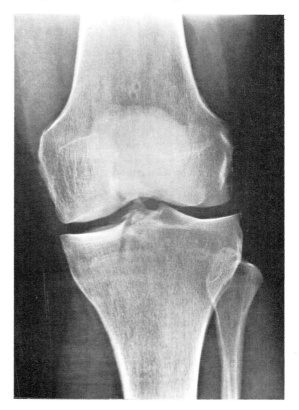

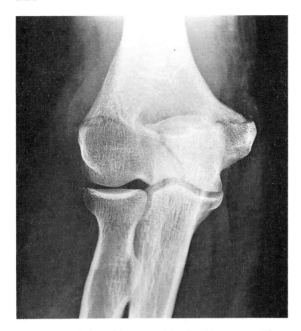

Fig. 7.16. 'Y' shaped fracture of the distal humerus with the fracture line undisputedly entering elbow joint.

tendon are stretched. The humeral head presses against the anterior glenoid rim, and if the dislocating force was severe or the head stays long in the dislocated position a compression fracture in the posterolateral aspect of the head will occur. X-ray examination is carried out to verify the diagnosis and to rule out fracture of the neck, or the tuberosity or the glenoid rim.

In orthopaedics it is always necessary to have roentgenograms of the injured part in two views at right angles to each other. AP X-rays of the shoulder in the frontal plane with the humerus in internal and external rotation are sufficient to study the humerus, but insufficient to study the glenohumeral joint.

In an acute dislocation of the shoulder a true AP view and a trans-scapular view are taken. The transthoracic view, which is difficult to interpret, has been dropped in the authors' department in favour of the trans-scapular view, which clearly shows the position of the humeral head (Fig. 7.19).

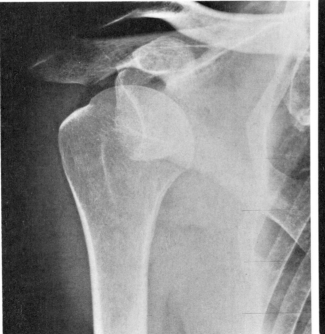
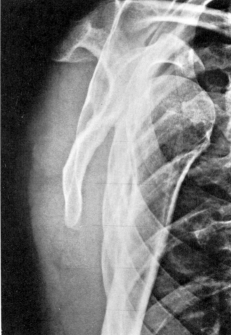

Fig. 7.17. Example of an anterior subcoracoid dislocation. This is the most common dislocation and often occurs without bony injury. It is prone to recurrence.

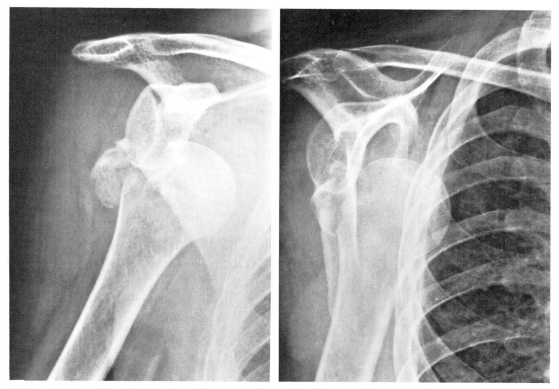

Fig. 7.18.   Anterior subglenoid dislocation with a commonly associated fracture of the greater tuberosity.

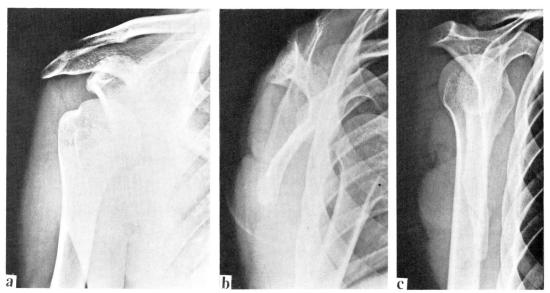

Fig. 7.19.   Anterior dislocation of the humeral head, easily seen on the trans-scapular view (b). After reduction the head lies in the triangle formed by the coracoid process anteriorly, the acromion posteriorly, and the glenoid inferiorly (c).

In the anteroposterior view the patient stands
at an angle of 45° with respect to the screen. In
this way the anterior and posterior glenoid rims
are superimposed. On the AP view it is possible
to diagnose a dislocation of the humeral head
but not to distinguish between an anterior or
posterior dislocation. In addition, an accompanying fracture of the glenoid rim, or a fracture of the greater tuberosity, can be seen in
this projection. In the authors' clinic arthrograms are no longer performed in dislocated
shoulders.

Posterior dislocation

The incidence of posterior dislocations is only
2% of all dislocations of the glenohumeral joint
(Fig. 7.20). Possibly there is some bony protection against posterior displacement by the fact
that the scapula is positioned on the thorax at
an angle of 45°. The glenoid cavity faces
anteriorly and a traumatic episode will tend to
result in an anterior, rather than a posterior,
dislocation. Twenty per cent of posterior dislocations are caused by an electric shock or a
convulsion (Fig. 7.21).

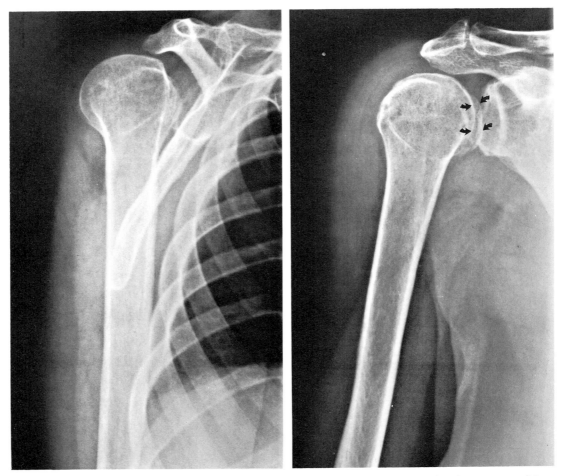

Fig. 7.20. Posterior dislocation of the humeral head—AP and trans-scapular views. Note the widened joint space and the
two parallel lines of cortical bone (arrows). One line represents the head while the other line represents the margin of a
trough-like impaction fracture.

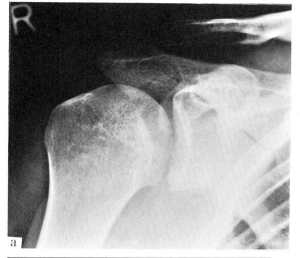

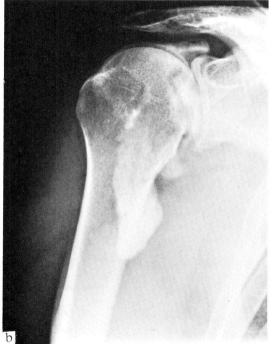

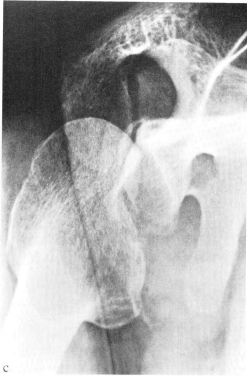

Fig. 7.21. A 30-year-old carpenter fell from a scaffolding while at work. He had no memory of what had happened and was brought to the casualty department. He had pain in both shoulders, but clinical and radiological examination failed to show any fracture. A diagnosis of cerebral concussion was made. A few weeks later he was followed up at out-patients' still complaining of discomfort of both shoulders. The radiology was repeated, and a compression fracture of the front part of the humeral head was seen. Because this was probably caused by a posterior dislocation, the patient was sent to a neurologist to ask if his fall from the scaffolding was caused by an epileptic convulsion. This in fact proved to be the case. (a) Routine anteroposterior view showing the two parallel margins of the head. (b) Arthrogram with contrast medium filling the trough-like impaction fracture. (c) 45° craniocaudal view with the patient supine and arm in supination. Note the large defect adjacent to the glenoid fossa.

There are different types of posterior dislocations. Subglenoid and subspinous dislocations should not be missed clinically or radiographically. The subacromial type is often missed. Of 194 patients with posterior dislocations collected from the literature the diagnosis was initially missed in 31 patients (Fig. 7.22).

X-ray examination is carried out to verify the diagnosis and to rule out a fracture. The incidence of fractures of the posterior glenoid rim, the minor tuberosity or the proximal humerus is over 30%. The subacromial type of dislocation is frequently missed on the AP film because it can look so deceptively normal.

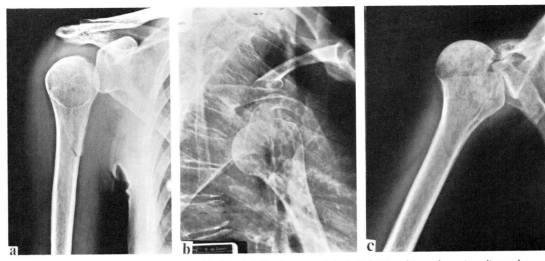

Fig. 7.22. Missed posterior dislocation. This elderly lady fell at home, and the initial AP and transthoracic radiographs were taken. The fracture of the humeral neck was seen and she was treated in a collar and cuff. After several out-patient visits when she complained of restricted painful movements an axial picture was taken showing the impacted humeral head dislocation (c). Several transthoracic films had been taken but nobody had spotted the posteriorly dislocated head!

On the anteroposterior view the following radiographic signs of posterior shoulder dislocation can be seen:

1 The posterior dislocated humeral head is fixed in an internal rotation and no external rotation view can be obtained.
2 The humeral head is displaced laterally by the posterior glenoid rim, and therefore the shoulder joint may appear widened in frontal views.
3 If the space between the anterior rim of the glenoid and the humeral head is greater than 6 mm then it is highly suggestive of a posterior dislocation.
4 The normal parallelism between the humeral head and the anterior rim of the glenoid fossa is lost.
5 In many patients with posterior dislocation two parallel lines of cortical bone may be identified on the superomedial aspect of the humeral head. One line represents the head and the other the margin of a trough-like impaction fracture.

The other view besides the AP is the transscapular view. The axial view is not only diagnostic of the dislocation, but will demonstrate the anterior head compression fracture as well as a fracture of the posterior rim of the glenoid.

The other view can be an axial view, a transscapular view or a transthoracic view. Because the dislocated shoulder is painful, and moving is severely limited, a good axial view is difficult and uncomfortable for the patient and the technician. A transthoracic view is an oblique view of the glenohumeral joint and the interpretation can be very difficult because of the superposition of the thoracic mass. The authors prefer a trans-scapular view, because it can be taken without having to move the upper extremity.

Fig. 7.23 shows the position of the X-ray tube, the scapula and the film. This picture can be taken with the patient standing, or if necessary supine, by placing a foam rubber triangle under the sound shoulder. It is diagnostic for the anterior and posterior dislocation.

Superior dislocation (Fig. 7.24) is rare but can be chronic. In patients with a recurrent anterior dislocation the authors take an AP view, an axial view and special views to demonstrate the posterolateral defect in the humeral head. In the AP view, especially on the internal

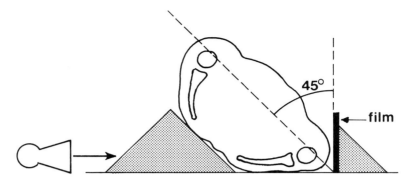

Fig. 7.23. Supine trans-scapular view.

rotation view, the defect can be seen when it is huge. The axial view is well known and will reveal anterior glenoid fractures or calcifications. The authors' routine view to visualize the posterolateral defect of the head and small avulsions or calcifications at the anteroinferior glenoid rim is the 45° craniocaudal view. The patient is supine with the arm in supination. The X-ray beam is directed caudally at a 45° angle.

The authors' second choice to show the defect is in the Stryker position. The patient is supine with the palm of the hand of the affected arm on top of the head, and the elbow pointing straight outwards. The X-ray beam is centered at a 45° angle cranially. The Didier view is also sometimes used, but the Hermodsson view seldom.

Arthrography

An arthrogram of the shoulder will reveal the soft-tissue lesions that accompany the dislocated shoulder. One might see a rupture of the musculotendinous cuff, or a large anterior capsular pouch due to detachment of the capsule, labrum and periosteum from the anterior glenoid rim. In the axial view one might see a small avulsion of the anterior glenoid rim.

FRACTURE OF THE PROXIMAL HUMERUS

Radiological examination is of great importance in these patients, not so much to demonstrate the fractures as to classify them, thereby en-abling the orthopaedic surgeon to formulate an appropriate treatment plan. The classification is based on the work of Neer (1970) who related the muscles to the fracture fragments to which they were bound. These muscles resulted, for a greater part, in the dislocation of fragments, and from an understanding of this a better insight into the position of the fracture is obtained. The most important fragment of a proximal humerus fracture is the humeral head: to the greater tuberosity is attached the supraspinatus tendon and infraspinatus (Fig. 7.25); to the minor tuberosity is attached subscapularis; and the shaft of the humerus is fixed to pectoralis major and latissimus dorsi.

The number of fragments determines if the fracture is a two-, three- or four-part fracture. The stability of the fracture can be judged by the displacement of the fragments. Apart from the fractures there can also be a dislocation of the head of the humerus, i.e. a 'fracture–dislocation' (Fig. 7.26).

Hip joint

The hip joint in the adult is, like the shoulder, subject to frequent dislocation. The ball and socket hip joint is strengthened by the ilio-femoral ligament in front and the ischiofemoral ligament behind.

The posterior dislocation is seen frequently following a 'head-on' car collision. The hip is in the partially flexed position and the knee is hit by the dashboard or back of the seat. The

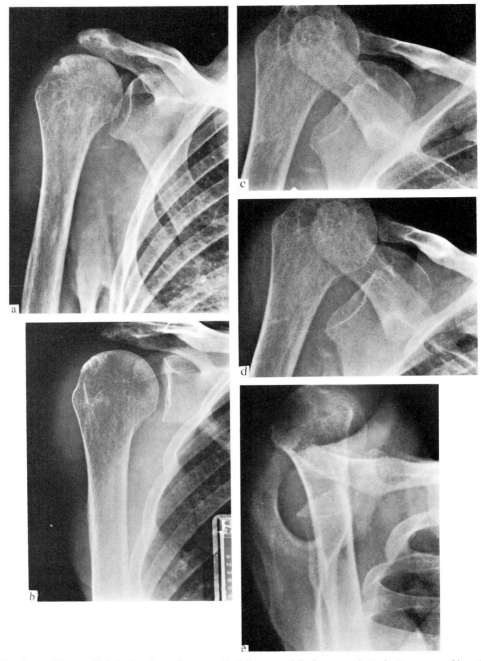

Fig. 7.24 (a–e). A 70-year-old dialysis patient, three months following a fall after anaesthetic for 'trouser-graft' prothesis, complaining of pain in the shoulder and unable to raise her arm unaided. The standard shoulder film is unremarkable, but on attempted abduction it is seen that the humerus subluxes and eventually dislocates in a superior anterolateral position. Pictures were achieved by screening. This type of superior dislocation is often accompanied by fracture of the acromion and/or clavicle. A considerable capsule rupture must have occurred.

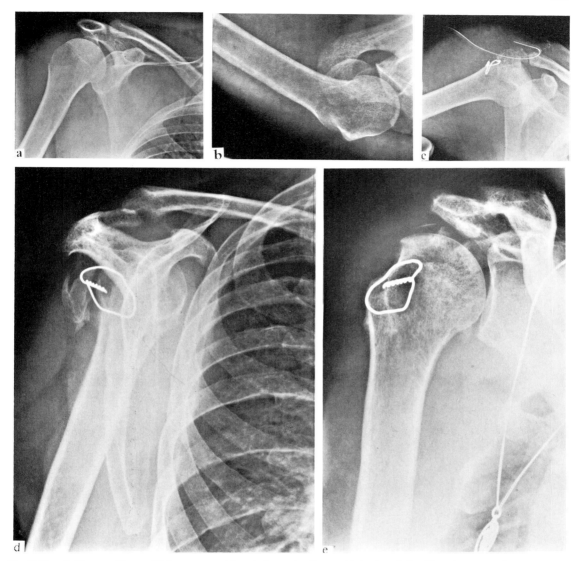

Fig. 7.25. A 41-year-old man fell from a second floor balcony, landing on his back and shoulder. He sustained two vertebral fractures and this shoulder injury. The greater tuberosity is torn off and lies behind the joint due to the pull of the supraspinatus tendon (a and b). Three weeks later a circle wire fixation was performed (c), but later films show shortening due to pull of the supraspinatus tendon and no consolidation of the greater tuberosity. (d) Anteroposterior and (e) trans-scapular views.

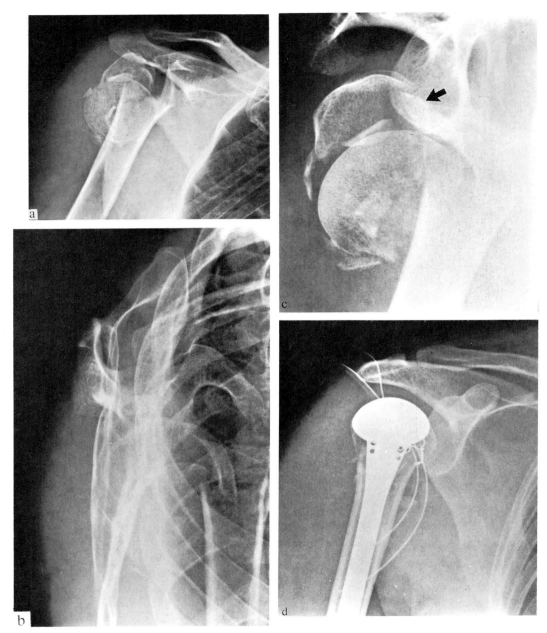

Fig. 7.26 (a–d). Four-part humerus fracture. A 40-year-old skier fell on the 'piste', sustaining a severe injury to the right shoulder. There is a comminuted fracture with multiple small bone fragments. This is a so-called four-part fracture–dislocation. The humeral shaft is pulled anteriorly and medially by pectoralis major. The greater tuberosity is retracted upwards and posteriorly by supraspinatus and rotator cuff. The lesser tuberosity (arrow) is pulled medially by subscapularis. The humeral head lies at 90° to the shaft and is posteroinferiorly dislocated. It was not possible at operation to reassemble all the fragments and so a total 'Neer' prothesis was inserted (d).

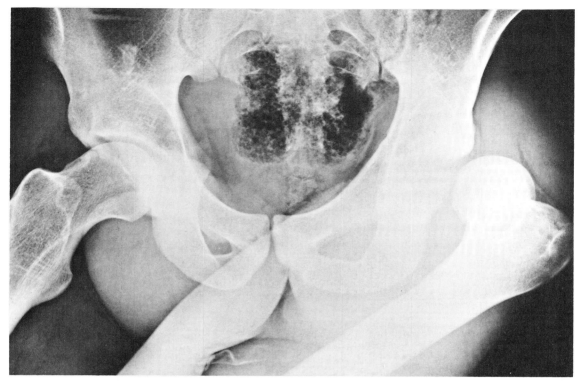

Fig. 7.27.   Posterior dislocation of the left hip without fracture. Note the position of the thigh in adduction and partial flexion.

femoral head, because of its shallow covering, is pushed backwards out of its socket (Fig. 7.27), the thigh coming to lie flexed and adducted. Posterior dislocation occurs in about 36% of cases of hip injury, and over 90% of these have an associated fracture of the posterior lip (Figs. 7.28 and 7.34). Sciatic nerve lesions are common, occurring in 15% of posterior hip fractures.

The opposite, anterior dislocation is rare, about 13%, and is caused by forced abduction and external rotation of the leg. The femoral head lies inferomedially and the femur is abducted (Fig. 7.29). Delayed reduction of all types of dislocation can result in femoral head necrosis in 50% of patients after 24 hours. Other complications of femoral head dislocation include arthritis from trapped fragments (Fig. 7.30), capsular ossification (Fig. 7.14), heterotopic new bone formation in missed dislocation

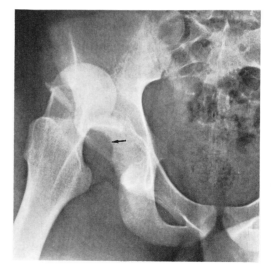

Fig. 7.28.   Posterior dislocation of the hip with fracture of the posterior acetabular lip. The fragment lies with the femoral head. Note the defect in the posterior acetabular rim (arrow).

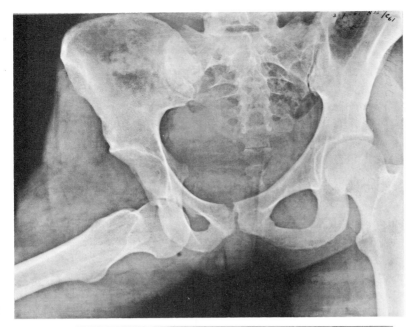

Fig. 7.29. Anterior dislocation, no fracture. The femoral head lies in the obturator foramen and the shaft is rotated and abducted.

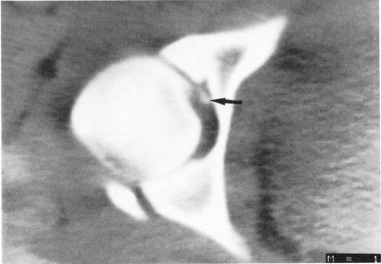

Fig. 7.30. CT scan showing small bony fragment (arrow) lying within joint, probably avulsed by the ligament of head of femur (ligamentum teres femoris) not seen on the conventional films. Note the fracture of the posterior acetabular lip. CT followed closed reduction of posterior dislocation–fracture.

(Fig. 7.31), and, as mentioned, sciatic nerve damage in posterior dislocations. A widening of more than 2 mm difference following reduction indicates interposition of tissues in the joint.

A third type is central dislocation of the hip and involves a fracture of the medial wall of the acetabulum (Fig. 7.32). A knowledge of the various lines around the acetabulum will help in appreciating the fracture more clearly (Fig. 7.33).

A variation of the anterior dislocation is the transobturator fracture–dislocation (Fig. 7.35). The authors have found that CT scanning is a useful adjunct to plain radiography of the acetabulum. It shows more clearly the fracture lines sometimes not seen on plain films. It also shows the presence of small bony fragments

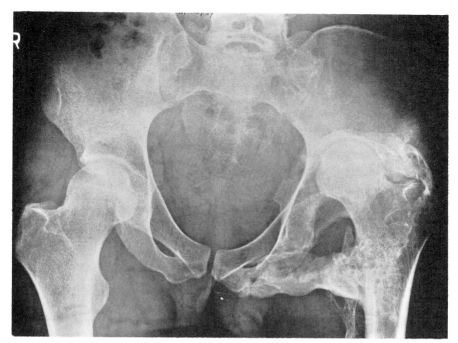

Fig. 7.31. Heterotopic new bone formation causing ankylosis of posteriorly dislocated hip. The patient lay in a coma for several weeks and the hip dislocation was missed.

Fig. 7.32. Central fracture–dislocation of the left femoral head in an elderly lady hit by a car on the left whilst crossing the road. There is protrusion of the left femoral head into the pelvic cavity. Note the 'straddle' fractures of both superior and both inferior pubic rami. A further fracture line from the acetabular roof runs up through the iliac wing. The patient was treated with a traction pin into the trochanter major. After four weeks she was gently mobilized with help from a physiotherapist with good results.

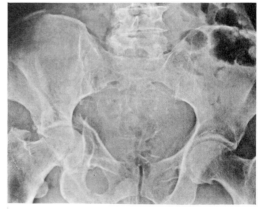

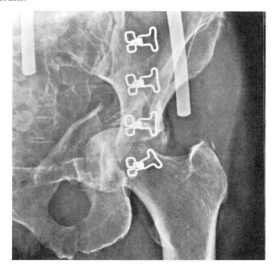

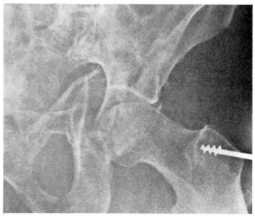

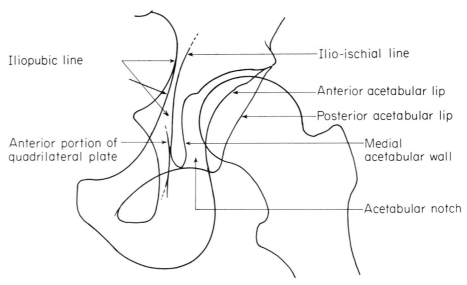

Fig. 7.33. A drawing of the various lines around the acetabulum.

within the joint space. A post-reduction CT is again helpful in assessing resulting displacement of fragments.

Fractures of the pelvis may be classified as stable or unstable for purposes of orthopaedic treatment. Injuries to the surrounding tissues are common and should be sought. Vascular lesions with a slow oozing extraperitoneal bleeding may be potentially fatal. A close watch should be kept on the patient's blood pressure and haemoglobin. If transfusion is insufficient after one hour, then surgery should be seriously considered. Angiography may occasionally be required (Fig. 7.36). However, immediate fixation of pelvic fractures often stops the bleeding, which is mainly venous and cannot be treated adequately by ligation or embolization.

Fractures of the sacrum may be difficult to see and can often have associated sacral plexus, vascular or rectal injuries. A rectal examination is mandatory in pelvic injuries to feel for rectal perforation, bone spicules or haematoma in the pre-rectal fossa or pouch of Douglas.

Stable fractures of the pelvis include fractures of the iliac wings, transverse sacral fractures, ischiopubic rami fractures, and avulsions of the anterior superior and anterior inferior iliac spines and ischial apophyses. Avulsion injuries are uncommon; patients are often young and frequently such injuries occur during sport. Iliac wing fractures have little orthopaedic significance, but bleeding can be severe with possible tearing or rupture of associated retroperitoneal soft tissues, i.e. ureters (Fig. 7.37).

Unstable fractures of the pelvis are usually caused by more dramatic and forceful trauma. The pelvic ring is disrupted in two or more places. These injuries will require some form of fixation, usually external. There may be a pure dislocation of the symphysis and one sacroiliac joint (Fig. 7.38). The force may cause the pelvis to be opened outwards like the leaves of a book, the so-called 'sprung-pelvis'; rarely the opposite may occur.

The other class of trauma is the vertical shearing force, resulting in a double vertical fracture or dislocation, first described by Malgaigne (1859) in his *Treatise on Fractures*, and

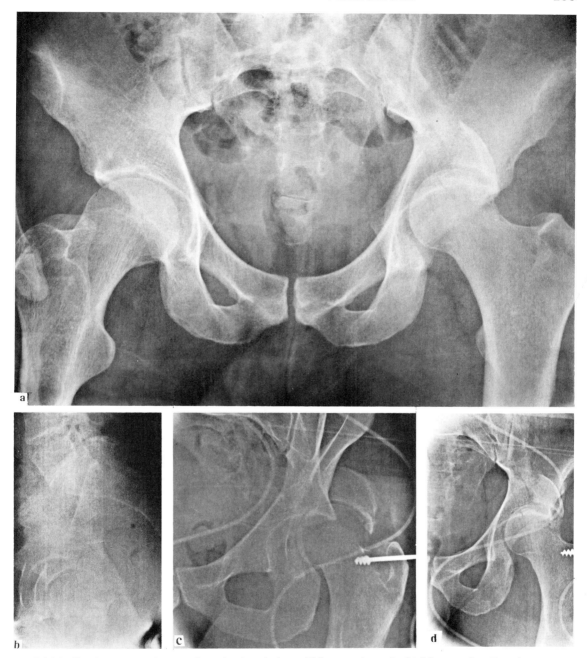

Fig. 7.34 (a–d). A young psychotic student who thought he could fly jumped out of a third floor window. Dorsal dislocation is difficult to appreciate on an AP pelvis film. The normal right femoral head is larger than the other, indicating that the dislocated head is closer to film. A loose posterior lip fragment lies behind the iliac wing. A fracture line runs from the acetabulum posteriorly and cranially, opening in the pelvic brim. An enhanced true lateral picture (b) shows the position of the left head of femur. Other abdominal injuries and laparotomy delayed full evaluation of the hip dislocation. Later oblique views (c, d), which the authors recommend instead of the lateral view, show the true nature of the pelvic and acetabular lip fractures. Note the temporary and obviously ineffective traction pin.

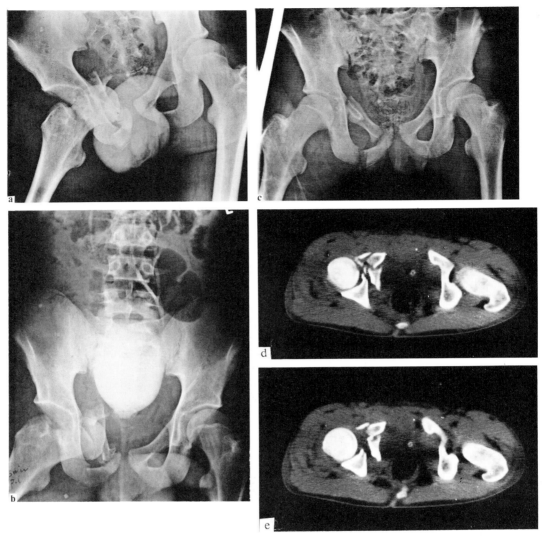

Fig. 7.35. Under the influence of alcohol this young male drove his car into a lamp-post. The gear lever hit into his abdomen. The plain film shows a transobturator fracture–dislocation of the right hip (a). The fractured superior pubic ramus and medial wall of the acetabulum have been pushed into the lesser pelvis. The excretion urogram (b) revealed two normal kidneys and ureters, but a greatly elevated bladder due to haematoma. Retrograde examination showed a total avulsion of the urethra at the bladder neck. The post-reduction film (c) shows a reasonable position of the fragments, but on the CT (d, e) there is still obvious medial displacement of acetabular wall fragments.

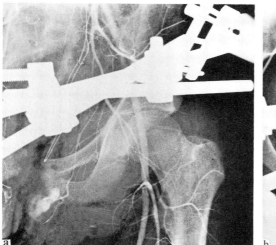
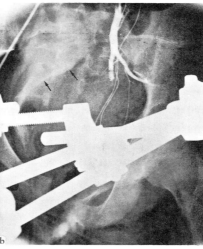

Fig. 7.36. A young man crashed his moped under a car. He had been drinking and was admitted in a state of shock. He had a haematoma of his scrotum, and a fractured left femur and tibia. He had a 'sprung-pelvis' (*see* Fig. 7.38) with a large pelvic haematoma. His pelvis was fixed externally, but he required 38 units of blood. The angiogram (a) shows extravasation from the left obturator artery. A wire-coil embolization of a branch of the internal iliac was performed (b). Note the bladder (arrows) pushed to the right by the large collection of blood.

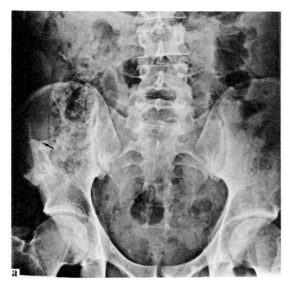
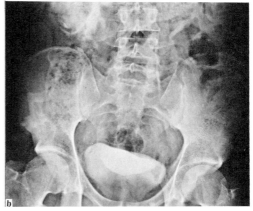
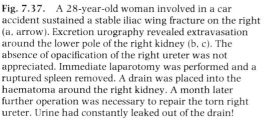
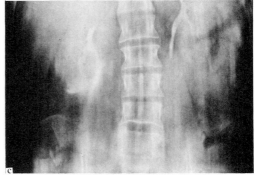

Fig. 7.37. A 28-year-old woman involved in a car accident sustained a stable iliac wing fracture on the right (a, arrow). Excretion urography revealed extravasation around the lower pole of the right kidney (b, c). The absence of opacification of the right ureter was not appreciated. Immediate laparotomy was performed and a ruptured spleen removed. A drain was placed into the haematoma around the right kidney. A month later further operation was necessary to repair the torn right ureter. Urine had constantly leaked out of the drain!

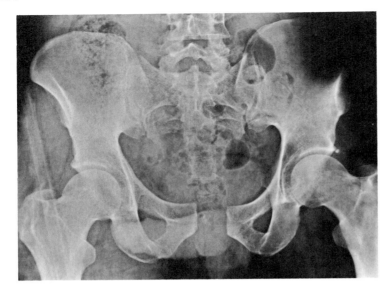

Fig. 7.38. A 42-year-old man whilst at work was squashed between a concrete pole and the bucket of a crane. He was admitted with low abdominal pain and could barely move. Careful scrutiny of the film shows, apart from the wide symphysis, a fracture of the right inferior pubic ramus, and a dislocated left sacroiliac joint with asymmetric folded-out left iliac wing—the so-called 'sprung-pelvis'.

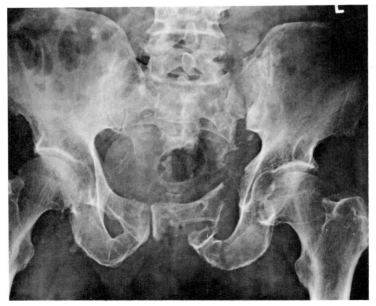

Fig. 7.39. Example of an unstable double vertical fracture of Malgaigne. The line of fracture runs through the inferior and superior pubic rami, the sacroiliac joint on the same side, and the fifth and fourth lumbar transverse processes.

to which his name has been ascribed. This may involve the superior and inferior pubic rami, together with the sacroiliac area on one side, known as the double vertical fracture (Fig. 7.39); or if the sacroiliac joint area on the opposite side is disrupted then it is called a 'bucket-handle' or contralateral double vertical fracture (Fig. 7.40). If missed and not properly immobil-ized there may be resulting dislocations and leg-shortening. Occasionally, there may be a combination of injuries. Having seen the ob-vious fracture–dislocation of the hip (Fig. 7.41) the observers' eyes are drawn towards the wide symphysis. The line of thinking should then be towards a second break in the ring and the sacroiliac joint provides the answer.

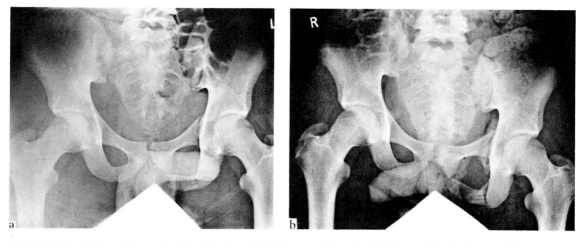

Fig. 7.40. 'Bucket-handle' or contralateral double vertical fracture–dislocation of Malgaigne (a). The fracture–dislocation of the right sacroiliac joint was missed and there was subsequent cranial subluxation of about 6 cm (b). This was non-reducible, resulting in leg-shortening.

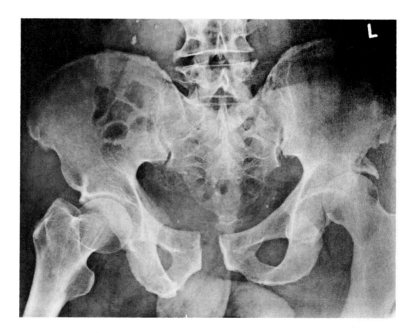

Fig. 7.41. Posterior dislocation of the left hip with fracture of the acetabular rim. The pubic symphysis is too wide, and notice the subtle dislocation of the left sacroiliac joint. Having seen the obvious lesions always look for the less obvious; this is the main role of the radiologist.

The authors have found that the use of excretion urography in blunt abdominal trauma and pelvic fractures is becoming so frequent as to be almost routine. Any severe jolt to the abdomen is likely to produce a moderate haematuria. It is clear that the urinary tract is susceptible to injury in this type of trauma. However, the authors try to insist on a reasonable indication, such as haematuria, anuria, or pain in the flanks, before performing excretion urography. In males a urogram is followed by retrograde urethrography with a water-soluble contrast medium before attempting catheterization (Fig. 7.42). Partial or total urethral ruptures

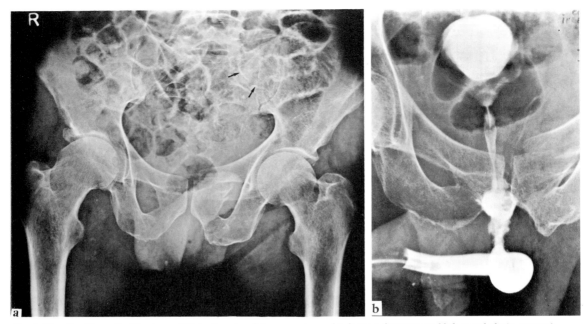

Fig. 7.42. Double vertical fracture of Malgaigne involving superior and inferior pubic rami and left sacral ala (a, arrows). A retrograde urethrogram (b), performed on the emergency room table, shows a partial urethral rupture. Careful catheterization by a urologist prevented a possible total rupture.

can be treated by a suprapubic cystostomy for three months, followed by urethral repair. Some urologists prefer immediate treatment by 'railroading' a catheter, controlled from above in the bladder and below through the penis. Trauma to the renal tract should be sought in the renal arteries, kidneys, ureters, bladder and urethra. Total arterial avulsion manifested by non-function of the kidney on the excretion urogram requires immediate surgery. Opacification of a normal kidney on the undamaged side is one of the most important functions of the excretion urogram, to prevent removal of the only kidney. Total ruptures of kidneys have been known to heal conservatively. The main indications for immediate surgical intervention are: arterial pedicle avulsion, as mentioned, continued bleeding, and disruption of the ureter. These are uncommon and generally a conservative approach to renal tract trauma predominates.

Bladder and urethral injuries occur in 10% of pelvic fractures. This figure rises to 27% of major fractures. In two-thirds of bladder ruptures there is no macroscopic haematuria (Fig 7.43). Eighty per cent of bladders will rupture extraperitoneally.

Cass and Ireland have stated that lesions are missed unless 400 ml contrast medium are run into the bladder and post-washout pictures are made. The authors run in up to 500 ml and then allow the patient to micturate himself if there is no obvious leakage during filling, urethral injury being excluded by a retrograde examination. A post-micturation film is then made. The authors have not found washout pictures to be of much help.

Carpal bone injuries

The wrist or carpus consists of eight interrelated bones between the distal radius and the meta-

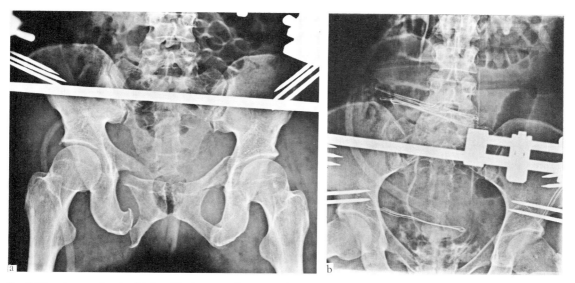

Fig. 7.43. A snowplough which suddenly reversed ran over the pelvis of a 32-year-old woman. The picture taken after insertion of a fixation frame shows a 'straddle' fracture of both superior and inferior pubic rami and a dislocation of the left sacroiliac joint (a). On the excretion urogram (b) there is extravasation of contrast medium around the bladder indicating rupture. At operation, there were three tears in the bladder containing splinters of bone. The urethra was severed and the vagina avulsed from the vulva. A subsequent urethrovaginal fistula occurred.

carpals, and these bones are connected to each other by strong ligamentous structures. The carpal bones act as a highly mobile pulley guiding the tendons while the hand is able to perform complex movements. Except for the pisiform, the carpal bones have no muscular or tendinous attachments, and movement of the wrist is dependent on the tendons that cross the carpus from the forearm to the hand. The stability of the carpus is dependent on the geometry of the carpal bones, and the ligamentous interconnections enable the transmission of forces from the hand to the forearm. When the forces become too great a carpal injury results. The most common cause is a fall where a force is applied to the outstretched extremity with the hand and wrist dorsiflexed. The magnitude of the force and its point of application determine the resulting injury: a scaphoid dislocation, a scaphoid fracture, a perilunate or lunate dislocation, or another carpal fracture. An injury of the carpus is clinically manifested by pain,

swelling and limited motion. Radiographs are extremely important to specify the type of carpal injury and to make the diagnosis, especially when obvious skeletal deformities are absent.

Recognition of a post-traumatic carpal instability requires some special views and an awareness by the physician of the condition.

SCAPHOID FRACTURE

Scaphoid fracture is the most common injury of the carpus and occurs at any place within the scaphoid: distal pole, mid-portion or proximal pole. Clinically, it is suspected on finding tenderness to direct pressure over the scaphoid. The diagnosis should be confirmed with a series of coned-down radiographs. Ulnar deviation of the hand is important, and in addition to a neutral posteroanterior and neutral lateral view the following are also recommended: 30° oblique; 60° oblique; posteroanterior making a fist with the

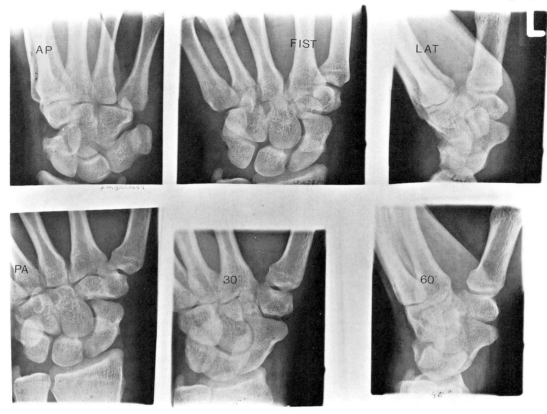

Fig. 7.44. Six routine views of the scaphoid: lateral; 30° oblique; 60° oblique; PA making a fist with the thumb turned in; PA; and lastly an AP view. Note that the fracture of the scaphoid in this patient is only seen on the AP view.

thumb turned in; and lastly, with the wrist the other way up, an anteroposterior view. Non-displaced or minimally displaced fractures may not be apparent on initial radiographs (Fig. 7.44).

If a fracture is suspected on clinical examination the diagnosis may be confirmed by scintigraphy (Fig. 7.5). Shortly after trauma, 24 hours or more, it is possible to have increased uptake at the site of the fracture. A less expensive way is to repeat the radiographs after two weeks, because the fracture may now be visible by the cortical resorption at the fracture line.

Displaced scaphoid fractures are often associated with other carpal injuries such as transscaphoid perilunate dislocation ('De Quervain's

fracture'). Because the scaphoid fracture is so obvious the perilunar dislocation is frequently missed (Fig. 7.45).

POST-TRAUMATIC CARPAL INSTABILITY

Post-traumatic carpal instability is caused by a traumatic disruption of the strong ligamentous structures of the carpus. When the influencing force is large, apart from a tearing of ligaments, there is also a dislocation of part of the carpus, such as in the perilunar dislocation. In this injury the capitate comes to lie dorsal to the lunate and the rest of the carpal bones remain

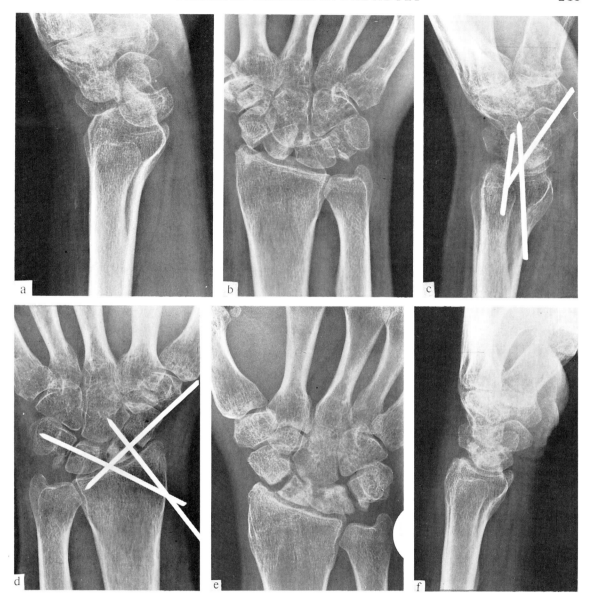

Fig. 7.45. Trans-scaphoid perilunar dislocation. A serviceman fell onto his wrist whilst playing football on the Island of Aruba. A fracture of the scaphoid was diagnosed and was treated in plaster. Several months later he was seen in Holland complaining that he could not lift with his right hand. Examination showed limited range of movements: dorsiflexion, 20°; palmar flexion, 0°; and radial deviation, 0°. Films (a) and (b) show a non-united scaphoid fracture and dorsal dislocation of the capitate and other carpal bones in relation to the lunate. The classic triangular appearance of the lunate in a true lunate dislocation is not seen here. (c) and (d) Wire-rod fixation of scaphoid and carpal bones. (e) and (f) End result with lunatomalacia and avascular necrosis of the un-united proximal pole of the scaphoid. A more prompt approach to treatment may have given a more satisfactory result.

bound to the capitate. It is also possible to have a lunar dislocation, where only the lunate is palmar dislocated. Reduction involves manipulating the lunate back onto the radius into a perilunar dislocation before reducing the capitate back into the cup of the lunate. The diagnosis of a lunar or perilunar dislocation is best made on a neutral lateral view.

Much more difficult to diagnose are the post-traumatic subluxations, where as a result of ligament tearing certain carpal bones do not take part in the normal carpal movements, but during moving they come to lie in a subluxed position. The diagnosis is frequently missed by the unwary observer, because the clinical and radiological findings may be quite subtle. If there is consideration of carpal instability, then the following six views of the wrist are made: a neutral posteroanterior view and a neutral true lateral, on which the diagnosis can usually be made; besides these, the authors also take extreme extension and flexion lateral views, and extreme radial and ulnar deviation PA views. Carpal instability can be recognized by locating central axes of the radius, lunate, scaphoid and capitate in the lateral view and by measuring the scapholunate angle (N 30–60°), the capitolunate angle (N 0–30°), and the radiolunate angle (N 0–12°) (Fig. 7.46). The central axes of capitate, lunate and radius are essentially parallel. The axis of the scaphoid bisects the other axes at an angle that may vary from 30 to 60° in a normal wrist. There are different forms of carpal instability, and because there is some confusion regarding their classification only two very frequently seen types of carpal instability will be discussed.

ROTATORY SCAPHOID SUBLUXATION

In this subluxation the proximal pole of the scaphoid dislocates proximally by disruption of the strong volar radiocarpal ligaments (radioscaphoid and scapholunate). Because the ligament between scaphoid and lunate also ruptures, the space between these two bones is widened, and

so scapholunate dissociation is another name for this type of instability. The roentgenographic findings seen on the anteroposterior view are the following:

1 A gap of greater than 2 mm between the scaphoid and the lunate.
2 A foreshortened appearance of the scaphoid due to an increased palmar flexion of the scaphoid in the neutral position of the wrist.
3 'Ring sign'. Due to the increased palmar flexion the cortical waist of the scaphoid projects as a ring. In the neutral lateral view the radioscaphoid angle is 60° or greater.

The radiographic findings may be quite subtle, so additional views, as already mentioned, might be necessary: a posteroanterior view in ulnar and radial deviation (Fig. 7.47) and a lateral view in flexion and extension. A clenched fist provides longitudinal compression and may widen the scapholunate gap on the PA view. Proof that the ligament between the scaphoid and lunate is ruptured can be obtained by arthrography (Fig. 7.48). The diagnostic finding is a communication between the radiocarpal and mid-carpal joint at the scapholunate junction.

OS LUNATUM SUBLUXATION

An instability of the os scaphoideum can be paired with an instability of the os lunatum. This instability can be expressed in various ways. In a normal wrist the axis of the lunate on the lateral view is parallel to the axis through the capitate and the radius. In cases of instability of the lunate there is a volar or dorsiflexion of the lunate present, and this is a result of a fracture or subluxation of the scaphoid, or as an end result of a reduced lunar or perilunar dislocation. The commonest instability is the so-called dorsiflexion instability. Fig. 7.49 shows this instability as an end result of a healed scaphoid fracture. The distal articular surface of the lunate faces dorsally and the capitate is dorsal to the mid-plane of the radius.

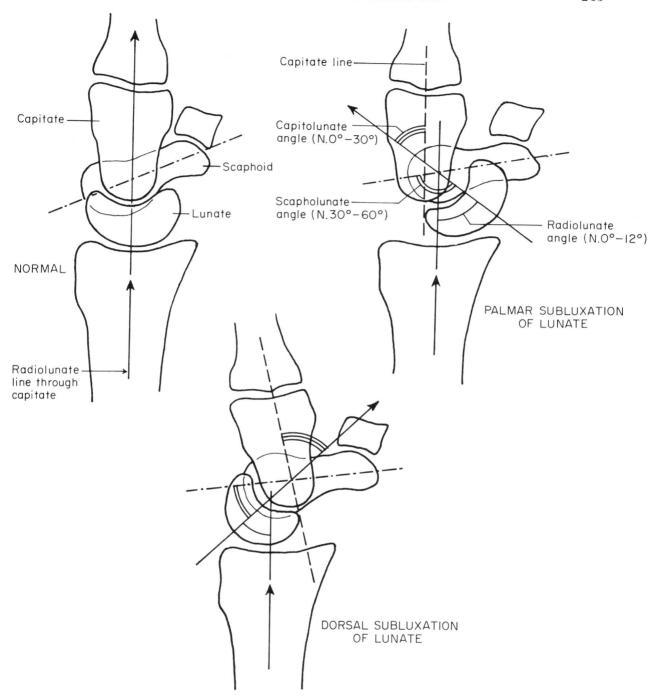

Fig. 7.46. Carpal instability recognized by locating the central axes of the radius, lunate, scaphoid, and capitate in the lateral view and measuring the scapholunate angle, the capitolunate angle, and the radiolunate angle.

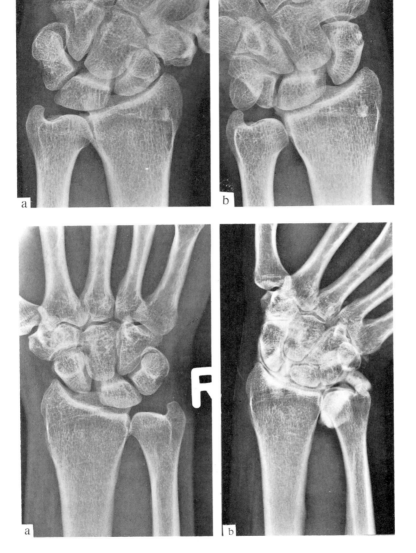

Fig. 7.47. Rotatory scaphoid subluxation. PA views in radial (a) and ulnar (b) deviation to show decreasing and increasing gap between the scaphoid and lunate.

Fig. 7.48. Rotatory scaphoid subluxation in a 52-year-old lady complaining of pain in the wrist, mainly on the radial side, for about four years. There was also limited movement of the wrist. The PA view (a) shows a widened gap betwen the scaphoid and lunate and a foreshortened scaphoid with 'ring sign'. In the arthrogram (b) the contrast medium is seen abnormally in the scapholunate space and the intercarpal space. There is also filling of the distal radioulnar joint, indicating a tear of the triangular cartilage.

Trauma of the knee

DISTAL FEMUR

Supracondylar and condylar fractures of the distal femur produce no problems for the radiologist. The osteochondral fracture of the knee during the acute stage is often missed because basically the diagnosis is not considered. These osteochondral fractures may be caused by impaction, avulsion or shearing forces. The fracture occurs through the surface layers of the bone, and the fragment contains cartilage and a small flake of bone which can be seen on the standard anteroposterior or lateral radiograph as a linear opacity lying in the joint space. The

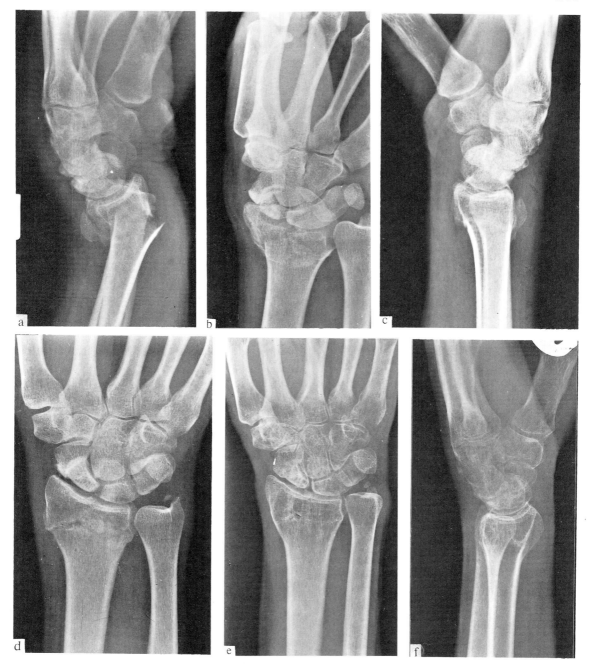

Fig. 7.49. Os lunatum subluxation. (a) and (b) Comminuted distal radius fracture with 'dinner fork' deformity of the wrist. The scaphoid fracture had occurred several weeks previously. (c) and (d) Post-reduction films; note already the anterior rotation of the lunate and dorsal position of the capitate on the lateral view. (e) and (f) End result with good healing of scaphoid and radius but unchanged lunate subluxation.

medial tangential osteochondral fracture of the patella is caused by the shearing forces exerted by the quadriceps during traumatic dislocation of the patella. Sometimes it is the edge of the lateral femoral condyle that is broken. The prominent margin of the lateral condyle is vulnerable to direct trauma, as from a kick or fall, and marginal fractures are common.

PROXIMAL TIBIA

Fractures of the proximal tibia affect the tibial condyles and the intercondylar eminence. Fractures of the lateral tibial condyle are often seen in pedestrians hit by cars, where the bumper hits the outside of the knee, affecting the femoral condyle and the lateral tibial plateau; hence the name 'bumper fracture'. This injury can also be caused by a fall from a height, usually with twisting of the leg.

A valgus, varus or rotation trauma can cause, apart from a fracture of the condyles, rupture of the collateral ligament and/or knee joint capsule. The place and size of the impressed part of the tibial plateau is more dependent on the flexed position of the knee at the moment of trauma. With the knee in flexion then the middle or posterior area of the plateau is impressed. A fracture of the medial and lateral condyles occurs more often following vertical compression trauma. There exist many classifications for tibial plateau fractures, mainly in order to make treatment plans easier for the orthopaedic surgeon. One of the more important criteria for operative intervention is the amount of condylar depression measured on the radiographs. Measurement of the amount of depression on a standard AP radiograph is not valid because the plane of the proximal articular surface of the tibia forms an angle of 76° with the tibial crest. The amount of depression of the posterior part of the tibial plateau tends to be magnified on a standard AP radiograph. The X-ray tube has to be angulated approximately 10–15° caudal in relation to the tibial crest to assess the depression accurately. Tomography appears to be a more reliable and useful tool in the assessment of tibial plateau fractures and provides the surgeon with the information he needs in planning the treatment. Tomography clearly demonstrates the position and the amount of depression, the degree of comminution and the displacement of the fragments, all important facts in planning the surgery (Fig. 7.50). In the authors' department adequate information is given with simple movement tom-

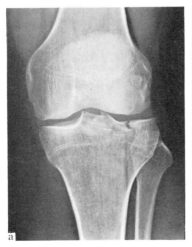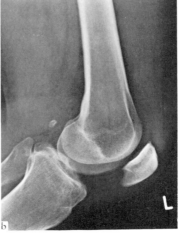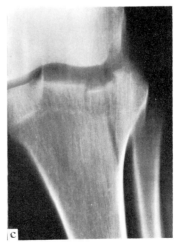

Fig. 7.50. A 50-year-old man fell from a first floor window, landing on his left leg and sustaining an injury to the knee. On the plain film (a and b) there is an obvious transcondylar lateral plateau fracture, but only on the tomogram (c) is it possible to assess the degree of comminution and depression of the articular fragment.

ography, usually ½ cm cuts in two planes at right angles. More complicated movements, such as spiral, circular, etc., provide beautiful pictures but little extra information.

FRACTURES OF THE INTERCONDYLAR EMINENCE OF THE TIBIA

Fracture of the tibial spine is predominantly seen in youth, although it may take place at any age. The anterior cruciate ligament attaches in front of the intercondylar eminence and the posterior cruciate behind it. The avulsed fragment of the intercondylar eminence often contains the piece of bone together with the attached anterior or posterior cruciate ligament (Fig. 7.51). So a fracture of the tibial spine indicates a probable cruciate ligament insufficiency. A common trauma is a bicycle accident in which a young person falls on the front of

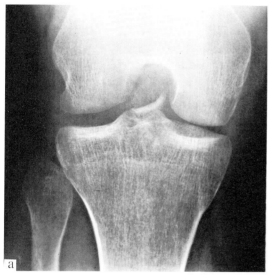

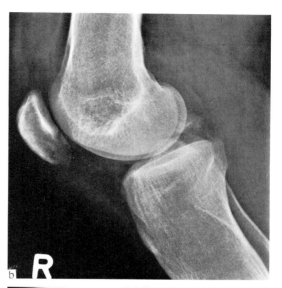

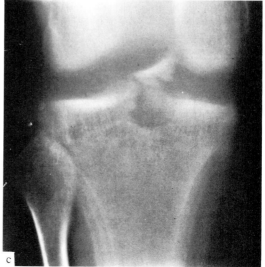

Fig. 7.51. A young woman fell from her moped, hitting her leg just below the knee against the towbar of a vehicle. Clinically there was a lesion of the posterior cruciate ligament. On the tunnel view (a) and lateral view (b) an avulsed fragment with attached posterior cruciate ligament lies posteriorly in the joint. The tomogram (c) shows the loose fragment with defect in the intercondylar area of the tibia.

the flexed knee. The femur is pushed posteriorly in relation to the tibia and an avulsion of the anterior part of the tibial spine with the anterior cruciate will result. The fracture is seen on the standard AP and lateral radiograph, but a tunnel view will help in visualizing the fragment. The treatment will depend upon the degree of displacement of the fragment. When the intercondylar fragment is completely dislodged from its bed or rotated, then open reduction and internal fixation are required.

DISLOCATION OF THE KNEE

Traumatic dislocation is, although a rare entity, a very serious injury because of neurovascular complications. Violent accidents with motor vehicles causing multiple injuries are the most common cause. Clinically the deformity is quite obvious, and because of the ease of reduction most of these are already reduced when seen in the emergency room. The dislocation is classified radiographically according to the position of the tibia in relation to the femoral condyles on the standard AP and lateral views. The types of classifications are anterior, medial, lateral and rotatory. A complete dislocation causes a major disruption of the soft tissues and ligaments of the knee, and frequently injures the popliteal artery or peroneal nerve (Fig. 7.52). The popliteal artery is fixed proximally and distally. Proximally it is anchored at the adductor hiatus to the femoral shaft, and distally beneath the tendinous arch to the tibia. Any major displacement of skeletal structures will stretch the artery. The incidence of vascular complications is high (± 30%) so the posterior tibialis and dorsalis pedis pulses should always be evaluated. A warm foot with no cyanosis is no proof of popliteal artery continuity. If there is any doubt as to the patency of the popliteal artery the authors perform an arteriogram not only to diagnose and locate any lesion, but also to show the extent of collateral circulation. Some feel that arteriography gives little additional information, since the location of the lesion should be well known, and prolongs the time interval between injury and surgery.

Injuries to the ankle and foot

When considering injuries in and around the adult ankle joint it is helpful to remember that the type of fracture or dislocation will depend upon the amount of force applied and the direction in which it acts. Thus, it is possible to have a simple classification based upon inversion or eversion injuries and an axial or vertical force such as jumping or falling from a height onto the feet. Other injuries will involve forced natural movements of plantarflexion and dorsiflexion. All these injuries can be modified by a rotational component. In assessing these injuries radiographically the radiologist can be helped by using a mental checklist: Is the proximal fibula intact (Maisonneuve fracture)? Is the syndesmosis between the tibia and fibula too wide? Rupture of the tibiofibular ligament can cause an unstable diastasis of the ankle joint — are the other tarsal bones intact? Look at the base of the fifth metatarsal (Jones' fracture) and the neck of the talus (Fig. 7.53). Most injuries can be adequately demonstrated by two views at right angles to the ankle.

Special care must be taken to project the malleoli over one another for the lateral view and to ensure that the fibula is projected free of the tibia on the AP mortise view. These views can be supplemented with both 45° oblique projections of the ankle joint. Further information regarding the articular cortex or position of loose bodies can be shown, preferably on spiral or hypocycloidal tomography. Sometimes the injuring force is conducted through into the subtalar area or calcaneus. The orthopaedic surgeon will want to know Böehler's angle if he is planning reduction surgery (Fig. 7.54). This is measured from a lateral calcaneal view and not a lateral ankle view. Böehler's angle is subtended by a line from the calcaneal tuberosity through the posterior articular facet, and a second line from the anterior process of calcaneum through the posterior articular facet. The normal angle is about 30–40° (Harty 1973). The axial calcaneal view is also necessary in all calcaneal fractures.

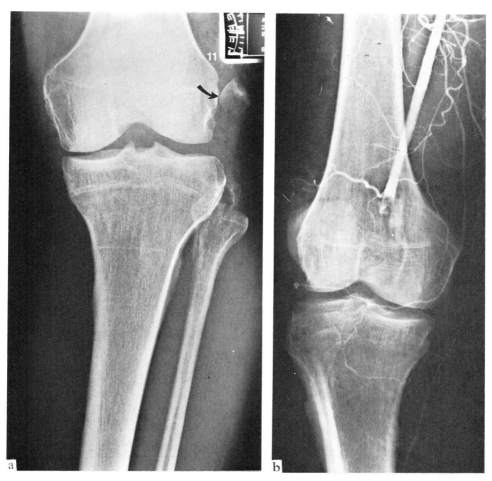

Fig. 7.52. A 67-year-old man was walking across a road when he was hit by a car. On arrival at the casualty department he could remember everything that had happened. He could not move his left foot very well and he had no feeling in the lateral side of his foot and lower leg. On clinical examination he had a severe instability of the posterolateral ligament apparatus of the knee. The knee could be easily excessively subluxated posterolaterally. The foot was warm and the relevant vessels, dorsalis pedis and tibialis posterior, were pulsating. Radiologically (a) there was no dislocation of the knee, but a fragment of the head of the fibula lay pulled up alongside the lateral femoral condyle (arrow). The diagnosis was made of a total tearing of the posterolateral ligaments and a lesion of the peroneal nerve. Surgical treatment was scheduled, but after a few hours the pulsations of the tibialis posterior became weak and the dorsalis pedis was negative. An angiogram was immediately performed (b) and this showed a complete stop in the proximal part of the popliteal artery. During the operation the continuity of the popliteal artery was intact but there was an obstruction due to an intimal dissection. A venous graft interposition was performed. Considering the severe ligament disruption, not only lateral and medial, but also posterior, a complete dislocation of the knee had probably occurred!

There are several very good classifications of ankle injury based on the movement causing the injury, i.e. supination/external rotation, pronation/abduction, etc. However, in practice, from the clinical history the most that the patient can tell you is that he fell with the foot turned in or out, or tripped on the point of his toes so that the foot was pulled back in excessive plantarflexion. Maybe he remembers falling on his leg in rotation and he heard a crack. The radiographs can then confirm the injury, and by working backwards it can be ascertained

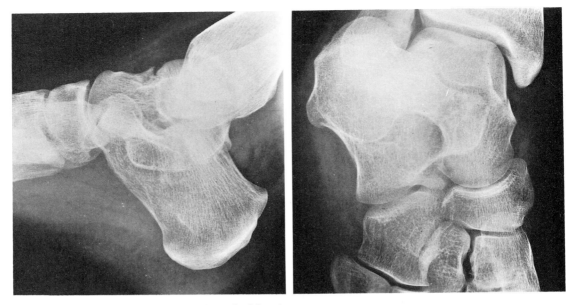

Fig. 7.53. Non-displaced fracture through the neck of the talus.

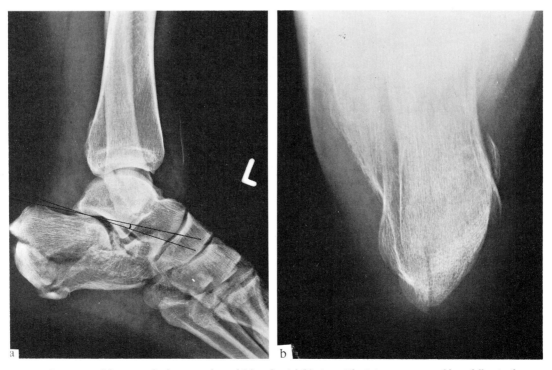

Fig. 7.54. Comminuted fracture of calcaneum, lateral (a) and axial (b) views. The injury was caused by a fall onto the feet from a height. Böehler's angle is considerably reduced to 2° (N. 30–40°).

how the injury was caused. The principle of treatment is then to reverse the direction of the precipitating force.

Dislocations of the ankle and foot usually occur at three main sites. The talus will dislocate out of the ankle mortise in all four directions: anterior, posterior, medial and lateral. Secondly, dislocation occurs below the talus in the subtalar and talonavicular joint areas. If the foot is displaced medially it is called a medial subtalar dislocation (Fig. 7.55), and if the foot moves laterally then it is known as a lateral subtalar dislocation. Thirdly, there is a tarsometatarsal dislocation named after Lisfranc who first described a mid-foot amputation through these joints whilst he was a field surgeon during the Napoleonic wars (Fig. 7.56). All these dislocations involve gross disruption of ligaments, joint capsules and vessels. Avascular necrosis of the talus, even following swift reduction, is not an uncommon result.

The myriad varieties of fractures of the ankle caused by inversion or eversion are well covered by the other textbooks. An important injury which the authors have seen missed on several occasions is the flake fracture of the articular cortex of the talus (Fig. 7.57), so-called osteochondral chip fractures. These can occur anywhere on the medial or lateral edge of the articular margin and sometimes have to be positively looked for with dorsiflexion or plantarflexion AP views. If undiagnosed these fractures may give rise to arthrosis (Fig. 7.61), or the flakes may break loose, becoming trapped or inverted in the joint (Fig. 7.59). Open removal or replacement and fixation may be necessary. Arthrograms can be helpful in localizing a loose fragment or in outlining a defect in the

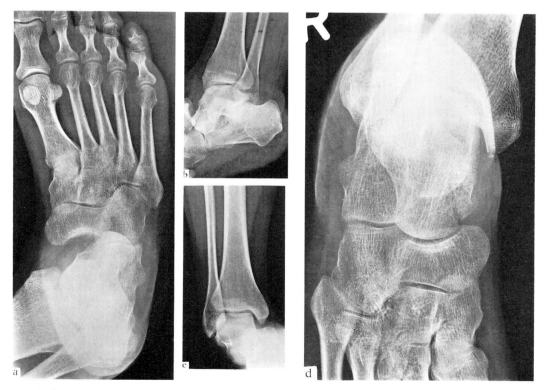

Fig. 7.55 (a–d). Medial subtalar dislocation occurring in a drunken man who fell whilst trying to climb curtains at a carnival party. Notice that the chip fracture of the head of the talus is only visible on the post-reduction film (d).

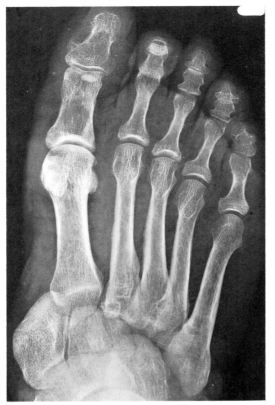

articular margin of the talus. A further impression injury may occur at the corner of the tibia and medial malleolus where the edge of the talus presses up into it during forced inversion. Again if clinical evidence is strong then look for a fracture in these 'hidden' areas.

Vertical force fractures of the ankle usually follow falls from heights or jumping. The tibia may act like a hammer on the talus, splitting it like a nut (Fig. 7.60). The opposite may also occur and the talus splits the tibia, with the fractures running lengthwise and intra-articularly (Fig. 7.61). If, as mentioned, the force is carried downwards into the heel then the subtalar joint and calcaneus will be injured.

Injuries to the lateral ligaments of the ankle deserve special consideration. Firstly, they are very common, especially in young people actively pursuing sports such as tennis, volleyball, basketball etc. Secondly, in the adult, fractures are less frequent in this area due to the relatively strong nature of the bony components of the ankle compared to its ligamentous support. Thirdly, effective treatment, depending on degree of injury, can considerably reduce the number of chronically unstable and painful ankles.

Fig. 7.56. Lisfranc tarsometatarsal dislocation. Unusually, in this case all five metatarsals are laterally dislocated. This occurred in a woman who literally fell off a chair whilst hanging out washing.

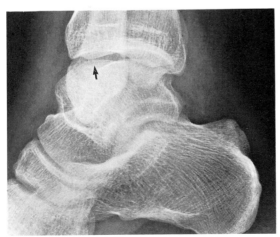
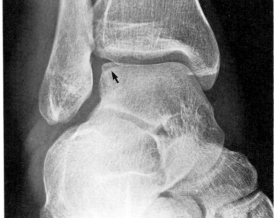

Fig. 7.57. Eversion injury with osteochondral flake fracture of lateral articular margin of talus (arrow).

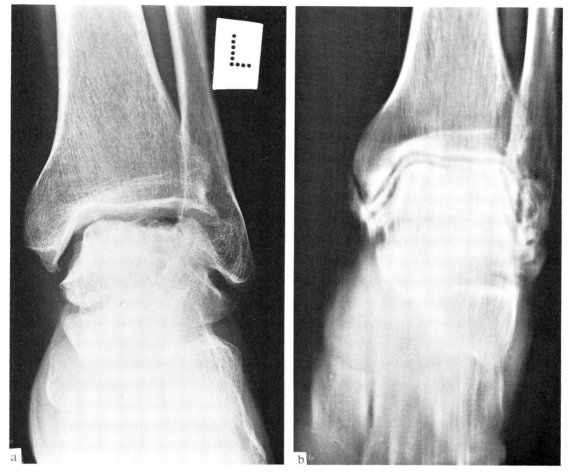

Fig. 7.58. Osteonecrosis of the talus and osteoarthrosis of the ankle joint following an old trauma (a). Arthrogram–planigram (b) showing irregular thinned cartilage laterally and irregular articular cortex.

There has been considerable discussion in the literature as to the treatment of choice for these ankle ligament injuries. It is the authors' practice to operate on all the major ligament injuries, i.e. two or more ruptured lateral ligaments, including the calcaneofibular ligament. The minor lesions, however, are conservatively treated in a plaster-cast for several weeks. This is usually for one ligament tear, the anterior talofibular ligament and joint capsule tears. There are three main ligaments binding the lateral side of the ankle. The anterior talofibular ligament from the anterior surface of the distal fibula passes anteriorly and medially to be inserted into the neck of the talus. The calcaneofibular ligament from the posterior aspect of the fibula passes posteriorly, medially, and inferiorly to insert into the superior aspect of the calcaneus. This ligament is also contiguous with the peroneus tendon sheath of longus and brevis. Thus any lesion of the calcaneofibular ligament also tears into this tendon sheath allowing it to fill with synovia, blood or contrast medium from the joint. The third supporting ligament is the posterior talofibular ligament from the posterior aspect of the fibula, passing up medially and

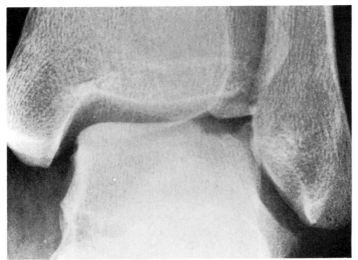
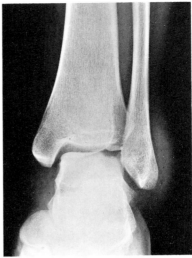

Fig. 7.59a. Osteochondral fracture of the lateral articular margin of the talus lying upside down in the joint.

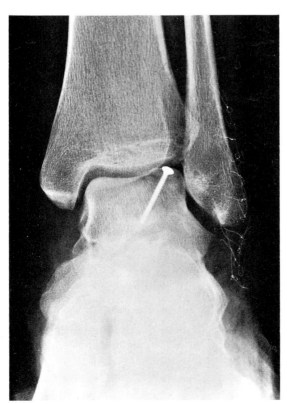

Fig. 7.59b. Open reduction with fragment fixed back in its place with a screw.

posteriorly to insert on the posterior aspect of the talus. All three ligaments run nearly horizontally.

It is well known that plain views, including stress inversion or talar tilt films, can give limited information. A talar tilt difference of more than 7° between both ankles is suggestive of acute or chronic ligamentous damage, but this is dependent on examiner variation and previous history of the 'good' ankle.

If there is clinical evidence of ankle instability occurring in a young patient, and if this occurs within 48 hours of injury, then the authors perform single-contrast arthrography of the ankle joint. The method is quite simple. Under sterile conditions the joint is entered anteriorly with a 19-gauge needle, avoiding the dorsalis pedis and medial to the anterior tibial tendon. Aim slightly upwards to avoid the lip of the tibia. 6–12 ml of 280–300 mg iodine-containing water-soluble contrast agent, together with 1 ml of 1½% lignocaine, is injected into the ankle joint under screening control, avoiding too much extravasation, which can obscure detail. Then, very importantly, the joint is vigorously exercised to spread the contrast medium, trying to fill the peroneus tendon sheath.

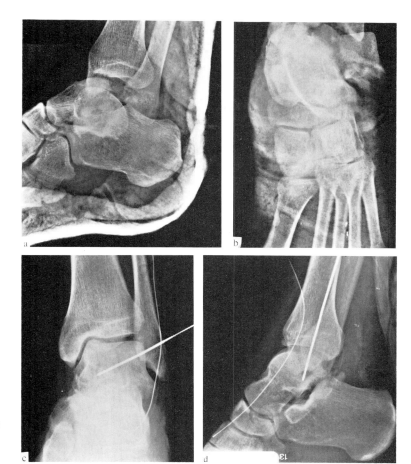

Fig. 7.60. A depressed young man jumped out of a window and fell 16 metres onto his feet. He sustained multiple injuries to the spine, pelvis, femur, tibia, and ankle. Films (a) and (b) show the talus to be split in two vertically and dislocated anterolaterally out of the ankle fork. There is an associated Jones' fracture of the base of the fifth metatarsal and a non-displaced tarsal navicular fracture. Open reduction and a pin through the fibula talus produced a good anatomical result (c and d).

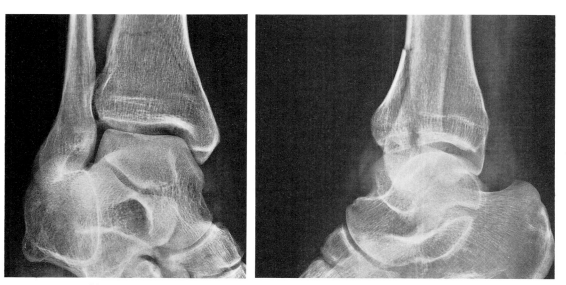

Fig. 7.61. Vertical force injury caused by jumping from a height. Intra-articular fracture of the distal anterior tibia. Similar force as patient in Fig. 7.60 with different result.

Routinely, the authors make an anteroposterior, a lateral, two obliques and two hand-stress pictures; the talar tilt and anterior draw. Filling of the various recesses and subtalar joint may occur and are all normal. Extravasation anterolateral to the joint is considered to be isolated talofibular ligament rupture and thus a minor lesion (Fig. 7.62). However, if there is also filling of the peroneal tendon sheath then this indicates a major lesion with rupture of the calcaneofibular ligament as well (Fig. 7.63). One pitfall is that should there be a largish tear in the joint capsule with a considerable extravasation then it may be difficult to force contrast medium into the peroneal tendon sheath. The authors have found it possible to obtain about 90% good correlation of arthrographic appearances with operation findings.

Stress injuries of bone

Stress lesions and stress fractures are fairly common in athletes and military recruits in training. Certain types of stress injury are related to various kinds of sport: long-distance runners and ballet dancers the mid-tibia; jumpers or hurdlers the groin and calcaneus; golfers the ribs; parachutists the proximal fibula; hitch-hikers with rucksack the first rib; hook of hamate fracture in golfers, tennis players and baseball players; wheelchair athletes (rotational activity) the ulna; and trapshooters the coracoid.

Breithaupt, a Prussian military surgeon, in 1855 was the first to describe clinically stress fractures in the swollen painful feet of soldiers after long marches. Stechow in 1897 made the

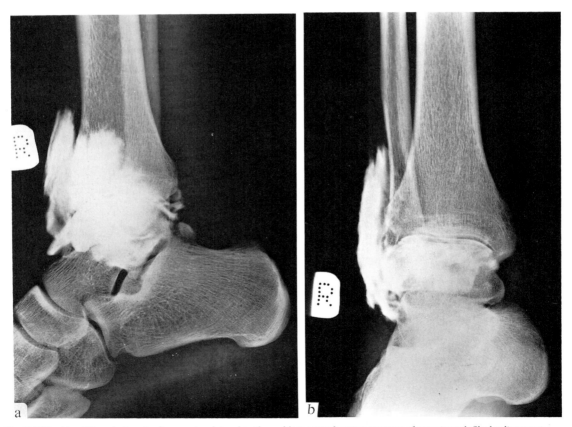

Fig. 7.62 (a, b). Minor lesion. Leakage anterolateral to the ankle joint indicating rupture of anterior talofibular ligament and capsule tear.

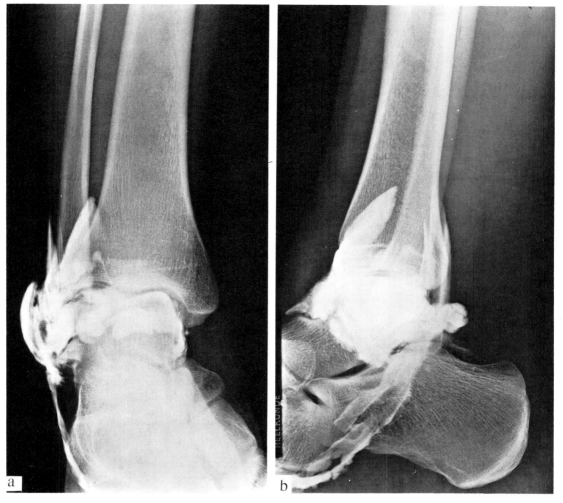

Fig. 7.63 (a, b). Major lesion. Apart from leakage anterolaterally there is also filling of the peroneal longus and brevis tendon sheaths, indicating rupture of the important calcaneofibular ligament.

first radiographic description of the condition. Precipitating factors causing stress lesions appear to be an intensifying of physical activity or change of training method. There is onset pain within the bone following exertion, and which is relieved by rest. The pain may be referred in nature. If the training is continued then a stress lesion may progress to an actual stress fracture. Initial radiographs may be negative, changes appearing from three weeks to three months after the onset of symptoms. X-ray changes include a thickening of cortical

bone from periosteal and endosteal apposition. If excessive activity occurs then osteoclastic activity will exceed osteoblastic activity and transverse stress fractures will occur (Fig. 7.64).

When trabecular bone is affected, as in the calcaneus (Fig. 7.65), there occur small impression fractures with apparent focal sclerosis. If stress injury is suspected and the radiographs are normal, then the authors perform a whole-body isotope scan, which allows for the fact that not all lesions are symptomatic and in some cases there may be referred pain. Scans are

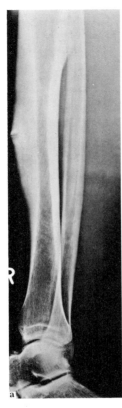
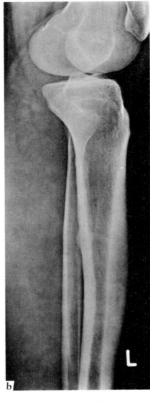

Fig. 7.64 (a, b). Stress lesion in both tibiae and a stress fracture on the right side in a marathon walker. A man aged 31 trained by walking 10 kilometres every day. He complained of pain in both shins. On examination there was also swelling on the anterior aspect of both tibiae. The stress fracture was originally mistaken to be an osteoid osteoma. The athletic history and double-sided effects of the condition do not support this diagnosis.

positive at an early stage before the X-rays. However, a normal bone scan excludes the diagnosis of a stress lesion. If unrecognized, a partial stress fracture may lead to a complete fracture such as may occur in the neck of the femur. If this happens internal fixation will be required. Most other stress lesions respond to rest or bedrest in cases affecting the femoral neck, and isotope scan changes often revert to normal. The bones most affected are the pelvis and lower limbs, i.e. femur, tibia, calcaneus and metatarsals. Most people are aware of the 'march fractures' occurring in soldiers.

Stress fractures have to be differentiated from ligamentous injury, chronic osteomyelitis, osteoid osteoma (often typical night pain, relieved by aspirin, and nidus lesion), osteogenic sarcoma (consider if strange periosteal appearance), osteomalacia (renal failure patients), ischaemic disorders (check circulation of elderly athletes) and arthritis.

There are a number of associated conditions which have little direct connection with the initial area of trauma. If you do not think of them they are likely to be missed. One is the fracture of the proximal fibula during a medial malleolus fracture, known as a Maisonneuve fracture. Also, cervical injury sometimes occurs in association with facial fractures. Three other associations, because of their unusual manifestations, deserve further consideration here. They include diaphragm rupture and pelvic trauma; minimal trauma and Sudeck's atrophy; and sternal fracture and cervicodorsal trauma.

Traumatic rupture of the diaphragm is not an unusual condition, however about half are missed initially. First described by Sennertus in 1541 it is caused by blunt or crushing injury to the thoracoabdominal area and is associated with fractures of the pelvis and long bones in about 50% of cases. Often there is multiple trauma affecting the liver, spleen and pancreas. Injury on the left side is more common; figures in the literature range from 4:1 to 9:1 in favour of the left. The liver tends to protect the diaphragm on the right.

Very often the signs are subtle with non-specific or no clinical findings. There may be elevation of the 'diaphragm' shadow on the affected side with, maybe, pulmonary contusion and haemothorax. Most commonly the stomach and a portion of omentum herniates, the stomach forming a 'pear shape' with its narrow lower end trapped in the tear. The dilated stomach can mimic a pneumothorax (Fig. 7.66) or aerated lung. Less commonly the spleen, colon or small bowel may herniate. Heart and mediastinum may be displaced. A barium meal or nasogastric tube may help to locate the stomach above the diaphragm. The oesophagogastric

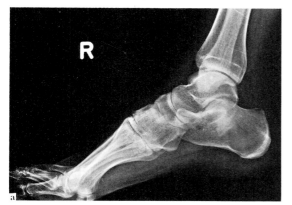

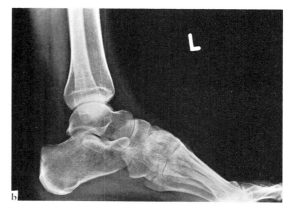

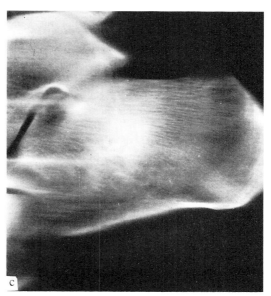

Fig. 7.65 (a–c). A 28-year-old woman complained of spontaneous pain in the right heel on the Monday following athletics training at the weekend involving jumping and hurdling. Stress fractures within the body of the calcaneus are also shown on the tomogram (c).

hiatus is usually in its normal place. The tear occurs in the dome or fibrous area. On the right side liver or kidney may herniate making diagnosis very difficult. Initial chest film may be normal, in 50% according to Ayella, a number of cases being found by exploratory laparotomy. If missed there may be a delayed obstructive phase in which bowel becomes obstructed; this may be many months or even years after the traumatic episode. Thankfully few patients die primarily as a result of the rupture of the diaphragm but rather from other, more severe, injuries.

Reflex sympathetic dystrophy syndrome (Sudeck's atrophy)

This is an unusual condition of unknown aetiology. About half of the cases present to casualty departments because of a preceding traumatic episode. The condition was described by Mitchell *et al.* in 1864, however Sudeck's description, with whose name it is associated, came in 1902. Onset occurs one week to several months after a precipitating factor. Diagnosis is usually made on a combination of clinical and radiological findings. All tissues are involved with,

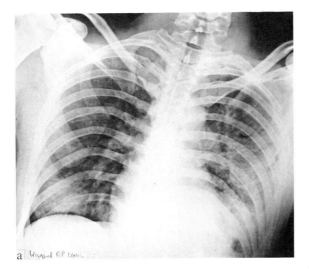

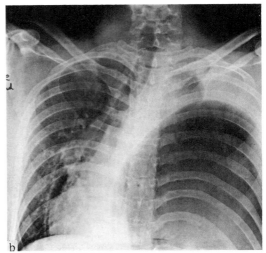

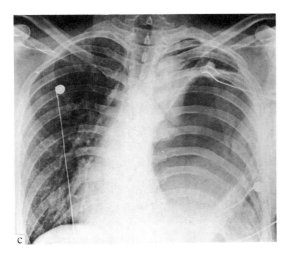

Fig. 7.66. Traumatic rupture of the diaphragm simulating tension pneumothorax. A 23-year-old man, under the influence of alcohol, crashed his car. There is closed contusion to the left side of the chest and abdomen and the left leg. There was an obvious fracture of the left femur treated directly by tibial snare traction. (a) shows contusion to the left lower lung field. There was no comment at the time that the left hemidiaphragm could not be seen. Nine days later the patient suddenly became breathless and there were asymmetrical chest movements. A tension pneumothorax on the left side was erroneously diagnosed (b). A low chest drain was introduced and stomach contents came out. A gastroscopy was performed and a hole was seen in the stomach. A second tube was introduced higher up the thorax (c). The patient then went into shock. At operation a large tear of the left hemidiaphragm was found and the hole in the stomach was also repaired.

characteristically, swelling, atrophic skin, cyanosis, and pain, which is sometimes severe. There may also be hyperaesthesia, vasomotor instability and joint stiffness. There is a history of trauma, usually minor, to the affected part, usually the hand but maybe the shoulder, or rarely the foot. The radiographs may be normal, but show a fracture in about 50%. There may be a diffuse spotty or patchy osteoporosis, which may be periarticular, simulating the appearance of primary articular disease (Fig. 7.67). The articular margins, however, are clearly defined and the joint spaces unaffected.

Appearance on X-ray alone cannot distinguish Sudeck's atrophy from disuse osteoporosis, thus the clinical presentation must be compatible before the diagnosis is made. Sudeck's atrophy is associated with other disorders such as infection, peripheral neuropathy, thrombophlebitis, cervical osteoarthritis, tendinitis and myocardial infarction. A painful shoulder and hand syndrome can occur after

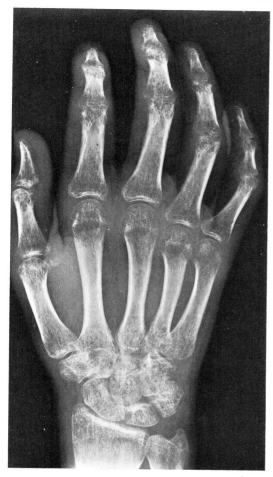

Fig. 7.67. Sudeck's atrophy in the hand of an 18-year-old girl. Note the extreme periarticular osteoporosis but no erosions. She complained of pain, especially at night, and swelling of the hand. Three weeks previously she had fallen onto the hand but no fracture was found. She was treated in a collar and cuff for the injury. The Sudeck's atrophy was treated with physiotherapy and stellate block before she had relief from the symptoms.

levels. Three stages of involvement have been described and the symptoms may return to normal at any time during these stages. At an early stage there is pain increased by movement or external stimuli and out of proportion to degree of injury. A second dystrophic stage occurs after about three months, with cold glossy skin, stiff joints and, on X-ray, osteoporosis. There may be spontaneous regression or it may be prolonged. Treatment, if symptoms are mild, is by immobilization; more severe symptoms may require sympathetic ganglion blocking.

One further association is that of sternal fracture and cervicodorsal spine injury. Flexion–compression trauma to the upper spine results in forward flexion of the spine, buckling the sternum and causing a fracture, together with a fracture or fracture–dislocation of the cervicodorsal spine. The spinal lesions may be clinically silent (Park *et al.* 1980) or there may be neck pain and a neurological deficit. However, it can be seen that an upper thoracic lesion (Fig. 7.68) can easily be overlooked, unless extra views such as supine obliques, 'swimmers' views or even arm traction pictures are obtained, often with considerable radiographic difficulty. It cannot be overemphasized that close liason between radiologist and radiographer is required for this type of patient and indeed for all severe neck injury patients. With help from the radiologist in positioning the patient the radiographer gains more confidence and produces pictures of better diagnostic quality. Again, linear tomography of the upper thoracic spine may help in delineating any damage.

The two types of injury are, firstly, a compression–flexion injury, such as a fall onto the head, or, secondly, a direct blow against the sternum with a continuing forward movement of the spine, causing a flexion injury. The cervicodorsal injury may be clinically silent, or there may be referred pain to the front of the chest, which may be explained away by the sternal fracture. In any patient with a sternal injury it is important to exclude a possible lesion of the cervicodorsal spine.

myocardial infarction in older people. The cause of this strange condition is unknown but there is often soft-tissue, nerve and vascular injury. Theories suggest that a chronic sensory stimulus leads to a circle of reflexes, with stimulation of efferent motor and sympathetic systems locally, causing hyperaemia, increased skin temperature, pain, and increased venous oxygen

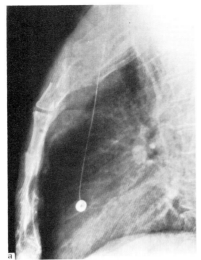

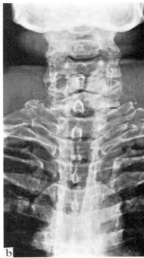

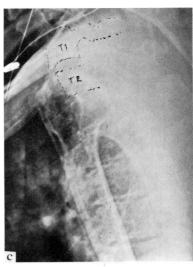

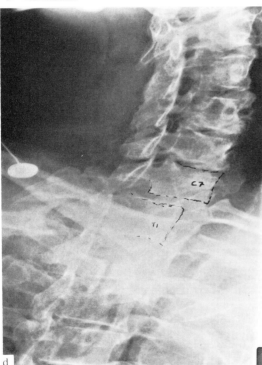

Fig. 7.68. Sternal fracture with cervicodorsal intervertebral subluxation. An elderly patient fell from a first floor window onto his head. There is a fracture of the manubrium (a) above the manubriosternal junction, the upper fragment being pushed backwards and downwards behind the lower fragment. There is a fracture of the first rib on the right, and the spinous processes of C7 and T1 are separated (b). The lateral view shows forward subluxation of C7 on T1 (c), and the supine oblique view shows more clearly the forward subluxation with impaction of the inferior facet of C7 locked on to and slightly in front of the superior facet of T1 (d).

Acknowledgements

We wish to thank Alice van der Weyden for typing the manuscript, J. Tinkelenberg for the fine drawings, and M. G. Popkes for the excellent photographs.

References and further reading

ARENDRUP H. C. & SKOV TENSER B. (1982) Traumatic rupture of the diaphragm. *Surg. Gynec. Obstet.* **154**, 526–30.

COLAPINTO V. & MCCALLUM R. W. (1977) Injury to the male posterior urethra in fractured pelvis: a new classification. *J. Urol.* **118**, 575–80.

DAFFNER R. H. (1978) Stress fractures: current concepts. *Skeletal Radiol.* **2**, 221–9.

DOBIJNS H. J., LINSCHEID R. L. & CHAO E. Y. S. (1975) Traumatic instability of the wrist. *A.A.O.S.: Instructional course lectures* **124**, 182–99.

ELSTROM J., PARKOVICH A. M., SASSOON H. & RODRIGUEZ J. (1976) The use of tomography in the assessment of fractures of the tibial plateau. *J. Bone Jt Surg.* **58A**, 551–5.

FORDHAM E. W. & RAMACHANDRAN P. C. (1974) Radionuclide imaging of osseous trauma. *Semin. nucl. Med.* **4**, October.

FRIEBERGER R. H. & KAYE J. J. (1979) *Arthrography*. New York: Appleton–Century–Crofts.

GIESECKE S. B., DALINKA M. K. & CLAYTON KYLE G. (1978) Lisfranc's fracture–dislocation: a manifestation of peripheral neuropathy. *Amer. J. Roentgenol.* **131**, 139–41.

GILULA L. A. & WEEKS P. M. (1978) Post-traumatic ligamentous instabilities of the wrist. *Diagn. Radiol.* **129**, 641–51.

GREEN N. E. & ALLEN B. L. (1977) Vascular injuries with dislocation of the knee. *J. Bone Jt Surg.* **59A**, 236–9.

GREEN D. P. & O'BRIEN E. T. (1980) Classification and management of carpal dislocations. *Clin. Orthop.* **149**, 55–72.

HARLEY J. D., MACK L. A. & WINQUIST R. A. (1982) CT of acetabular fractures: comparison with conventional radiography. *Amer J. Roentgenol.* **138**, 413–17.

HARTY M. (1973) *Orthop. Clin. N. Amer.* **4**, 180.

KARAHARJU E. O. (1983) Blunt abdominal trauma in patients with multiple injuries. *Injury: the British Journal of Accident Surgery* **4**, 307–10.

MILGEAM J. W., ROGERS L. F. & MILLER J. W. (1978) Osteochondral fractures: mechanisms of injury and fate of fragments. *Amer. J. Roentgenol.* **130**, 651–8.

MOORE T. M. & HARVEY J. P. (1974) Roentgenographic measurement of tibial-plateau depression due to fracture. *J. Bone Jt Surg* **56A**, 155–60.

NEER C. S. (1970) Displaced proximal humeral fractures. Part I. Classification and evaluation. *J. Bone Jt Surg.* **52A**, 1077–89.

NORFRAY J. F. *et al.* (1980) Early confirmation of stress fractures in joggers. *J. Amer. med. Ass.* **243**, 1647–9.

O'CARROLL P. F., DOYLE J. & DUFFY G. (1982) Radiography and scintigraphy in the diagnosis of carpal scaphoid fractures. *Irish J. med. Sci.* **151**, 211–13.

PARK W. M., MCCALL I. W., MCSWEENEY T. & JONES B. F. (1980) Cervicodorsal injury presenting as sternal fracture. *Clin. Radiol.* **31**, 49–53.

PRATHER J. L. *et al.* (1977) *J. Bone Jt Surg.* **59A**, 869–74.

PRINGLE R. G. (1983) Missed fractures. *Injury* **4**, 311–16.

SHIRKHODA ALI, BRASHEAR H. R. & STAAN E. V. (1980) Computed tomography of acetabular fractures. *Radiology* **134**, 683–8.

SOLHEIM K. (1983) Closed diaphragmatic rupture. *Injury* **4**, 301–6.

Chapter 8
General Orthopaedic Disease

Z. MATĚJOVSKÝ

Neoplasm

There is hardly another orthopaedic condition in which early and exact diagnosis is of such importance as in bone tumours. A correct and early diagnosis of the character of the lesion, and its benign or malignant nature, is important, particularly for the prognosis, loss or preservation of an extremity, and the survival of the patient. Therefore all the available diagnostic investigations have to be used, and interpreted in conjunction with clinical symptoms, in order to reach the correct diagnosis as soon as possible and start proper treatment without delay. The localization of the lesion in the skeleton and the age of the patient may be helpful in diagnosis. In some patients the true nature of the tumour may be recognized from standard radiographic examination, whilst in other cases special techniques such as tomography, computed tomography, arteriography, lymphography, and scintigraphy may be necessary to specify the extent and character of the disease. Even if the evaluation of clinical symptoms in combination with radiological and other diagnostic techniques will in most cases produce a proper diagnosis, definite confirmation must be obtained from histological examination. In the following discussion of bone tumours note that the classification of the World Health Organization is used (Schajowicz et al. 1972). The extent of this chapter does not allow a full description of the radiological appearance of all the bone tumours in all their variation. For further information references are listed at the end of the chapter.

BENIGN BONE TUMOURS

The orthopaedic surgeon, confronted with a benign bone tumour, will discuss the case with the radiologist in order to define the extent and localization of the lesion, and to confirm its benign character. Therapy, in most cases, will entail complete removal of the tumour, either by curetting or by block excision. The surgical procedure has to achieve safe boundaries, completely removing the affected tissue, but should not be too extensive and unnecessarily impair the function of the extremity.

Osteoid osteoma

Osteoid osteoma is a benign osteoblastic tumour, characterized by a small oval or round mass, usually about 1 cm in diameter, called a nidus. Histologically the nidus consists of highly vascularized cellular tissue with osteoid and immature bone formation. It is frequently found in cortical bone, producing a zone of reactive sclerosis, which surrounds the nidus. Osteoid osteoma arises most often in patients in the first three decades of life. Long bones of extremities are affected most often, but exceptional localizations have been described in almost all parts of the skeleton. The most common symptom is pain, which often disturbs the patient's sleep, and may be relieved by salicylates. The pain is sometimes referred to sites away from the tumour and to adjacent joints. This may mislead the radiologist into taking an X-ray of the wrong part. Therapy consists of excision of the nidus, although it is not necessary to resect the reactive sclerotic zone, which will disappear one or two years after the nidus has been excised.

264

Radiological diagnosis is easy in cases with a clearly visible nidus and surrounding sclerotic bone formation. In plain radiographs, however, the nidus may be indistinguishable, being covered by a thick layer of sclerotic bone (Fig. 8.1). Tomography, and especially computed tomography, is of great importance in these instances. The tissue of the nidus is highly vascularized, which may be demonstrated on arteriography. Because of the thick layer of sclerotic bone special techniques such as subtraction arteriography are often necessary to demonstrate the vascularization of the nidus. Diagnostic problems may arise in localization of osteoid osteoma in cancellous bone, where surrounding bone sclerosis may be less developed. Spinal localizations, because of their rarity, are often difficult to diagnose (Fig. 8.2).

Differential diagnosis. Some forms of chronic or subacute osteomyelitis in bone may present with a similar roentgenographic pattern with bone sclerosis and a centrally rarefied focus. Histologically these lesions should be clearly distinguished.

Benign osteoblastoma
Benign osteoblastoma is a rare tumour; histologically its structure is very similar to that of osteoid osteoma, but usually the lesion is larger in size. Some authors consider the size of these two osteoblastic tumours to be important in establishing the diagnosis, and classify lesions over $1\frac{1}{2}$ cm in diameter as osteoblastomas. A benign osteoblastoma does not show the limited growth potential of osteoid osteoma and patients with aggressive growth of tumour and even malignant change have been reported. Patients in the first three decades of life are affected most often, and the lesion occurs more frequently in the spine than in the bones of the extremities. The tumour is characterized by slow development, the main symptom being pain, which may be due to pressure on adjacent tissues. In the spine, compression of the spinal cord and nerves occurs, resulting sometimes in

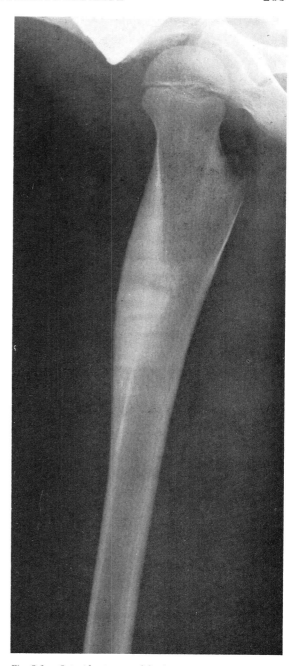

Fig. 8.1. Osteoid osteoma of the femur in a 7-year-old girl. The patient had one year of lasting intermittent pain in the hip, disturbing sleep. The roentgenograph shows extensive cortical thickening; the nidus is covered by newly formed bone and is not clearly visible.

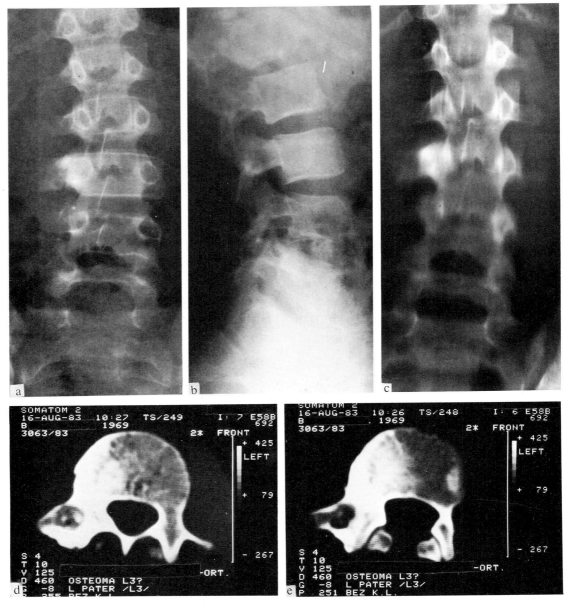

Fig. 8.2. Osteoid osteoma of the third lumbar vertebra in a 14-year-old boy who presented with eight months' duration of pain and developing scoliosis. In the anteroposterior view (a) sclerosis of the lateral part of the vertebral body and transverse process is seen. The findings in the lateral projection (b) are poor. (c) Tomography confirmed the extent of bone sclerosis but did not reveal the nidus. (d and e) Two layers of computed tomography clearly visualize the nidus and the surrounding sclerotic zone in the transverse process and vertebral body.

paraplegia. Therapy consists of complete surgical removal of the tumour. This may be technically difficult in certain situations, such as when the tumour is in the spine or sacrum. If part of the tumour has been left, it usually continues to grow, although favourable results have been reported even after incomplete removal.

The radiological pattern of benign osteoblastoma is not characteristic. Sometimes only a lytic lesion is observed, without the sclerotic bone formation. Other lesions resemble osteoid osteoma with ample surrounding bone sclerosis, but the nidus is larger than in osteoid osteoma. In lesions persisting for a longer period the tumorous tissue becomes ossified. In the spine computed tomography is of greatest help in assessing the extent of the tumour and the degree of spinal cord compression (Fig. 8.3). In arteriography, the unossified part of the tumour usually demonstrates increased vascularity, but without the actual signs of malignancy.

Osteochondroma—osteocartilaginous exostosis

The neoplastic nature of osteochondromas is questionable, but because of rare malignant transformation and some clinical features most authors classify them as benign bone tumours. This most common lesion is formed by enchondral ossification of a proliferating cartilaginous cap. The majority of affected patients are in the second decade of life, and the metaphyses of long bones, especially around the knee, are most often affected. The growth of osteochondromas is usually finished with closure of the epiphyseal plates, and the osteochondroma may persist unchanged for the rest of the patient's life. Small lesions are often asymptomatic and can be diagnosed during radiographic examination for other reasons. On achieving a certain size the swelling becomes evident, and in some areas, such as the upper fibula, the tumour growth may result in compression of adjacent structures. Surgical removal of the tumour brings, in most instances, a definite cure, and recurrences are extremely rare.

Roentgenological diagnosis in most cases is simple, and anteroposterior and lateral radiographs are sufficient for the diagnosis and exact localization of the lesion. In large osteochondromas with compression of the adjacent tissues, further techniques such as arteriography or computed tomography may be helpful in planning the surgical intervention. These investigations are also useful in showing the exact extent of the cartilaginous cap of the tumour, which in plain radiographs is not properly visualized (Fig. 8.4).

Multiple osteocartilaginous exostosis, also denoted as chondrodysplasia, diaphyseal aclasis, or dyschondroplasia, is a hereditary systemic disorder of skeletal development, characterized by two or more lesions histologically and anatomically identical with solitary osteochondromas. In addition, depending on the severity of the disorder, all bones pre-formed in cartilage may show abnormality and sometimes severe deformity. Malignant change in one of the affected bones, usually into chondrosarcoma, is much more frequent than in solitary exostosis. Radiographically it is important to be able to evaluate the early signs of malignant change, such as growth of one of the exostoses, a changing and irregular structure, destruction of the osseous stem, proliferation and calcification of the cartilaginous cap, and invasion of soft tissues.

Chondroma

Chondromas are relatively common tumours, and histologically they are characterized by the formation of mature hyaline cartilage. The occurrence is almost equally divided in all age groups, and most often the short tubular bones of the hands and feet are involved. The lesions are usually located centrally in bones, 'enchondromas', but less frequently juxtacortical or periosteal chondromas are also to be encountered. Chondromas grow slowly, and very often they are asymptomatic, especially in short tubular bones, and then are diagnosed when a pathological fracture occurs. Pain is the most common symptom in large lesions of long bones.

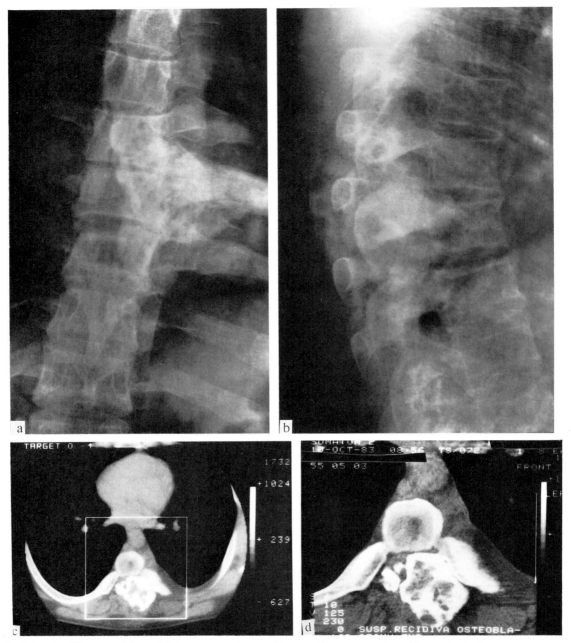

Fig. 8.3. Osteoblastoma of the eighth thoracic vertebra in a 28-year-old man presenting with paraplegia after two years of pain and worsening neurological symptoms. (a) The anteroposterior view shows an osseous mass laterally over the eighth thoracic vertebra. (b) The lateral view shows the tumour involving the spinal canal and protruding dorsally. (c) Whole-body computed tomography at the level of T8 localizes exactly the extent of the tumour. (d) Computed tomography—target area—illustrates in detail the invasion of the spinal canal by tumour and medullary compression.

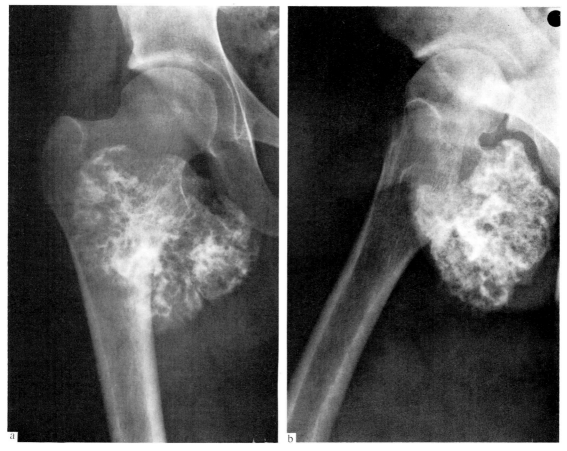

Fig. 8.4. Solitary osteocartilaginous exostosis (osteochondroma) of the proximal femur in a 15-year-old boy who presented with limited movement of the right hip. (a) The anteroposterior view shows the extent of tumour with a typical structure of osteochondroma. (b) The roentgenograph in 80° of external hip rotation illustrates the tumour originating from the posterior aspect of the trochanteric part of the femur. The exact localization of the tumour will advise the surgeon to choose the posterior approach to the hip.

Curetting and bone graft to fill the defect brings a cure in most instances. Incomplete removal of the tumour tissue is the cause of recurrences, which may become evident several years later. Malignant change is rare in short tubular bones of hands and feet, but is more frequent in enchondromas of long bones and the vertebrae, where surgery needs to be more radical.

Roentgenological diagnosis. The most common picture of chondroma is that of a well-circumscribed osteolytic lesion. Different degrees of calcification may be seen, especially in large lesions in long tubular bones and in slowly developing tumours. The overlying cortex may be expanded. A large lesion with destruction of the cortex, soft-tissue invasion, and rapid progression of the tumour are signs of malignant change. Radiographs in two planes are usually sufficient to localize a lesion of the extremity, whilst vertebral column localization by computed tomography is essential. In arteriography, chondromas are avascular, except in cases with destruction of cortex or in cortical localization, when increased vascularization without actual signs of malignancy may be observed (Fig. 8.5).

Multiple enchondromatosis represents a rare inborn, but not hereditary, disorder of skeletal development, characterized by enchondromas affecting at least several bones pre-formed in cartilage. The extent of the disorder is variable; the author has seen patients with two or three lesions, but also with almost general involvement of the skeleton and with severe deformity. Malignant change is estimated to occur in about 30% or more of the patients affected. Radiologically the diagnosis of the disorder is not difficult, but it is essential to evaluate the early radiographic signs of malignant change, as surgery may be curative, or at least substantially prolong the patient's life.

Benign chondroblastoma

Benign chondroblastoma is a rather rare tumour, characterized by highly cellular tissue formed by chondroblast-like cells, with occasional multinucleated giant cells, and by production of intercellular cartilaginous matrix with areas of focal calcification. Young patients in the second and third decade of life are affected most often, and most of the tumours are located in epiphyses of long bones. Pain and impaired function of the adjacent joint are constant symptoms. Curetting and grafting in most cases brings a definite cure, but malignant change has been reported. Roentgenologically the tumour is seen as a lytic lesion in the epi-

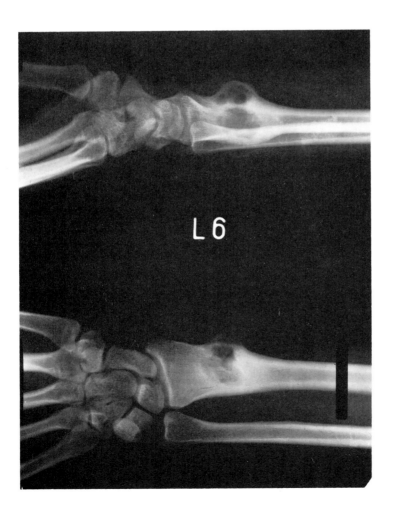

Fig. 8.5. Chondroma localized eccentrically in the radius of a 23-year-old female patient. The roentgenographs show a lytic lesion with borders marked by reactive sclerosis. The extraosseously protruding part of the tumour is covered by a thin layer of newly formed periosteal bone.

physis, usually with a sclerotic rim. During the slow growth of the tumour the intercellular cartilage becomes calcified, manifesting as mottled areas of density. Large chondroblastomas may cause thinning of the cortex and may eventually break through or cause a pathological fracture. In the femoral head deformation and compression may be the result of tumour growth (Fig. 8.6).

In the differential diagnosis, chondromas and chondromyxoid fibromas may be considered, but they rarely affect the epiphysis. Roentgenologically and histologically a clear-cell chondrosarcoma may easily be misinterpreted as benign chondroblastoma, but it usually appears in adult patients. Cystic changes in idiopathic femoral head necrosis may be similar to the picture of a benign chondroblastoma, and the age of the patient is helpful in considering the diagnosis.

Chondromyxoid fibroma
Chondromyxoid fibroma is a very rare benign bone tumour. Histologically it consists of lobules of spindle or stellate cells, producing chondroid and myxoid intercellular matrix. Multinucleated giant cells or large pleomorphic cells may be present, sometimes causing diagnostic confusion with giant cell tumour or chondrosarcoma. The tumour most often affects patients in the second and third decade of life, the most frequent localization being in the diaphyses of long bones, especially of the tibia, but any bone may be affected. Curetting and grafting is usually successful, although some authors advise block excision to avoid possible recurrence. Malignant change is extremely rare.

Roentgenologically the tumour usually appears as an osteolytic, well-circumscribed area, sometimes with a thin sclerotic border, located eccentrically in the bone. Tumours located in small bones may cause expansion of the bone. The tumour may break through the cortex and expand into overlying soft tissue. On arteriography these tumours usually appear avascular, with slightly increased reactive vessel formation, in those with soft-tissue invasion. The tumour is very rare, but it should be always

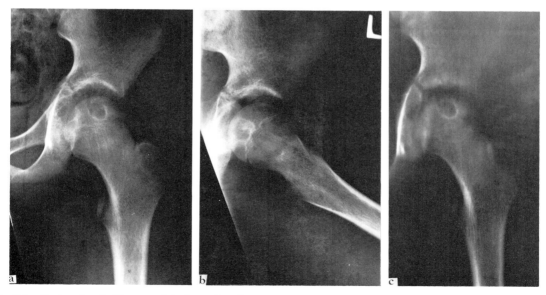

Fig. 8.6. Benign chondroblastoma of the femoral epiphysis in a 10-year-old boy who presented with slight pain and a limp in the left hip. A small osteolytic lesion with distinct partly sclerotic margins involves the femoral epiphysis. (a) The axial view in external rotation and abduction of the hip helps to localize the lesion precisely. (b) Tomographs confirm the exact localization and eventually show the tumour breaking through the articular surface of the femoral head.

considered in the differential diagnosis of benign osteolytic bone tumours, especially as the histological diagnosis may suggest the possibility of other benign tumours and even chondrosarcoma.

Haemangioma

Haemangiomas are benign tumours composed of newly formed vessels of capillary or cavernous type. Some of these lesions are probably malformations and remain stable throughout the patient's life, causing no clinical symptoms. Most vertebral haemangiomas are discovered incidentally during roentgenological investigation of the spine performed for other reasons. Therefore most haemangiomas do not require treatment. Occasionally a lesion may show growth and then surgical intervention may become necessary. Haemangiomas are most often located in the vertebrae and in the cranium, and usually they are found in adults.

Roentgenological features are typical in the vertebrae and skull. The affected vertebral body shows rarefaction of bone with distinct vertical striation or a coarse honeycomb picture. Vertical striation, a 'sun-ray' pattern, is typical in skull lesions. In the extremities, haemangiomas may appear as lytic, sometimes lobulated, areas. Arteriography is positive in most haemangiomas, and may be different in capillary and cavernous types. Subtraction arteriography may be helpful in demonstrating these findings. Arteriography should be undertaken in cases requiring surgery; in asymptomatic cases the typical radiograph is sufficient to establish the diagnosis.

Cases of multiple haemangioma, 'haemangiomatosis', have been described. A rare condition known as massive bone osteolysis, disappearing bone disease, or Gorham's disease is possibly related to haemangiomatosis. It is usually characterized by progressing osteolysis of one or more adjacent bones.

Desmoplastic fibroma

Desmoplastic fibroma is a rare tumour, and histologically it is poorly cellular, the tumour cells forming an abundance of collagen fibres. Age predilection is not clearly specified, even if most patients in the published series are under 30 years of age. Pain, sometimes with functional disability, is the most common symptom. In some patients a pathological fracture may be the first sign of the disease. Because of possible recurrence segmental resection and graft replacement is preferred by most authors.

Radiographically the tumour appears as a radiolucent lesion, which is sometimes trabeculated, though the borders may be well delineated and sometimes sclerotic. Large lesions may break through the cortex. With arteriography the tumour tissue is usually avascular.

Giant-cell tumour of bone

Giant-cell tumour of bone is a locally aggressive tumour, consisting histologically of richly vascularized tissue with spindle-shaped or ovoid stromal cells and numerous multinuclear giant cells. A great majority of these tumours are of a benign character, but exceptionally the development of lung metastases has been described in these otherwise benign tumours. A malignant variant of a giant-cell tumour is extremely rare. It is still under discussion whether it develops primarily as malignant or arises from pre-existing benign giant-cell tumours. Middle-aged patients in the third and fourth decade of life are affected most often; occurrence in young patients before the closure of the epiphyseal plates is very exceptional, and a female preponderance has been reported in most series. The typical localization is in the epiphyses of long bones; about 50% are localized around the knee. The vertebrae are less often affected. Multiple occurrence has been reported, but such cases need to be examined thoroughly for the possibility of a systemic disease, such as hyperparathyroidism. The main symptom is pain, later there is swelling, and treatment, in the first place, is surgical. Some lesions may be cured by thorough curetting and grafting, but because of high incidence of local recurrence most authors recommend resection with either graft or prosthetic replacement. Radiation therapy may be applied for inoperable positions, but the risk of late development of radiation sarcoma seems to be rather high.

Roentgenologically giant-cell tumours appear as osteolytic lesions localized eccentrically in the epiphyses, sometimes expanding the affected bone, with ill-defined margins without any reactive sclerosis. Destruction of cortex and soft-tissue invasion may be found in advanced or recurrent cases. With arteriography most giant-cell tumours show a high degree of vascularization with abundant tumour vessel formation, confluent stain and early venous filling. This picture may easily lead to the mistaken diagnosis of malignancy, although no correlation has been reported between the roentgenological findings and later behaviour of the tumour. Computed tomography is indispensable in localizing the extent of tumours of the vertebrae (Figs. 8.7, 8.8, & 8.9).

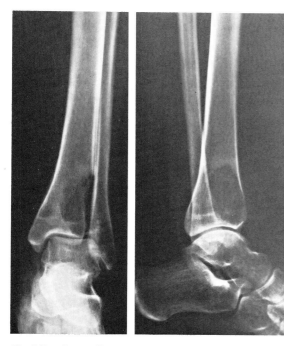

Fig. 8.7. Giant-cell tumour of the distal tibial epiphysis in a 15-year-old girl. A purely osteolytic lesion is located eccentrically. The cortex is destroyed, and the borders towards the medullary cavity are ill-defined.

Differential diagnosis of giant-cell tumour is difficult: historically many other bone conditions containing giant cells and appearing as lytic lesions, such as aneurysmal bone cyst, benign chondroblastoma, chondromyxoid fibroma, fibrous tumours, and the brown tumour of hyperparathyroidism, were classified as giant-cell tumours. At present exact histological, clinical and roentgenological examination should differentiate all these lesions. The clinical and roentgenological diagnosis of early stages of malignancy or malignant change is extremely difficult, and unless clear signs of malignancy are found on histology it is almost impossible to predict the behaviour of the tumour.

MALIGNANT BONE TUMOURS

In malignant bone tumours, diagnostic procedures are more complex, as not only the diagnosis but also the grade and stage of the tumour have to be established (Enneking *et al.* 1980, Lodwick *et al.* 1980). For planning therapy it is necessary to know the grade of malignancy of the tumour, which should be interpreted from both radiological and histological examination, and the extent of the tumour, i.e. whether it is still confined to one anatomical compartment, or has already involved more than one compartment. In assessing the local extent of the tumour, radiographs will show the bone changes, whereas the extraosseal component will be better shown by computed tomography. Even with the use of computed tomography, arteriography brings valuable information about the soft-tissue extent of the tumour and its vascularization, and is one of the essential methods to confirm the malignant state of the lesion. In staging it is essential to look for possible metastases, which in bone tumours most often occur in the lungs, and less often in lymph nodes. A lung radiograph and lung tomography should be performed in every patient with a malignant bone tumour. The use of computed tomography has provided evidence that more patients have lung metastases at the time of diagnosis of the primary tumour than has been reported in older

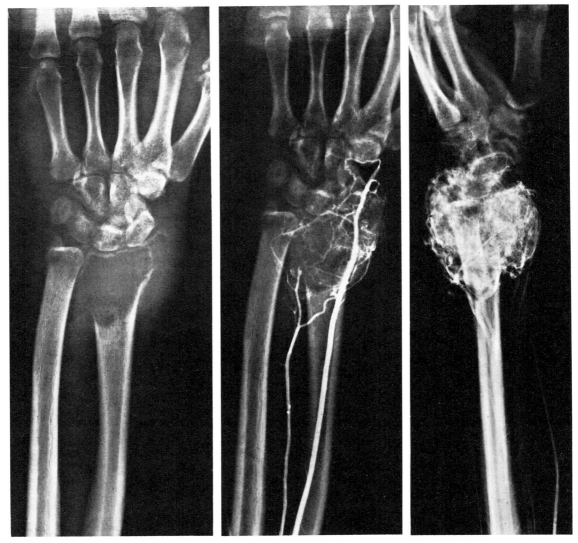

Fig. 8.8.   Giant-cell tumour of the distal radius in a 29-year-old man. The roentgenograph illustrates an osteolytic lesion, breaking through the cortex on both sides. Biplane arteriography clearly shows the soft-tissue extension of the tumour. Intensive new vessel formation and confluent stain are typical of most giant-cell tumours, but are not signs of malignancy. The tumour healed after marginal excision and bone graft and the patient was recurrence-free for five years.

series. Some clinical reports on lymphography and lymphatic scintigraphy have shown that the incidence of lymph node metastases in malignant bone tumours is substantially more frequent than has previously been expected. In some patients with osteosarcoma and Ewing's sarcoma, multifocal skeletal involvement has been reported. Whether this is due to early metastasis to bone, or whether the disease is multifocal from the beginning, is not clear. Therefore, a whole-body scintigram is recommended, to exclude further skeletal involvement, in patients with malignant bone tumours. In recent years complex treatment, including sur-

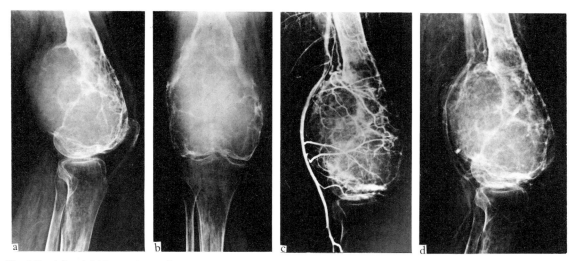

Fig. 8.9. (a) and (b) Large giant-cell tumour in a 36-year-old woman who presented with several years' duration of symptoms, having previously several times refused a proposed amputation. An osteolytic trabeculated lesion expands into the popliteal region with almost complete destruction of cortex, but does not invade the knee joint. The tibia shows clear signs of reactive osteoporosis. (c) In arteriography the arterial phase shows increased vascularization of the tumour with new vessel formation. (d) The late capillary and venous phase shows less intensive stain of the tumour, which after resection was found to be substantially necrotic with cystic degenerative changes.

gery, radiation and chemotherapy, has substantially improved the prognosis in osteosarcoma and Ewing's sarcoma. In patients who are diagnosed early and do not have clinically evident metastases, the percentage of survival has greatly increased, thus underlining the importance of early and exact diagnosis.

Osteosarcoma

Osteosarcoma is the most common malignant bone tumour and histologically it is characterized by direct formation of bone by the tumour cells. Besides this basic quality, the histological pattern shows considerable variation: the degree of osteoid ossification may be variable; and the tumour cells sometimes produce cartilage or fibrous tissue, although some areas may be completely undifferentiated. Osteosarcoma is a tumour of young people, the maximum incidence being in the second decade, and males are more often affected. The metaphyses of long bones are a common site, particularly the distal femur, the proximal tibia and the proximal humerus. The usual, or 'classical', osteosarcoma

arises centrally in the bone and expands and invades surrounding tissue.

The most common symptom is pain, not dependent on stress and present during the night, along with swelling. Formerly the treatment was radical surgery or radiation, or sometimes a combination of both, but this did not bring a substantial improvement in prognosis and 80–90% of patients died from metastases after 2–3 years. The present system of treatment, including radical removal of the primary tumour and adjuvant chemotherapy for elimination of micrometastases, has increased survival to well over 50% of patients. Depending on the degree of osteoid calcification, the radiological picture of osteosarcoma is variable. Completely osteolytic or highly sclerotic tumours may be encountered, but most osteosarcomas exhibit a combination of lytic and sclerotic changes. Ossification may also be present in the soft-tissue component of the tumour, sometimes arranged in spicules, appearing as a 'sunburst pattern'. At the border of the tumour under the elevated periosteum reactive bone production forms the 'Codman's triangle', which although characteristic of osteosarcoma may also be found in other conditions. Almost all osteosarcomas show hypervascularization and signs of malignancy on arteriography. Osteoblastic and undifferentiated zones have a higher degree of vascularization than chondroblastic and well-differentiated parts. The extraosseal component of the tumour and its borders are usually well demonstrated in arteriography (Figs. 8.10, 8.11 & 8.12).

Subtypes of osteosarcoma. The roentgenological differentiation of lytic, sclerotic and mixed types has not been found to influence prognosis. In the same way, no prognostic difference was found between tumours which histologically were predominantly osteoblastic, chondroblastic or fibroblastic. On the other hand, telangiectatic osteosarcoma, characterized by a purely lytic radiological appearance, has an extremely poor prognosis. Osteosarcoma of the jaw has a better prognosis than the common type of this tumour. Many of the osteosarcomas arising in later age are secondary to pre-existing lesions, such as Paget's disease, or originate in irradiated bones as radiation sarcomas. Juxtacortical osteosarcoma is another variant originating on the external surface of bone. Histologically it shows a high degree of differentiation. The growth of this tumour is much slower, the tendency to form metastases is much less expressed and the prognosis is substantially better than in the usual osteosarcoma. In these patients radical surgical removal is considered adequate

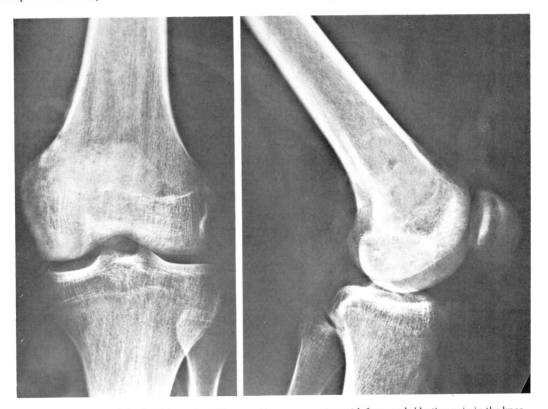

Fig. 8.10. Osteosarcoma of the distal femur in a 22-year-old man presenting with four weeks' lasting pain in the knee. The roentgenographs show an exceptionally early stage of the tumour. A slight periosteal elevation and a small soft-tissue extension of the tumour are the only signs seen over the medial aspect of the metaphysis. In addition, on close examination compared to the other side of the metaphysis some slight destruction of the regular pattern of bony trabeculae can be seen.

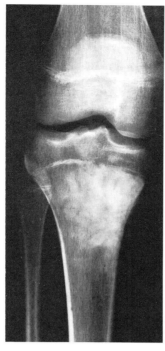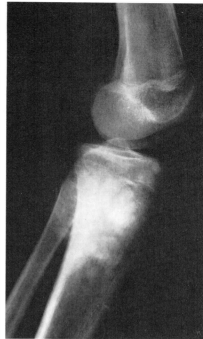

Fig. 8.11. Osteosarcoma of the proximal tibial metaphysis in a 16-year-old girl, with prevalent sclerotic changes, minimal periosteal reaction and no soft-tissue invasion, which was proved in arteriography. Such findings, similar to those in Fig. 8.10, suggest the possibility of a limb-saving operation.

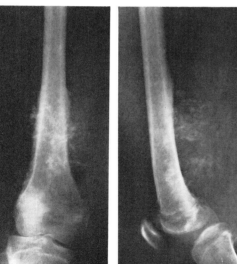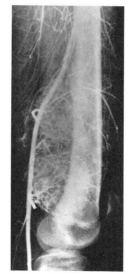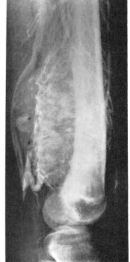

Fig. 8.12a. Large osteosarcoma of the distal femur in a 14-year-old girl. Anteroposterior and lateral roentgenographs show an extensive extraosseal component of the tumour with tumorous bone formation in soft tissue.

Fig. 8.12b. Lateral views of arteriography show typical signs of malignancy with new vessel formation, intensive blush of tumorous tissue and accelerated venous return. Note that in the venous phase there is compression of the popliteal vein by tumour nodules which is not seen in the arterial phase. Because of the close vicinity of the tumour and vessels the arteriography clearly indicates the necessity of amputation.

treatment. Some authors differentiate a parosseal and periosteal form of juxtacortical osteosarcoma. Roentgenologically osseous tissue localized on the surface of bone is typical. As these tumours show a tendency to encircle the shaft of the affected bone, tomography and especially computed tomography is essential to prove the absence of medullary involvement (Fig. 8.13).

Differential diagnosis. Several lesions may be misinterpreted as osteosarcoma, usually with drastic consequences if subjected to radical surgery. Among these are abundant callus formation, especially in stress fractures, and benign osteoblastoma. Some large proliferating osteo-

chondromas and myositis ossificans may be misdiagnosed as juxtacortical osteosarcoma. Even haematogenous osteomyelitis in certain stages may be difficult to distinguish. Occasionally even histology can be confusing.

Chondrosarcoma

Chondrosarcoma is a malignant bone tumour in which tumour cells produce cartilage. In contrast to benign chondroma the tumour tissue is more cellular and pleomorphic, the tumour cells having large, irregular or double nuclei. The histological differentiation of early signs of malignancy in cartilaginous tumours may be difficult. Chondrosarcoma is a tumour of middle age

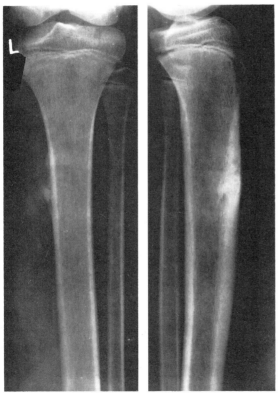

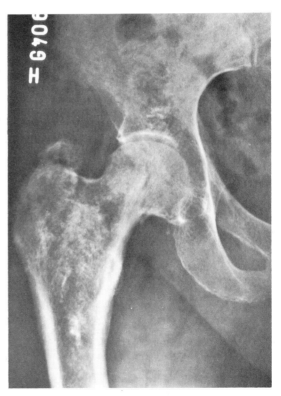

Fig. 8.13. Periosteal osteosarcoma of the tibia in a 13-year-old boy, who presented with two months' lasting pain and swelling under the knee. The anteroposterior roentgenographs show periosteal elevation (Codman's triangle). On the lateral view there is increased density in the anterior aspect of the tibia. Resection and graft replacement was performed with lasting favourable result.

Fig. 8.14. Chondrosarcoma of the proximal femur in a 68-year-old woman. The lesion appears partly osteolytic, extending from the trochanteric part into the neck and diaphysis, and partly formed by coarse granular calcifications. The cortex is minimally destroyed except for the greater trochanter. An excision with safe margins and prosthetic replacement resulting in eight years' recurrence-free survival was performed.

and is rare below the age of 20 years. The pelvis, the femur and the humerus are the most frequent sites. Most of these tumours grow slowly, swelling, pain and sometimes even a pathological fracture being the main symptoms. Radical surgical removal of the tumour may be curative in around 50% of patients, and the extent of surgery should be dependent on the grade and stage of the tumour. Tumours of low-grade malignancy without cortical destruction may be cured in over 90%. On the other hand, high-grade malignant chondrosarcomas with soft-tissue involvement have a survival rate of some 20–30%. Perforation of the tumour during surgery almost always results in later development of local recurrence from implantation metastases.

Chondrosarcomas are usually subclassified in to primary and secondary types. The radiographic appearance of a primary chondrosarcoma is very often of diagnostic importance, and is characterized by bone destruction combined with mottled sclerotic changes, representing areas of calcification or ossification. Cortical destruction is an important prognostic factor and is decisive for planning the extent of the surgery. Soft tissue involvement will best be visualized by computed tomography (Figs. 8.14 & 8.15).

With arteriography most chondrosarcomas show a low degree of vascularity, but occasionally in tumours of high malignancy angiographic features of highly vascularized malignant tumours are present. Secondary chon-

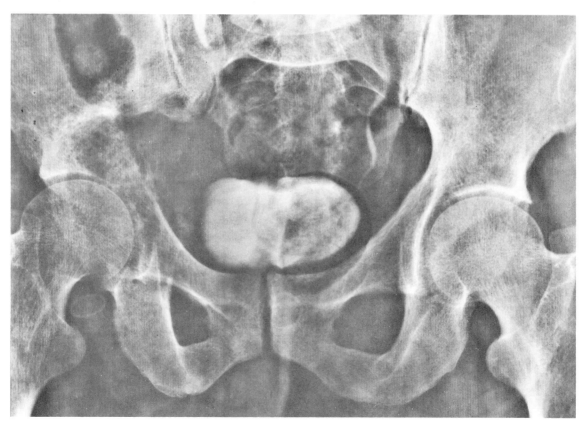

Fig. 8.15. Chondrosarcoma of the right ilium in a 52-year-old man. The lesion appears to be predominantly osteolytic, with some border sclerosis in the ilium. Cystography is helpful in establishing the soft-tissue extension of pelvic tumours. Urinary bladder compression or displacement is an important sign in evaluating the operability of the tumour.

drosarcomas originate in pre-existing benign cartilaginous lesions, such as osteochondromas, solitary or multiple, chondromas, solitary or multiple, synovial chondromatosis and others. The radiographic diagnosis of malignant change is difficult but extremely important. Every change in structure, i.e. signs of growth, or especially bone destruction, should be carefully evaluated (Fig. 8.16). Juxtacortical chondrosarcoma is a variant arising from the external surface of the bone, characterized by well-differentiated tumour cells and areas of ossification and calcification. A highly malignant variant is the mesenchymal chondrosarcoma, which appears radiographically as a lytic lesion with areas of calcification. On the other hand, clear-cell chondrosarcoma is characterized by a favourable prognosis, is most often localized at the end of a long bone, and appears as a lytic lesion, sometimes with sharp sclerotic margins.

Fibrosarcoma of bone

Fibrosarcoma of bone is a rare malignant bone tumour, formed histologically by spindle-shaped cells which produce variable amounts of collagen. There is no special age or sex prevalence, and localization is similar to that of osteosarcoma. Radical surgery is the preferred treatment. Radiographically it appears as a lytic lesion with various degrees of bone destruction. Computed tomography is essential for investigating the soft-tissue involvement. The arteriographic picture varies according to the degree of malignancy and extent of the tumour.

Malignant fibrous histiocytoma

The tumour of histiocytic origin has been recognized only in recent years, some tumours formerly classified as fibrosarcomas, osteosarcomas or undifferentiated sarcomas being reclassified into this new entity. Reported series

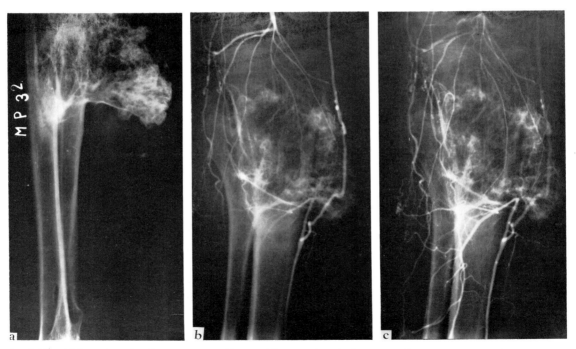

Fig. 8.16. (a) Secondary chondrosarcoma in a 18-year-old man with multiple osteocartilaginous exostoses, who complained of gradual enlargement of a proximal tibia exostosis during the last six months. The lateral roentgenograph shows a large exostosis protruding dorsally. (b) and (c) Arteriography shows complete occlusion of the popliteal artery with well-developed collateral circulation. Arteriography provides the surgeon with important information, showing the possibility of tumour removal with safe margins, the occluded artery and vein being included in the resection specimen.

are not yet numerous, and there seems to be no special age predilection, but long bones are affected more often. The tumour should be removed by radical surgery. Radiographically the tumours are osteolytic, with ill-defined borders, and destruction of cortex and soft-tissue invasion are usual. The diagnosis of a malignant tumour may be ascertained, but further differentiation is hardly possible (Fig. 8.17).

Ewing's sarcoma

Ewing's sarcoma is a tumour arising from the bone marrow, histologically characterized by solidly packed, small and rather uniform cells with round nuclei. Patients in the first three decades of life are affected most often, and maximum occurrence is in the second decade. All bones and every part of each bone may be affected, the most frequent localization being in the femur and in the pelvic girdle. Pain is usually the first symptom, followed by swelling. Some patients have an elevated temperature, an increased erythrocyte sedimentation rate and anaemia, and leucocytosis may be encountered. Ewing's sarcoma was considered to be the most lethal of bone tumours and neither surgery nor radiation has improved the poor prognosis. Recently, systemic chemotherapy in combination with surgery and radiation has increased the survival rate to over 60% in some of the reported series. Radiological features are variable. Osteolytic changes are most common, but areas of reactive bone formation may be found. The gradual elevation of the periosteum by tumour growth produces layers of reactive bone, called 'onion-skin' periosteal appositions, which are considered to be pathognomonic of Ewing's tumour. In the author's experience, other conditions, such as haematogenous osteomyelitis, eosinophilic granuloma and other bone lesions, may manifest in the same way. The soft-tissue extension of the tumour, which is present in a majority of patients at the time of diagnosis, can be visualized by computed tomography or arteriography. Most Ewing's sarcomas with soft-tissue extension show a high degree of vascularization with signs of malignancy, but occasionally large tumours may be partly necrotic, and in these areas arteriographic findings are negative. Computed tomography, arteriography and eventually lymphography may be helpful in assessing the effect of therapy (Figs. 8.18, 8.19 & 8.20). Differential diagnosis is difficult and almost impossible from plain roentgenographs. Haematogenous osteomyelitis may present with very similar clinical, laboratory and roentgenographic findings. Eosinophilic granuloma, malignant lymphoma, metastases of childhood tumours of organs and soft tissues, and even osteosarcoma may present with similar pictures. Arteriography helps in many cases to establish the malignancy of the

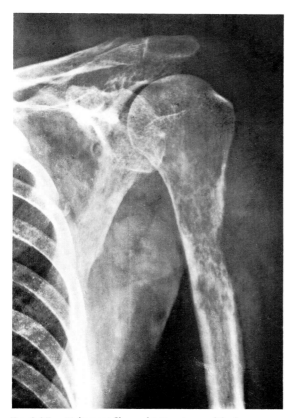

Fig. 8.17. Malignant fibrous histiocytoma of the humerus in a 65-year-old man who presented with pain and swelling of his left arm. The roentgenograph illustrates an osteolytic lesion with cortex destruction. The multiple areas of bone destruction give a mottled appearance.

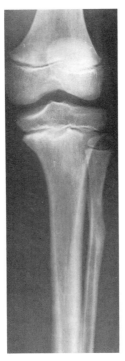
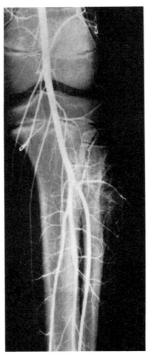
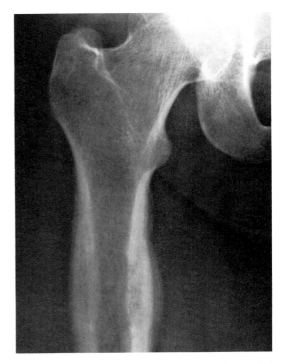

Fig. 8.18. Ewing's sarcoma of the fibula in an 11-year-old boy, presenting with two months' lasting symptoms of pain under the knee. The anteroposterior roentgenograph shows minimal changes of bone structure, except for a cortical erosion from the lateral side and periosteal apposition from the medial side of the affected upper fibula. Arteriography illustrates the soft-tissue extension of the tumour. The formation of new irregular vessels suggests malignancy.

Fig. 8.19. Ewing's sarcoma of the femur in a 19-year-old girl, who had several months' lasting pain in the right hip. The tumour was still localized intraossally. The roentgenograph shows a lytic lesion extending from the medullary cavity and eroding the cortex. 'Onion-skin' periosteal bone formation is visible.

lesion. In all suspicious cases histology should be performed: treating Ewing's sarcoma on the basis of radiological diagnosis only is not justified.

Malignant lymphoma of bone
The classification of neoplasms of the reticuloendothelial system is still developing. Some varieties of malignant lymphomas may be primarily localized in bone; most of these were formerly classified as reticulum cell sarcomas. There seems to be no special age or localization predilection in these tumours. Most malignant lymphomas are sensitive to radiation and chemotherapy; surgery is indicated in solitary lesions and may become necessary in lesions of

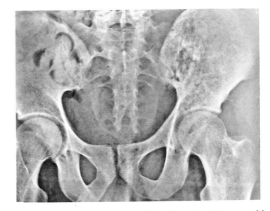

Fig. 8.20a. Ewing's sarcoma of the ilium in a 20-year-old man presenting with symptoms of slight pain in the lumbosacral region of one year duration. Finally a swelling developing over the iliac crest was the reason for medical examination. The roentgenograph illustrates mixed lytic and sclerotic changes in the ilium.

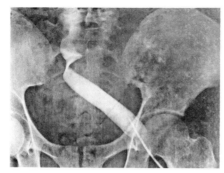

Fig. 8.20b. Because of impaired venous return of the left lower extremity, venography was performed, showing displacement, dilatation and compression of the left iliac vein.

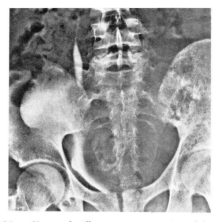

Fig. 8.20e. Urography illustrates compression of the right ureter and displacement of the urinary bladder.

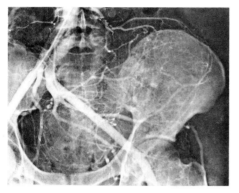

Fig. 8.20c. Arteriography shows extensive displacement of the iliac arteries, illustrating the large intrapelvic extent of the tumour. Note the increased diameter of the left lumbar and internal iliac artery, supplying the tumour.

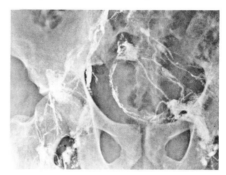

Fig. 8.20f. Lymphography shows displacement of the pelvic lymphatic vessels and enlarged lymph nodes, suggestive of metastatic involvement. The combination of the above-mentioned radiological examinations is extremely helpful in assessing the extent of involvement and operability of pelvic tumours.

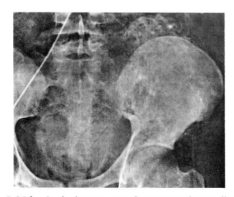

Fig. 8.20d. In the later stages of arteriography capillary blush of low intensity was found only in the periphery of the tumour, as most of the large tumour mass was necrotic.

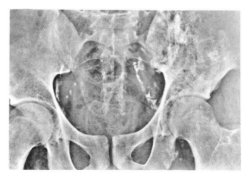

Fig. 8.20g. The persisting blush of lymph nodes is useful in evaluation of treatment. Six months later, following irradiation and chemotherapy, the position of left iliac lymph nodes testifies to a substantial reduction of tumour size.

the extremity with extensive bone destruction
and soft-tissue involvement. Prognosis is considered better than in Ewing's sarcoma, for
about 50% of patients survive five years, even
if some of them relapse and succumb later.

Roentgenologically, malignant lymphoma in
bone is characterized by small areas of osteolytic
changes, giving a mottled appearance of bone.
Later these become confluent and the tumour
destroys the cortex and invades the soft tissue.
In order to plan treatment the radiologist has to
assess the stage of the disease, and the involvement of other systems, especially of the lymph
nodes. Lymphography is essential in the staging
of malignant lymphoma, and scintigraphy provides information about multiple skeletal involvement. The roentgenological picture of
malignant lymphoma in bone is not typical, and
differential diagnosis from other malignant bone
tumours such as Ewing's sarcoma, myeloma,
metastatic carcinoma and even osteomyelitis is
hardly possible.

Myeloma

Myeloma is the most common malignant bone
tumour, and usually presents with multiple or
diffuse bone involvement, and the presence of
abnormal protein in the blood and urine. Occasionally solitary myeloma without abnormal
laboratory findings may occur. Histologically
the tumour is formed by plasma cells with varying degrees of immaturity. Myeloma rarely
affects patients under 50 years of age. Although
any bone may be involved, localization is most
frequent in the spine, ribs, skull and pelvis. In
generalized disease the main treatment consists
of systemic chemotherapy, although irradiation
may be helpful in achieving remissions of some
foci. Surgery is indicated only in exceptional solitary bone involvement, or as palliative treatment of frequent pathological fractures (Fig.
8.21).

Roentgenologically, numerous round and
oval, osteolytic 'punched out' lesions are typical
of multiple myeloma. The involvement of the
skull is almost pathognomonic in developed disease. Vertebral localizations often manifest as

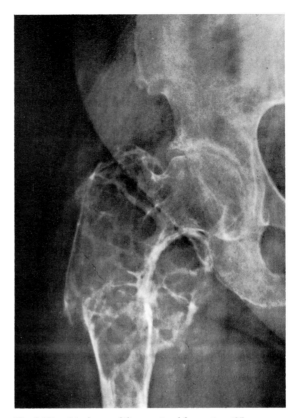

Fig. 8.21.   Myeloma of the proximal femur in a 65-year-
old female patient complaining of pain and instability of
the right hip. At the time of diagnosis the femoral lesion
appeared to be solitary; two years later the disease became
generalized. The roentgenograph shows a lytic, expanding
and trabeculated lesion with a pathological fracture. The
tumour was resected and replaced by a special long-stem
prosthesis.

pathological fractures with compression of vertebral bodies. Exceptionally, myelomas producing bone sclerosis have been described. Periosteal bone formation and sclerosis of a lesion
may appear as a result of radiation and chemotherapy. The differential diagnosis in developed
disease with multiple bone involvement and positive laboratory findings causes little difficulty;
in solitary lesions only biopsy will confirm the
diagnosis.

Adamantinoma

Adamantinoma of long bones is a rare slowly
growing tumour, usually of low malignancy

and uncertain histogenesis. Most reported cases are localized in the shaft of tibia. Segmental resection is the treatment of choice, but some authors advocate amputation because of possible recurrence and metastases. The roentgenological appearance is characterized by multilocular osteolytic defects, expanding the affected bone. The defects are well-delineated, and the borders sclerotic, forming a trabeculated pattern (Fig. 8.22).

Chordoma

Chordoma is another rare tumour of low malignancy, arising from notochordal remnants. The two most frequent sites are in the sacrococcygeal and spheno-occipital region; the tumour rarely occurs below the age of 30 years. Because of the localization, radical surgery in most cases is impossible. Exceptionally small sacral tumours may be totally resected, but even partial removal may sometimes prolong the patient's life. Positive effects of radiation therapy have been reported in some cases. Roentgenologically, sacral tumours are characterized by irregular bone destruction; occasionally calcification may be seen in the tumour area. A soft-tissue mass extending anteriorly can be visualized by computed tomography. In spheno-occipital sites some degree of bone destruction is evident on radiographs, but the exact extent of the lesion will best be determined by cranial arteriography and computed tomography (Fig. 8.23).

TUMOUR-LIKE LESIONS OF BONE

The group of tumour-like lesions of bone includes several conditions which show clinical, radiological and sometimes even histological similarity to bone tumours. These lesions should always be considered in differential diagnosis, because they are characterized by a favourable prognosis and usually do not require radical surgical treatment.

Juvenile bone cyst

The juvenile bone cyst, also called unicameral, is a lesion of unknown origin affecting children and adolescents. The most frequent localization is in the metaphyses of long bones, especially of the proximal humerus and proximal femur. Very often these cysts develop asymptomatically and are diagnosed when a pathological fracture occurs. Although spontaneous healing following fracture has been described, curetting and filling the defect with a bone graft is the treatment of choice. Recently positive results from conservative treatment by intralesional injection of corticosteroids have been reported.

Roentgenologically, the cysts appear as central lytic lesions of bone, expanding and thinning the cortex. In some cysts reactive formation of bony trabeculae produces a multilocular pattern. Arteriography does not demonstrate an increased vascularity.

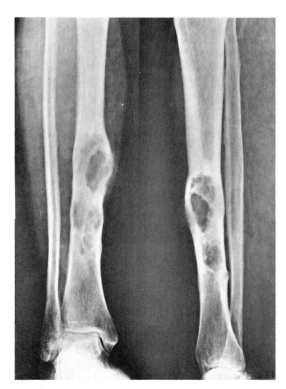

Fig. 8.22. Adamantinoma of the tibia in a 67-year-old woman. The biplane roentgenographs show a multiloculated lytic lesion, partly expanding and thinning the cortex. Segmental resection, bone graft replacement and osteosynthesis were performed.

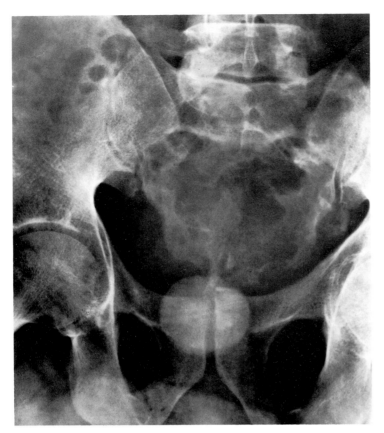

Fig. 8.23. Chordoma of the sacrum in a 58-year-old man. The roentgenograph shows a lytic lesion with ill-defined margins involving all sacral segments. Because of the extent of involvement radical surgical treatment was not possible.

Aneurysmal bone cyst

The aneurysmal cyst is an osteolytic lesion of bone, usually affecting patients under 30 years of age, involving all parts of the skeleton, with a predilection for the shafts of long bones and the vertebral column. The cysts consist of blood-filled spaces surrounded by soft tissue, which on histology appear very similar to the structure of a giant-cell tumour of bone. Surgical treatment is successful in most cases, even if recurrences occur.

Roentgenologically, an eccentric, or less often central, lytic lesion is seen, expanding the affected bone and sometimes even extending into soft tissue. Septa and ridges producing a trabeculated pattern are often present. The extraosseal expansion is covered by newly formed periosteal bone. With arteriography aneurysmal

cysts usually show increased vascularity due to the blood-filled spaces (Fig. 8.24).

Metaphyseal fibrous cortical defect

This lesion of uncertain origin, also called non-ossifying fibroma or fibrous xanthoma, is mostly found in growing children and adolescents. Very often it is asymptomatic and is detected in radiological examination for another reason. It may disappear spontaneously after some months or years; exceptionally progression leading to pathological fracture may occur. Small lesions do not require surgical intervention. In cases of progression curetting and filling with bone graft is the treatment of choice.

The roentgenological findings are characteristic and diagnostic. An osteolytic, sometimes trabeculated, lesion with distinct sclerotic bor-

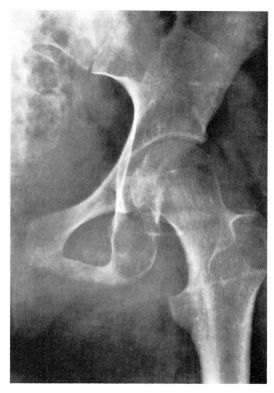

Fig. 8.24. Aneurysmal bone cyst of the ischial bone in a 15-year-old girl presenting with slight pain in the left hip. A lytic lesion with thinned cortex and well-delineated margins involves the whole circumference of the affected bone. Arteriography was negative except for a slight blush in the capillary phase. The lesion was healed after curetting and grafting.

ders is located eccentrically in the metaphysis of a long bone.

Eosinophilic granuloma

Eosinophilic granuloma may occur as solitary or multiple bone involvement. Lichtenstein (1972) considers them to be a stage of histiocytosis X, which is a common denominator for different types of reticuloendothelioses. The foci of eosinophilic granuloma are histologically and radiologically identical whether they occur singly or multiply, or as part of Letterer–Siwe or Hand–Schüller–Christian disease. Any part of the skeleton may be affected.

Spontaneous regression of eosinophilic granuloma is possible. Intralesional or systemic corticosteroid treatment accelerates the healing; low-dose radiation is recommended for inaccessible localizations. In biopsied lesions curetting and filling with bone graft results in cure.

Radiographically, eosinophilic granulomas appear as osteolytic, 'punched out', round and oval lesions of different size, without peripheral sclerosis; sometimes a periosteal reaction may be evident. Vertebral body localization is probably responsible for the compression of vertebral bodies in young patients.

Myositis ossificans

Ossification of muscles may occur as a systemic disease or as a localized defect. Localized types, arising either following trauma of the muscle or spontaneously (idiopathic or pseudomalignant myositis ossificans), should be considered in the differential diagnosis with osteosarcoma. The pseudomalignant type usually starts with painful swelling of the affected muscle, with negative radiological findings. A few weeks later fast-developing ossification and periosteal reaction of the adjacent bone are visualized (Fig. 8.25).

'Brown tumour' of hyperparathyroidism

In about one-third of patients with hyperparathyroidism there are changes in the skeleton. Subperiosteal resorption of the middle phalanges of the hands is a constant sign, followed by general skeletal demineralization. Solitary or multiple lytic lesions of bone, 'brown tumours', may be present. Histologically and roentgenologically they may be very similar to giant-cell tumours of bone. Localization outside the epiphyses of long bones, negative arteriographic findings, and especially laboratory findings of a raised serum calcium, will be helpful in differential diagnosis (Fig. 8.26).

Fibrous dysplasia

Fibrous dysplasia may show solitary or multiple skeletal involvement. Histologically both types are identical: the affected bone is destroyed and

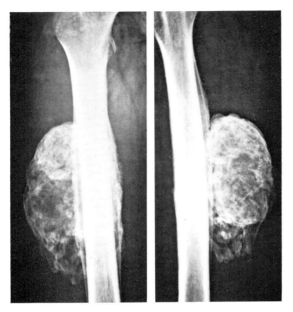

Fig. 8.25a. Pseudomalignant myositis ossificans of femoral muscles in a 12-year-old boy. First roentgenographs taken one week after beginning of symptoms of pain in the thigh and elevated temperature, without a history of trauma, did not reveal any changes. The pictures taken five weeks after the beginning of symptoms show an extraosseal, oval calcified mass adjacent to the femur, with a distinct periosteal reaction.

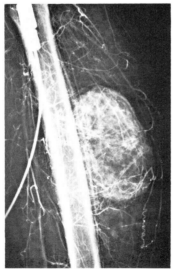

Fig. 8.25b. The later arterial phase of arteriography shows increased vascularity with new vessel formation, but without clear signs of malignancy. A marginal excision was performed, resulting in a permanent cure.

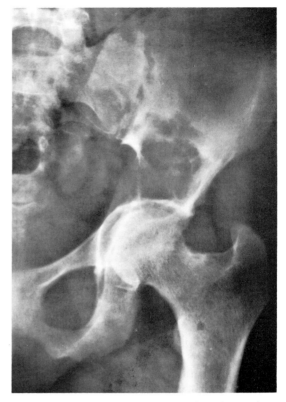

Fig. 8.26. Brown tumour of hyperparathyroidism in the ilium of a 20-year-old woman who was admitted because of a suspected malignant tumour. Laboratory and other radiological examinations helped to establish the diagnosis, and a parathyroid adenoma was surgically removed. The roentgenograph shows a lytic lesion with ill-defined margins and destruction of the inner cortex. After removal of the adenoma the pelvic lesion was curetted, filled with bone graft, and healed without complications.

replaced by fibrous connective tissue. Roentgenological features are variable, depending on the size and localization of the lesion. Small lesions appear as lytic well-delineated foci, and larger ones with secondary bone formation in the fibrous tissue show a ground-glass appearance. Extensive involvement of entire bones, often seen in polyostotic forms, causes severe deformity of the affected bone, which is enlarged by confluent osteolytic foci. In these cases the bone bends, and pathological fractures are frequent. Treatment is difficult and the bones often heal with severe deformity.

METASTATIC TUMOURS OF BONE

Metastatic tumours are certainly the most common form of malignant disease affecting the skeleton. Any malignant tumorous disease may form skeletal metastases, which may involve the skeleton before the primary tumour is diagnosed. In children such conditions are rare, but the author has seen early skeletal metastases from neuroblastoma and other childhood tumours which were considered to be primary bone tumours. In old age the most frequent malignancies in bone are metastatic carcinomas. Roentgenologically, the majority are characterized by bone destruction, with variable osteolytic changes, and usually without distinct borders. Some, such as prostatic carcinoma metastases, may be distinctly sclerotic. The differentiation of individual metastasis types from roentgenographs is hardly possible. Using arteriography, most skeletal metastases show a vascularization typical of the primary tumour. In the author's experience the highest degree of vascularization was found in skeletal metastases of hypernephroma, followed by thyroid and bronchogenic carcinoma, whereas prostatic carcinoma metastases exhibited no increased vascularization. Solitary or multiple metastatic skeletal involvement is best demonstrated with scintigraphy, which will show lesions not yet visible on radiographs. In adult patients with suspected malignant bone lesions, the possibility of metastases should be always considered, and possible primary sites of tumour such as lungs, kidneys, breast, prostate and other organs should be examined.

SOFT-TISSUE TUMOURS

A great variety of both benign and malignant soft-tissue tumours may affect the musculoskeletal system. Whereas plain roentgenographs show only secondary skeletal changes caused by soft-tissue tumours developing in joints or in the vicinity of bone, arteriography and computed tomography are indispensable in evaluating the character and extent of these tumours (Figs. 8.27 & 8.28).

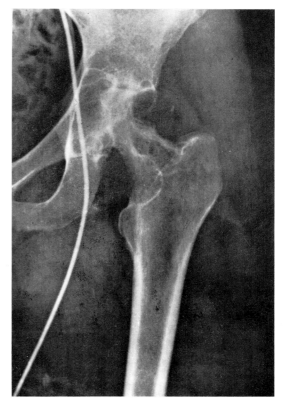

Fig. 8.27. Pigmented villonodular synovitis affecting the hip joint of a 48-year-old woman. Deep erosions of both the femoral head and acetabulum may be seen in roentgenograph. The hip was resected because of severe damage of the joint cartilage and replaced by a total hip prosthesis.

Infection of bone

Infection of bone, or osteomyelitis, may be caused by various organisms, the most frequent being staphylococcus and streptococcus. Even though the use of antibiotics has diminished the occurrence of this disease, cases are still encountered. A bone may be infected through external wounds from injuries, or even occur as complication of surgery. A clear case history and clinical symptoms seldom cause diagnostic difficulties. More problematical is the diagnosis of blood-borne osteomyelitis, in which the initial symptoms and the roentgenological picture can be very similar to those of a neoplastic bone

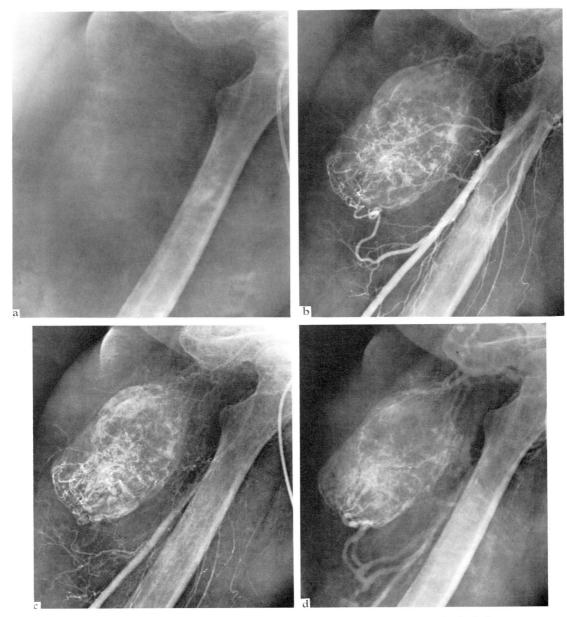

Fig. 8.28. (a) Soft-tissue sarcoma of the thigh in a 56-year-old woman. In plain roentogenographs the findings are negative. (b) The arterial phase of arteriography shows increased vascularization of the tumour with formation of pathological vessels, which are irregular in their course and calibre. (c) The late arterial and capillary phases show blood pools, arteriovenous shunts and distinct blush of tumour, which except for the proximal pole shows well-delineated borders. (d) The venous phase demonstrates large abnormal draining veins on both poles of the tumour, a proof of accelerated arteriovenous flow caused mainly by arteriovenous shunts. Signs of malignancy are present in all phases of arteriography. Although a wide excision was performed, the patient soon died of distant metastases.

disease. In haematogenous osteomyelitis, often occurring in children and adolescents, first radiological change usually shows some 10 days after the onset of symptoms. The metaphyses are the primary site in most cases, but any part of bone may be affected. The cartilaginous epiphyseal plates form a barrier and therefore joint involvement is rare, in contrast to tuberculosis, in which arthritis is more common than osteitis. Small cancellous bone abscesses form well-delineated osteolytic foci, which later become confluent. Periosteal reaction is another early radiological sign, and may be indistinguishable from that seen in malignant tumours of bone. The differential diagnosis between Ewing's sarcoma and haematogenous osteomyelitis is extremely difficult in some cases: plain radiographs are inconclusive and further diagnostic procedures have to be applied. Ongoing infection of bone may cause bone necrosis and sequestrum formation. The sequestrum should be surgically removed, therefore its radiological identification and exact localization is an important guide for the orthopaedic surgeon. Sometimes the sequestrum is surrounded by sclerotic bone formation, and tomography or computed tomography will be helpful in visualizing its exact extent (Figs. 8.29 & 8.30).

Chronic osteomyelitis of long duration may result in bizarre roentgenological pictures, based on mixed lytic and sclerotic changes, which reflect simultaneously both the ongoing infection and the reparative process. Especially difficult is the diagnosis of osteomyelitis affecting the spine. Destruction of bone, sometimes with surrounding sclerosis, will eventually result in

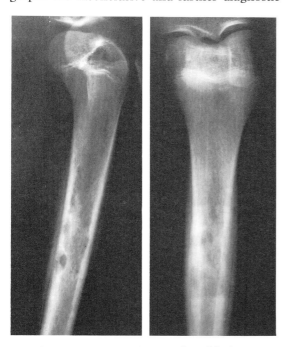

Fig. 8.29. Haematogenous osteomyelitis of the femur in a 14-year-old girl, who three weeks after follicular tonsillitis started to complain of pain above the knee. Several small lytic areas in the medullary cavity, partly eroding the cortex, are seen in the femoral diaphysis. 'Onion-skin' periosteal appositions are indistinguishable from those in a malignant bone tumour. Arteriography was negative, and no increased vascularization or signs of malignancy were found.

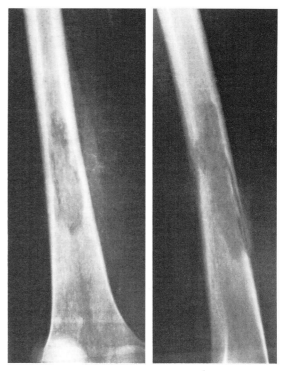

Fig. 8.30. Haematogenous osteomyelitis of femur in a 19-year-old girl following an infectious disease with high temperature. A large confluent lytic lesion involving the medullary cavity and partly destroying the cortex is seen in the femoral shaft, with periosteal bone formation not arranged in layers shown in the anteroposterior view.

compression fractures of the vertebral bodies, and this is difficult to differentiate from tumour involvement. A paraspinal soft-tissue mass may represent an abscess formation, but neoplastic soft-tissue invasion may present a very similar picture.

Skeletal tuberculosis

Skeletal tuberculosis has become a rare disease in Europe and North America, but is still common in many countries with insufficient health care and a low standard of nutrition. Osseous lesions most often affect vertebral bodies (Pott's disease). They have a destructive character, and occasionally reactive bone may be formed. Large paraspinal abscesses with eventual secondary calcification are typical. Joint tuberculosis is second in frequency, and the hip and knee joints are the sites of predilection.

Miscellaneous

PAGET'S DISEASE

The pathogenesis of this skeletal disorder, also called osteitis deformans, is still entirely unknown. It has a remarkable racial and geographical incidence, and males are more often affected. Histologically, bone destruction followed by new bone formation is characteristic, providing a 'mosaic' structure. The newly formed bone is arranged in a different pattern, which is usually less strong and is the reason for bone bending and for the occurrence of pathological fractures. The extent of the disease varies from a single bone to an almost complete skeletal involvement. Pelvis, spine, long bones and the skull are the most frequent localizations, but any bone may be affected. The disease is sometimes diagnosed incidentally; in some cases pain or deformation is the reason for roentgenological examination. In advanced stages of Paget's disease complications such as pathological fractures, protrusio acetabuli, neurological symptoms due to skull or vertebral involvement, and even sarcomatous transformation may occur.

Radiographically, three stages can be distinguished. In the first, mostly lytic changes within areas of bone destruction are seen. The second stage is characterized by new bone formation, which obliterates the demarcation of the cortex and cancellous bone and increases the size of the bone. In the third stage, new bone formation causes a diffuse increase in bone density within the enlarged bone. All three stages may be evident in one patient and even in one bone. The early stages of malignant changes are difficult to diagnose, and the prognosis for sarcoma arising in Paget's disease is very poor. A marked increase of the serum alkaline phosphatase level is a leading symptom in Paget's disease and is of diagnostic value in differentiating it from skeletal involvement in prostatic cancer (Figs. 8.31 & 8.32).

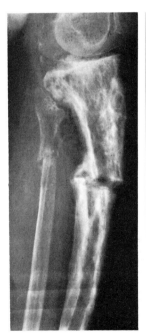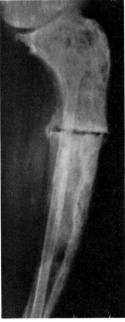

Fig. 8.31.   Paget's disease of tibia in a 78-year-old woman suffering for two years from progressive leg deformity. The roentgenographs show a mixed phase of Paget's disease, with lytic changes next to new bone formation. The demarcation of cortex and medullary bone is obliterated, and the affected bone is enlarged. A pathological fracture is one of the frequent complications of Paget's disease.

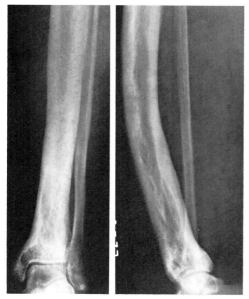

Fig. 8.32a. Monostotic Paget's disease of the distal tibia in a 62-year-old woman who complained of bending of the leg. New bone formation with irregular thickening of cortex is prevalent in this stage of disease.

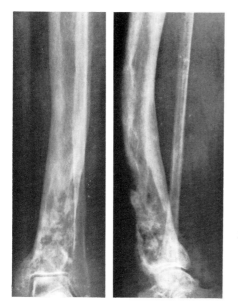

Fig. 8.32b. Three years later the patient was examined because of severely increased pain and swelling in the lower leg. The roentgenographs show a changed pattern of osseous structure with increased lytic changes in the affected bone.

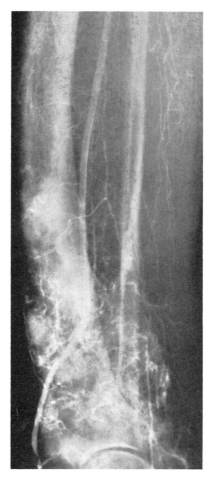

ig. 8.32c. Arteriography confirmed the suspicion of malignancy. Signs of malignancy and soft-tissue involvement by tumour are shown in the picture. Above-he-knee amputation was performed, and histological examination confirmed an osteosarcoma developing in aget's disease.

RESS FRACTURES

Stress fractures, also called fatigue fractures, occur in normal bones of healthy individuals without any trauma. They are caused by repeated stressing of the bone by minor mechanical insults, resulting from loading and muscle activity. They are frequently seen in young athletes with a strongly developed skeleton, but different types of stress fractures may occur in

children and elderly people. Intensive or unusual physical activity is most often the aetiological factor. The diagnosis is dependent on a
proper history, which should assess the activity
preceding symptoms. Pain produced by activity
and occurring at the site of the stress fracture
is the first symptom, followed later by swelling.
Roentgenological findings are usually negative
at the time of first symptoms and develop several weeks later. Stress fractures may be divided
into two groups, compression and distraction
types. A great variety of roentgenological
features of stress fractures occurring in different
parts of the skeleton has been described by
Devas (1975).

Most stress fractures heal easily, rest from the
activity which caused the pain usually being
sufficient treatment. Exceptionally for some
types of fractures plaster fixation is necessary.
These fractures are often misinterpreted as tumorous or inflammatory lesions, because of the
absence of a history of trauma, and because of
the radiological changes. Abundant periosteal
and endosteal callus formation may cover the
line of fracture, which adds to diagnostic difficulties (Fig. 8.33).

OSTEOMALACIA

Osteomalacia is a systemic disease of the skeleton, characterized by inadequate mineralization
of osteoid tissue. The mineral content of bones
is decreased, which results in the bones having
an abnormally translucent appearance on radiological examination. The term 'rickets' is
used to describe the defect of osteoid mineralization in the immature skeleton.

Osteomalacia may be caused by a great variety of disorders of calcium and phosphate metabolism, the two main groups being those due to
an insufficient supply of these minerals, and
those arising from failure of absorption. Besides
general demineralization the radiological
appearance of developed osteomalacia is characterized by secondary signs such as fractures
and deformities from bending bones, most frequently encountered in the pelvis and lower ex-

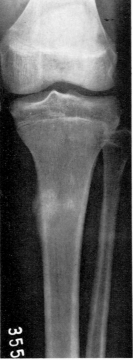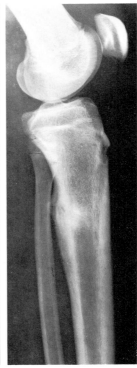

Fig. 8.33. Stress fracture of the tibia in a 16-year-old boy
who complained of pain under the knee after intensive
sports training. Bone sclerosis and periosteal callus
formation without a distinct history of trauma is
sometimes the reason for diagnostic difficulties, and may
be misinterpreted for roentgenological signs of a tumorous
lesion.

tremities. Kyphosis, especially of the thoracic
spine, is a frequent symptom. Stress fractures
with little tendency to healing develop in the
weakened bones; these fractures with seams of
unmineralized osteoid are known as Looser's
zones (Figs. 8.34 & 8.35).

Recognition of osteomalacia is of great importance to the orthopaedic surgeon, as bone surgery in affected patients is connected with delayed and uncertain healing, and the results of
osteosynthesis and other surgical procedures
are seldom satisfactory.

The skeletal manifestations of rickets due to
malnutrition are nowadays rarely seen in North
America and Europe, but they may develop due
to malabsorption syndromes or renal disorders.
Particularly affected are the metaphyses, in

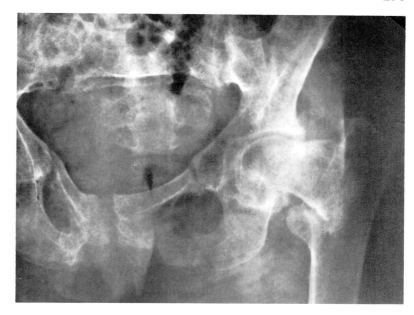

Fig. 8.34. Advanced osteomalacia in a 63-year-old woman suffering from renal insufficiency who was admitted because of a fracture of the femoral neck, which occurred without adequate trauma. In the roentgenograph generalized demineralization of the skeleton is visible. In addition to the femoral neck fracture multiple Looser's zones are present in both pubic bones.

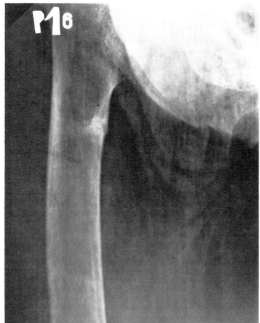

Fig. 8.35. Advanced osteomalacia in a 66-year-old woman suffering from a malabsorption syndrome, who was examined because of pain in the right hip. The roentgenograph shows excessive demineralization of the femur with a Looser's zone below the lesser trochanter. The cortex is demineralized to such an extent that the borders of cortex and medulla are not distinguishable.

which irregularities of ossification and resulting bone deformities are observed.

OSTEOPOROSIS

Osteoporosis is a generalized or localized skeletal disorder resulting from deficient osteoid matrix formation. The radiographs show diminished bone density, and the differentiation from osteomalacia may be difficult in some stages of the disease, but histological examination of bone biopsies can usually clearly differentiate these two disorders.

Localized osteoporosis appears in the vicinity of lesions causing hyperaemia, such as osteomyelitis and arthritis or even tumours (Fig. 8.9), and it occurs frequently after plaster immobilization of fractures.

Generalized osteoporosis is common in advanced age, but may also be the result of metabolic disorders, such as vitamin C deficiency, or endocrine glands malfunction, such as sex hormone deficiency or hypercorticosteroidism. In radiology, methods of quantitative densimetric assessment of osteoporosis have been described, but many circumstances make such measurements rather difficult. The changes may be unevenly distributed throughout the skeleton and it is difficult to estimate a standard mineral content according to age, as age-dependent osteoporosis develops differently in each individual. Fractures develop easily in the weakened skeleton, the vertebral bodies and the femoral neck being most often involved. As these fractures often occur with minimal trauma, differential diagnosis with pathological fractures in tumorous lesions may be difficult.

Sudeck's atrophy, also called painful osteoporosis, is an often seen post-traumatic complication of unclear pathogenesis. It usually occurs in the extremities, and is accompanied by pain, oedema and vascular changes, especially venous congestion. Radiographs show a diffuse or more often spotty decrease in bone density, usually around the joints.

References

DAHLIN D.C. (1978) *Bone Tumors*, 3rd Edition. Springfield Ill: Charles C. Thomas.

DEVAS M. (1975) *Stress Fractures*. Edinburgh: Churchill Livingstone.

ENNEKING W.F., SPANIER S.S. & GOODMAN M.A. (1980) A system for the surgical staging of musculoskeletal sarcoma. *Clin. Orthop.* **153**, 106.

HUVOS A.G. (1979) *Bone Tumors*. Philadelphia: W.B. Saunders Co.

JAFFE H.L. (1959) *Tumors and Tumorous Conditions of the Bones and Joints*. Philadelphia: Lea & Febiger.

LICHTENSTEIN L. (1972) *Bone Tumors*. St Louis: The C.V. Mosby Co.

LODWICK G.S., WILSON A.J., FARRELL C., VIRTAMA P. & DITTRICH F. (1980) Determining growth rates of focal lesions of bone from radiographs. *Radiology* **134**, 577.

MIRRA J.M. (1980) *Bone Tumors*. Philadelphia; J.B. Lippincott Co.

MURRAY R.O. & JACOBSON H.G. (1971) *The Radiology of Skeletal Disorders*. Edinburgh: Churchill Livingstone.

SCHAJOWICZ F. (1981) *Tumors and Tumorlike Lesions of Bone and Joints*. Berlin: Springer Verlag.

SCHAJOWICZ F., ACKERMAN L.V. & SISSONS H.A. (1972) *Histological Typing of Bone Tumors*. Geneva: World Health Organization.

SPJUT H.J., DORFMAN H.D., FECHNER R.E. & ACKERMAN L.V. (1971) *Tumors of Bone and Cartilage*. Washington D.C.: Armed Forces Institute of Pathology.

WILNER D. (1982) *Radiology of Bone Tumors and Allied Disorders*. Philadelphia: W.B. Saunders Co.

YAGHMAI I. (1979) *Angiography of Bone and Soft Tissue Lesions*. Berlin: Springer Verlag.

Chapter 9
Common Paediatric Problems

H. CARTY & J. F. TAYLOR

NORMAL VARIANTS

One of the most difficult problems facing the orthopaedic surgeon or radiologist with a small paediatric practice is the recognition of normality. There are an almost infinite variety of unusual appearances seen on radiographs that are nothing more than normal variants, and have no pathological significance. Many, such as the fragmented dense tarsal navicular or dense calcaneal epiphysis, are sufficiently common that most ought to recognize them. Pseudosubluxation of C2 on C3 continues to cause problems in cases of cervical trauma (Fig. 9.1). Casualty officers ought to be aware of the problems. Standard X-ray textbooks are fairly comprehensive, but as the problem is infinite not all variations will be included. When doubt still persists,

check with the clinical history to see if this is the precise site of complaint. If the lesion is asymptomatic then one is justified in treating the abnormality expectantly. In difficult cases X-rays of the opposite side may also be taken for comparison but must be exposed in the same projection. The practice of obtaining routine views of the opposite side is to be condemned. It causes unnecessary irradiation of the population and is expensive.

In non-urgent situations a second opinion can be obtained from a specialized centre.

BONE AGE

Skeletal maturity and, therefore, the capacity for growth is assessed by comparing the state of development of the patient's epiphyses with a

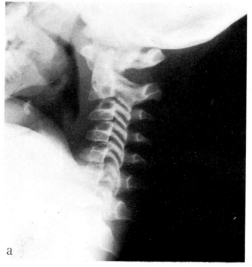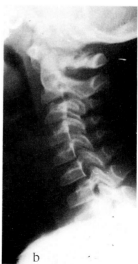

Fig. 9.1. Pseudosubluxation of C2 on C3. (a) The neck is held slightly flexed and there is apparent forward slip of C2 on C3. The posterior surfaces remain in alignment and the prevertebral soft tissues are normal. (b) Repeat film with a little straightening of the neck. The spine is now clearly normal.

297

standard reference atlas (Greulich & Pyle 1959, Tanner *et al.* 1975). An AP X-ray of the non-dominant hand and wrist is required, the elbow being no longer used in the routine assessment. Before the appearance of the carpal epiphyses at three months, one should use an AP view of a knee. The distal femoral epiphysis appears at approximately 36 weeks of fetal development and the proximal tibial at 38 weeks. Prior to this the calcaneal epiphysis which appears at 24 weeks is the reference point. Its shape gradually matures. As well as noting the presence of knee epiphyses one should note their structure, as fragmentation must raise the question of hypothyroidism.

Bone age is retarded in failure-to-thrive states, growth hormone deficiency, Perthes' disease, hypothyroidism, renal failure (where it may be accompanied by rickets) and some skeletal dysplasias. It is also retarded in Meyer's dysplasia and in some cases of brachydactyly syndromes. Bone age advancement is found in untreated or inadequately treated adrenogenital syndrome, hyperthyroidism and hypersecretion of cortisol. It may also be advanced where there has been joint hyperaemia secondary to trauma or arthritis, but it is a local phenomenon in this situation.

It is important to realize that the standard reference texts relate to the bone age of the reference community. The standards will vary somewhat in different racial communities with a different socioeconomic structure. The assessment of bone age is a useful guide to skeletal maturity and height prediction, but is used in conjunction with other clinical parameters.

SKELETAL DYSPLASIAS

Abnormalities of bone growth or development due to genetic factors are a fairly frequent problem in paediatric practice. Numerous attempts to classify the dysplasias have been made this century. The classification currently in use is known as the Paris nomenclature (Maroteaux 1979). The bone dysplasias are divided into five broad categories:

1   The osteochondrodysplasias. These include those lesions in which there is a primary abnormality of bone growth and cartilage. This group includes many of the classically recognized dysplasias, e.g. SED, achondroplasia.
2   The dysostoses. There is a skeletal malformation occurring singly or in a group of bones in combination, e.g. cleidocranial dysostosis.
3   The acro-osteolyses.
4   Chromosomal abnormalities.
5   Metabolic enzymatic disorders, which include disorders of metabolism of calcium, phosphorus, lipids, amino acids, and mucopolysaccharides.

It is beyond the scope of this book to discuss the diseases individually. Guidelines as to how the problem should be approached are all that can be offered.

Dysplasia may first be recognized in the neonatal period because of proportionate or disproportionate short stature and an unusual facies in the viable child. Many present at birth and are lethal. An accurate diagnosis based on skeletal radiographs and autopsy should be attempted to enable genetic counselling. A further group of children with dysplasias will present at 1–2 years and are noticed because of locomotion difficulties, i.e. a waddling gait, knock knees. The others will present randomly throughout childhood (Fig. 9.2). Some will escape notice until adult life when they present with premature osteoarthritis. Myopia, deafness and dentition problems are frequent associations of the dysplasias, and the children may first be noticed because of these complications. Others are referred to growth clinics because of short stature.

When a dysplasia is suspected a radiographic skeletal survey should be undertaken. The views required are AP and lateral of the skull. The lateral skull film should include a detailed view of the atlantoaxial articulation to assess its stability. AP and lateral views of the spine, AP of chest, pelvis, one hand and wrist, and AP of knees and a detailed view of any area of particular clinical interest should also be taken. If there is an abnormality of bone modelling, an

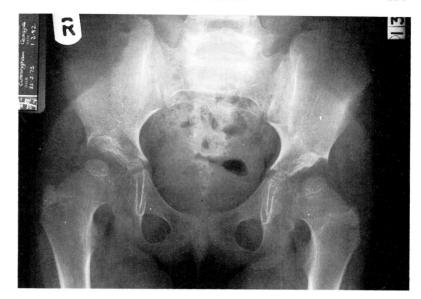

Fig. 9.2. The pelvis of a nine-year-old girl who waddled into the orthopaedic department complaining of left hip pain. No previous abnormality was noted or reported. The acetabuli are irregular and poorly formed. The femoral heads are small and there is broadening of the femoral neck. X-rays of the hands, knees and shoulders showed classical changes of multiple epiphyseal dysplasia.

AP view of the whole of a long bone on a single radiograph should also be included. If the diagnosis can be confidently made by the initial survey and clinical assessment, follow-up films of areas of clinical abnormality, i.e. a knee undergoing corrective surgery, are all that are required. If the diagnosis remains uncertain then a repeat full survey should be undertaken, initially at three-year intervals and increasing to five years as the child grows older and the rate of evolution of changes slows down as the skeleton approaches maturity.

Where possible the radiologist should see the patient, or at least clinical photographs, before attempting a diagnosis. When studying the radiographs one should determine the area of dominant involvement, i.e. epiphysis, metaphysis or diaphysis, or if it is a mixed lesion. Then decide on the presence or absence of spinal involvement. This gives a broad idea of the nature of the disorder and the X-rays and clinical details can be compared with reference texts. If one cannot accurately define the abnormality it is better to admit this than to misdiagnose a dysplasia. Incorrect diagnosis will lead to misleading prognostic information being given to parents and patient. The correct diagnosis may become apparent with time, hence

the value of serial radiographs. The number of children with dysplasias who accurately match the textbook descriptions is significantly fewer than children who either have variations of the classical disease or have entirely new and as yet unclassified dysplasias.

Most dysplasias are due to new mutations or are autosomally recessively inherited. Genetic counselling has to be based on this. A few, however, are due to embryopathy (thalidomide, fetal alcohol syndrome), and a history of drug ingestion in pregnancy is essential if new teratogens are not to be missed.

There are, however, other reasons for accurate diagnosis of a dysplasia. Parental fear of mental retardation is allayed once they know that this is not an association. In general, mental retardation is only a feature of dysplasia associated with chromosomal abnormalities and certain of the metabolic dysplastic diseases. Eye and ear complications can be detected early and the educational problems caused kept to a minimum. In some instances surgery can minimize the harmful effects. Eventual height, manual dexterity and locomotor disability can be predicted and arrangements for special school facilities made. Counselling as to eventual occupation can be instituted early and may well spare the family a great deal of heartbreak. A knowledge of the evolution of the disease permits appropriate timing of corrective orthopaedic surgery and will prevent unnecessary hospital stays and operations.

One also needs a detailed family history and radiographs of other affected family individuals. Care, however, has to be taken not to cause a guilt complex in the affected parent or to distress other affected members who obviously had been unaware of their condition.

It is also always worth seeking a second expert opinion. Most authorities on dysplasias have a collection of undiagnosed conditions, and may well have in their possession details of a similar patient to the referred case. In this way details of new dysplasias are constantly reported and longitudinal studies will show the natural history.

Registers of dysplasias are kept in several centres throughout the world and help and advice can be sought from these. Ultimately a central cross-referenced computerized bank of information of both classified and unclassified conditions may be possible, but much work remains to be done before it is a practical reality.

NON-ACCIDENTAL INJURY (NAI, BATTERED BABY SYNDROME, CAFFEY'S DISEASE)

Many synonyms are used to describe the condition of deliberate trauma to an infant. Superficial signs on physical examination that should alert the clinician are excess bruising, often at different stages of resolution, bruising in the distribution of a hand or palm, scratches, cuts, cigarette burns, and scalds. A torn frenulum of the lip and conjunctival haemorrhages are almost diagnostic. Repeated visits to hospital with apparently trivial complaints should alert the clinician, as this is often a reflection of a cry for help from the parents. Some infants who are the victims of assault may be undernourished and ill-kempt, but this is not universal. The condition, while commoner in socioeconomic groups 4 and 5, is found in all social classes.

Apart from superficial and skeletal trauma, visceral injury due to punching the abdomen or trampling on it may occur. Sexual abuse also occurs. The child may be dead or moribund on presentation. If it is moribund this is almost invariably due to cranial trauma with subdural haematomas and raised intracranial pressure, the injuries having occurred either by vigorous shaking or in association with skull fractures. In the less severely ill child listlessness and terror are common. Once suspected the child should be undressed completely for examination, all lesions should be photographed, and the patient referred for a skeletal radiographic survey. It is safest to admit the child for observation and it is important to see the other siblings.

Occasionally diagnostic confusion can arise between mild cases of osteogenesis imperfecta (OI) and NAI. Children with OI will sustain long-bone fractures, but the presence of cranial fractures, conjunctival haemorrhages and subdural haematomas is unlikely in this condition.

Radiology of NAI

A full skeletal survey is essential if the condition is suspected. AP views of the axial skeleton, together with an AP and lateral skull, are done initially. These are supplemented with detailed views of joints and lateral views as indicated following initial survey. Soft-tissue swelling may be seen in areas of recent injury. The finding of fractures at different stages of repair is diagnostic of the condition in the normally ossified skeleton. Characteristically the fractures occur in the metaphyses of the long bones and are due to excessive rotation or twisting of a joint. Corner metaphyseal fractures (Fig. 9.3) are almost diagnostic. These are subtle and heal rather unobtrusively, and are easily overlooked. Other common fractures are in the ribs, seen in a linear distribution, frequently along the axilla, and are due to the child falling forcibly against a hard surface. Squeezing of the rib cage may also produce posterior rib fractures close to the spine.

Rib fractures are very rare in young children in the absence of deliberate trauma. The pos-

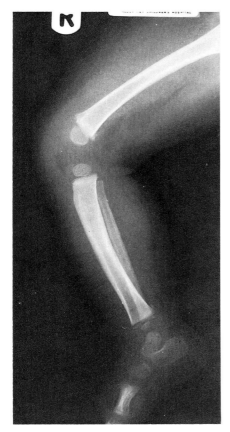

Fig. 9.3. Right lower leg of child who has been the victim of child abuse. There are classical metaphyseal fractures at the distal femur and distal tibia.

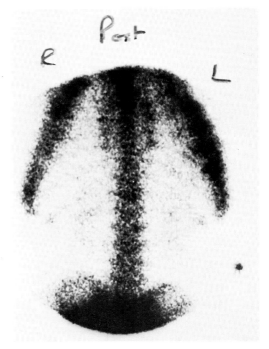

Fig. 9.4. Isotope scan of the thorax of a three-month-old infant. There is symmetrical increase in uptake of the isotope at the fractures of the posterior ends of ribs in the upper and mid-thorax.

terior rib fractures, easy to overlook on the X-ray, are more easily detected by nuclear scanning (Fig. 9.4). Periosteal reaction along the long bones due to a subperiosteal haematoma is common and may be seen when no fracture line is visible. It has to be distinguished from the normal physiological 'periostitis of infancy'. This latter is not seen before one month and is maximal at six months. When present it is always symmetrical in the limbs and may only be seen on one projection.

Other causes of periosteal reaction such as osteomyelitis, scurvy, infantile cortical hyperostosis, trauma, vitamin A intoxication, leukaemia and neuroblastoma are less likely to cause confusion due to a different appearance and distribution.

Skull fractures are also common, occurring in about 20% of cases, and may be of the linear or depressed variety, depending on the nature of the trauma. The radiologist should look for suture diastasis due to underlying subdural haematoma. Ultrasound and CAT scanning are used to supplement radiology in the cranium. Coexistent visceral injury may also be detected by ultrasound or isotope techniques. Isotope scanning is also used to supplement skeletal X-rays in some children. It helps to determine the fractures and is more sensitive than X-rays in the detection of rib fractures. The authors do not use it routinely but reserve it to help resolve these problems. There is great controversy at present in the literature as to the role of the two techniques. In the authors' opinion the X-ray survey is the correct initial investigation.

BONE DISEASE IN THE PREMATURE

As smaller premature infants are surviving due to intensive neonatal care, neonatologists and paediatric radiologists are seeing increasing numbers of tiny babies with a severe osteopenia, periostitis and changes of rickets in both long bones and ribs. This is known by a variety of names—rickets of the premature, ventilator bone disease, and incubator bone disease. The radiological changes develop slowly and are easily overlooked in the infant whose serial X-rays are compared only with the one taken the previous day (Fig. 9.5). The changes are easily appreciated if one compares the current films with the early neonatal ones. The disease is important, as respiration is made more difficult by the flail chest associated with rickets and pain associated with fractures. There may also be long-term orthopaedic sequelae of any rickety deformity. The disease develops in spite of apparently adequate prophylaxis with vitamin D. The infants require calcium supplements as well as vitamin D prophylactically. There may well be a deficiency of trace elements such as copper or magnesium.

THE SPINE

Radiography of the cervical spine

The initial X-rays in all cases are an AP and lateral view. The X-rays are done in the supine position. Horizontal-beam lateral views are done in cases of injury. The standard views are supplemented by flexion and extension views where instability is suspected clinically. This is mainly in cases of injury and cervical movement is supervised by the orthopaedic staff. Oblique views are required for diagnosing facetal subluxation and dislocations. If congenital vertebral abnormalities are not clearly identified on the simple views these are supplemented by tomography and pictures taken under screen control.

The twisted neck

In the infant a twisted or bent neck is usually painless. The commonest cases are due to congenital torticollis, in which the pathology is in the sternomastoid muscle, or there may be cervical vertebral segmentation defects causing a cervicothoracic scoliosis. X-rays will demonstrate these if present. Other causes include Sprengel's shoulder and the Klippel–Feil

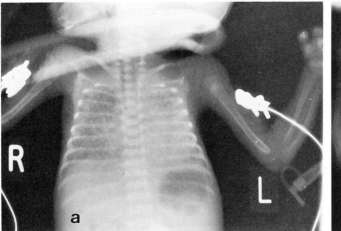 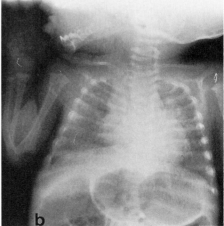

Fig. 9.5. Premature infant born at 30 weeks' gestation. (a) Chest X-ray shortly after birth with severe changes of hyaline membrane disease. The bones are normal. (b) Chest X-ray at four months of age. There are changes in the lungs of bronchopulmonary dysplasia. There are now several rib fractures, a fracture of the shaft of the right ulna, periosteal reaction on the ribs and humeri and changes of rickets at the wrist.

syndrome. Soft-tissue masses, i.e. cystic hygroma, may also cause secondary torticollis.

In the older child acquired neck deformities are usually painful. Traumatic torticollis is probably the commonest cause. X-rays will demonstrate the muscle spasm and tilt and exclude bony injury. Calcifying discitis or a bony or neurogenic neoplasm will also be identified if this is the underlying cause of the pain. Cervical neuroblastomas may present with a Horner's syndrome as well as pain (Fig. 9.6). A retropharyngeal abscess may lead to subluxation of the upper cervical vertebrae. A 2-mm distance between the odontoid peg and the arch of atlas is generally accepted as the maximum in the older patient. In normal infants this distance can be 5 mm. Confirmatory evidence of trauma or inflammation is seen in widening of the prevertebral soft tissues.

Klippel–Feil syndrome (brevicollis)
Congenital failure of cervical vertebral segmentation and disorders of soft tissues coexist. Clinically the neck is short, and cervical movements limited. Lateral webbing may involve the face and shoulders. Cleft palate and cardiothoracic defects may coexist. Typical radiological changes are fusion of cervical vertebrae, which are flat and wide, with obliteration of intervertebral discs. However, because of the short neck the face overlaps the cervical spine on the AP view and tomographs may be required to delineate the precise abnormality. Hemivertebrae and cervical spina bifida may coexist (Fig. 9.7).

There is an increased incidence of renal abnormalities in children with the Klippel–Feil syndrome. These range from renal agenesis to horseshoe kidney and other congenital malformations. All children should have ultrasound of the renal tract to be followed by IVU if an abnormality is detected.

Brevicollis must be differentiated from Sprengel's shoulder. Other causes of vertebral fusion such as previous fracture or infection may be excluded by the history. Fusion and growth disturbances of the vertebral bodies secondary to Still's disease develop late in childhood.

Minor degrees of congenital vertebral fusion can also occur and are often discovered incidentally. The condition has no clinical significance.

Sprengel's shoulder—congenital high scapula
Failure of normal scapular descent, from a cervical to a thoracic position, results in Sprengel's

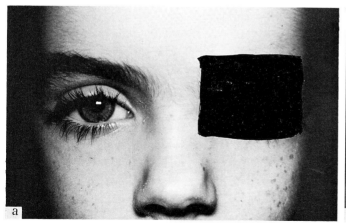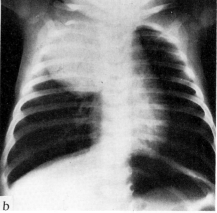

Fig. 9.6. Cervical neuroblastoma. (a) There is ptosis of the right eye and a small right pupil. (b) Chest X-ray of same child. There is a large well-defined soft-tissue mass in the right upper chest. There is no rib or vertebral erosion or calcification. The mass lay posteriorly on a lateral view. There are no specific radiological diagnostic features, but the combination of Horner's syndrome, raised VMA and the mass is virtually diagnostic of a cervical or high thoracic neuroblastoma.

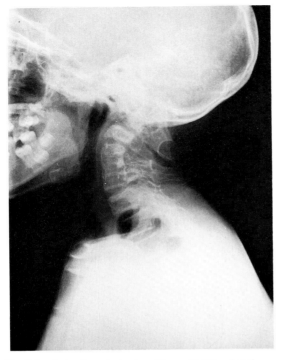

Fig. 9.7. Lateral cervical spine of boy with Klippel–Feil syndrome. There is fusion of both the bodies and the posterior elements of C3, 4, 5 with shortening of the neck. Tomography would be required to assess the atlantoaxial articulation.

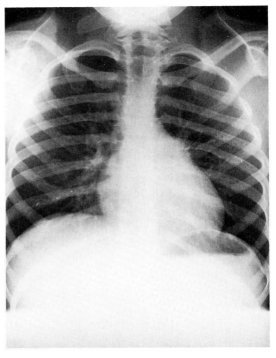

Fig. 9.8. Chest X-ray of a child with bilateral Sprengel's shoulder. The shoulders are elevated. There is an omovertebral bone on the right.

shoulder. Though it may be noticed at birth, many are now referred for advice in areas with scoliosis school-screening programmes. There is upward and forward displacement of the hypoplastic scapula, more usually the left. There is ipsilateral shortening of the neck. A bony bar, the omovertebral bone, may be palpable running from the superomedial border of the scapula to a lower cervical vertebra. The trapezius, rhomboid and other muscles of the chest may be hypoplastic. Scapular rotation is diminished (Fig. 9.8). Congenital scoliosis or costal anomalies may coexist. Clinically the condition is differentiated from acquired scoliosis by bending the child forward. In the uncomplicated patient with Sprengel's shoulder the spine is straight.

Radiography. Anteroposterior views are required of both shoulders, and should include films taken with active abduction of the arms to demonstrate limited scapular rotation. Views of the cervical and dorsal spine are taken to exclude the Klippel–Feil disorder. The omovertebral bone is present in over 30% of patients, but on occasions this structure is fibrous or cartilaginous and not seen on X-ray.

Cervical trauma

Cervical trauma is discussed in the chapter on trauma. One special paediatric problem needs to be emphasized: pseudosubluxation. One often sees apparent subluxation of the body of C2 or C3 in the spine of a young child referred for an X-ray because of trauma when there is, in fact, no instability or spinal injury. This is often accompanied by buckling of the trachea and widening of the soft tissues. It is due to the radiograph being taken in a degree of flexion.

The posterior spinous processes remain in alignment and the difficulty can be resolved by a further view taken in extension (Fig. 9.1).

Intervertebral disc calcification

This is a well-recognized syndrome in children. Its peak incidence is about 6–7 years but has been described in those as young as one year. It is commoner in males. The presenting complaints are pain, stiffness and torticollis, which are accompanied by pyrexia, and a raised ESR and white cell count. The lesion is probably inflammatory in origin. Calcification is seen in the intervertebral discs, most commonly in the low cervical and upper thoracic spine (Fig. 9.9). Two discs are commonly affected. It can occur in the lumbar spine but rarely in children. The condition clinically resolves in 2–3 months with symptomatic management. The calcium is gradually resorbed over a period of months to years. Some loss of disc height is frequent.

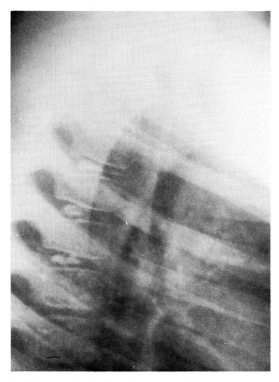

Fig. 9.9. Calcific discitis in the proximal thoracic spine.

Spinal pain

Pain in the back in childhood can usually be localized fairly accurately by the history and clinical palpation. Generalized back pain should lead one to think of systemic illness, i.e. Still's, rheumatic fever, leukaemia or metastatic disease. The common causes of back pain in the thoracic and lumbar spine are juvenile discitis, infective spondylitis, and, in addition, in the lumbar spine, spondylolysis or spondylolisthesis. A rarer cause will be an intraspinal tumour. Occasionally renal or GI pathology may present as back pain, and the possibility of urinary tract infection or appendicitis must be remembered in children presenting with a painful back and fever, if disasters are to be avoided. Conversely, a child with an infective discitis may present as an acute surgical abdomen and languish on a surgical ward. Clinical awareness and scrutiny of radiographs in both instances will help to avoid trouble.

Another clinical manifestation of vertebral or disc pathology is an alteration in activity—for example the toddler previously potty-trained who refuses to squat, or the infant previously sitting upright who insists on lying down.

Another clue to underlying spinal pathology is the onset of a scoliosis—painful or painless. This is a frequent sign of a vertebral tumour.

Investigation of spinal pain

A good clinical history and physical examination are vital and may be diagnostic, as in trauma. Physical examination must include assessment of local pain, tenderness, and postural change, and a search for motor, sensory or reflex changes in the legs, and signs of foot tension. Most cases will need at initial investigation a full blood count, ESR and radiographs. Supplementary investigations will include a Mantoux test, urine examination, salmonella agglutinins and a brucella complement fixation test. Good-quality plain radiographs are essential. It is the authors' practice to take standard AP and lateral views of the affected area of spine. These are then reviewed, and coned views and tomographs are taken where indicated. Isotope scanning will often localize a lesion and is indicated when the back pain persists for two weeks or more and is X-ray negative. Even when radiographs are positive it should still be done to exclude further lesions. In cases of spondylolysis it will aid in assessing healing—a hotspot indicating attempted bony repair of the defect.

If there is uncertainty about the diagnosis of a lesion a biopsy is indicated. This may be a needle or open biopsy, the decision resting on the experience of the clinician and on the site and presumptive diagnosis of the lesions.

Common causes of cord compression are intrathecal tumours, both benign and malignant, and an extradural abscess, which may exist without obvious clinical evidence of infection. The plain radiographs will often be normal, and in the presence of signs of cord compression urgent myelography is indicated. In infants a general anaesthetic is required, and the radiology should be undertaken in a centre with neurosurgical facilities so that any necessary decompression can take place under the same anaesthetic. The CSF must be sent for examination, as a negative radiculogram may lead to either polyneuritis or myelitis being considered as a cause of paralysis. CAT scanning will give information about the extent of a tumour, accurate demonstration of infiltration and soft-tissue extension.

Infective spondylitis (non-tuberculous)
Frank infective spondylitis with destructive changes in the discs and vertebral bodies is becoming a rare condition in western society. The symptoms in the older child are pain, fever and considerable toxicity. Muscle spasm is severe. When associated with an extradural abscess root pain and signs of cord compression may be present. Spinal percussion will yield local tenderness. In the young infant symptoms are less obvious and may be limited to listlessness and spinal deformity. Spondylitis is a complication of sickle cell disease, immune deficiency states and chronic granulomatous disease, but most commonly it occurs in children with no known predisposing factor.

The earliest radiological change is local paravertebral soft-tissue swelling. This progresses to loss of disc space, erosion of the anterior vertebral body and vertebral end-plates, and vertebral collapse. Reactive bone sclerosis takes place with repair. Some residual vertebral deformity is inevitable and ankylosis common. Isotope scanning with Tc MDP in acute cases may be normal as there is insufficient reactive change to render the scan positive. In chronic cases the scan will be positive, indicating the extent of the disorder but not the aetiology. Scanning with indium-labelled white cells may prove more sensitive than MDP in both the initial diagnosis and in diagnosing reactivation of infection. It may also distinguish infective spondylitis from inflammatory juvenile discitis, but there is insufficient experience as yet to assess its reliability.

Clinical and radiological diagnostic difficulty occurs in trying to distinguish this condition from inflammatory juvenile discitis, also called non-specific spondylitis. The clinical symptoms of pain and fever are the same. The child with juvenile discitis will have a raised ESR and leucocytosis. The radiographs are variable and usually one sees loss of disc height with progressive erosion of the adjacent vertebral end-plates. The anterior vertebral body is spared (Fig. 9.10). Juvenile discitis is found in the lumbar spine in about 80% of cases and is most common in the 4–6 year age group. The aetiology is unknown but is now thought to be viral. It is a self-limiting condition with gradual resolution of the radiological changes, but some loss of disc space height is a usual sequel. Bony ankylosis does not occur.

The more benign clinical presentation—lower ESR, normal blood culture, Widal reaction and antistaphylococcal titres, the absence of paravertebral abscess and the slower evolution of radiological change—and the site of the lesion and the age at presentation, coupled with an awareness of its existence, leads one to make the diagnosis and to distinguish this from the more sinister infective spondylitis. It is impossible to distinguish the two conditions on radiological

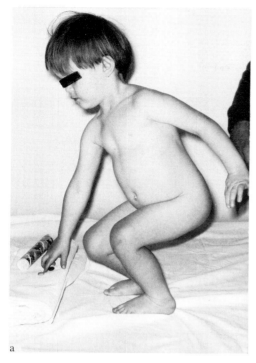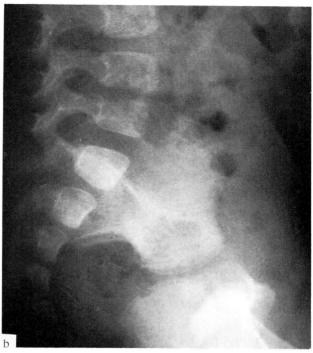

Fig. 9.10. A 2-year-old girl with juvenile discitis. Note the spinal posture as she bends to pick up the sweets. This rigidity would also be seen in other conditions causing spinal pain. (b) There is a narrow disc space at L4/5 with a little erosion of the proximal end-plate of L5. This appearance is not specific for non-infective spondylitis. An infective spondylitis could have a similar appearance. The diagnosis is suggested by the combination of the clinical presentation, haematology and X-ray changes.

grounds alone. If it is imperative to establish a positive diagnosis a biopsy of the affected disc space will resolve the issue. Where possible this should be by needle biopsy. Failure to culture an organism from the biopsy material favours the more benign diagnosis.

Spinal tuberculosis
Limitation of movement precedes pain, and the patient may rarely present with a psoas abscess or sinus. Systemic symptoms include listlessness, anorexia and loss of weight. The incidence is higher in immigrants. A positive family history is rare in Britain, cases being sporadic.

Radiology. The radiological changes are those of a destructive discitis but are not pathognomonic. T9–L3 are the most commonly affected vertebrae. Loss of disc space with destruction of the vertebral end-plates is seen in pyogenic discitis. Paravertebral abscesses are slightly commoner than in pyogenic lesions. Destruction of the anterior vertebral body may occur and the disease may involve the vertebral appendages, in contrast to pyogenic lesions. It is necessary to differentiate Scheuermann's disease (adolescent kyphosis), in which vertebral wedging occurs, but in which fragmentation and patchy deossification is restricted to the upper and lower ring epiphyses. The diagnosis of TB is based on the clinical symptoms, Mantoux testing, the elevated ESR and if necessary a biopsy. Coincident pulmonary TB is rare in Britain. Healing takes place with chemotherapy. If vertebral destruction has occurred healing will lead to bony ankylosis and an acute angular kyphos (Fig. 9.11).

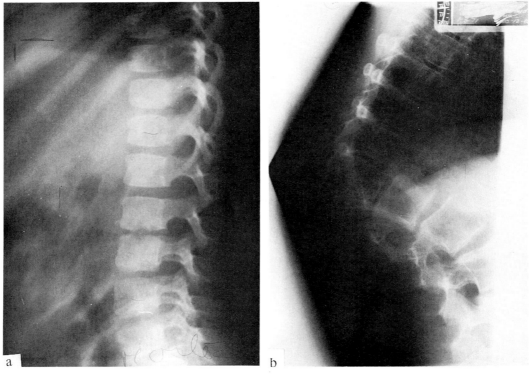

Fig. 9.11. (a) Early change of spinal TB. There is narrowing of the disc space at L3/4 with a central destructive lesion. The destruction is more localized than that seen in pyogenic discitis but this is not invariable and the X-ray is not diagnostic of TB. (b) X-ray of another patient. There is an angular kyphosis at the site of the previous tubercular infection and bony ankylosis has taken place.

Spondylolisthesis

In children spondylolisthesis may result from congenital deficiencies in the lumbosacral area (dysplastic type), or from a defect in the pars interarticularis (isthmic type), which may be congenital or traumatic. If congenital, then the subluxation of one vertebra on another causes tension in the sacral nerves and hamstring spasm, the patient presenting with a stiff waddling gait and loss of the normal spinal curvature. In traumatic cases the child, often very athletic, presents with backache and local muscle spasm. A substantial proportion of patients seen within a week of fracture will heal after plaster-jacket immobilization, and early diagnosis is therefore important. Isotope scanning is useful, as a hotspot indicates increased bone activity as attempted repair takes place.

The condition may also be associated with scoliosis. Supine and lateral X-rays are supplemented by lateral views with the patient erect to measure the extent of the slip. A minor defect in the pars interarticularis may only be seen on oblique views. If the defect is unilateral, reactive sclerosis may be seen in the contralateral pedicle or lamina.

In determining the need for surgical stabilization, the angle of slip, that is the measurement of the kyphotic relationship of the fifth lumbar to the first sacral vertebra, is important. The angle is formed by a line drawn parallel to the inferior aspect of the fifth lumbar body, and a line drawn perpendicular to the posterior aspect of the body of the first sacral vertebra. The amount of slip may be measured by the grading system of Mayerding, the scoring system of

Newman, or the percentage of slip as described by Boxall *et al.* (1979). Anterior erosion of the first sacral vertebra and the trapezoidal shape of the fifth lumbar make measurement imprecise.

Radiculography may be desirable in severe cases with signs of neural involvement, to exclude a cause other than the slip in the aetiology of the neural deficit. It is also important if the surgeon is contemplating vertebral fusion without decompression as the method of stabilization.

Intervertebral disc prolapse
Rare in children, this may occur with only moderate flexion of the loaded spine. Spinal pain and spasm is usually accompanied by sciatica and neurological deficit. However, in children presentation is frequently atypical and large hernias may cause pain with little motor or sensory loss. The prognosis is less favourable than in adults. Plain radiographs may reveal loss of lordosis, or a scoliosis secondary to muscle spasm. Disc space narrowing is rare but the prolapse will usually be demonstrable by radiculography. At the L5/S1 level a posterior prolapse may only be diagnosed by epidurography, CT scan or operation.

Tumours
Primary vertebral bone tumours are commoner in the appendages than in the bodies. Secondary deposits can occur in either, but vertebral collapse is the most frequent manifestation. Intrathecal lesions will lead to pressure erosion of the pedicles with expansion of the interpedicular distance.

Severe spinal pain and immobility, with no obvious radiographic lesions in the vertebral bodies, should lead to a search for lesions in the vertebral arches. Coned local views and tomography of the lesion are required. Isotope scanning will help to localize a lesion. Urgent myelography is indicated where there are signs of compression, commoner with intraspinal lesions, and where there may be no plain film changes.

Aneurysmal bone cyst. There is local pain and muscle spasm in the spine or affected long bone. Progressive enlargement of a spinal lesion may cause a sensory or motor defect. Radiologically these benign tumours have characteristic soap-bubble radiolucencies. There is local expansion of bone, with a scalloped border, and slight reactive sclerosis. Fine calcified septae are seen within the lesion, which in long bones is eccentric in the metaphysis.

They occur in the vertebral appendages and may extend into the body. Local excision is curative, but in the cervical spine diagnostic biopsy may need to be followed by radiation therapy if excision is too dangerous. In a long bone the child frequently presents with a pathological fracture. The tumour is in the metaphysis and is often eccentric. They can look very aggressive (Fig. 9.12).

Osteoblastoma. The neural arches are common sites of this rare tumour, though long bones and

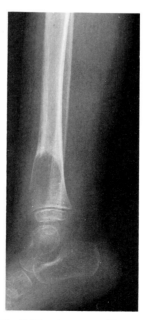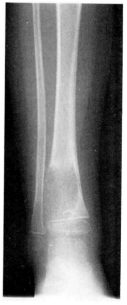

Fig. 9.12. Aneurysmal bone cyst. There is an expansile mainly lucent lesion eccentrically placed in the metaphysis of the distal tibia with a few septae seen on the AP view. Periosteal reaction is present on the medial tibial shaft due to a healing fracture.

the bones of the hand and foot may be involved.

Clinically there is local pain, and in palpable bone a localized swelling. In the neural arch intraspinal expansion may compress the cord. The child may thus present with backache, nerve root pain, or paraplegia.

Radiographs reveal a radiolucent lesion with areas of radio-opacity (Fig. 9.13). The cortex may be perforated by the soft-tissue mass. In the spine the tumour occurs in the vertebral appendages. In the lateral view a small elevated flake of cortex may be the earliest sign of the expansile lesion. Small osteoid osteomata or osteoblastomata are notoriously difficult to locate. A hotspot will usually be present on isotope bone scanning, localizing the lesion, which can then be further assessed by coned radiographs. These lesions are benign and a localized excision effects a cure.

Eosinophilic granuloma (Calvé's disease). Varying degrees of vertebra plana are seen in the spine of children who are X-rayed for spinal pain. It can occur at any age. At its most severe the vertebral body is flattened to a thin disc but the disc spaces are maintained (Fig. 9.14). The lesion can occur at any level and it is now accepted that there is an eosinophilic granuloma as the underlying cause. The pedicles may also be destroyed. The lesion is usually solitary and is not part of more generalized histiocytosis. The lesion is mildly hot on bone scanning. It has such a characteristic appearance at its most severe that biopsy is not required, but in lesser degrees of collapse and destruction a biopsy is necessary. Though some resolve spontaneously, healing may be hastened by curettage and the insertion of bone chips. Radiation therapy is used as an alternative.

Metastases. It is unusual for a child to present with metastatic disease without an obvious primary tumour. Spinal metastases manifest themselves as pain or may present with signs of cord compression. Generalized vertebral collapse with osteoporosis may be seen in leukaemic infiltration. The common neoplasm which metastasizes to the spine is neuroblastoma, but this tends to destroy both vertebral appendages and body. More classical metastases will first destroy the pedicle before involving the vertebral body.

Osteoid osteoma. This most commonly occurs in the adolescent's long bones. Characteristically the severe pain responds to aspirin. When the history is suggestive and radiographs are negative an isotope scan will usually be positive

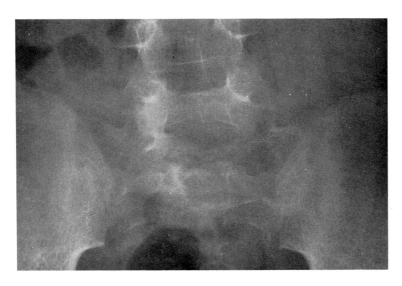

Fig. 9.13. X-ray of sacrum of an eight-year-old boy complaining of pain in the left hip. There is a destructive lesion in the proximal left sacrum extending into the articular facet. This lesion was purely destructive and no dense areas were visible. The diagnosis of osteoblastoma was made on the histology. An aneurysmal bone cyst or eosinophilic granuloma could also have a very similar appearance.

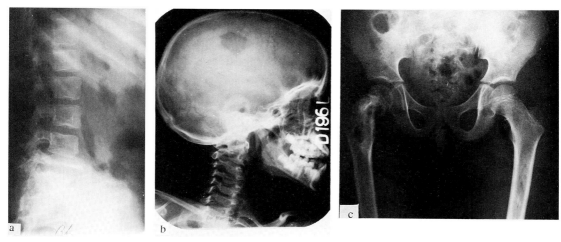

Fig. 9.14. (a) There is a vertebra plana at L5. The appearance is characteristic of eosinophilic granuloma. (b) and (c) Further lesions are present in the skull, right ilium and right femur of this child.

and will localize the lesion. The typical X-ray change in the long bone is of dense consolidated periosteal reaction around a central nidus, but the nidus is rarely seen in the dense reactive bone.

In the spine the osteoma is usually seen in the appendages as a localized area of increased bone density. It may be associated with scoliosis and the lesion is then located by seeking bony expansion on the concave side of the apical vertebrae.

Local curettage, provided the nidus is removed, is curative.

Developmental spinal anomalies
The vertebrae develop from three main primary centres of ossification, one for the body and one on each side of the vertebral arch. The arch is incomplete until after the second fetal month, when the two sides unite and enclose the cord. The vertebral appendages grow from the edges of the arch. The body, although having only one ossification centre, forms as two cartilaginous centres. Unilateral failure of chondrification leads to a hemivertebra, and failure of fusion to the butterfly vertebra.

Spina bifida and myelomeningocele. Failure of fusion of the posterior arches, or absence of these

elements with widening of the spinal canal, is the cause of spina bifida. When associated with a myelomeningocele it is clinically obvious.

The sac is usually dorsal, but may on occasion may protrude anteriorly through the vertebral bodies, to present in the chest, abdomen or pelvis.

The more distal the sac the more likely it is that it encloses neural elements.

Examination should include palpation of the bony defect to determine the extent, and transillumination of the sac for neural tissue. The head is examined for evidence of hydrocephalus. The limb and anal reflexes are examined, and motor loss determined by stimulating areas of skin to produce withdrawal.

Plain radiographs should be obtained of the whole spine. These will reveal the extent of the principal defect and the presence of obvious vertebral abnormalities such as hemivertebrae. Prognosis is based on the clinical and radiological findings, and an interdisciplinary treatment plan is formulated. Ultrasound of the head is required for the assessment of hydrocephalus. Renal tract assessment by ultrasound and IVP is required initially as a baseline, and regular monitoring for neuropathic change is also necessary. Active surgical management of kyphosis and scoliosis may be required in later years, as may iliopsoas tendon transplants and corrective foot surgery. All surgical procedures are designed to improve postural stability and locomotion. Radiological assessment of continuity of valve systems is essential before spinal surgery. Renal stones should be actively looked for when assessing spinal films in these children.

A characteristic defect in the wing of the ilium is seen following Sharrard's posterolateral iliopsoas transplantation, when the psoas muscle is detached from the lesser trochanter, drawn into the pelvis through the iliac blade and resutured to the greater trochanter (Fig. 9.15).

Associated hip dislocation is common in children with spina bifida. The iliopsoas is innervated by the first and second lumbar nerves, the hip flexors and adductors principally by the

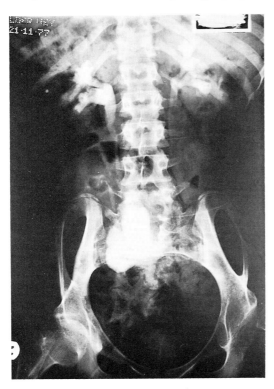

Fig. 9.15. Child with low lumbar and sacral myelomeningocele repaired at birth. The ureters have been transplanted into an ileal loop. Characteristic defects are present in both iliac wings following iliopsoas transplantation.

second and third, and the abductors and extensors by the fourth and fifth lumbar and first sacral. Dislocation occurs when the first and second lumbar nerves are spared, with strong flexors and adductors, function in the abductors and extensors being impaired. Clinically the affected baby presents with flexed and adducted hips and extended knees. Dislocation of the hip is inevitable unless measures are taken to balance the power of the abductors and adductors.

If there is subluxation at birth the position may be maintained by passive abduction exercises, and abduction splints. These are contraindicated if dislocation has occurred, as the bones are fragile and may easily be fractured.

After three months open reduction and adductor tenotomy is performed. A posterior or posterolateral psoas transfer may be undertaken simultaneously in the older child, or as a separate procedure in the infant.

An AP radiograph shows the high femoral head, with lateral rotation, the greater trochanter facing the acetabulum. Unlike CDH the acetabulum is well developed, the acetabular angle being low. Manipulation of the leg into flexion (to relax the psoas) and internal rotation at the time of arthrography will often show that the head can be reduced, a limbus being rare.

The lower limb in spina bifida.   Poor lower limb development with rigidity and talipes is an accompaniment of spina bifida and is due to muscular imbalance and neuromuscular dysplasia. Neuropathic skin changes with trophic ulcers are common. Fractures present with either obvious deformity or soft-tissue swelling and some local increase in heat. The bones are thin and osteoporotic. The fractures are often metaphyseal. Osteomyelitis is frequently found in bone under a trophic ulcer. Fractures in patients with spinal dysraphism heal with superabundant callus.

Spina bifida occulta.   This anomaly may present as an incidental radiological finding, or the clinician may notice abnormal hair or skin dimples over the lower lumbar spine. Fusion of the vertebral arches commences after birth but is completed in adolescence. Thus incomplete bony fusion seen on an X-ray of an infant's spine may not be due to a developmental anomaly but may represent a normal stage of ossification.

Where there is objective evidence of weakness, reflex changes, loss of bladder control or the development of foot deformities such as pes cavus or pes varus, and particularly where progression is noted, a radiculogram is indicated to identify filling defects due to lipomata, intraspinal meningoceles or dermoid cysts, diastematomyelia or distal tethering of the dura and cord. The cord is attached by the filum terminale to the third sacral vertebra. At birth the conus lies at the level of the disc space at L3/L4, and normally is seen to ascend with differential growth, being at the level of L1 at maturity. Tethering of the filum or dural plaques produces neurological symptoms due to excessive tension on the cord (Fig. 9.16).

Diastematomyelia. This congenital malformation is a spicule of bone, or more usually fibrocartilage, projecting posteriorly from a vertebral body through the spinal cord and dura. It produces a form of cord tethering, and may present with signs of neurological deficit as described above. Arnold–Chiari malformation may be associated. In thoracic lesions there may be physical signs of an upper motor neurone lesion. Excision of the bar is indicated in the presence of progressive disability, or prior to correction of a scoliotic curve.

Plain radiographs in diastematomyelia may be normal. A little widening of the interpedicular distance may be present. The bony spicule if seen will be in the middle of the canal with its long axis vertical on the AP film. The usual level is between T11 and L2. A fibrocartilaginous bar will only be seen on myelography or CT scan, which are indicated when there is objective evidence of a neurological lesion in the presence of normal straight film.

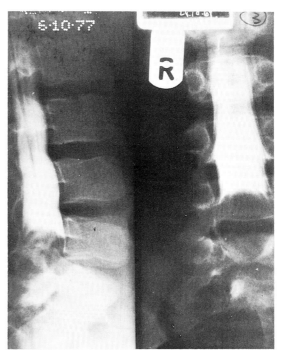

Fig. 9.16. Radiculogram of an eight-year-old boy who presented to the orthopaedic department with pes cavus. The lumbar X-ray was normal. At radiculography the filum was tethered to the level of L5 and to an intrathecal dermoid.

Other congenital vertebral anomalies. Hemivertebrae, butterfly vertebrae and complex segmentation defects are discussed in Chapter 11. It should, however, be mentioned that complex segmentation defects when balanced may not result in scoliosis and are occasionally found incidentally. There may be no associated neurological signs and when they are thoracic there are no bladder or bowel problems. The trunk may be somewhat shortened and disproportionate stature results. They are also seen in spondylocostal dysplasia where there are associated rib abnormalities.

Vater anomalad. This term has been coined to describe an association of anomalies involving the skeleton, and renal and alimentary tracts. Vater is mnemonic and stands for vertebral, anal, tracheo-oesophageal, renal and radial anomalies. Cardiac lesions are also a frequent accompaniment. The vertebral anomalies found in association with rectal atresia and tracheo-oesophageal fistula are non-specific and range from hemivertebrae, block vertebrae and butterfly vertebrae to complex lesions, sacral deficiency and sacral tilt.

All children require an initial full spinal X-ray survey to establish the presence of a lesion, and, if one is present, subsequent clinical monitoring to assess scoliosis. Renal anomalies which are also non-specific and range from simple duplex kidneys to very complex lesions leading to early renal failure are detected, assessed and monitored by ultrasound, IVU and nuclear studies.

Sacral agenesis and lumbosacral agenesis. In this condition there is congenital absence of sacral segments which range from minor lesions with loss of a single sacral segment to complete absence of sacrum and a varying number of vertebral bodies with midline fusion of the iliac bones. Sacral anomalies are associated with ano-rectal malformations and urinary tract abnormalities. In the presacral anomalies the agenesis may be unilateral. Renshaw (1978) classifies the lesions as follows: type I, total or partial unilateral sacral agenesis; type II, partial agenesis but with a bilateral symmetrical defect; type III, variable lumbar and total sacral agenesis with the ilia articulating with the sides of the lowest vertebra present; type IV, total sacral and variable lumbar agenesis with the caudal end-plate of the lowest vertebra resting above either fused ilia or an iliac amphiarthrosis.

Complete absence of the sacrum can be diagnosed clinically, producing flat buttocks, a short gluteal cleft, and narrow pelvis. The neurological abnormalities are symmetrical, except in hemiagenesis of the sacrum, which is also characterized by pelvic obliquity. However, most patients will become ambulant to some extent.

Lumbosacral deficiency is associated with parenteral insulin therapy in the mother, and profound neurological disturbances. There is a spinal 'gibbus', and frequently scoliosis, knee and hip flexion contractures, and foot deformity.

Amputation may be required. Spinal X-rays will determine the extent of the spinal defect. The associated renal and cloacal abnormalities will also need assessment and monitoring.

CONGENITAL DISLOCATION OF THE HIP

Most children with dislocated hips present in the neonatal period. Limited abduction, a clunk on performing Ortolani's test, or inequality of the buttock skin creases having been noted at a post-natal examination. The clinician must then determine whether he is dealing with a normal child, a child who had a transient dislocation for physiological reasons, CDH, or dislocation occurring as part of neuromuscular or ligamentous disorders, such as arthrogryposis, cerebral palsy or Larsen's syndrome. A small number of children still present late—either because of a missed lesion in the neonatal period, or true late onset.

A normal child may have a click in the hip on forced abduction, without any dislocation. The click may represent movement of the ligamentum teres or other ligamentous structures. The sensation noted by the clinician is distinguishable from the 'clunk' of the dislocating hip. Transient reducible dislocation may occur due to laxity of the muscles on which hip stability depends. Such weakness is seen in premature babies and those subjected to prolonged labour, or where mothers were given relaxant drugs shortly before delivery. Immediately after birth firm pressure by the paediatrician on the baby's adducted leg will produce dislocation. However, the hip is inherently stable, and if held in a reduced position by double nappies for a few weeks will develop normally.

A careful history and systematic examination of the newborn may permit differentiation of CDH from neuromuscular disorders. CDH is commoner in female infants and there is often a positive family history. It is also more frequent following breech delivery.

It is taught that CDH may be accompanied by characteristic signs. Asymmetry of the skin folds on the inner thigh can indicate telescoping of one leg, but is present in a third of all new-born babies. Limitation of hip abduction may be present in the neglected dislocation, but is inconsistent in the newborn. Progressive reduction of abduction is a useful sign of impending dislocation in cerebral palsy. A correctly performed Ortolani test is the most reliable clinical test for dislocation. The baby lies supine and the examiner holds the legs with the knee and hips flexed. The hips are slowly abducted. The dislocated head lies posteriorly, and during abduction may return to the acetabulum with a clunk. However, some heads are irreducible and a negative Ortolani test does not exclude CDH. The clinician will also examine for arthrogryposis and other neuromuscular disorders. Spinal anomalies will also require an X-ray for their identification. The older child often presents with delay in walking or a wadddling gait.

Pathology

The hip joint in CDH is said to be dysplastic, which implies that even if in the newborn the hip is reduced, development may be retarded. Dislocation is associated with a loose capsule. In the absence of early treatment, relocation may be prevented by a capsular constriction at the acetabular rim, by a long hypertrophied ligamentum teres or by a limbus. This term is used to describe the labrum acetabulare, which in the normal hip is everted to clasp the head, but which, in prolonged dislocation, inverts to form a barrier to reduction. Persistent pressure on the ilium from the displaced femoral head leads to the development of a false acetabulum.

Treatment may fail due to malalignment, where the femoral head and neck do not point into the acetabular sockets when the child's legs are in the anatomical position. This malalignment may be due to an abnormal acetabulum, femoral neck or both.

The normal acetabulum faces partly downwards, the angle of inclination of the acetabular roof being less than $30°$ to the horizontal. In subluxation the acetabulum is shallow and the defective roof leads to a greater acetabular angle, as seen on X-ray. The acetabular alignment also varies with respect to the coronal plane. In the normal child it faces forward at about $6°$ (McKibbin 1978), but this increases to $23°$ in CDH.

The normal femoral neck–shaft angle is increased in established dislocation. However, CDH is also accompanied by anteversion of the femoral neck. By this is meant that with respect to the bicondylar plane, or the greater trochanter, the neck and head do not point directly medially but to some extent anteriorly.

Treatment

It is thought that development of the hip and resolution of dysplasia is promoted by holding the leg so that the femoral head is directed at the acetabulum. In the neonate, if competent examination has revealed a dislocatable hip, most surgeons recommend splintage of the legs in abduction and possibly some rotation for a period. Whatever the method, regular clinical examination and imaging by ultrasound or radiology are required to determine that the reduction is achieved in the splint and that the capsule is becoming less loose. Arthrography is not generally indicated.

In the older child, soft-tissue contracture occurs as the femoral head migrates proximally. It is then necessary to ensure that congruent reduction can be obtained, or to determine the soft-tissue barrier to obstruction by arthrography.

The child is admitted to hospital and traction applied to pull the leg distally. Radiography will be required to demonstrate that the femoral head has reached the level of the acetabulum. If abduction has been applied after traction (Lloyd Roberts & Swann 1966) reduction may be achieved. Prolonged traction leads to osteoporosis or damage to the growth cartilages, and if reduction is not effected after two weeks operative reduction is advisable. During the open reduction the surgeon will estimate femoral anteversion and the acetabular inclination. Because of the inevitable movement between closure of the wound and completion of the subsequent spica, a radiograph of the hips to check that reduction is maintained should be taken prior to discontinuing the anaesthetic.

Late diagnosis or continuing subluxation may lead to the need for acetabular realignment or reconstruction. The innominate (Salter) osteotomy divides the ilium horizontally above the acetabulum, and places a triangular bone graft in the ilium, so directing the acetabulum anteriorly and downwards (Fig. 9.17c, d). The graft is often held in place by wires. The osteotomy (Chiari) divides the ilium horizontally immediately above the acetabulum, the plane of the division being so designed that on medial displacement of the distal fragment the wing of the ilium forms a buttress above and lateral to the dysplastic acetabulum. This operation provides no anterior cover (Fig. 9.17e, f). If radiographs reveal rotation of one fragment on the other, proper cover of the acetabulum may be lacking.

Shelf procedures are those on which free bone grafts are inserted into selected sites above the acetabulum. They may be followed by resorption of the graft. Acetabuloplasty refers to the operation in which the roof of the acetabulum is turned downwards by partial iliac osteotomy. The gap so created is filled with bone, which may on occasion collapse, causing late failure of the operation.

Radiology

In the newborn treatment is based on the history and clinical findings. Reliance must not be placed on the X-ray for the diagnosis. A transient dislocation is often reduced by positioning for the X-ray, and a normal X-ray may lead to a failure to treat. However, an AP X-ray should be taken to assess the acetabular angle. Unrecognized spinal or sacral anomalies may also be detected. In frank dislocation proximal and lateral femoral displacement and a steep acetabulum are seen. The dislocation is sometimes easier to see on the Von Rosen (1968) view, in which the legs are extended, internally rotated and abducted to 45°. Dislocation is indicated when a line projected medially along the long

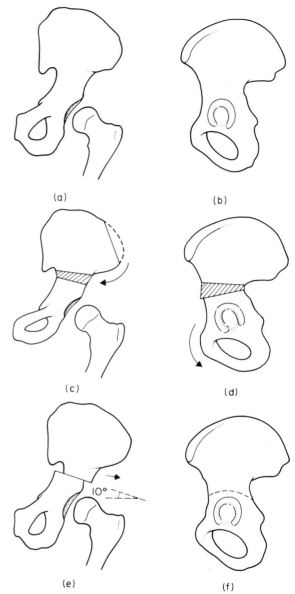

(a)   (b)

(c)   (d)

(e)   (f)

Fig. 9.17. (a) and (b) Displacement of the femoral head leads to a shallow acetabulum. (c) and (d) show the AP and lateral views of a Salter osteotomy. A bone graft has been excised from the region of the anterior superior iliac spine and is inserted with its base anteriorly to rotate and direct the acetabulum downwards in both the sagittal and coronal planes. (e) and (f) In the Chiari procedure the pelvic osteotomy is seen on the AP X-ray to be angled inferiorly at about 10°. Medial displacement of the distal fragment results in effective 'cover' for the femoral head by the proximal fragment. In the lateral view the osteotomy should be curved to prevent anteroposterior displacement.

axis of the femur runs above the acetabulum and crosses the line from the opposite side above the lumbosacral junction. However, failure to abduct the leg to 45° produces a false-positive.

Plain X-rays are of more use after three months, as bony outlines become more distinct. Gonadal radiation must be restricted. The hip dislocates upwards, outwards and posteriorly, but this latter movement cannot be detected on a plain AP X-ray.

The ossification centre for the femoral head appears at about six months. In dislocation it is delayed, and remains smaller if dysplasia persists. The normal acetabulum as seen on a correctly positioned X-ray is curved and has a slight central concavity. In acetabular dysplasia the acetabulum is steep, small and shallow (Fig. 9.18).

To enable an assessment of the relationship of the unossified femoral head to the acetabulum, numerous lines and angles have been proposed. The most important of these are as follows.

Hilgenreiner's lines. A line is drawn horizontally through the triradiate cartilages. A perpendicular parasagittal line then drawn through the anterior inferior iliac spines or the outer lip of the acetabulum (Perkins' line) forms four quadrants. The normal femoral head lies in the medial and inferior quadrant.

Acetabular angle. A line is drawn from the centre of the triradiate cartilage to the outer lip of the acetabulum, forming the acetabular angle with Hilgenreiner's horizontal line. This angle can be measured in the newborn, and should be less than 30°.

Shenton's line. This is projected from the medial femoral shaft along the inferior surface of the femoral neck. It should form a continuous curve with the inferior surface of the superior pubic ramus.

Simon's line. This is also a curve from the lateral margin of the ilium and outer lip of the acetabulum to the upper margin of the femoral neck.

In doubtful cases the application of these lines may be helpful but the usefulness of all of them is dependent on a correctly positioned X-ray. The radiological features of hip dislocation in the older child are proximal displacement of the femoral head, delay in ossification and size of the femoral head compared to the normal side, acetabular dysplasia and the development of a false acetabulum. However, proper planning of treatment will require clinical and radiological estimation of acetabular and femoral alignment.

Acetabular alignment
The inclination of the acetabulum is properly measured on a PA X-ray, because it varies with the tilt of the pelvis. In the PA view the anterior iliac spines and pubis are all in the same plane relative to the film. Acetabular anteversion may be estimated by the method of Lloyd Roberts *et al.* (1978). Using the plain X-ray the antero-

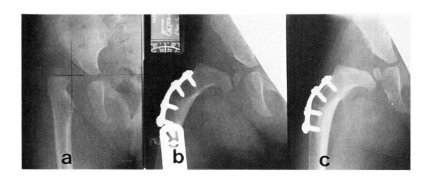

Fig. 9.18. (a) Patient who presented at eight months with right hip dislocation. The acetabulum is steep and shallow and the femoral head is dislocated. (b) and (c) Following osteotomy the head is now contained in the joint but remains small and slightly sclerotic. This suggests vascular compromise.

lateral and posterolateral acetabular margins are outlined. If the acetabulum faces laterally these two are superimposed, but increasing anteversion correlates with increasing distance between the two. More refined methods of measuring acetabular anteversion require the use of X-ray stereoscopy or the CT scan.

Femoral alignment

The inclination of the femoral neck is measured on an AP X-ray, the normal neck–shaft angle being 150°. With 90° of femoral anteversion the neck–shaft angle will appear to be 180°, as the neck points at the X-ray beam. Ideal measurement necessitates screening in increasing internal rotation until the greatest length of femoral neck is seen. This is the position in which the neck–shaft angle should be measured.

Femoral anteversion has been measured in the same way. The patient is placed in the prone position under the image intensifier, with the knees flexed. The length of the femoral neck is observed in varying degrees of internal rotation. The femoral anteversion is the degree of internal rotation beyond which the length of the neck is not seen to increase. The use of ultrasound in measuring femoral anteversion has recently been demonstrated by Moulton and Upadhjay (1982). The value of this technique as a routine requires further assessment. Many other methods are described in the literature, and have been reviewed by Tachdjian. However, the computerized tomography (CT) scan has superseded radiography, but only limited information can be gained until adequate ossification occurs after 18 months. Scan time and radiation dose depend on the scanner used. The dose per slice varies from 1 to 4 rads. For this reason the scan is not recommended for routine assessment of femoral anteversions, but may be reserved for a complicated situation in the older child (Peterson *et al.* 1981).

Shands and Steele found in the normal child 39° of femoral anteversion during the first year of life. It decreases by 1–2° yearly, being 24° at the age of 10 and 16° in the adult.

Hip arthrography

Satisfactory reduction is usual in the neonate and arthrography is rarely indicated. When there is failure of concentric reduction after early diagnosis and some months of effective conservative treatment in a splint, or in the patient who presents late, soft tissues may be an obstruction to reduction, and arthrography is indicated (Fig. 9.19).

The procedure is done under GA and with screen control. The usual aseptic precautions are observed. A 22-G spinal needle which has a short bevel is used for puncture of the joint. A medial approach is used. The ischial tuberosity is identified and the needle is passed lateral to this and advanced at an oblique angle into the joint until it rests on bone. The position is checked on the screen and a test dose of contrast is injected. Very small quantities of dye, i.e. about 0·1 ml, are used for the test injection, otherwise the joint will become obscured by extra-articular dye if repeated test injections have to be made. When contrast is in the joint, it flows freely over the head and around the

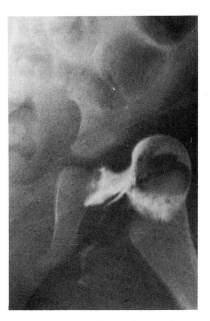

Fig. 9.19. Arthrogram of left hip. There is a large limbus preventing reduction of the femoral head.

capsule. This is easily checked by gentle rotation of the femur with the needle left *in situ*. Once a satisfactory position is obtained further contrast is injected, 2–5 ml being required, depending on the capacity of the joint. A double-contrast arthrogram can be achieved by the injection of air through the same needle, but in very capacious joints bubbling can be a problem, and air embolism has been reported. Films are taken in neutral and abducted positions, to determine the optimum position for reduction. This is usually in the abducted internally rotated position if there is anteversion of the femoral neck.

Following the initial diagnosis of dislocation and subsequent reduction in plaster or spica,

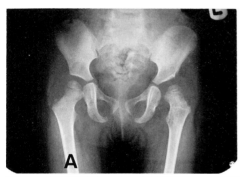

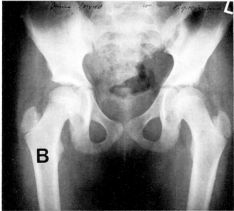

Fig. 9.20.   CDH of the left hip with late presentation. (a) The left acetabulum is dysplastic, the femoral head small and the neck broad. X-ray taken following six months in plaster. (b) X-ray of pelvis. Seven years later there is minimal residual acetabular irregularity. Excellent result of treatment.

serial radiographs are required at three-monthly intervals to observe that reduction is maintained, the acetabulum develops and the femoral head ossifies. Gonadal protection should be applied. It is often impossible to see the hips through the heavy plaster, a little easier through resin casts, but the best time to take the X-ray is at plaster change following the removal of the old one.

The femoral head should be examined for fragmentation, sclerosis or a cessation of epiphyseal growth which might indicate iatrogenic ischaemic necrosis (Fig. 9.18). Late sequelae of treated CDH may include the development of coxa vara, premature fusion of the growth plate, flattening of the femoral head and premature osteoarthrosis at the hip (Fig. 9.20), however efficient treatment can produce excellent results.

The greatest care must be exercised in examination of the film requested by a surgeon after supposed closed reduction and spical fixation. The dislocated head may lie exactly behind the acetabulum and appear reduced. If there is the slightest doubt, screening, tomography or CT scan must be ordered.

Ultrasonography

Ultrasound is of great value in detecting subluxation and dislocation of the infantile hip prior to the development of the ossific nucleus of the femoral head. It is in precisely this group of children that radiographs are most difficult to interpret.

Graf (1983) used a fixed arm unit. Screening in two planes he demonstrated that the sonograms detected deformities of both the femoral head and the acetabulum. However real-time ultrasound is portable, much simpler to operate, and reveals transient displacements (Clarke *et al.* 1985). It can also be used while reduction of a previously displaced hip is maintained in an abduction brace. The technique requires expertise and an examination in two defined planes. However it is non-invasive and a useful adjunct to radiography, both for screening infants at risk and for follow-up studies.

THE PAINFUL HIP

The infant
The commonest cause of pain in the neonatal hip is sepsis, either osteomyelitis, septic arthritis or both. While the mother may notice crying as the nappy is changed or immobility of the affected leg which lies in flexion and abduction, commonly the patient presents to a paediatrician as an ill baby with pyrexia, vomiting, icterus or convulsions and few local signs. Other possible causes of pain at this age are birth fractures, fractures due to osteogenesis imperfecta, haemophilia, neoplastic disorders, and in the older infant Caffey's disease. The diagnosis depends on a high degree of suspicion in a baby with an immobile leg and radiological evidence of widening of the joint space. Oedema in the inguinal region appears only after irreversible destruction has taken place. Treatment includes antibiotics, but decompression debridement of the joint should be undertaken at operation (Griffin & Green 1978). If there is no pus in the joint the femoral neck should be drilled to exclude osteomyelitis.

Radiology
The first sign is swelling due to soft-tissue oedema. Brown (1975) demonstrated that the so-called capsular line seen on the AP film is intermuscular. Later there is widening of the joint space and subluxation. Cervical periostitis indicates that the primary focus is in the bone (Fig. 9.21).

The effects of the infantile infection include delay in femoral capital ossification. Isotope scanning may be useful, as the infection becomes quiescent, in demonstrating the presence of a viable femoral head. At the time of presentation the scan may reveal pelvic or femoral neck osteomyelitis not seen on X-ray. It is imperative to effect a precise diagnosis if cervical pseudarthrosis has occurred as a result of the infection (Lloyd Roberts 1978). Surgery is required if the head and shaft are dissociated. Arthrography and simultaneous manipulation and screening may assist the diagnosis. Demon-

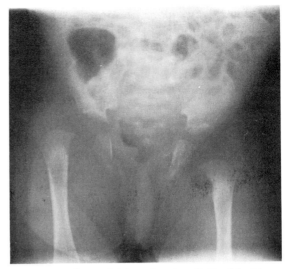

Fig. 9.21. Infant with bilateral septic arthritis of the hips. The right hip is dislocated, the left subluxes inferiorly. There is metaphyseal destruction on the medial borders of both femoral necks due to osteomyelitis.

stration of cervical pseudarthrosis will lead the surgeon to contemplate stabilization, but if the femoral head is totally destroyed osteotomy may be required.

A late sequel of neonatal infection is the development of a dense and irregular femoral head simulating Perthes' disease. Previous sepsis may be diagnosed on noting trabecular irregularity and increased radiodensity in the metaphysis and acetabulum, but these are not always present. If the growth plate was affected there will be prominence of the greater trochanter and shortening of the neck.

Pyogenic arthritis in childhood
The hip is painful flexed and lies in external rotation, and the child is usually ill. An acute onset and high fever differentiate this from tuberculous arthritis. There is focal tenderness with anterior pressure over the hip joint. Radiographs must be carefully searched for widening of the joint space or metaphyseal osteomyelitis (Fig. 9.21). There may also be displacement of muscle surrounding the joint by the capsular distension, or subluxation. However, in the early case the radiographs are normal.

Early drainage is indicated. Late sequelae include avascular necrosis and premature fusion, but are less common than in neonatal infection. Bone scanning during the acute infection occasionally shows a cold joint due to compromised vascularity from the pressure of pus within the joint. This is prognostically serious and very urgent decompression is indicated.

The painful hip in childhood
A very painful hip in the older child is most often due to sepsis, but tuberculosis, traumatic and toxic synovitis, arthralgia of rheumatic fevers, capital necrosis as in sickle cell disease, haemarthrosis, juvenile rheumatoid disease and hysteria must all be considered. When the pain is less severe the child will present mainly with a limp. The irritable hip syndrome, Perthes' disease and slipped upper femoral epiphyses are the three most common causes.

Irritable hip syndrome
This is the term used by clinicians to describe the painful hip with associated muscle spasm and restricted movement and sometimes pain to the knee. The underlying cause is a synovitis which is sometimes traumatic. The disease is idiopathic and self-limiting, but is occasionally recurrent but without long-term sequelae. It occurs in children aged 3–10, and is a little commoner in boys. Radiographs are either normal or have some swelling of the muscles around the joint. Nuclear scanning with pinhole images will show either a normal scan or some general increase in uptake through the joint relative to the normal side. Long-term follow-up is not indicated.

PERTHES' DISEASE (LEGG–PERTHES DISEASE)

Avascular necrosis of the femoral capital epiphysis of unknown origin is known as Perthes' disease. The children present with pain, limp, limitation of movement, especially of internal rotation and abduction, and on occasion wasting of the thigh muscles. There is a 4:1 male to female ratio. Girls have a worse prognosis than boys. Thirteen per cent of cases are bilateral. The children present between three and 12 years, with a peak occurrence around five years. Anthropometric measurement has revealed that affected children have diminished stature, and diminished breadth at the shoulders and pelvis. Disproportionate growth has been noted, the forearm growth being more impaired than the upper arms, and the children have delayed skeletal maturation. Perthes'-type changes are seen in some of the skeletal dysplasias, especially multiple epiphyseal dysplasia and the osteochondrodystrophies, and there is a known association with brachydactyly. Avascular necrosis of the femoral head is also seen in sickle cell disease, Gaucher's disease, hypothyroidism, renal failure, steroid arthropathy and secondary to treatment for congenital dislocation of the hip.

In Perthes' disease the form of treatment is currently the subject of controversy and debate. The principle of treatment is to contain the femoral head within the acetabulum, thus preventing deformity. Those not requiring treatment include children under five years of age, and those with limited involvement of the femoral head as defined by radiography, such patients having a uniformly good prognosis. Containment may be achieved by braces which hold the hip or hips in flexion, abduction and internal rotation, or by upper femoral osteotomy. Brace therapy may be complicated by diminution in growth rate of the immobilized limb. The clinician may require both limb-length radiographs to act as a baseline and an X-ray in the brace to demonstrate that treatment has in fact achieved containment.

Radiology
At presentation AP and frog lateral or Lowenstein lateral X-rays are indicated, the AP view to include both hips. Gonadal protection should be omitted in girls for the first film but should

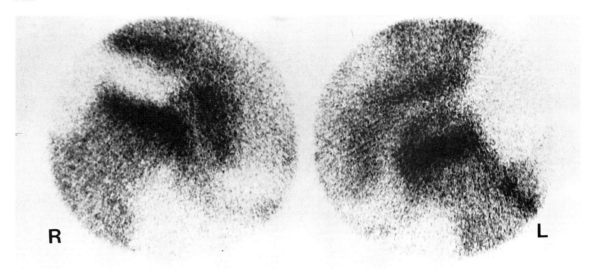

Fig. 9.22. Pinhole view of the hips of a child with Perthes' disease. On the right there is a cold anterolateral two-thirds of the right femoral head, a classical appearance of Perthes' disease. The normal left hip is shown for comparison.

be included on follow-up radiographs. If there is any abnormality of shape or epiphyseal modelling, other than the Perthes' changes, which might suggest a dysplasia then further skeletal X-rays are taken as indicated. Serial follow-up examinations take place at three- to four-monthly intervals, extending to six months and

yearly as clinical symptoms resolve and the rate of radiological change slows. At the time of presentation the radiograph may be normal. Isotope bone scanning will, however, show the classical Perthes' changes of a cold anterolateral two-thirds of the femoral head even at this stage (Fig. 9.22). The earliest radiological signs are a

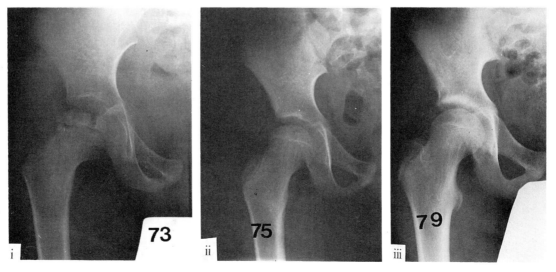

Fig. 9.23a. (i, ii, iii) Serial X-rays of a boy with Perthes' disease of the right hip. At presentation there is fragmentation of the femoral head which resolves to virtual normality in four years.

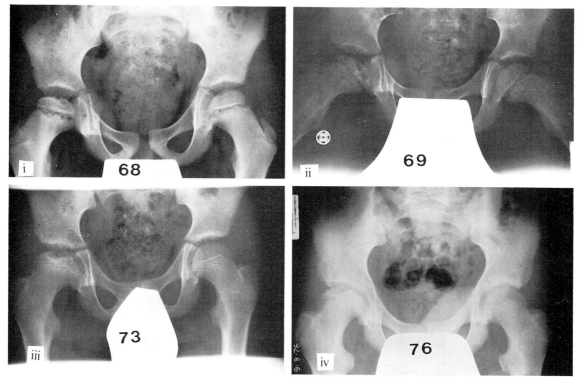

Fig. 9.23b. (i, ii, iii, iv) At presentation there is a widened joint space, slight increase in density of the femoral head and fissuring of the epiphysis on the right. (ii), (iii) and (iv) show the evolution of the changes over an eight-year period. There is still a sequestrum present. The child is currently asymptomatic.

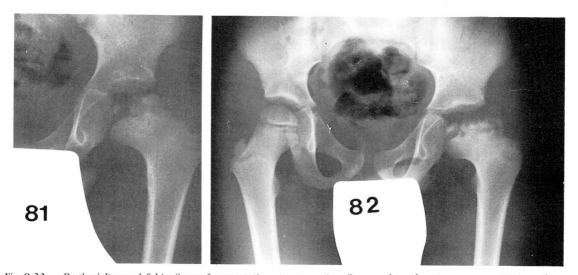

Fig. 9.23c. Perthes' disease, left hip. Severe fragmentation at presentation. One year later there is some reconstitution of the head but it has become flattened and is subluxing laterally. The acetabulum has become flat, the femoral neck broadened and shortened. These changes carry a poor prognosis.

slight increase in joint space, which is the cartilaginous overgrowth of the femoral head,
some relative osteoporosis of the hip, and a subchondral fissure, best seen in the lateral view.
As the disease progresses, the ossified epiphysis
becomes smaller in the vertical diameter than
its counterpart, and it increases in density and
fragments (Fig. 9.23). The increased radiodensity represents new bone ensheathing dead trabeculae (McKibbin & Ralis). Growth of vessels
and removal of dead bone are indicated by
radiolucent areas.

Metaphyseal cysts develop in approximately
one-third of patients. These are most frequently
found laterally, just under the growth plate.
They may be multiple. The fragmentation of the
femoral head is due to resorption of the dead
epiphysis and the reossification. During this
phase lateral extrusion of the head may be seen
on X-ray and confirmed by arthrography (Fig.
9.24). The extrusion is accompanied by broadening of the femoral neck and growth plate,
and the acetabulum enlarges in an attempt
to contain the broadened head and cartilage.

The radiological extent of the disease may be
defined using the Catterall (1971) grouping and
the concept of the 'head at risk' (Lloyd Roberts
et al. 1976).

The Catterall grouping requires good-quality
AP and lateral X-rays of the hip:

Group 1. Only the anterior epiphysis is involved. There is no collapse and no sequestrum
formation.
Group 2. More involvement and collapse of
the femoral head and sequestrum formation.
Group 3. Most of head involved. There is a
central sequestrum. Normal bone laterally may
appear as specks of calcification, which subsequently displaces in an anterolateral direction.
Group 4. Total epiphyseal sequestration,
showing as a dense line.

The head-at-risk signs are: lateral subluxation; speckled calcification lateral to the epiphysis with a translucency in its lateral margin;
a diffuse metaphyseal reaction; and a horizontal
growth plate.

Nuclear imaging. Scanning gives dynamic information about the state of vascularization of
the femoral head. It is frequently positive when
the X-rays are normal. There is, however, no
close correlation between the appearance of the
hips on scanning and Catterall grading. Scan
abnormalities fall into three main patterns:

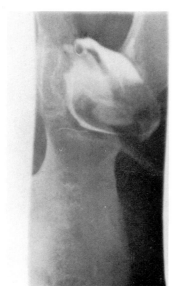 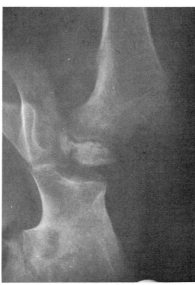

Fig. 9.24. The flattened
cartilaginous head and lateral
subluxation are well shown on
the arthrogram.

1 The classical appearance of a cold lateral two-thirds of the femoral head.

2 A generalized increase in uptake throughout the epiphysis and growth plate which represents repair.

3 A mixed scan pattern with cold areas interspersed with hot areas which is intermediate and may represent repeated insults.

A scan is indicated at presentation, as it is both diagnostic and gives a guide to the state of vascularity of the head. The authors do not routinely re-scan unless there is a clinical problem.

Arthrography in Perthes' disease. Containment is contraindicated or impossible if there is spreading of the capital epiphysis sufficient to cause it to abut on the acetabular margin in abduction. This can only be determined by arthrography and screening on abduction and internal rotation to confirm that the lateral cartilaginous epiphyseal margin can be contained within the acetabulum.

The arthrogram is done in the X-ray department with an aseptic technique and with screen control. The hip is manipulated and films taken in abduction with varying degrees of internal and external rotation to determine the degree of containment of the femoral head and degree of cartilaginous flattening (Fig. 9.24) and the relationship of the flattened cartilage to the underlying ossified area.

The long-term prognosis in Perthes' disease is variable and can range from return to virtual normality to residual flattening of the femoral head with coxa vara, coxa magna and broadening of the acetabulum.

In the adolescent who previously had the disease, pain is rare but does occur. Grossbard (1981) showed that the cause of the pain could be established using plain films and arthrography, and included osteochondritis dissecans, a torn labrum, and hingeing of the enlarged femoral head on the outer lip of the acetabulum.

It is current practice to advise containment, by operation or splintage, in patients over the age of four years with Catterall grade 3 or 4

involvement, or signs of a head at risk. The presence of these signs indicates destruction of the epiphysis or metaphysis. It is preferable to make the diagnosis prior to fragmentation of the head, assessing avascularity with a bone scan, and advising containment if more than a third of the caput is 'cold'.

SLIPPED UPPER FEMORAL EPIPHYSIS

Displacement of the proximal femoral epiphysis may occur suddenly or gradually. The acute slip is a fracture–separation of the epiphysis and growth plate from the metaphysis. This follows severe trauma or septic arthritis, and may be seen at any age.

In adolescents the gradual slip occurs typically between 12 and 15 years, being twice as common in boys. The patient complains of pain in the thigh and knee and has a limp with an external rotation deformity of the leg. Examination excludes underlying disorders which lead to a broad growth plate. The boy is usually fat with impaired sexual development. Associated endocrinopathies include hypopituitarism secondary to intracranial tumours, the Kleinefelter syndrome, and hypothyroidism. Epiphysiolysis may also complicate mongolism, hypothyroidism, and osteodystrophy, or follow radiotherapy or be a familial condition.

Once the diagnosis is made, management in the child with a relatively undisplaced unfused epiphysis consists of pinning the epiphysis to prevent further slip. When the epiphysis later fuses, the pins are removed and any deformity may be corrected by osteotomy. If the epiphysis is fused at presentation, osteotomy to correct limb posture may be undertaken at once. In the untreated child continuing medial slip of the epiphysis takes place and severe osteoarthritis and avascular necrosis may result. Avascular necrosis of the head may occur spontaneously or be a complication of manipulation.

Radiology
Standard frontal and lateral radiographs of the affected hip are mandatory once the lesion is

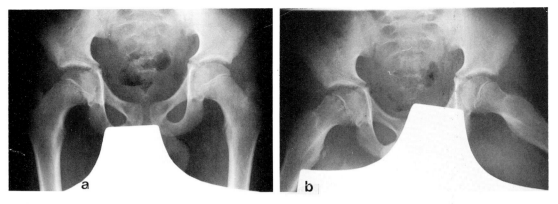

Fig. 9.25. (a,b). AP and lateral view of the hips in a boy with a slipped femoral epiphysis on the right. There is osteoporosis of the right hip seen well on the AP view. A line extended along the femoral neck does not pass through the epiphysis. The slip is easier to appreciate on the lateral view.

suspected. The slip is easier to see on the lateral view. The 'frog' lateral must be used with care as further displacement may occur. On the frontal view the lesion can be suspected, as there is usually some osteoporosis of the hip, apparent decreased vertical height of the epiphysis, and widening of the metaphysis, and a line extended through the femoral head with the superior aspect of the femoral neck will be medial to the femoral capital epiphysis (Fig. 9.25). In normal hips some of the epiphysis will lie lateral to this line. Another sign is that the femoral metaphysis on the affected side fails to overlap the lower medial aspect of the acetabulum. When assessing minimal slip of the contralateral hip, it may be wise to obtain an AP view in which the X-ray beam passes in the same plane as the

growth plate. This is effected by internally rotating the femur until the femoral neck lies in the coronal plane. In chronic cases periosteal new bone will be seen buttressed along the posteromedial aspect of the femoral neck. In gross cases—most commonly in children with renal osteodystrophy—the lateral femoral neck may even articulate with the acetabulum.

Pinning of the adolescent hip is technically difficult (Turner *et al.* 1984). Radiation can be reduced using image intensification linked to an image storage device. The problem is that in cross-section the epiphysis is crescent-shaped, and to hold it pin-tips must be placed a few millimetres from the articular surface. However, a pin that transgresses the joint posteriorly will appear to be in the head on a standard AP view

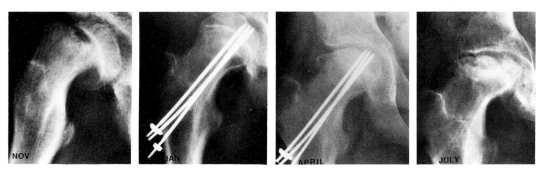

Fig. 9.26. Severe slip of the right femoral capital epiphysis. A good reduction was achieved with pinning. The tip of the pins, however, protrude into the joint space. Five months after surgery the epiphysis is flattened due to necrosis of the head and by eight months there is complete avascular necrosis of the femoral head.

(Fig. 9.26). Proper placement may be seen by rotating the C-arm with the leg fixed on an orthopaedic table, but it is only ensured by leaving the leg free and rotating it whilst screening.

Post-operative radiological screening may be advisable if there is doubt about the pin position obtained at operation. Follow-up radiographs are required at six-monthly intervals to assess fusion of the growth plate, the contralateral hip being observed for any predisposition to slip.

Avascular necrosis leads to a sequential change in femoral head density (Dunn & Angel 1978) and may occur within two years of the onset. Chondrolysis may be seen as a narrowing of the cartilage space within six months of operation. It is accompanied by osteoporosis and foveal erosion and predisposes to early growth plate closure and coxa magna. Both complications have been noted in the absence of treatment.

Protrusio acetabuli

Medial displacement of the inner wall of the acetabulum with medial displacement of the femoral head is a rare condition in childhood (Fig. 9.27). It can occur in bone-softening conditions, secondary to trauma or arthritis. It is occasionally seen as an apparently idiopathic condition. The differential diagnosis includes monarticular seronegative arthritis and adolescent idiopathic chondrolysis (Bleck 1983). The severe form, with medial intrapelvic displacement of the femoral head, is very rare. The child presents with pain and severe limitation of movement.

Femoral dysplasia

Development anomalies of the femur include proximal focal femoral deficiency and congenital coxa vara. These conditions have been fully reviewed by Lloyd Roberts (1978).

Coxa vara

The angle formed by the femoral neck with the shaft is around 150° at birth decreasing to 120–130° in adult life. The difference in the two age groups is due to relative increased growth of the subcapital growth plate medially in the infant which changes to greater growth in the lateral position as the child grows older. Coxa vara can be primary or may be secondary to disturbance of the normal growth plate. Causes will include trauma, infection and avascular necrosis. In these situations the femoral neck is underdeveloped while trochanteric growth continues. The actual angle of neck on the shaft remains normal so the coxa vara is apparent rather than a true one.

True coxa vara in which there is a genuine reduction of the angle occurs as a primary condition—infantile coxa vara—but is also seen

Fig. 9.27. There is bilateral protrusio acetabuli in this 16-year-old boy. The protrusio is more severe on the left. He presented to the orthopaedic clinic complaining of left hip pain. He had been treated with steroids in the past for asthma. The protrusio could be due to bone softening due to the steroids, but there was no other stigma. The precise aetiology of his lesion is not known.

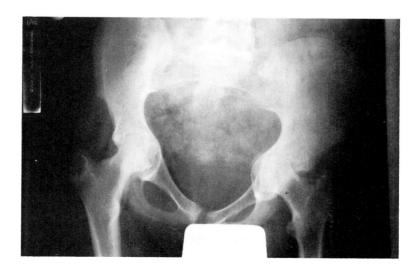

associated with a congenital short femur, bone-softening conditions and some skeletal dysplasias. A combination of clinical and radiological examination will usually ascertain the cause.

In infantile coxa vara the child presents with a painless limp, noticed shortly after he starts to walk. The sex incidence is equal. About one-third of cases are bilateral. The aetiology is unknown. The radiological changes are a widened growth plate which lies vertically rather than obliquely, a decrease in the angle of the femoral neck and shaft and characteristically a triangular metaphyseal fragment at the medial femoral neck. Complete slip of the epiphysis can also occur.

Proximal focal femoral deficiency

The condition is one in which there is variable failure of development of the femur. The mildest form is characterized by a short thigh, bowed laterally, often associated with fragmentation of the upper femoral epiphyses. These children have stable hips and the condition may be detectable at birth. At its most severe there is only a stub of distal femur remaining. There is no articulation with the pelvis and there is no acetabulum. Between these extremes are other degrees of severity. The classification is based on the presence and location of the femoral head. Limb-shortening is obvious and the limb is unstable on the pelvis. Ipsilateral fibular hemimelia occurs in about 50% of cases (Fig. 9.28).

Radiology

The surgeon must decide whether instability exists and if reconstructive procedures can lead to a mobile, stable joint. In the first year of life, if there is no ossification in the position normally occupied by the femoral head, an arthrogram will be required to determine if a head exists. However, reduction or absence of the acetabulum usually implies absence of the femoral head. Where an unossified head is present, the radiological characteristics of the most proximal

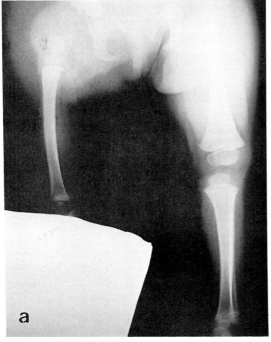 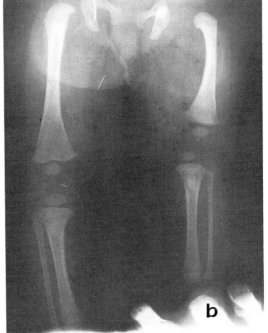

Fig. 9.28. Two children with proximal focal femoral deficiency. (a) Only a tiny stub of distal femur remains. There is ipsilateral fibular amelia. (b) There is only mild deficiency and the acetabulum is well formed. The prognosis is good.

area of ossified femur are important. A pointed sclerotic end indicates imminent disintegration of the junction between the bone and cartilage. However, a broad rounded end with sclerosis in the central shaft indicates a good prognosis in which progressive ossification of the cartilage model will occur.

Genu varum—bow legs

A degree of varus deformity of the knees is common in the newborn. This is a normal developmental appearance, but it can be very exaggerated and appear almost pathological. The normal varus appearance of the knee in the newborn decreases with growth until the more adult slightly valgoid appearance occurs slowly after the age of two. It is important to recognize the developmental genu varum as it does not require active treatment. Radiologically the tibia is seen to be adducted on the femur. There may be a degree of accompanying tibial torsion. The medial aspects of the distal femoral and proximal tibial epiphyses are accentuated and often beaked. The medial cortex of the tibia is thickened (Fig. 9.29). A more severe degree of genu varum is seen in Blount's disease, rickets, or secondary to damage to the growth plates of the knee by infection or trauma.

Blount's disease (tibia vara)

This is an entity distinct from the physiological genu varum. The infantile form is more severe, but the disorder can occur in adolescents. The child is seen to have progressive bowing of the legs, with internal tibial torsion. Radiographs show a depression of the medial tibial plateau, and widening of the medial joint space. There is deficient ossification of the medial tibial epiphysis and irregular metaphyseal ossification, radiolucent zones separating islands of bone with a curved prominence or beak on the postero-medial part of the proximal metaphysis (Fig. 9.30). Premature fusion of the medial growth plate may follow. Tibia vara may be difficult to distinguish from severe physiological bowing. Lack of bowing in the distal femur and the formation of a 'beak' favour tibia vara, which is most frequent in Finnish, Hungarian and Negro children. A full-length weight-bearing film of the legs is used to calculate the angular deformity. Treatment is by corrective osteotomy, which may need repetition during growth.

Knock-knee (genu valgum)

Physiological knock-knee occurs in the toddler as he learns to stand on a wide base. Physiological knock-knee, often associated with apparent flat feet, will resolve after 2–3 years, and detailed investigation is not required. When an infant is brought to the clinic he is examined walking and standing. The severity of the condition is determined by measuring the distance between the malleoli, the intermalleolar separation (IMS). A torsional deformity should be excluded as many have internal femoral torsion, the internally rotated patellae being the cause of the parents' concern.

More severe genu valgum occurs secondary to rickets, trauma, osteomyelitis and bone

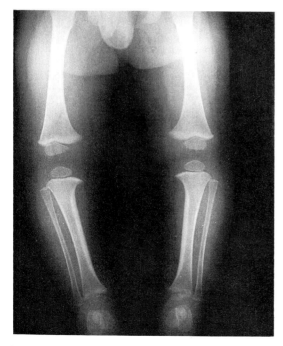

Fig. 9.29. Infantile genu varum on the right. The beaking of the proximal tibia and thickening of the medial cortex of the tibia are well demonstrated.

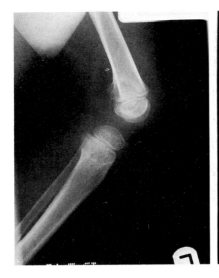 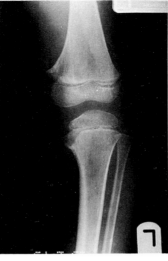

Fig. 9.30. Blount's disease. The flattening of the medial tibial epiphysis and the defective ossification of the proximal tibial metaphysis are well seen. There is also some beaking of the distal femoral metaphysis.

dysplasias including the Ellis van Creveld syndrome, in which there is patellar hypoplasia.

The limb bones—aplasia and dysplasia

Reduction deformities may result in absence of the whole limb, partial or complete absence of the long bones, the foot being attached to the pelvis, or a longitudinal defect with, for instance, loss of the medial foot, the tibia and the femur. The malformations of the lower limbs are similar to those of the upper limb but there are some differences. In the upper limb the abnormalities progress from the distal portions proximally, whereas in the lower limb femoral abnormalities occur alone or with only minimal involvement of the tibia. Fusion abnormalities are rare in long bones of the leg.

Complete femoral aplasia occurs but is rare. Bifurcation of the distal femur is another rare anomaly. Tibial aplasia is rarer than fibular aplasia. It is often associated with a claw hand and CDH.

Radiology will identify the absent bones and enable assessment of limb stability and function to be made.

Angular and rotational deformity and discrepancy of length

Angular deformity—congenital tibial bowing.

Mild physiological bowing of the legs is common in the infant and resolves spontaneously. It is usually an isolated lesion, may be bilateral, and is probably due to positional abnormalities *in utero*. The bowing is usually posterior and medial. Radiologically a thickened cortex is found along the concavity of the curvature.

Anterior tibial bowing carries a less favourable prognosis, and when associated with a narrow medullary canal may proceed to fracture and pseudarthrosis. These children frequently suffer from neurofibromatosis.

Tibial bowing of both varieties is seen in association with bone-softening conditions such as osteogenesis imperfecta, rickets and hypophosphatasia. It is also a feature of campomelic dwarfism and thanatophoric dwarfism. The conditions are easy to identify by their other features. It is frequent in fibrous dysplasia, especially the monostotic variety.

Rotational deformity (torsion). A bone has a torsional deformity if it is twisted in its longitudinal axis. Whereas an angular deformity can be detected radiologically, a torsion is more difficult to detect by conventional radiography. The diagnosis is, therefore, clinical. The majority of torsional problems relate to intoeing produced by internal femoral or tibial torsion. External rotation of the foot is seen in a few infants and is due to external torsion in the limb bones, as an acute deformity after femoral fracture, or in an adolescent with a slipped upper femoral epiphysis.

Anteversion of the femoral neck is a torsional deformity which has been discussed in dealing with CDH. Children who present with intoeing usually have an internal torsion in the femoral diaphysis. It is thought to be clinically measurable by an increased range of internal rotation of the femur (estimated by observing the patella) and a decreased range of external rotation. (This supposition is not always true, as in cerebral palsy increased internal rotation results from inward turning of the whole bone consequent upon the activity of the hamstrings.) However, palpation of the greater trochanter allows clinical estimation of the position of the upper femur.

In the tibia an internal twist is measured by observing the relationship of the bicondylar plate (at right angles to the direction in which the patella points) and the bimalleolar plane. Normally these lie at $45°$ to each other, but in internal tibial torsion the malleoli are rotated round and may come to lie in the same (normal) plane as the condyles.

The infant with torsion is normally a toddler brought to the clinic because of intoeing. Watch him walk. If his patellae point inwards this indicates femoral anteversion. In the normal four-year-old the midpoint between internal and external rotation is in the sagittal plane and the amount of femoral torsion can thus be measured. Radiographs are not generally helpful, but as dysplasia of the hip is often accompanied by an internal torsion in the upper femur an AP X-ray of the hips is wise. Measurement of femoral torsion can be made using the radiographic and ultrasound scanning techniques mentioned when discussing femoral anteversion. Ultrasound has been reported to be of value in estimating tibial torsion. Treatment is generally not required, but the condition changes little after the age of eight years, and very occasionally derotation osteotomy is required.

If on walking the intoeing infant's patellae point forwards, then examine the tibiae for torsion. If tibial torsion is absent then the cause is in the foot, i.e. forefoot adduction, which is an angular deformity. In this case radiography defines the level of the deformity as described for talipes.

Limb length discrepancy can occur due to overgrowth of the affected limb or shortening, either congenital or acquired. Minor degrees may require no treatment. Major discrepancies may lead to pelvic tilt, scoliosis and osteoarthrosis. Successful management depends upon accurate diagnosis and meticulous surgical care, and both of these require considerable collaboration between radiologist and surgeon. The causes of limb length inequality include:

Congenital soft tissue anomalies—causing overgrowth of the limb.
1 Arteriovenous fistulae and Klippel–Trenaunay syndrome.
2 Haemangiomata and lymphangiomata.
3 Fibrous dysplasia.
4 Neurofibromatosis.
5 Congenital hemihypertrophy.
6 Beckwith–Wiedemann syndrome.

Causes of decreased growth include:
(a) *Congenital bone anomalies and dysplasias*
1 Congenital short femur and/or coxa vara.
2 Congenital dislocation of hip or knee.
3 Congenital absence of tibia or fibula.
4 Talipes equinovarus.
5 Dyschondroplasia.

(b) *Neurological disorders*
1 Anterior poliomyelitis.
2 Cerebral palsy.
3 Developmental anomalies of the spine and spinal cord.

(c) *Trauma and infection*
1 Growth plate injuries. These may include premature fusion after prolonged immobilization.
2 Malunion of diaphyseal fractures with excessive overlap. Accurate reduction and

union may be followed by relative lengthening.

If the discrepancy was present at birth, congenital soft-tissue or bone anomalies are likely. With acquired lesions there is an appropriate clinical history. The lower limb is the usual cause of concern, but the clinical examination must include measurements of the upper limbs. Detailed anthropometry including skin thickness may lead to a diagnosis of unilateral hypoplasia of gigantism. External signs of spinal dysraphism are excluded, and the skin examined for naevi and haemangiomata.

Radiography

When the discrepancy is discovered the initial X-rays will include an AP X-ray of thoracic and lumbar spine and pelvis, and AP and lateral X-rays of the bones found short on clinical examination. These films will exclude gross spinal defects and dysplasia of the hip.

Further investigation depends on the clinical diagnosis. Apart from measurement, films of the limbs are seldom indicated. Radiculography is required if intraspinal lesions are suspected, arteriography if an A/V malformation is suspected.

Accurate measurement of leg length is required and several methods are available:

1 *Teleroentgenography.* A single exposure of both lower limbs with a radio-opaque ruler placed between patient and film is taken, but some magnification is inevitable.

2 *Slit scanography.* The X-ray source is a moving slit and traverses the length of the limb. This produces no linear magnification, and measurements are made from the film. It is used with long films and gives pictures of considerable bone detail, but requires a suitably designed room.

3 *Interrupted ruler (grid) films.* The X-ray exposure is confined to the joints. A rigid, continuous radio-opaque ruler lies between patient and film. A convenient method of arranging this

is to make a wooden cassette tunnel on which the patient lies, and to place transverse wires at 1-cm intervals on the upper surface. Separate exposures are made for each joint. For accuracy the tube must be centred over each joint. If there is marked inequality of length, separate films may be required for each leg. Sandbags maintain alignment between the exposures. This is the method the authors favour. The length of each bone is calculated to assess the site and degree of shortening.

An accurate prognosis of the final discrepancy may be difficult. In poliomyelitis the discrepancy may not increase if the patient becomes mobile. In neurological disorders such as spina bifida the discrepancy is likely to be progressive. In childhood it is, therefore, wise to arrange repeat examinations at six-monthly intervals over 2–3 years before calculating the final outcome. The clinician then plots the bone length so obtained on a growth chart, originally described by Anderson *et al.* (1963). Under some circumstances the straight-line graph may be preferred (Moseley 1977).

Treatment

It is possible to retard or stop growth on the longer limb or shorten it surgically, but these are usually unacceptable to the patient. Moderate stimulation of long-bone growth is possible by circumferential periosteal division on the diaphysis, and this technique may be used in cerebral palsy or talipes at the time of other operations, the maximum gain being less than 2 cm. Discrepancy of up to 2·5 cm can be corrected by altered footwear. Between 2·5 and 15 cm limb lengthening is possible. The procedure is complicated and dangerous and the parent should be warned that there is a risk that complications may necessitate amputation.

Lengthening may be delayed until near puberty when the final outcome is more certain. However, if it is likely that two bones may need lengthening, one operation may be undertaken some years earlier. The Anderson frame, which confined the patient to bed, is used less than the Wagner or Orthofix apparatus, which permit mobility. These are distraction devices, fixed to bone at each end by two screws. Femoral lengthening is performed by fixing two screws proximally and two distally. Some surgeons then make a transverse osteotomy in mid-diaphysis. The bones are distracted over several weeks and the gap fills with new bone. More rapid healing occurs if a Z-osteotomy is made, the vertical limb of the Z being 2 cm longer than the desired lengthening. Distraction is undertaken at 1·5 mm per day, and at completion two opposing tongues of bone are in contact over 2 cm.

Radiography is required in the intraoperative or post-operative period to check that the bone alignment is parallel. At the end of distraction the final lengthening and new bone formation is confirmed, and films repeated at about three-monthly intervals. When there is sufficient bone at the distraction site the device is removed and a weight-relieving brace used for a few months. In tibial lengthening, fibular osteotomy precedes tibial osteotomy.

Neurological and vascular complications do not often require radiography, but a cessation of distraction for a period. However, subluxation at nearby joints is a constant hazard and in femoral lengthening check AP films should include the hip. Non-union requires bone grafting and the application of a plate.

THE KNEE

Congenital anomalies of the patella
Isolated congenital absence of the patella is rare. It has been described in familial cases. The commonest cause of its complete absence is as part of the nail–patella syndrome. A small sclerotic dysplastic patella is also commonly seen in this syndrome. Congenital absence cannot be diagnosed until after three years, when the ossification centre appears. Hypoplasia of the patella also occurs in congenital dislocation and quadriceps contracture. Bipartite and tripartite patellae are common incidental findings. When present they are usually bilateral, which serves to distinguish them from fractures in cases of doubt.

Patellar dislocation
Recurrent dislocation at intervals of days or weeks, or habitual dislocation in which the displacement occurs at each flexion movement, has a familial tendency and usually affects girls. Primary causes may include the ligamentous laxity associated with arachnodactyly, and connective tissue disorders such as the Ehlers–Danlos and Ellis–van Creveld syndromes. Secondary laxity of the medial capsule occurs after the initial displacement. There are a few documented cases of patellar dislocation following injections into the quadriceps, Patellar dislocation may occur if the vastus lateralis or intermedius is involved. The high patella and genu valgum with lateral rotation of the tibia and a hypoplastic lateral femoral condyle are secondary effects of habitual dislocation, as is the wasting of vastus medialis. This concept is supported by the fact that these features are seen in patellar dislocation secondary to muscle imbalance of the neurological disorders such as cerebral palsy, poliomyelitis and myelomeningocele.

The first episode of dislocation in subluxation and recurrent dislocation of adolescents is usually precipitated by trauma and is very painful. The patella dislocates laterally and the medial quadriceps expansion is torn. The pain over the medial joint line and effusion may thus lead to the mistaken diagnosis of meniscal tear. Hypermobility of the patella or apprehension on attempted lateral displacement leads to the true diagnosis.

Radiography
AP and lateral views with 30° of flexion and skyline views at 30°, 60°, 90° of flexion are the standard radiographs required in assessing the patella. In normal extended knees the patella is subluxed laterally, the medial facet rarely being in contact with the femoral condyle, congruity being attained during flexion. In recurrent dislocation or subluxation the patella rides high and is displaced or rotated laterally during flexion. On the skyline views the medial space is wider than the lateral and the patella may move laterally as flexion is increased. Small erosions

may be seen on the medial patellar facet or on the lateral femoral condyle. Patella alta may be demonstrated by the method of Blackburne and Peel (1977). A lateral radiograph is taken with the knee flexed 30°. A vertical line is drawn across the posterior surface of the patella, and curved downwards to cut a line projected forward from the tibial plateau. The height from the lower articular surface of the patella to the tibial plateau (A) and the length of the posterior articular surface (B) allow the patellar index to be calculated from A/B. In the normal knee the value is 0·80, values above 1·0 representing patella alta. Jakob *et al.* (1981) have reviewed other methods of measurement.

Treatment

After the first dislocation a period of splintage and rest precedes exercises to develop the medial quadriceps. Continuous episodes, or the development of cartilage degeneration and retropatellar pain, is an indication for arthroscopy prior to corrective surgery. In children muscle balancing is obtained by a lateral release and a tightening or transfer of the medial capsule. In adolescents realignment of the patellar tendon may be achieved by medial and inferior transfer of the insertion.

Hyperextension of the knee

Mild hyperextension with a normal flexion range may occur with ligamentous laxity. Severe genu recurvatum with anterior dislocation of the tibia on the femur may be secondary to neuromuscular disorders such as meningomyelocele or arthrogryposis, and is also seen in connective tissue diseases and Larsen's syndrome. There is other clinical evidence of these lesions. Conservative therapy may be initiated by passive flexion and splintage, but lack of an infrapatellar pouch on arthrography is an indication for surgical release of the extensor mechanism.

Arthrogryposis

Clinically the infant has featureless extremities, rigidity and dislocation of joints, fibrosis of muscle groups and a normal intellect. Spina bifida may be associated, and a similar condition occurs in the legs of patients with congenital absence of the sacrum.

At the hip, flexion deformity may occur without dislocation. When one or both hips are dislocated, deformity is rare. In the knee fixed flexion or extension deformities occur. The foot may present with equinovarus, or with a congenital vertical talus. The former is treated by serial manipulation and plaster of Paris splinting for the first six months of life. Failure of correction may require excision of the talus, and following this procedure there may be spontaneous fusion between tibia and calcaneus. Long, thin, poorly modelled bones, poor muscle development and joint subluxation are noted on X-rays.

Snapping or clicking of the knee

Clicking of the knee may be palpable in the infant and usually resolves without treatment. In the older child it may be caused by a discoid meniscus or a snapping popliteus tendon. A more definite click and sensation of giving way should lead the clinician to exclude patellar dislocation.

Discoid meniscus

In this condition the meniscus is larger than normal and lacks the normal tapering. The patient usually presents at 6–8 years complaining of pain. Palpation reveals a clunk during the last 20° of extension, and there may be fullness in the lateral joint line. Radiography shows relative widening of the lateral joint space but may be normal. Arthrography and arthroscopy confirm the diagnosis (Nathan & Cole 1969). If symptoms are severe, a partial meniscectomy may be necessary.

Meniscal cysts

Usually in the lateral meniscus, these present as hard lumps on the outer side of the knee, most prominent in mid-flexion. The child may complain of mild aching. Radiologically a soft-tissue shadow may be seen on the AP film in relation to the lateral joint line, but usually the X-ray is normal.

Popliteal cysts

These are larger swellings, some 2–3 cm in diameter, usually appearing posteriorly on the medial aspect of the knee. They may be a distended bursa or, on occasion, a herniation of joint synovium, a feature which can be demonstrated by arthrography. They transilluminate and are prominent on hyperextension. Radiographs reveal a soft-tissue swelling, and ligaments. Aneurysms and an abscess should be considered in the differential diagnosis but can be excluded by ultrasound examination. Most settle spontaneously, but some are excised.

The painful knee

In the older child and adolescents, knee pain frequently affects those involved in sporting activities and presents a challenge of diagnosis. A history of a violent twisting injury followed by locking and effusion points to a meniscal injury, cruciate tear or fracture of the tibial spine, but ripping of fat pads, synovial plicae and dislocation of the patella must also be considered. AP and lateral X-rays are indicated in all such cases and will demonstrate fractures or dislocations but may be normal in meniscal or synovial lesions. Fractures of the patella are difficult to diagnose in young children because the distal fragment may be so small as not to be detectable by radiography. The diagnosis may be suggested if a high-riding patella is seen in the presence of an effusion. Houghton and Ackroyd (1981) emphasize the importance of early operative repair of this fracture.

Pain also occurs in inflammatory conditions such as acute septic arthritis, rheumatoid disease and more rarely in the haemarthrosis of bleeding disorders.

Osteochondritis of the tibial tubercle is the common cause of chronic pain in athletic boys and the diagnosis is made by asking the patient to point with one finger to the site of the discomfort. Patellofemoral pain may be due to chondromalacia patellae with or without de-tectable incongruity, osteochondritis dissecans and synovial plicae and synovial chondromatosis.

Sinding–Larsen disease

This condition is one in which there is traumatic avulsion of fragments of the lower border of the patella with associated soft-tissue swelling. The condition must be distinguished from the normal variant in which there is an accessory ossification centre lying anterior to the lower patella and parallel to it. Children with Sinding–Larsen disease present with pain. The lesion often co-exists with Osgood–Schlatter disease. The disease is self-limiting and requires only supportive treatment.

Osteochondritis dissecans

A segment of articular cartilage and underlying bone appears to undergo avascular necrosis following a subchondral fracture, the fragment then detaching to form a loose body. Though usually seen in adolescent males this condition is described at all ages from five years into adult life. The knee is most frequently affected but it also occurs in the capitellum at the elbow, the medial and superior aspect of the talus, and more rarely the superior pole of the proximal femoral epiphysis. The lesion is almost certainly traumatic initially.

At the knee the patient first experiences intermittent aching in the joint on activity, with some swelling. Later, if the fragment detaches the knee may click or lock. Typically the fragment is on the lateral surface of the medial femoral condyle (Fig. 9.31). Examination with the knee flexed reveals tenderness over the lesion. If the knee is flexed and then internally rotated pain will be experienced at the affected area when the knee is extended to 30°.

Radiography

AP and lateral and tunnel views are obtained. A radiolucent line delineates the separating fragment of dense bone. The lesion is normally clearly outlined and saucer-shaped. It must be differentiated from irregular ossification in the

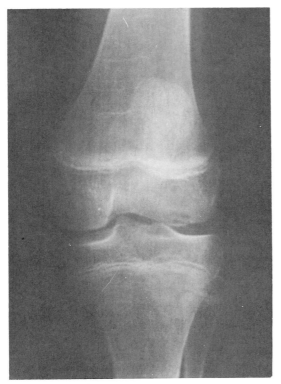

Fig. 9.31. There is a defect on the lateral femoral condyle which is the typical appearance of osteochondritis dissecans. It occurs more frequently on the medial femoral condyle.

normal distal femoral epiphysis or the irregular outline observed aged 2–6 years. A posterior lesion may only be seen on the tunnel view. Arthroscopy or arthrography will reveal interruption of the articular surface, and a small loose body may be removed under arthroscopic guidance.

Treatment

If the fragment remains *in situ* relief from weight-bearing may permit revascularization. If a plaster-cast is to be used the surgeon may request weight-bearing lateral radiographs in varying degrees of flexion to demonstrate the angle at which pressure is removed from the lesion. The knee is then immobilized in that position for some months. Alternatives include a weight-relieving caliper. With partial separation, surgical drilling of the fragment may hasten revascularization. More advanced lesions may be excised if small. If they comprise a large area of weight-bearing articular surface they are refixed using Smillie's small metal pins.

Osteochondritis of the tibial tubercle (Osgood–Schlatter disease)

This is a condition in which there is traumatic avulsion of fragments of bone at the site of insertion of the quadriceps meniscus into the tibial tuberosity. This disorder occurs in athletic children during a period of rapid adolescent growth. Boys are affected seven times more frequently than girls. There is pain and swelling at the junction of the patellar tendon and tibial tubercle. On occasion there is a history of sudden onset during sport; more usually the onset is gradual. Radiography reveals elevation of part of the apophysis which has been avulsed from the underlying tibia. A lateral radiograph is all that is required.

A lateral radiograph of a normal tubercle may reveal irregular ossification. In osteochondritis there is prominence and irregularity of the tibial tubercle with overlying soft-tissue swelling. Sometimes a small free fragment of bone is seen anterior and superior to the tuberosity. Symptoms resolve in the absence of strain and as the growth rate decreases. A splint or plaster-cast will enforce rest, and occasionally acute pain justifies a local steroid injection.

Meniscal tear

Torn menisci are much rarer in children than adults but increase in incidence during adolescence. They, like most knee lesions, are more frequent in athletic children and occur as a result of twisting or flexion injuries. The child may present acutely following trauma or may present with a history of intermittent locking and effusions. If suspected, arthrography will demonstrate the lesion. Plain X-rays are usually normal.

Patellofemoral pain

The patient localizes the pain to the region of the medial and/or lateral border of the patella. Firm pressure on the patella during flexion of the knee exacerbates the pain, and in chondromalacia there is palpable crepitus. When the knee is extended and the quadriceps relaxed, pushing the patella distally and backwards reproduces the pain, and the medial surface is tender on direct pressure. These features may be due to articular cartilage degeneration (chondromalacia patellae), synovial plicae or more rarely synovial osteochondromatosis or pigmented villonodular synovitis.

Chondromalacia patellae

Chondromalacia may be regarded as two disorders, one idiopathic in which no cause can be detected. In other patients the normal articular pressure leading to cartilage degeneration and secondary chondromalacia may result from the conditions predisposing to patellar subluxation, including muscle imbalance, or misalignment due to genu valgum, torsional deformity, or tightness of the central or lateral quadriceps.

The basic disorder is a softening of the articular cartilage. Outerbridge (1961) described four grades:

1 Localized softening, swelling and fibrillation.
2 Fragmentation and fissuring less than 1·3 cm in diameter.
3 The area is greater than 1·3 cm in diameter.
4 Erosion of cartilage to expose subchondral bone.

The condition is frequent on the medial facet, but is probably asymptomatic until it progresses to an area of habitual patellofemoral contact. The patient presents with retropatellar pain, a feeling of instability of the knee or locking. Pressure on the patella produces pain and a grating sensation. The sex incidence is equal. The disease is often insidious but there may be a clear history of trauma. Patients can present at any age between 10 and 30 years. There is a high incidence in service personnel.

Radiography

Routine views show no abnormality in chondromalacia in children. Their value is in excluding other causes of knee pain. Axial skyline views at 30, 60 and 90° with simulated weight-bearing may reveal incongruity in secondary chondromalacia. In primary chondromalacia comparison of medial and lateral facet lengths will show relative lengthening of the lateral facet, indicative of lateral patellar rotation. A positive technetium bone scan is thought to confirm the presence of a grade 4 lesion.

Treatment

A large proportion of patients with primary chondromalacia settle after months · or years without therapy and with no evidence of an increased risk of late osteoarthrosis. Those that do not settle are given a course of an anti-inflammatory drug (e.g. aspirin) and straight-leg raising quadriceps exercises for some months. Failure to resolve is an indication for arthroscopy, which will also exclude occult meniscal lesions and plicae. Grade 2 and 3 lesions may then be treated by excision of the affected area and drilling of the subchondral bone as described by Goodfellow et al. (1976). Alternatively patellofemoral pressure may be reduced by elevating the tibial tubercle and insertion of the patellar tendon by a bone graft. However, patients treated in this way are unable to kneel for long periods. Secondary chondromalacia is commonly due to relative tightness of the lateral quadriceps which may be relieved by a lateral release (Osborne & Fulford 1982).

Synovial plicae

These are bands of synovium which lie transversely across the knee. They may be found above or below the patella, or run so that they become interposed between the articulating surfaces of the patellofemoral joint. They are diagnosed at arthroscopy and excision effects a cure.

Other rare causes of knee pain in childhood are synovial chondromatosis, pigmented villonodular synovitis, chronic synovitis, synovial haemangioma or tumour. Still's disease and haemophilia will be discussed in general bone disorders.

Cortical defect.   A common site for this lesion is the distal femoral metaphysis posteriorly. This must be recognized or failure to do so will lead to unnecessary investigation. They are usually discovered as an incidental finding.

Irregular ossification variants.   The epiphysis of the knee and metaphysis of the distal femur during the normal development are very irregular. Failure to appreciate this leads to errors in diagnosis of tumours, osteochondritis dissecans and epiphyseal dysplasias. A full description of these variants can be found in Keats (1980).

THE FOOT

Foot deformities
Congenital flexed toes.
Congenital hyperextension.
Metatarsus adductus.
CTEV.
CTCV.
Pes cavus.

Terminology
The terminology to describe foot deformities is not standardized. For instance varus, as in congenital talipes equinovarus, is used by some to describe an angular deformity—medial deviation of the forefoot at the mid-tarsal joint; by others to describe a rotational deformity—an inversion of the forefoot so that it points medially; and by others to describe both of these. If manipulative or surgical correction is to be properly used the clinician must know the deformity and at what level it occurs. Discussion is simplified by the following usage.

At the ankle
Equinus or plantar flexion describes downward movement.
Calcaneus or dorsiflexion describes upward movement.

At the subtalar joint
Varus—a medial deviation of the calcaneus.
Valgus—a lateral deviation of the calcaneus.

At the mid-tarsal joint and intertarsal joints
Abduction to describe an angular deformity in which the forefoot is bent outwards, the sole remaining flat on the floor.
   Adduction is the opposite, with the forefoot bent inwards.
   Inversion (or supination) is rotational or torsional deformity in which, with the heel on the floor, the sole of the forefoot rotates to face medially.
   Eversion (or pronation), also rotational, in which the sole of the forefoot twists to face outwards.

At the first metacarpophalangeal joint
Traditionally hallux valgus refers to a disorder in which there is principally an angular deformity, the great toe deviating away from the midline.

Congenital flexion contractures of the toes
Often a familial complaint and bilateral, the patient presents in infancy with toes, usually the third and/or fourth, flexed at the PIP joint and rotated so that the tip points medially. The clinician excludes anomalies elsewhere in the foot and spine as flexion of the toes may be seen in spinal dysraphism, but in that condition there is increased tension in the long flexor muscles. Radiographs merely confirm the deformity. If treatment is indicated the toes are strapped in dorsiflexion but many correct spontaneously.

Congenital dorsiflexion of the fifth toe
The little toe of the infant is seen to lie dorsally, the plantar aspect being rotated medially, and radiographs reveal that this is due to dorsal subluxation at the metatarsophalangeal joint.

Deformed feet
A clinical diagnosis of a flat foot is a common cause for referral to orthopaedic clinics. The

patient is usually just commencing to stand, and at this time the infant obtains greater stability by abducting his legs. This is accompanied by slight eversion of the whole foot. A longitudinal arch is not seen due to the infantile fat pad in that position. The condition is bilateral and the normal shape of the foot is palpable. There is usually spontaneous resolution.

A small proportion of infantile flat feet do not improve. There may be a familial predisposition, femoral or tibial torsion, genu valgum, a tight tendoachilles or obesity. In the older child painful flat feet may be due to tarsal coalition. A standing lateral radiograph, normal in the flexible flat foot, may show some subluxation at the talonavicular joint, but there is not frank dislocation and the talocalcaneal angle is normal, unlike congenital convex pes cavus. The range of dorsiflexion and plantar flexion is equal, thus differentiating this condition from talipes calcaneovalgus.

Talipes calcaneovalgus

Many of these patients are referred in the neonatal period, the obstetrician having noted a decreased range of plantar flexion, the feet being held in dorsiflexion and eversion. As with the flexible form of talipes equinovarus, there is a greater incidence among first-born children, and this is probably an example of intrauterine restriction and malposture. Clinical examination will confirm normal muscle function in the flexor muscles. A lateral radiograph is of importance in determining the talocalcaneal angle, which should be normal, with no suggestion of a vertical talus. The condition is treated by intermittent passive manipulation.

Congenital vertical talus

In this condition the talus is plantarflexed, and the navicular articulates with the dorsal aspect of the talar head. Though the condition may appear as an isolated deformity, it may be associated with spinal dysraphism, arthrogryposis, CDH and neurofibromatosis.

Clinically the forefoot is abducted. The sole is convex, with loss of the normal arch, and in the older child the head of the talus may be palpable inferiorly.

A lateral radiograph reveals an increase in the talocalcaneal angle due to the plantar flexion of the talus relative to calcaneus. Both are held in equinus relative to the tibia. The navicular will not be seen until the age of three years, but its position can be gauged between the medial cuneiform and head of the talus.

Treatment may be attempted by manipulation and cast correction. As the foot is placed in inversion and forefoot equinus, radiographic confirmation of reduction is almost impossible. Operative correction includes a lengthening of the tendoachilles to correct the hindfoot equinus. It is useful to check complete release with a lateral radiograph. The navicular is replaced in a normal position after extensive freeing of contracted structures, the position being maintained by K wires.

Metatarsus adductus

There is increased adduction and possibly inversion of the forefoot, but the heel is normal, or in slight valgus. An AP radiograph reveals that the forefoot is deviated medially about a vertical axis at the level of the tarsometatarsal joints. The navicular does not show medial subluxation and may be lateral in relation to the head of the talus.

Radiographs are important in monitoring the effect of treatment, restoration of the normal shape being by manipulation or surgery.

Talipes equinovarus (TEV)

Equinovarus deformity may be associated with mesenchymal disorders such as arthrogryposis multiplex congenita, or with neuromuscular defects. Occult spina bifida lesions may require radiological confirmation. Having excluded other disease, talipes equinovarus may be subdivided as flexible or rigid.

Flexible or physiological TEV. An otherwise normal foot is temporarily deformed *in utero*. The condition is commoner in first-born children, and if treated in the neonatal period resolves in a few weeks.

Rigid TEV. A dysplasia of muscles, bones and ligaments leads to a progressive and intractable condition. The muscles are dysplastic below the knee leading to a wasted calf. Replacement of muscle by fibrous tissue results in an inability of the muscles to elongate with growth and tethering, which is most marked in the long flexor muscles which lie on the medial aspect of the ankle. This explains the recurring deformity, which has three basic components, radiology being required to determine the level at which they occur.

1 Forefoot adduction occurs at the tarsometatarsal, intertarsal and talonavicular joints.
2 Inversion, a medial rotation of the sole, may occur at all those joints and at the subtalar joint.
3 Equinus deformity is largely at the ankle, but additional plantar flexion of the calcaneus occurs at the subtalar joint.

The abnormalities seen on radiographs of the patient with severe talipes can only be resolved if the deformity is considered in three dimensions. The anterior aspect of the normal lateral calcaneus and the cuboid cannot be deviated medially, as the former lies against the lateral aspect of talus, the latter against the navicular. However, in TEV the tension in the tendoachilles causes plantar flexion of the calcaneus relative to the talus. The anterior aspect of the calcaneus and attached cuboid are therefore displaced downwards, carrying with them the fourth and fifth metatarsals. With inversion of the foot the anterior calcaneus comes to lie inferior to the talar neck, the cuboid below the navicular and cuneiforms (Fig. 9.32a, b).

Adaptive changes occur during growth, and the bones themselves deform. The neck of the talus deviates medially, contributing to forefoot adduction. Such cartilaginous and bony deformity increases if correction is not rapidly obtained in the neonatal period. If present, soft-tissue release alone will not produce correction.

Most authorities believe that TEV is associated with internal tibial torsion. This is best estimated clinically but rarely requires treatment. Forced eversion of the foot during treatment may lead to posterior displacement of the fibula and some degree of external torsion. Forced dorsiflexion may damage the top of the talus which becomes flat, or lead to inhibition of growth in the lower tibial growth plate.

The forefoot is inverted and adducted at the tarsal and tarsometatarsal joints.

X-rays
These are important for both diagnosis and treatment to assess the relationship of the tarsal bones and adequate reduction. The distinction between flexible and rigid TEV is usually made clinically. In the rigid form the wasting of the calf muscles is more pronounced and there is diminution in the size of the calcaneus. In the older child there is reduction in size of the whole foot. For assessment of severity and progress the position of the foot must be standardized.

In the infant, strapping should hold the foot as near to the neutral position as possible. In the older child, standing films are requested in order properly to evaluate fixed equinus. The anteroposterior view is taken with the tube angled at 45° to the sole, aiming at the hindfoot. The lateral film should be placed parallel to the hindfoot (Fig. 9.32b). With severe forefoot adduction the radiographer may be tempted to place the film against the forefoot, in which case the ankle is seen laterally rotated with an apparent flattening of the top of the talus.

Anteroposterior view
The projection of the long axis of the talus runs through the first metatarsal making a normal angle of 30° with a line parallel to the lateral border of the calcaneus (Fig. 9.32a). In talipes this talocalcaneal (TC) angle (Fig. 9.32b) is reduced due to the inferior and medial displacement of the anterior calcaneus beneath the head of the talus.

Talonavicular subluxation is always seen to be accompanied by a diminished talocalcaneal

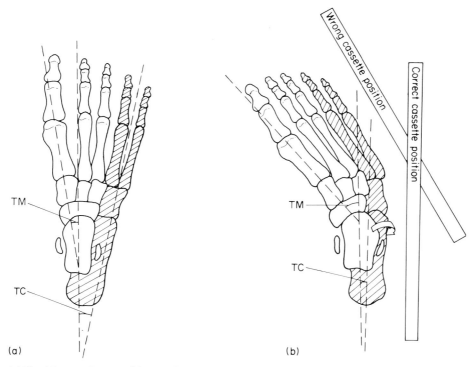

Fig. 9.32. (a) The AP view of a normal foot. In the infant the navicular does not ossify until the age of three years. An axial line projected forwards from the talus will fall between the first and second metatarsals, and make an angle of about 30° with an axial line along the calcaneus (TC angle). (b) In talipes equinovarus the lateral rays of the foot (shaded) have been displaced inferiorly and medially so that the TC angle is almost zero. The radiographer will usually position the cassette for a lateral view along the lateral aspect of the forefoot. The resulting oblique view of the hindfoot will show an apparent flat-topped talus and posterior displacement of the fibula. These structures are accurately displayed if the cassette is aligned parallel to the hindfoot.

angle but the reverse is not true. Detection of medial navicular subluxation is important for the surgeon. Though it does not ossify until three years, Simons (1978) has demonstrated that the subluxation can be inferred radiologically. Normally the axes of first metatarsal and talus almost coincide, the angle between them (TM) being small. However, in talipes the forefoot and metatarsals deviate medially, increasing the TM angle. Simons showed that in the presence of a talocalcaneal (TC) angle of less than 15° a TM angle of greater than 15° indicates talonavicular subluxation (Fig. 9.32).

Lateral view
Fixed equinus at the ankle joint may be demonstrated by examining the relationship of the

tibia and talus. Plantar flexion of the calcaneus at the subtalar joint is evidenced by a reduced talocalcaneal angle, the normal being 30°. The angle between the axis of the calcaneum and fifth metatarsal is normally 150°. Excessive pressure on the forefoot during attempts to correct equinus may lead to dorsal displacement of the forefoot relative to the hind foot, the 'mid-tarsal break'. One sign of this is an increased angle between the calcaneus and the fifth metatarsal.

Treatment
Correction of the deformity is commenced at birth by manipulation. Maintenance is by strapping, splints or cast. At 4–5 weeks AP and lateral radiographs are obtained in the corrected position. The presence of a mid-tarsal 'break' is

an indication for operative release of tethering structures. In mild cases this may only be a posterior release with Z-lengthening of the tendoachilles, posterior ankle capsule, or flexor tendons. Radiographs are usually not required, but Simons (1978) recommends an intraoperative lateral radiograph to confirm that there is no residual fixed equinus.

If the clinical and radiological studies have indicated persistent inversion, the superficial layers of the deltoid ligament may be divided. Forefoot adduction and cavus deformity necessitate division of the plantar aponeurosis, talonavicular and plantar ligaments. The corrected position may be maintained by K-wires or retentive casts.

Calcaneal osteotomy. Dwyer (1963) described this operation for persistent heel inversion (Fig. 10.33). It is appropriate for the child over four years with heavy lateral heel wear but with a normal relationship between forefoot and hindfoot. An axial radiograph of the calcaneus shows that this remains small and inverted. Dwyer described the operation through a medial incision with insertion of a tibial graft. Many surgeons now operate from the lateral side and excise from the calcaneus a wedge based laterally. This is then reinserted with the base me-

dial, and the lateral cortex closed with a staple. Alternatively, or in addition, the proximal end of the calcaneus may be displaced laterally, this position then being held with a longitudinal pin.

Calcaneocuboid arthrodesis. This operation is used in the child over four years with persistent forefoot inversion and adduction. An AP radiograph will have demonstrated the site of the deformity as principally at the mid-tarsal joint. Evans, the originator, showed that the procedure required a medial release to mobilize the navicular which will subsequently be replaced laterally. Through a lateral incision the calcaneocuboid joint is excised. The forefoot is then replaced in a normal relationship to the hindfoot. Evans used two lateral staples to maintain the correction, but a talonavicular wire may also be required.

Tarsometatarsal release and metatarsal osteotomy. Mild forefoot adduction at the tarsometatarsal joints is an indication for freeing of these joint capsules and correction in a cast as described by Heyman *et al.* in 1958. In more severe cases basal metatarsal osteotomy is undertaken on the lateral four toes.

Radiology
An AP radiograph at the age of three will show all bones ossified except the navicular. On the lateral aspect of the foot the cuboid extends across both the first and second rows of tarsals. The axis of the talus, projected anteriorly runs through the first metatarsal and forms the talocalcaneal (TC) angle with the axis of the calcaneus. In Fig. 9.32(a) the axes of talus and first metatarsal almost coincide.

An AP radiograph in talipes equinovarus shows a decreased TC angle due to the anterior aspect of the calcaneus moving down and medially (Fig. 9.34). There is medial translation and supination of the proximal tarsal bones, the sole facing medially. Talonavicular subluxation is present, as manifest by a TC angle of less than 15° and a talo-first metatarsal angle (TM) of more than 15°.

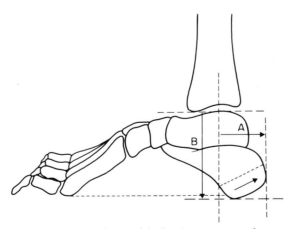

Fig. 9.33. A lateral view of the foot in pes cavus to show how the increased height of the arch may be corrected by calcaneal osteotomy with posterior displacement of the distal fragment.

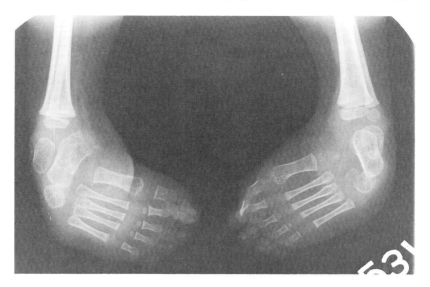

Fig. 9.34. Severe degree of talipes equinovarus bilaterally.

The correct position of the cassette for the lateral radiograph is shown (Fig. 9.32b). Radiographers may try to align the cassette along the adducted forefoot. This results in the dome of the talus appearing oblique and 'flat topped' and the fibula appears to be displaced posteriorly. These findings have led to the erroneous diagnosis of external tibial torsion in some patients.

Pes cavus

The forefoot is plantarflexed at the mid-tarsal joint, the metatarsophalangeal joints are hyperextended and the interphalangeal joints flexed, resulting in a foot with a high arch. Often the forefoot is broad. Usually there is some muscle imbalance, with either overactivity in the long flexors and extensors, or weakness in the intrinsic muscles. This imbalance may occur in Friedreich's ataxia, poliomyelitis and spinal dysraphism, but in a few patients no neurological disorder is detected. An AP radiograph of the lumbar spine must be obtained before labelling the condition idiopathic.

The calcaneocavus foot is the most intractable form of pes cavus, in which weakness of the triceps surae leads to a progressive calcaneal deformity. This causes a decreased distance between the axis of movement of the ankle joint and the posterior aspect of the calcaneus. By shortening the lever arm on which the triceps acts, there is a further decrease in the effect of the already weak triceps. Surgical correction is by posterior displacement osteotomy of the calcaneus (Fig. 9.33). Bradley and Coleman (1981) have shown that the effectiveness of the procedure can be judged by an increase in the ratio:

$$\frac{\text{Centre of tibia to posterior end of calcaneus}}{\text{Ankle joint to bottom of calcaneus}}$$

as seen on a lateral radiograph (A/B on Fig. 9.33).

Calcaneocavus deformity may be corrected by a posterior and proximal displacement of the posterior calcaneus. The deformity progresses because the lever arm (A) on which the triceps acts becomes shortened as the height of the heel (B) increases. Surgical correction can thus be assessed by measuring A, the mid-tibial axis to posterior calcaneus, and B, ankle joint to inferior calcaneus. An improvement will show an increase in the ratio A/B.

Hallux valgus

The deformity, which is a lateral deviation of the great toe, is usually associated with an increase in the angle between the first and second metatarsals (the intermetatarsal angle). The patient, usually female, presents in adolescence. The condition may be familial or associated with increased length of the first ray.

Radiographs are primarily of value in estimating the effect of treatment. Houghton and Dickson (1979) recommend a standing AP, the tube being 36 inches above the plate. The beam is directed at the mid-tarsal joint and angled 15° posteriorly. These authors describe:

(a) The hallux valgus angle—between the long axes of the first metatarsal and the proximal phalanx.
(b) The intermetatarsal angle—the angle formed at the intersection of lines drawn through the long axes of the first and second metatarsals.
(c) The angle of metatarsus primus varus—between the long axes of the medial cuneiform and the first metatarsal.

They found no true varus of the first metatarsal. The intermetatarsal angle is said to be abnormally increased if it is greater than 10°. There is correlation between the hallux valgus angle and the first intermetatarsal angle. The sesamoids may be seen to be deviated laterally.

Treatment may be by soft-tissue release of the muscles acting on the lateral side of the proximal phalanx, but this operation may be followed by hallux varus. Osteotomy of the first metatarsal shaft is also described at the neck and in the mid-shaft, the distal fragment being displaced laterally, with restoration of great toe alignment, and this is the preferred treatment. In the presence of a long first ray the first metatarsal should also be shortened.

Painful feet
Painful heels are commonly seen at about the age of 10, often in athletic boys. This is thought to be either a traction apophysitis similar to apophysitis of the tibial tubercle, or to an inflammatory disorder in a bursa associated with the tendocalcaneus. A radiograph may show increased density and patchy osteoporosis in the apophysis. Treatment is by sponge inserts to the shoes or elevation of the heel. Older adolescents, especially girls, present with a painful swelling on the posterolateral aspect of the calcaneus. A lateral radiograph confirms the prominence, probably due to periostitis from shoe pressure. Excision of the prominence may be required.

Pain in the mid-tarsal region in a 5-year-old is usually due to osteochondritis of the navicular. The child has a limp and tenderness and some swelling over the bone. Radiographs reveal increased density and subsequently fragmentation. The condition resolves spontaneously. In the adolescent, pain in the mid-foot may be due to tarsal coalition.

Tarsal coalition
In this disorder, tarsal bones are united by a bridge. Symptoms occur in adolescence, probably due to ossification of a fibrous or cartilaginous bar. The patient complains of pain in the subtalar or mid-tarsal area of the foot, especially after activity.

Examination reveals some loss of the longitudinal arch and prominence of the navicular. There is restricted movement at the affected joints; subtalar or mid-tarsal and peroneal spasm may be detectable.

Radiography
Calcaneonavicular coalition. Oblique projections at varying angles may be required to demonstrate the bar. The patient stands on the cassette, and the beam is directed from lateral to medial side at 45°. A complete bar is readily seen. Close proximity of the calcaneus and navicular and hypoplasia of the talar head should lead the clinician to suspect a cartilaginous bar (Fig. 9.35). The adjacent cortical surfaces are irregular and poorly defined.

Talocalcaneal coalition. The bridge is usually medial, being due to union of the sustentaculum tali to the middle facet of the talus, or partial union posteriorly to the sustentaculum. Rarely the anterior or posterior facets may be involved.

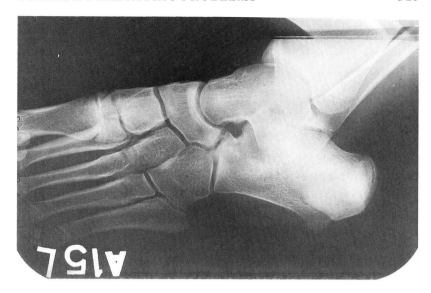

Fig. 9.35. Calcaneonavicular coalition. An incomplete bar is present between the calcaneus and the navicular. The irregular margins suggest a cartilaginous portion.

Irregular movement between the calcaneus and adjacent bones may lead to degenerative change. Mid-tarsal instability may be associated with talar beaking seen on the lateral radiograph.

Treatment
Support for the sole with an inner heel-raise may assist, or the foot may be immobilized for some weeks in a cast. In calcaneonavicular coalition in the adolescent, excision of the bar gives excellent results. Complete medial talocalcaneal bar is treated by talonavicular fusion, but incomplete lesions require a triple arthrodesis.

Metatarsalgia
Osteochondritis of the metatarsal head. The patient, who is usually a teenage girl, presents with focal pain at the metatarsal head, usually the second or third, which is tender and enlarged. Movement is diminished at the affected joint. AP radiographs reveal the head to be wide and there is a flat articular surface. The neck is thickened and the joint space increased.

Treatment is by an insole support and avoidance of sport for a few weeks.

Stress fracture. The patient complains of pain over the metatarsal shafts, usually the second or third. It most frequently occurs in adolescents after unusual activity. Clinically the affected bone is tender and a swelling may be palpable.

Radiographs may be normal in the first two weeks; later periosteal reaction along the shaft and callus becomes visible. The fracture is frequently never seen.

Morton's metatarsalgia. This is due to a painful neuroma in the second or third interdigital clefts, where plantar pressure at the level of the metatarsal head causes shooting pain. It may be seen in adolescents, especially after exercise in narrow football boots. There are no X-ray findings.

THE ARM DEFORMITIES

Congenital dislocation of the radial head
This may occur as an isolated deformity or in association with anomalies such as arthrogryposis. The child presents with limited extension and supination and the radial head is palpable.

Reduction deformity

The term amelia is used when the whole limb is absent. Phocomelia occurred in thalidomide embryopathy and describes the situation where there are no long bones between the axial girdle and the digits. Ectromelia describes the situation in which there are varying degrees of hypoplasia of the humerus and radius together with its peripheral rays. Ectromelia may be proximal or distal. It may also be axial which implies both distal and proximal shortening. Reduction deformities lead to degrees of disability of manual dexterity. The lesion is clinically obvious, but radiology is required to define the precise deformity, so that orthopaedic management may be planned to encourage maximal manual dexterity and grip. In the neonate all ossification centres will not be present, so a precise description of the extent of the aplasia may not be possible. The lesions are isolated and are not part of recognized syndromes.

'Lobster-claw hand'

Congenital absence of the metacarpals and digits leading to the lobster-claw hand is the commonest serious segmentation defect of the hand. Function is usually excellent using the thumb against the palm, and surgery is rarely required.

Radial dysplasia (radial club hand—radial aplasia)

The term radial dysplasia is used to describe the condition in which there is maldevelopment of the radius with associated abnormality of nerves, blood supply and adjacent joints. Approximately 60% of affected individuals have total aplasia, and 20% partial aplasia, which is usually of the distal portion. The remainder have hypoplasia of the radius which is small in size but with no true segmental defect. Associated absence of the radial carpal bones and the thumb are found with the most severe lesions. About 50% of cases are bilateral. Radial dysplasia is part of the vater anomalad (*see* p. 313). It is also an association of Fanconi's syndrome, congenital thrombocytopenia, the Holt–Oram syndrome, and of some other cardiac defects.

The radial deformity is identified on X-rays. When partial aplasia is present the distal portion is absent. The hand is deviated to the radial side due to the muscle contractions. Ulnar bowing and shortening is also present. The distal ulnar epiphysis often fuses prematurely. The humeroulnar articulation is often abnormal, both laxity and contractions being reported. The wrist joint is distorted due to absence of the radial carpal bones. The thumb is always abnormal in severe cases, absent in 75% and with varying degrees of hypoplasia in the remainder. The digits are usually normal.

Ulnar dysmelia

Ulnar dysmelia is a rare lesion, occurring only approximately one-third as frequently as radial dysplasia. It is occasionally associated with fibular abnormality but is not part of other syndromes. The lesion is usually unilateral. The ulnar carpal bones may be small or absent and the ulnar metacarpals and digits absent or fused. The radius is bowed and often dislocated at the elbow.

Ulnar dimelia

This rare anomaly has been described. There are usually seven fingers but no thumb and reduplication of the triquetral, capitate and hamate bones.

Segmentation defects

Errors in segmentation of the skeletal primordium occur early in fetal life and lead to important orthopaedic lesions. Radiology is required to define the lesion prior to surgery.

Polydactyly

Polydactyly is due to oversegmentation. The additional digit is commonly the thumb. Radiographs will identify the less well-formed digit which will require excision and show any additional metacarpal abnormality.

Polydactyly is an association of the Ellis–van Creveld syndrome and Lawrence–Moon–Biedl syndrome.

Syndactyly

Failure of segmentation leads to failure of separation of the fingers. Radiographs will distinguish those joined by skin bridges as opposed to bony junction. The latter is more serious and leads to greater disability. In the hands the proximal interphalangeal joint is more commonly affected, while in the foot the distal joint is affected.

The most complex deformities are seen when there is irregular segmentation, leading to syndactyly of rudimentary digits. Similar lesions occur in the feet. Syndactyly is associated with many syndromes, most notably acrocephalo-syndactyly. It is also familial being inherited as an autosomal dominant condition. There may be associated fusion of carpal and tarsal bones.

Congenital radioulnar synostosis

The commonest segmentation error in the long tubular bones is fusion of the proximal ends of the radius and ulna. The forearm is held in pronation. It is associated with XXY and occasionally XYY chromosomal abnormalities, and is also inherited as an autosomal dominant condition without any other associated lesions.

Radiology

The radius is bowed, and the head defective or absent. This distinguishes the condition from traumatic radioulnar synostosis which may occur as a complication of fracture or a posterior surgical approach to the elbow, and in which the radial head is well formed. The congenital variety is usually bilateral.

At X-ray. The capitellum is hypoplastic and the radial head dome-shaped. These features distinguish the condition from that occurring after a compression injury to the distal radial growth plate, or malunited forearm fracture, such as occurs with osteitis fragilitans.

Madelung deformity

There is a growth disturbance of one or both distal radial epiphyses. Typically the radius is bowed and short, the dislocated distal ulna presenting as a prominence. Wrist extension is limited, as is supination. It can occur as an isolated lesion. In congenital dyschondrosteosis (Leri–Weill syndrome) there is Madelung deformity, shortening of the fibula and tibia and mesomelic dwarfism. The condition is inherited as an autosomal dominant. The rest of the skeleton is normal. Madelung-type deformity is also seen in diaphyseal aclasis, but there will be exostoses visible on the radiographs allowing easy differentiation.

Radiography

The wedge shape of the distal radial epiphysis as seen on an AP film is accentuated, the ulnar part being abnormally thin. The distal radius is bowed, convex dorsally (Fig. 9.36). The lunate is wedged in the V between the distal radius and ulna. The condition must be differentiated from traumatic Madelung's deformity in which the radial bowing is absent. Rickets, though causing bowing, has a wide growth plate and the levels of the radial and ulnar styloid processes are equal.

Congenital bands and amputations

Annular bands around a limb, often with distal oedema, are due to intrauterine amniotic bands. The most severe lesion caused by these bands is that of intrauterine amputation when the severed portion of the limb may be delivered separately. Osseous or cutaneous syndactyly may also result, as may hypoplasia of the distal limb due to ischaemia. Digital curvatures, brachydactyly and macrodactyly are discussed in Chapter 12.

Congenital pseudarthrosis of the clavicle

Usually presenting in the neonate, a swelling is noted lateral to the mid-clavicle. There is no history of trauma and no functional disability.

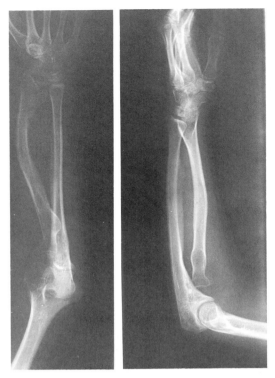

Fig. 9.36. Congenital Madelung deformity, AP and lateral views. The wedging of the lunate in a V formed of the distal radius and ulna is seen. The bowed radius distinguishes this from a post-traumatic lesion and the absence of exostoses from diaphyseal aclasis.

Radiography

The adjacent ends of the clavicular fragments are enlarged. The larger sternal fragment is above and medial to the lateral fragment. Unlike fracture of the clavicle, no callus is seen (Fig. 9.37). No other skeletal abnormalities are seen, unlike cleidocranial dysostosis, where defective clavicles are associated with skull deformities, persistent metopic suture and Wormian bones, pelvic deficiency and epiphyseal abnormalities of the hands and feet.

The painful arm—pulled elbow

Occurring in children under five years of age, the condition is commoner in the left arm of boys. It is caused by longitudinal traction on the extended and pronated arm, as when attempting to save a falling child. Anatomical

studies have shown that in this position a pull causes a partial tear in the orbicular ligament, the radial head slipping distal to the annular ligament which may become partly interposed between the radial head and the capitellum. Following the injury there is local pain, the elbow is held flexed, pronated, immobile and to the side. Treatment is a rapid supination of the flexed elbow under GA.

Radiography

Radiographs may be therapeutic, in that as the AP film is obtained the radiographer supinates the forearm, noting a click as reduction is effected. The child immediately uses the arm normally. The diagnosis depends on the history and, if correct, radiographs will reveal no abnormality. However, they should be taken to exclude fractures of the radial head.

The painful limb—pseudoparesis

Ceasing to use a limb due to pain is called pseudoparesis and is a common reason for casualty attendance in paediatrics. Causes of this will include trauma, osteomyelitis and septic arthritis. The clinical history and careful clinical assessment of the limb searching for oedema or local increase in heat and point of maximal tenderness may yield a diagnosis. A raised temperature and white cell count point to infection. It is often difficult to localize the lesion clinically, and X-ray of the whole upper limb to include the clavicle is indicated to search for an underlying cause. The X-rays are frequently normal. In septic arthritis the X-rays will probably be normal; some swelling of the joint capsule and surrounding soft-tissue oedema may be the only signs. It is rare to find destructive changes of infection or periosteal reaction with such a presentation. A bone scan may localize an infective focus in bone or show generalized increase of uptake around a joint; a negative scan does not exclude infection.

Pathological fractures through bone cysts and metaphyseal fractures of non-accidental injury are occasionally seen. The commonest fracture is probably a hairline supracondylar frac-

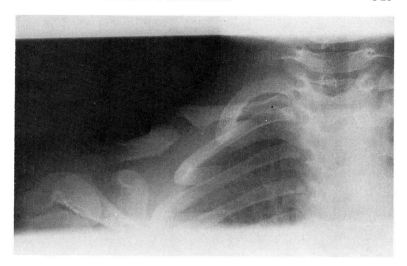

Fig. 9.37. Congenital pseudarthrosis of the clavicle in an 8-year-old boy. The edges of the clavicle at the pseudarthrosis are enlarged. The sternal fragment is medial and above the lateral fragment.

ture of the elbow. Most children with normal X-rays will recover use of the arm in a few days without specific treatment.

Osteomyelitis

Osteomyelitis usually occurs by haematogenous spread. Staphylococci are perhaps the organisms most frequently found in the older child, but streptococci and coliform bacteria are common in neonatal infection and in trophic ulcers. Salmonella is a frequent infection in the population with sickle cell disease. The child presents with malaise, fever, pain and severe tenderness in the affected area. The infection usually localizes in the metaphyses. There may be overlying cellulitis. It must be stressed that X-rays in the acute case are almost invariably normal—soft-tissue oedema may not even be apparent. The diagnosis is clinical, as the white blood count and the mandatory blood culture may be unhelpful and the ESR is non-specific. Bone scanning with Tc MDP in the acute phase may show hyperaemia and a focal lesion in the metaphysis, but is negative in about 12% of all reported series, especially in the neonate.

Management of acute infection

Active treatment must be given to all children if a presumptive diagnosis of acute osteomyelitis or septic arthritis is made. The authors believe

that the need to obtain pus for culture and to relieve pain makes emergency incision and drainage mandatory in favourable circumstances. If surgery is hazardous parenteral antibiotics are commenced, based on knowledge of likely organisms, and following the removal of blood for culture.

While radiographs are negative in acute osteomyelitis they are important in follow-up. If the lesion was near a growth plate a careful watch must be kept for premature fusion of part or whole of the epiphysis and consequent limb length discrepancy (Fig. 9.38). The development of avascular necrosis of an epiphysis evidenced by increasing density must also be sought. If reactivation of infection is suspected isotope scanning with MDP or more particularly with indium-labelled white cells is more sensitive than radiographs. If limb discrepancy develops the difference can be accurately measured on grid films.

GENERALIZED BONE DISORDERS IN CHILDHOOD

Osteogenesis imperfecta (OI)

OI, as its name implies, is a disease of defective development of bone which leads to soft brittle bones with multiple fractures and limb deformity. The bone lesions are frequently accom-

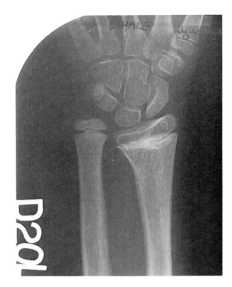 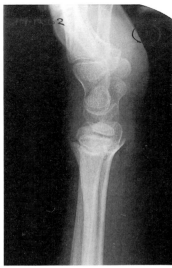

Fig. 9.38. Previous history of trauma at the distal radius. There has been damage to the growth plate with consequent shortening of the radius and premature fusion. This can also result from infection or arthritis.

panied by dental, eye, ear and ligament abnormalities, some of which are secondary to bone softening. The severity of clinical manifestation is variable and the disease is subdivided into congenital and tarda forms. Blue sclerae, once thought to be an invariable accompaniment of the disease, are not a prerequisite for the diagnosis.

Congenital form

Multiple fractures may be seen in the fetus *in utero*. Many infants are stillborn or die soon after birth. The disease is inherited as an autosomal recessive trait. Clinically the children appear to have large heads, have lax mobile joints, deformed limbs, and short stature due to a combination of fractures and bone softening. They also have abnormal dentition and bruise easily. The fractures occur with only minimal stress. There is a tendency for improvement as the patient approaches puberty.

The radiological changes are characteristic in the classical case—multiple fractures, often at different states of healing, wide, osteoporotic, poorly modelled bones, platyspondyly and poorly ossified skull vault with Wormian bones. The rib fractures may lead to thoracic constriction (Fig. 9.39).

OI tarda

The range of severity of the tarda form is very variable, and clinical and radiological features will depend on this. The child is brought to clinical attention because of the fractures. A wrong diagnosis of non-accidental injury is often made and causes great parental distress. The two can be distinguished radiologically by noting the osteopenia of OI tarda, which is often accompanied by long slender bones which are bowed. There may be mild compression of the vertebral bodies and in the skull Wormian bones are usually present. Fractures heal either normally or with rather florid callus. Non-union and pseudarthrosis can occur in the long bones. These children are more normal in stature than those with the congenital form, but some evidence of softening such as bowing, genu valgum or scoliosis will usually be clinically apparent.

Arthrogryposis

Long, thin gracile bones that are seen in OI tarda also occur in arthrogryposis. The condition is thought to be related to prenatal motor dysfunction. The patient presents clinically with muscular atrophy, joint contractions and dislocations. In about half the patients all four limbs

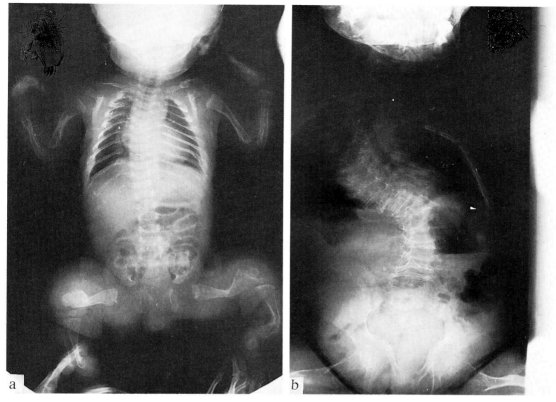

Fig. 9.39. Osteogenesis imperfecta. (a) X-ray of the skeleton of a two-month-old girl with severe osteogenesis imperfecta. There are multiple fractures of the long bones and poor modelling. (b) Now aged eight, she has developed severe scoliosis, platyspondyly and pelvic constriction.

are involved. The disease always affects the lower limbs and the involvement is fairly symmetrical. There is an increased incidence of congenital heart disease, undescended testes, hernia and other non-specific genitourinary abnormalities. Intellectual development is normal. Life expectancy after the first two years is normal but before that there is an increased incidence of death. No new lesions appear after birth but increasing contractures may take place. Treatment is aimed at preventing this and improving function of the limbs.

Radiologically one sees diminished subcutaneous and muscular development, long, thin gracile bones, and flexion deformities which may be associated with soft-tissue webbing. Fractures are frequent. Carpal coalition of some

degree is present in about 40% of patients. Hip dislocation occurs in up to two-thirds of the patients and may be bilateral. Equinovarus deformity occurs in three-quarters of the patients and scoliosis in about one-third.

None of the radiological features is specific for arthrogryposis and the diagnosis is mainly clinical.

Neurofibromatosis
Neurofibromatosis is a hamartomatous dysplasia of all three germ layers, congenital in origin, and with widespread and varied clinical manifestations. 70–80% of patients have skin manifestations, *café au lait* spots and skin tumours being the commonest. Other features include scoliosis, localized gigantism, neurogenic

tumours and pseudarthrosis. Deafness and blindness occur due to involvement of the optic and acoustic nerves. Intracranial lesions can cause hydrocephalus and epilepsy. Hypertension can occur due to renal involvement. Malignant degeneration in the neurofibromata is reported in about 5% of cases but this is mainly in adult life.

A family history is present in two-thirds of patients. The transmission is by autosomal dominant inheritance.

Radiology
The radiological features vary with the site of the lesion.

Spine and ribs
Scoliosis occurs in up to 50% of affected patients. Classically the curve is sharply angulated and may have a kyphotic element with associated rib dysplasia and 'ribbon' ribs (Fig. 9.40). It may be associated with paravertebral neurogenic tumours or an anterior thoracic meningocele. Posterior scalloping of the vertebral bodies is common. Congenital vertebral anomalies, i.e. hemivertebra, are frequent but not specific to neurofibromatosis. Tumours or hyperplasia of the nerves cause widening of the intervertebral foramina (Fig. 9.41). The ribs, as well as being thin and twisted, are often irregular and notched.

Skull
The skull vault tends to be large. Hydrocephalus can occur secondary to obstructing neurogenic tumours but is not a primary manifestation. Asymmetry of the cranial fossae, sphenoid wing elevation or aplasia, and osseous overgrowth and deformity of the facial bones are seen in some patients. Enlargement of the foramina due to tumours of the optic, acoustic and trigeminal nerves is also relatively common.

Limbs
The commonest limb manifestation is reported to be pseudarthrosis, but not all patients with

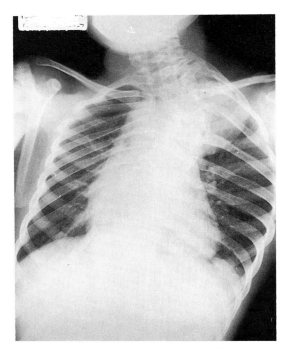

Fig. 9.40. A nine-year-old girl with neurofibromatosis. There is an acute kyphoscoliosis of the proximal thoracic spine with associated ribbon ribs on the right and a large paravertebral neurogenic tumour.

tibial or fibular pseudarthrosis have neurofibromatosis. It also occurs in fibrous dysplasia and secondary to trauma. In neurofibromatosis sclerosis of the bone and narrowing of the medullary canal and cortical irregularity are also found in the long bones. Hypertrophy of a limb and its soft tissue may be seen and must be differentiated from other causes. Bony deformity secondary to soft-tissue fibromata also occurs. Sudden increase in size of a neurofibroma suggests malignant degeneration.

Gastrointestinal and genitourinary involvement
Neurofibromatous masses may involve any organ. The symptoms will depend on the precise nature of the involvement. Dysplasia of the renal arteries is a cause of hypertension in children and can be diagnosed arteriographically. There is an increased incidence of phaeochromocytoma.

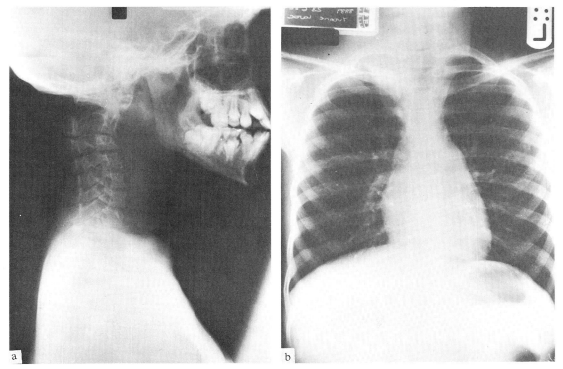

Fig. 9.41(a, b). A 13-year-old girl with neurofibromatosis. There is a large tumour in the neck extending into the upper thorax. There is anterior and lateral displacement of the trachea. Intraspinal extension is present—note widening of the foramina.

Haemophilia

The term haemophilia is used to describe the abnormal bleeding tendency with failure of blood clotting that occurs with deficiency of clotting factors. Factors VIII and IX are the two most commonly deficient, the former being four times more frequent. The disease is of variable severity. Its genetic transmission is X-linked recessive. For practical purposes the disease can be considered to be confined to the male population. A few very rare cases have been described in females. The clinical manifestations are due to bleeding into joints and muscles. Palpable abdominal haematomas presenting as pseudotumours, neurological signs from compression by haematomas, and paraplegia secondary to haemorrhage into the spinal cord are well-known complications. Synovitis due to both the direct effect of blood on synovia and later haemosiderin deposition is the first joint manifestation. With repeated bleeds synovial hypertrophy occurs, leading to impaired cartilage nutrition with subsequent erosion. The long-term effects can be severe joint derangement, articular and capsular fibrosis, and even joint ankylosis.

Radiology. Soft-tissue haemorrhage is recognized by an alteration in density of the tissues and distortion of the fat planes. Ultrasound is particularly helpful in diagnosing retroperitoneal bleeds. The child with a psoas bleed may present with hip pain or even present with acute abdominal symptoms mimicking appendicitis.

Haemarthrosis. The initial bleed can be seen as a joint effusion and it has no distinguishing features. Any joint can be involved but the knees and the elbows are most frequently affected. With repeated bleeds loss of cartilage ensues, recognizable initially by loss of joint space. Subsequent changes are cortical irregularity, cortical erosions and subcortical cysts. Occasionally haemosiderin deposition in the joint is noted as a fine increase in soft-tissue density. The intracondylar notch in the knee becomes widened and irregular (Fig. 9.42) and the patella more square. The signs are not specific as they can also be seen in juvenile rheumatoid disease. Epiphyseal overgrowth due to hyperaemia is a frequent occurrence, as is premature epiphyseal fusion. Intraosseous haemorrhage, both subperiosteal and deeper, occurs, leading to the formation of cysts of various sizes. When large they earn the name pseudotumours. Particularly in the iliac blade they can attain a very great size (Fig. 9.43).

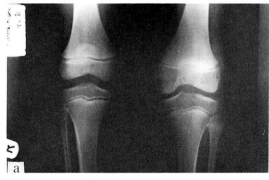

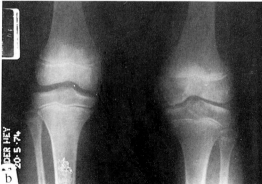

Fig. 9.42(a, b). This boy had repeated bleeds into his left knee joint. Slight enlargement of the epiphyses is seen on the early film. Four years later there is narrowing of the joint space and erosive change. The intercondylar notch is widened.

Fractures can occur through these cysts. Long-term sequelae of haemarthrosis will include limb length discrepancy due to premature epiphyseal fusion and secondary osteoarthrosis.

Management of haemophilia is by early replacement of the missing factor as soon as a bleed occurs, or prophylactic administration prior to elective procedures. With aggressive management the more severe joint destruction can be avoided.

Rickets

Primary nutritional rickets due to deficient vitamin D intake is increasingly rare in western society. Rickets due to chronic renal disease is the most frequent of the secondary causes. The bony changes may be complicated by secondary hyperparathyroidism. Familial hypophosphataemic rickets is inherited as a dominant disorder and is due to failure of resorption of phosphate in the renal tubules.

Chronic pancreatic insufficiency and coeliac disease may also be complicated by rickets. Rickets can also be induced by drugs due to interference with the normal enzymatic pathways for vitamin D absorption. Biochemical analysis will aid in differentiating the different causes.

Radiology. The hazy, cupped, irregular, widened growth plates of rickets are diagnostic (Fig. 9.44). Bowing of the long bones of the legs due to bone softening can also occur. Rarely, thickening of the parietal and frontal bones of the skull will lead to 'bossing'. In severe cases the anterior rib ends also become hazy and cupped. Slipping of the femoral capital epiphysis is a complication of the rickets of renal osteodystrophy.

An AP X-ray of the hand and knee is used for monitoring the response to treatment. As the condition improves the haziness is lost and calcification of the zone of provisional ossification occurs, with gradual incorporation into the normal bone.

In metaphyseal chondrodysplasia type, Schmidt changes very similar to rickets occur,

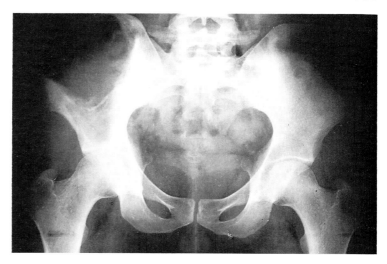

Fig. 9.43. A 16-year-old boy with haemophilia. A large pseudotumour is present in the right iliac blade.

particularly in the knees. The biochemistry is normal, allowing for easy differentiation (Fig. 9.44c).

Irregularity of the growth plates with fraying of the metaphysis and corner fractures are also found in Menke's kinky hair syndrome and rubella osteitis, but the other features of these diseases are diagnostic and confusion should not occur.

Diaphyseal aclasis (multiple exostoses, osteochondromatosis)

The disorder is characterized by exostoses protruding from the bones. The exostoses are osteochondromata and are covered by a cartilaginous cap. They occur throughout the skeleton but tend to be largest near the joints, and the knees are always involved. They can occur in an area of previous irradiation. The condition is inherited as an autosomal dominant. The child presents clinically either with a palpable mass at the site of the lesion, or with impaired joint movement due to interference by the exostosis. Treatment is by excision of the lesions where they cause clinical symptoms. In severe cases the lesions are so numerous that it will be impossible to remove all symptomatic lesions. More detailed descriptions of the disorder will be found in Gideon *et al.* (1975).

Fibrous dysplasia

Lesions of fibrous dysplasia are fairly frequently found as an incidental finding on radiographs. The radiological changes are variable and range from a soap-bubble cystic pattern to areas of

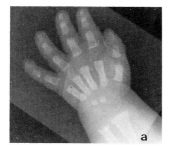
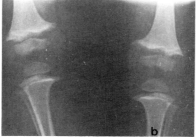
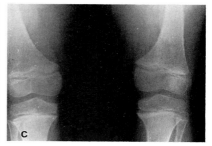

Fig. 9.44. (a) This child has congenital hypophosphataemic rickets. The fraying of the metaphyses is classical. (b) This child had renal failure. More severe changes of rickets are seen. Corner metaphyseal fractures occur and should not be confused with the lesion of non-accidental injury. (c) Mild changes of 'rickets' at the knees. This boy has metaphyseal chondrodysplasia and is biochemically normal.

sclerosis and rarefaction classically described as a ground-glass appearance (Fig. 9.45). The clinical presentation of a lesion depends on the site. In the skull vault with affection of the sphenoid bone, facial or skull asymmetry is the presenting complaint. Pain and deformity are more frequent problems in peripheral lesions. A pseudarthrosis may develop when the lesion is in the tibial shaft. The lesion of fibrous dysplasia may be monostotic or polyostotic. The polyostotic form when associated with precocious puberty and skin pigmentation is called the McCune–Albright syndrome.

Malignant infiltration

Classical bone metastases as seen in the adult population are rare in children and very rarely are the presenting complaint. Widespread skeletal infiltration may occur in neuroblastoma, rhabdosarcoma, medulloblastoma and leukae-mia and the child may present with bone pain (Fig. 9.46). This type of osteoporosis must be distinguished from the rare idiopathic juvenile osteoporosis, the osteoporosis of Cushing's disease, and disuse. The peripheral blood film or bone marrow will prove diagnostic in the case of malignant infiltration.

Juvenile chronic arthritis

Joint pain in children has many causes, of which traumatic synovitis and infection are the most frequent. Both these lesions are usually monoarticular. The commonest cause of polyarthropathy in childhood is rheumatoid arthritis. It is important to remember that this can also be monoarticular. When the polyarthritis is associated with lymph node enlargement and splenomegaly it is called Still's disease. Skin eruptions may also occur. Most children with juvenile chronic arthritis present at about 3–5

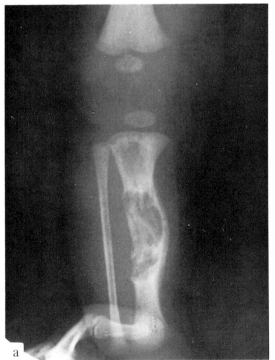
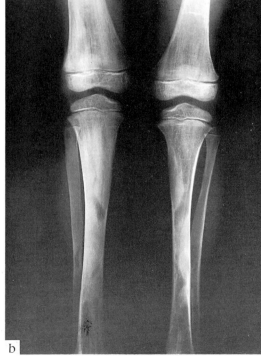

Fig. 9.45.   (a) Right tibia of a young infant with monostotic fibrous dysplasia. The cystic changes are well shown. (b) Polyostotic fibrous dysplasia. The areas of mixed sclerosis and amorphous bone are shown.

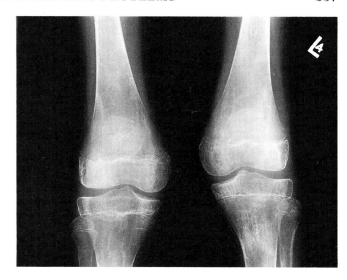

Fig. 9.46. Leukaemic infiltration of bone in a 13-year-old girl. There is severe osteoporosis with destruction of the normal trabecular pattern. Widespread skeletal infiltration with neuroblastoma could look very similar.

years. They complain of pain and stiffness of the spine or the affected joint. This is accompanied by general malaise. In children the disease is frequently seronegative. Diagnosis is clinical initially, and is confirmed by the subsequent course, radiological change and synovial biopsy when this is indicated. The large joints and spine are frequently most severely affected in children. The radiological changes will depend on the stage at which the lesion is seen. Initially soft-tissue swelling and effusion are seen. As synovial overgrowth and cartilage destruction progresses, narrowing of the joint space, and cartilage and bony destruction with erosion of the growing ends of the bone and osteoporosis occur (Fig. 9.47). Bony ankylosis is a frequent end result. Because of hyperaemia, accelerated skeletal maturation takes place, and premature bony fusion can lead to discrepancy in bone length. In severe cases crippling deformities occur, but the active disease tends to burn out in the early teens.

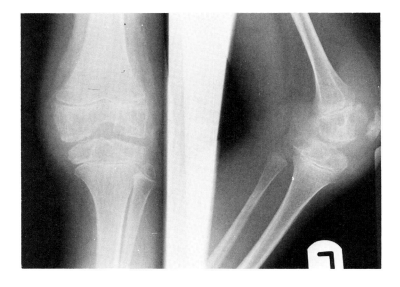

Fig. 9.47. Severe arthropathy of Still's disease in a six-year-old girl. The child had symptoms for three years. The destruction, soft-tissue swelling and epiphyseal enlargement are all clearly seen. The widened irregular intercondylar notch is a frequent finding.

References and further reading

Normal variants

CAFFEY J. (1985) *Pediatric X-ray Diagnosis*, 8th Edition, Section 11. Chicago: Year Book Medical Publishers.

KEATS T.E. (1984) *An Atlas of Normal Roentgen Variants that may Simulate Disease*, 3rd Edition, Chicago: Year Book Medical Publishers.

KOHLER A. & ZIMMER E.A. (1968) *Border Lines of the Normal and Early Pathologic in Skeletal Roentgenology*, 3rd Edition. New York: Grune & Stratton.

Bone age

GREULICH W.W. & PYLE S.I. (1959) *Radiographic Atlas of Skeletal Development of the Hand and Wrist*, 2nd Edition: Stanford: Stanford University Press.

MEYER J. (1964) Dysplasia epiphysealis capitis femoris. *Acta orthop. scand.* **34**, 183–92.

TANNER J.M., WHITEHOUSE R.H., MARSHALL W.A., HEALEY M.J.R. & GOLDSTEIN H. (1984) *Assessment of Skeletal Maturity and Prediction of Adult Height* (TW2 Method, 2nd Edition). London: Academic Press.

Skeletal dysplasia

BERGSMA D. (ed.) (1979) *Birth Defects Compendium*, 2nd Edition. The National Foundation March of Dimes. McMillan Press.

CREMIN B.J. & BEIGHTON P. (1978) *Bone Dysplasia of Infancy*. Berlin: Springer–Verlag.

McKUSICK V.A. (1972) *Heritable Disorders of Connective Tissue*, 4th Edition. St Louis: The C. V. Mosby Co.

MAROTEAUX P. (1979) International Nomenclature of constitutional disease of bone. Revision, May 1977. In *Bone Disease of Children*, pp. 6–11. Philadelphia: J.B. Lippinott.

SPRANGER J.W., LANGER L.O. & WIEDEMANN H.R. (1974) *Bone Dysplasias—an Atlas of Constitutional Disorders of Skeletal Development*. Philadelphia: W.B. Saunders.

TEMTAMY S., & McKUSICK V. (1973) *The Genetics of Head Malformations*. The National Foundation March of Dimes, New York.

Non-accidental injury

ADAMS P.C., STRAND R.D., BRESNAN M.J. & LUCKY A.W. (1974) Kinky hair syndrome: serial study of radiological findings with emphasis on the similarity to the battered child syndrome. *Radiology* **112**, 401–7.

AKBARNIA B., TORG J.S., KIRKPATRICK J. & SUSSMAN S. (1974) Manifestations of the battered child syndrome. *J. Bone Jt Surg.* **56A**, 1159–66.

ASTLEY R. (1979) Metaphyseal fractures in osteogenesis imperfecta. *Brit. J. Radiol.* **52**, 441–4.

CAFFEY J. (1985) *Pediatric X-ray Diagnosis*, 8th Edition, pp. 780–5. Chicago: Year Book Medical Publishers.

CREMIN B., GOODMAN H., SPRANGER J. & BEIGHTON P. (1982) Wormian bones in osteogenesis imperfecta and other disorders. *Skeletal Radiol.* **8**, 35–9.

KOGUTT M.S., SWISCHUK L.E. & FAGAN C.J. (1974) Patterns of injury and the significance of uncommon fractures in the battered child syndrome. *Amer. J. Roentgenol.* **121**, 143–9.

KOZLOWSKI K. & McCROSSIN C. (1979) Menke's kinky hair syndrome. *Paediat. Radiol.* **8**, 191–4.

MERTEN D.F., RADKOWSKI M.A. & LEONIDAS J.C. (1983). The abused child: a radiological reappraisal. *Radiology* **146**, 377–83.

Bone diseases in the premature

BOSLEY A.R.J., VERRIER-JONES E.R. & CAMPBELL M.J. (1980) Aetiological factors in rickets of prematurity. *Arch. Dis. Childh.* **55**, 683–6.

GEFTER W.B., EPSTEIN D.M., ANDAY E.K. & DALINKA M. K. (1982) Rickets presenting as multiple fractures in premature infants on hyperalimentation. *Radiology* **142**, 371–5.

KOO W.K., GUPTA J.M., NAYANAR V.V., WILKINSON M. & POSEN S. (1982) Skeletal changes in preterm infants. *Arch. Dis. Childh.* **57**, 447–52.

STEICHEN J., KAPLAN B. & EDWARDS N. (1976) Bone mineral content in full term infants measured by direct photon absorptiometry. *Amer. J. Roentgenol.* **126**, 124–5.

STEICHEN J.J.J., GRATTAN J.L. & TSANG R.C. (1980) Osteopenia of prematurity: the cause and possible treatment. *J. Pediat.* **96**, 528–34.

The neck

BLOMQUIST H.K., LINDQUIST M. & MATTSSON S. (1979). Calcification of intervertebral discs in childhood. *Paediat. Radiol.* **8**, 23–6.

CATTELL H.S. & FILTZER D.L. (1965) Pseudosubluxation and other normal variations in the cervical spine in children. A study of one hundred and sixty children. *J. Bone Jt Surg.* **47A**, 1295–309.

CAVENDISH M.E. (1972) Congenital elevation of the scapula. *J. Bone Jt Surg.* **54B**, 395–408.

EYRING G.J., PETERSON C.A. & BJORNSON D.R. (1964) Intervertebral disc calcification in childhood. A distinct clinical syndrome. *J. Bone Jt Surg.* **46A**, 1432–41.

FIETTI V.G. & FIELDING J.W. (1976) The Klippel–Feil syndrome: early roentgenographic appearance and progression of the deformity. *J. Bone Jt Surg.* **58A**, 891–2.

HEUSINGER R.N., LANG J.E. & McEWAN G.D. (1974) Klippel–Feil syndrome. A constellation of associated anomalies. *J. Bone Jt Surg.* **56A**, 1246–53.

McCLURE J.G. & RANEY R.B. (1975) Anomalies of the scapula. *Clin. Orthop.* **110**, 22–31.

MELVICK J.C. & SILVERMAN F.N. (1963) Intervertebral disc calcification in childhood. *Radiology* **80**, 399–408.

SWISHUK L.E. (1977) Anterior displacement of C2 in children: physiologic or pathologic? A helpful differentiating line. *Radiology* **122**, 759–63.

Inflammatory disease of the spine

BAILEY H.L., GABRIEL M., HODGSON A.R. & SHIN J.S. (1972) Tuberculosis of the spine in children; operative findings and results in one hundred consecutive patients treated by removal of the lesion and anterior grafting. *J. Bone Jt Surg.* **54A**, 1633–57.

BOSTON H.C., BIANCO A.J. & RHODES K.H. (1975) Disc space infections in children. *Orthop. Clin. N. Amer.* **6**, 953–64.

BREMNER A.E. & NELIGAN G.A. (1953) Benign form of acute osteitis of the spine in young children. *Brit. med. J.* **1**, 856–60.

CAFFEY J. (1975) *Pediatric X-Ray Diagnosis*, 7th Edition, 1628–30. Chicago: Year Book Medical Publishers.

CLEVELAND R.H. & DELONG G.R. (1981) The relationship of juvenile lumbar disc disease and Scheuermann's. *Paediat. Radiol.* **10**, 161–4.

GRUNEBAUM M., HORODNICEANU C., MUKAMEL M., VARSANO I. & LUBIN E. (1982) The imaging diagnosis of non pyogenic discitis in children. *Paediat. Radiol.* **12**, 133–9.

HARWOOD NASH D.C. (1981) Computer tomography of the pediatric spine, a protocol for the 1980s. *Radiol. Clin. N. Amer.* **19**, 479–94.

HENSEY O., COAD N., CURTY H. & STILLS J. (1983) *Arch. Dis. Childh.* **58**, 983–7.

JAMISON R.C., HEINLICH E.M., MIETHKE J.C. & O'LOUGHLIN B.J. (1961) Non-specific spondylitis of infants and children. *Radiology* **77**, 355–67.

LASCARI A.D., GRAHAM M.H. & McQUEEN J.C. (1967) Intervertebral disc infection in children. *J. Pediat.* **70**, 751–7.

MURPHY W.A., DESTOUET J.M. & GYILALEN L. (1981) Percutaneous skeletal biopsy 1981. A procedure for radiologists. *Radiology* **139**, 545–9.

PETERS A.M., KARIMJEE S., SAVERYMUTTU S. & LAVENDER J.P. (1982) Indium 111 oxine and indium 111 acetylacetone labelled leucocytes in the diagnosis of inflammatory disease. *Brit. J. Radiol.* **55**, 827–33.

WENER D.R., BOBECHKO W.P. & GILDAY D.L. (1978) The spectrum of IV disc space infection in children. *J. Bone Jt. Surg.* **60A**, 100.

Spondylolisthesis

BLACKBURNE J.S. & VELIKAS E.P. (1977) Spondylolisthesis in children and adolescents. *J. Bone Jt Surg.* **59B**, 490–4.

BOXALL D., BRADFORD D.S., WINTER R.B. & MOE J.H. (1979) Management of severe spondylolisthesis in children and adolescents. *J. Bone Jt Surg.* **61A**, 479–95.

CYRAN B.M., HUTTON W.C. & TROUP J.D.G. (1976) Spondylolytic fractures. *J. Bone Jt Surg.* **58B**, 462–6.

FULLENLOVE T.M. & WILSON J.G. (1974) Traumatic defects of the pars interarticularis of the lumbar vertebrae. *Amer. J. Roentgenol.* **122**, 634–8.

LOWE R.N., HAYES T.D., KAYE J., BAGG R.G. & LUEKENS C.A. (1976) Standing roentgenograms in spondylolisthesis. *Clin. Orthop.* **117**, 80–4.

MAYERDING H.W. (1932) Spondylolisthesis. *Surg. Gynec. Obstet.* **54**, 371–7.

NATHAN H. (1959) Spondylolysis. *J. Bone Jt Surg.* **41A**, 303–20.

NEWMAN P.H. (1965) A clinical syndrome associated with severe lumbosacral subluxation. *J Bone Jt Surg.* **47B**, 472–81.

OAKLEY R.H. & CURTY H. (1984) Review of spondylolisthesis and spondylolysis in paediatric practice. *Brit. J. Radiol.* **57**, 877–85.

SHERMAN F.C., WILKINSON R.H. & HALL J.E. (1977) Reactive sclerosis of a pedicle and spondylolysis in the lumbar spine. *J. Bone Jt Surg.* **59A**, 49–54.

WILTSE L.L. & JACKSON D.W. (1976) Treatment of spondylolisthesis and spondylolysis in children. *Clin. Orthop.* **117**, 92–100.

WILTSE L.L., NEWMAN P.H. & MACNAB I. (1976) Classification of spondylolisthesis. *Clin. Orthop.* **117**, 23–9.

Disc prolapse

BULLOS S. (1973) Herniated intervertebral lumbar disc in the teenager. *J. Bone Jt Surg.* **55B**, 273–8.

KEY J.A. (1950) Intervertebral disc lesions in children and adolescents. *J. Bone Jt Surg.* **32A**, 97–102.

NELSON C.L., JANECKI C.J., GILDENBERG P.L. & SAVA G. (1972) Disc protrusions in the young. *Clin. Orthop.* **88**, 142–50.

O'CONNELL J.E.A. (1960) Intervertebral disc protrusions in childhood and adolescence. *Brit. J. Surg.* **47**, 611–16.

OZONOFF M.B. (1979) Intervertebral disc prolapse. *In paediatric Orthopaedic Radiology*, p. 59. Philadelphia: W.B. Saunders.

Spinal tumours

BONAK DARPOUR A., LEVY W.M. & AEGENTEN E. (1978) Primary and secondary aneurysmal bone cyst. A radiological study of 75 cases. *Radiology* **126**, 75–83.

DAHLIN D.C. & McLEOD R.A. (1982) Aneurysmal bone cyst and other non-neoplastic conditions. *Skeletal Radiol.* **8**, 243–51.

FREIBERGER R.H. (1960) Osteoid osteoma of the spine. A cause of backache and scoliosis in children and young adults. *Radiology* **75**, 232–5.

JACKSON R.P., RECKLING F.W. & MANTZ F.W. (1977) Osteoid osteoma and osteoblastoma. Similar histologic lesions with different natural histories. *Clin. Orthop.* **128**, 303–13.

McLEOD R.A., DAHLIN D.C. & BEABOUT J.W. (1976) The spectrum of osteoblastoma. *Amer. J. Roentgenol.* **126**, 321–5.

MEHTA N.H. & MURRAY R.O. (1977) Scoliosis provoked by painful vertebral lesions. *Skeletal Radiol.* **1**, 223–30.

OZONOFF M.B. (1979) *Pediatric Orthopaedic Radiology*, p. 67, Philadelphia: W.B. Saunders.

WINTER P.F., JOHSON P.M., HILAL S.K. & FELDMAN F. (1977) Scintigraphic detection of osteoid osteoma. *Radiology* **122**, 177–8.

Developmental spinal anomalies

ANDERSON F.M. (1975) Occult spinal dysraphism. A series of 73 cases. *Pediatrics* **55**, 826–35.

ANDERSON F.M. & BURKE B.L. (1977) Anterior sacral meningocele. A presentation of three cases. *J. Amer. med. Ass.* **237**, 39–42.

BANTA J.V. & NICHOLS O. (1969) Sacral agenesis. *J. Bone Jt Surg.* **51A**, 693–703.

DONALDSON W.F. (1974) Neural spinal dysraphism. In *Spinal Deformity in Neurological and Muscular Disorders* (ed. Hardy J.H.). St Louis: C.V. Mosby.

DUNCAN A.W. & HOARE R.D. (1978) Spinal arachnoid cysts in children. *Radiology* **126**, 423–9.

FITZ C.R. & HARWOOD NASH D.C. (1975) The tethered conus. *Amer. J. Roentgenol.* **125**, 515–23.

GOLD L.H.A., KIEFFER S.A. & PETERSON H.O. (1969) Lipomatous invasion of the spinal cord associated with spinal dysraphism. *Amer. J. Roentgenol.* **107**, 479–85.

GRYSPEERDT G.L. (1963) Myelographic assessment of occult forms of spinal dysraphism. *Acta radiol.* 1, 702–17.

HALL J.E. & POITRAS B. (1977) The management of kyphosis in patients with myelomeningocoele. *Clin. Orthop.* 128, 33–40.

HARWOOD NASH D.C. (1981) Computer tomography of the pediatric spine: a protocol for the 1980s. *Radiol. Clin. N. Amer.* 19, 479–94.

HILAL S.K., MARTON D. & POLLACK E. (1974) Diastematomyelia in children. Radiographic study of 34 cases. *Radiology* 112, 609–21.

HOTSON S. & CARTY H. (1982) Lumbosacral agenesis: a report of three new cases and a review of the literature. *Brit. J. Radiol.* 55, 629–33.

JAMES C.C.M. & LASSMAN L.P. (1962) Spinal dysraphism. The diagnosis and treatment in spina bifida occulta. *J. Bone Jt Surg.* 44B, 828–40.

LOHKAMP F., CLAUSSEN C. & SCHUMACHER C. (1976) CT demonstration of pathologic changes of the spinal cord accompanying spina bifida and disastematomyelia. In *Skull, Spine and Contents*, part II. (ed. Kaufman H.G.) *Progr. pediat. Radiol.* 6, 200.

RENSHAW T.S. (1978) Sacral agenesis: a classification and review of twenty-two cases. *J. Bone Jt Surg.* 60A, 373–83.

RICKHAM P.P., LISTER J. & IRVING I.M. (1978) *Neonatal Surgery*, 2nd Edition, pp. 519–39. London: Butterworths.

SCHEY W.L. (1976) Vertebral malformations and associated somaticovisceral abnormalities. *Clin. Radiol.* 27, 341–53.

SHARRARD W.J.N. (1971) *Paediatric Orthopaedics and Fractures*. Oxford: Blackwell Scientific Publications.

Congenital dislocation of the hip

BENSON M.K.D. & JAMESON-EVANS D.C. (1976) The pelvic osteotomy of Chiari. *J. Bone Jt Surg.* 58B, 164–8.

BROWNING W.H., ROSENKRANTZ H. & TARQUINIO T. (1982) Computed tomography in congenital hip dislocation. *J. Bone Jt Surg.* 64A, 27–31.

CHIARI K. (1963) Ergebnisse mit der Beckenosteotomie als pflannen dach plastir. *Z. Orthop.* 87, 14–26.

CHIARI K. (1974) Median displacement osteotomy of the pelvis. *Clin Orthop.* 98, 55.

CLARKE N.M.P., HORCKE H.T., McHUGH P., LEE M.S., BORNS P.F. & MacEWEN G.D. (1985) Real-time ultrasound in the diagnosis of congenital dislocation and dysplasia of the hip. *J. Bone Jt Surg.* 67B, 406–12.

GORE D.R. (1974) Iatrogenic avascular necrosis of the hip in young children. A review of 6 cases. *J. Bone Jt Surg.* 56A, 493–502.

GRAF R. (1983) New possibilities for the diagnosis of congenital hip joint dislocation by ultrasonography. *J. Paediat. Orthop.* 3, 354–9.

GRECH P. (1977) *Hip Arthrography*. London: Chapman & Hall.

LLOYD ROBERTS G.C. & SWANN M. (1966) Pitfalls in the management of congenital dislocation of the hip. *J. Bone Jt Surg.* 48B, 666–81.

LLOYD ROBERTS G.C., HARRISON H. & CHRISPIN A.R. (1978) Anteversion of the acetabulum in congenital dislocation of the hip. *Orthop. Clin. N. Amer.* 9, 89–93.

McKIBBIN B. (1978) Anatomical factors in the stability of the hip in the newborn. *J. Bone Jt Surg.* 52B, 148–9.

MOULTON A. & UPADHJAY S.S. (1982) A direct method for measuring femoral anteversion using ultrasound. *J. Bone Jt Surg.* 64B, 469–72.

OGDEN J.A. & JENSON P.S. (1976) Roentgenography of congenital dislocation of the hip. *Radiology* 119, 189–92.

ORTOLANI M. (1937) Un segno poconto e sua importanza per le diagnosi di prelussazione congenita del anca. *Paediatrica* 45, 129–36.

PETERSON H.A., KLASSON R.A., McLEOD R.A. & HOFFMAN A.D. (1981) The use of computed tomography in dislocation of the hip and femoral neck anteversion in children. *J. Bone Jt Surg.* 63B, 198–208.

SALTER R.B. (1961) Innominate osteotomy in the treatment of congenital dislocation of the hips and subluxation of the hips. *J. Bone Jt Surg.* 43B, 518–39.

SHANDS A.R. & STEELE M.K. (1958) Torsion of the femur. A follow-up report on the use of the Dunlop method for its determination. *J. Bone Jt Surg.* 40A, 803.

SHARRARD W.J. (1964) Posterior iliopsoas transplantation in the treatment of paralytic dislocation of the hip. *J. Bone Jt Surg.* 46B, 426–44.

STAHELT L.T., LIPPERT F. & DENOTTEN P. (1977) Femoral anteversion and physical performance in adolescent and adult life. *Clin. Orthop.* 129, 213–16.

TACHDJIAN M. (1972) *Pediatric Orthopaedics*. Philadelphia: W. B. Saunders.

TREVOR D., JOHNS D.L. & FIXON J.A. (1975) Acetabuloplasty in the treatment of congenital dislocation of the femur. *J. Bone Jt Surg.* 57B, 167–74.

VON ROSEN S. (1968) Further experience with congenital dislocation of the hip in the newborn. *J. Bone Jt Surg.* 50B, 538–41.

WEINTROUB S., BOYD A., CHRISPIN A.R. & LLOYD ROBERTS G.C. (1981) The use of stereophotogrametry to measure acetabular and femoral anteversion. *J. Bone Jt Surg.* 63B, 209–13.

WESTIN G.W., ILFELD F.W. & PROVOST J. (1976). Total avascular necrosis of the femoral capital epiphysis in congenital dislocated hips. *Clin. Orthop.* 119, 93.

The painful hip

BROWN I. (1975) A study of the capsular shadow in disorders of the hip in children. *J. Bone Jt Surg.* 57B, 175–9.

GRIFFIN P.P & GREEN W.T. (1978) Hip joint infection in infants and children. *Arch. Clin. N. Amer.* 9, 123–34.

LLOYD ROBERTS G.C. (1978) Pyogenic arthritis of the hip. In *Hip Disorders in Childhood* (eds. Lloyd Roberts G.C. & Ratcliff A.H.C.). London: Butterworth.

NELSON J.D. & KOONTZ W.C. (1968) Septic arthritis in infants and children. A review of 117 cases. *Pediatrics* 38, 966–71.

Perthes' disease

CAFFEY J. (1968) The early roentgenographic changes in essential coxa plana: their significance in pathogenesis. *Amer. J. Roentgenol.* 103, 620.

CARTY H., MAXTED M., FIELDING J.A., GULLIFORD P. & OWEN R. (1984) Isotope scanning in the 'irritable hip syndrome'. *Skeletal Radiol.* 11, 32–7.

CATTERALL A. (1971) The natural history of Perthes' disease. *J. Bone Jt Surg.* 53B, 37–53.

DANGIELIS J.A. (1976) Pinhole imaging in Legg–Perthes disease: further observations. *Semin. nucl. Med.* **6**, 69–82.

DOUGLAS J.A., FISHER R.L., OZONOFF M.B. & SZILKAS J.J. (1975) ⁹⁹Tcᵐ polyphosphate bone imaging in Legg–Perthes disease. *Radiology* **115**, 407–13.

GIRDANY B.R. & OSMAN M.Z. (1968) Longitudinal growth and skeletal maturation in Perthes' disease. *Radiol. Clin. N. Amer.* **6**, 245–51.

GOLDMAN A.B., HALLEN T., SALVATI E. & FREIBERGEN R.H. (1976) Osteochondritis dissecans complicating Legg–Perthes disease. A report of 4 cases. *Radiology* **121**, 561–6.

GROSSBARD G.D. (1981) Hip pain during adolescence after Perthes' disease. *J. Bone Jt Surg.* **65B**, 572–4.

KATZ J.F. (1968) Arthrography in Legg–Calvé–Perthes disease. *J. Bone Jt Surg.* **50A**, 467–72.

KEMP H.S. & BOLDERO J.L. (1966) Radiological changes in Perthes' disease. *Brit. J. Radiol.* **39**, 744–60.

LLOYD ROBERTS G.C., CATTERALL A. & SALAMON P.B. (1976) A controlled study for the indications and the results of femoral osteotomy in Perthes' disease. *J. Bone Jt Surg.* **58B**, 31–6.

MCKIBBIN B. & RALIS Z. (1974) Pathological changes in a case of Perthes' disease. *J. Bone Jt Surg.* **56B**, 438–47.

MORLE N.J. & GOLDING J.S.R. (1974) Idiopathic chondrolysis of the hip. *Clin. Radiol.* **25**, 247–51.

O'HARA J.P., DAVIS N.D., GAGE J.R., SINDBERG A.B. & WINTER R.R. (1977) Long term follow up of Perthes' disease treated non-operatively. *Clin. Orthop.* **125**, 49–56.

Slipped upper femoral epiphysis

CHAPMAN J.A., DEAKIN D.P. & GREEN J.H. (1980) Slipped upper femoral epiphysis after radiotherapy. *J. Bone Jt Surg.* **62B**, 337–9.

CRAWFORD A.H., MCEWAN G.D. & FORTE D. (1977) Slipped capital femoral epiphysis and coexistent hypothyroidism. *Clin. Orthop.* **122**, 138–40.

DUNN D.M. & ANGEL J.C. (1978) Replacement of the femoral head by open operation in severe adolescent slipping of the upper femoral epiphysis. *J. Bone Jt Surg.* **60B**, 394–403.

EL-KHOURY G.Y. & MICKLESON M.R. (1977) Chondrolysis following slipped capital epiphysis. *Radiology* **123**, 327–30.

HEATLEY F.W., GREENWOOD R.H. & BOASE D.L. (1976) Slipping of the upper femoral epiphysis in patients with intracranial tumours. *J. Bone Jt Surg.* **58B**, 169–75.

HOLDMAN A.B., SCHNEIDER R. & MARTEL W. (1978) Acute chondrolysis complicating slipped capital femoral epiphysis. *Amer. J. Roentgenol.* **130**, 945–50.

KELSEY J.L., ACHESON R.M. & KEGGI K.J. (1972) The body build of patients with slipped capital femoral epiphysis. *Amer. J. Dis. Child.* **124**, 276–81.

NIXON J.R. & DOUGLAS J.F. (1980) Bilateral slipping of the upper femoral epiphyses in end stage renal failure. *J. Bone Jt Surg.* **62B**, 18–21.

RENNIE A.M. (1967) Familial slipped upper femoral epiphysis. *J. Bone Jt Surg.* **49B**, 535–9.

TURNER A., TAYLOR J.F., CARTY H. & OWEN R. (1984) The radiological evaluation of multiple pin fixation of the femoral head. *Brit. J. Radiol.* **57**, 887–90.

Protrusio acetabuli

ALEXANDER C. (1965) The aetiology of primary protrusio acetabuli. *Brit. J. Radiol.* **38**, 567–80.

BLECK E.E. (1983) Idiopathic chondrolysis of the hip. *J. Bone Jt Surg.* **65A**, 1266–77.

MCDONALD P. (1971) Primary protrusio acetabuli. Report of an affected family. *J. Bone Jt Surg.* **53B**, 30–6.

OZONOFF M.B. (1979) In *Pediatric Orthopedic Radiology*, p. 153. Philadelphia: W.B. Saunders.

Proximal focal femoral deficiencies and coxa vara

AITKEN G.T. (1968) Proximal femoral focal deficiency. Definition, classification and management. In *Proximal Focal Femoral Deficiency, a Congenital Anomaly*. A symposium edited by G.T. Aitken. National Academy of Sciences: Washington D.C.

CALHOUN J.D. & PIERRET G. (1972) Infantile coxa vara. *Amer. J. Roentgenol.* **115**, 561–8.

LEVINSON E.D., OZONOFF M.B. & ROYON P.M. (1977) Proximal focal femoral deficiency. *Radiology* **125**, 197–204.

LLOYD ROBERTS G.C. (1978) Congenital femoral deficiency. In *Hip Disorders in Children* (eds. Lloyd Roberts G.C. & Ratcliff A.H. C.), pp. 1–34. London: Butterworth.

PANTING A.L. & WILLIAMS P.F. (1978) Proximal focal femoral deficiency. *J. Bone Jt Surg.* **60B**, 46–52.

Genu varum, genu valgum, Blount's disease and limb length discrepancy

ANDERSON M.T., GREEN W.T. & MESSNER M.B. (1963) Growth and predictions of growth in the lower extremities. *J. Bone Jt Surg.* **45A**, 1–14.

BATESON E.M. (1968) The relationship between Blount's disease and bow legs. *Brit. J. Radiol.* **41**, 107–14.

BLOUNT W.P. (1937) Tibia vara. Osteochondrosis deformans tibiae. *J. Bone Jt Surg.* **19**, 1–29.

GOLDING J.S.R., BATESON E.M. & MCNEIL-SMITH J.D.G. (1969) Infantile tibia vara (Blount's disease or osteochondrosis deformans tibiae). In *The Growth Plate and its Disorders* (ed. Rang M.), pp 109–19. Baltimore: Williams & Wilkins.

GREENBERG L.A. & SWARTZ A.A. (1971) Genu varum and genu-valgum. Another look. *Amer. J. Dis. Child.* **121**, 219–21.

HOLT J.F., LATOURETTE H.B. & WATSON E.H. (1954) Physiological bowing of the legs in young children. *J. Amer. med. Ass.* **154**, 390.

KHERMOSH O., LIOR G. & WEISSMAN S.L. (1971) Tibial torsion in children. *Clin. Orthop.* **79**, 25–31.

MCEWAN D.W. & DUNBAR J.S. (1958) Radiologic study of physiologic knock-knee in childhood. *J. Canad. Ass. Radiol.* **W**, 59–64.

MOSELEY C.F. (1977) A straight line graph for leg length discrepancies. *J. Bone Jt Surg.* **59A**, 174–9.

OZONOFF M.B. (1978) *Pediatric Orthopedic Radiology* pp. 222–34. Philadelphia: W.B. Saunders.

STAHELI L.T. & ENGEL G.M. (1972) Tibial torsion. A method of assessment and survey of normal children. *Clin. Orthop.* **86**, 183–6.

Patella and painful knee

BERNHANG A.M. & LEVINE S.A. (1973) Familial absence of the patella. *J. Bone Jt Surg.* **55A**, 1088–90.

BLACKBURNE J.S. & PEEL T.E. (1977) A new method of measuring patellar height. *J. Bone Jt Surg.* **59B**, 241–2.

BOSE K. & CHONG K.C. (1976) The clinical manifestation and pathomechanisms of contracture of the exterior mechanism of the knee. *J. Bone Jt Surg.* **58B**, 478–84.

BURGAN D.W. (1971) Arthrographic findings in meniscal cysts. *Radiology* **101**, 579–82.

FONG E.E. (1946) Iliac horns (symmetrical bilateral central posterior iliac process). A case report. *Radiology* **47**, 517.

GOODFELLOW J., HUNGERFORD D.C. & WOODS C. (1976) Patello femoral joint mechanics and pathology. *J. Bone Jt Surg.* **58B**, 291–3.

HALL F.M. (1977) Arthrography of the discoid lateral meniscus. *Amer. J. Roentgenol.* **128**, 993.

HOUGHTON G.R. & ACKROYD C. (1981) Sleeve fractures of the patellae in children. *J. Bone Jt Surg.* **62B**, 165–8.

INSALL J., GOLDBERG V. & SALVATI E. (1972) Recurrent dislocation and the high riding patella. *Clin. Orthop.* **88**, 67–9.

JAKOB R.P., VON GUMPPONBERG S. & ENGELHARDT P. (1981) Does Osgood Schlatter's disease influence the position of the patella? *J. Bone Jt Surg.* **63B**, 579–86.

KEATS T.E. (1985) *An Atlas of Normal Roentgen Variants that may Simulate Disease*, 3rd Edition. Chicago: Year Book Medical Publishers.

LINDEN B. (1977) Osteochondritis dissecans of the femoral condyles. A long term follow up study. *J. Bone Jt Surg.* **59A**, 769–76.

MILGRAM J.W. (1978) Radiological and pathological manifestations of osteochondritis dissecans of the distal femur. A study of 50 cases. *Radiology* **126**, 305–11.

NATHAN P.A. & COLE S.C. (1969) Discoid meniscus a clinical and pathological study. *Clin. Orthop.* **64**, 107–13.

OSBORNE A.H. & FULFORD P.C. (1982) Lateral release for chondromalacia patellae. *J. Bone Jt Surg.* **64B**, 202–8.

OUTERBRIDGE R.E. (1961) The aetiology of chondromalacia patellae. *J. Bone Jt Surg.* **43B**, 752–7.

OUTERBRIDGE R.E. & DUNLOP J. (1975) The problem of chondromalacia patellae. *Clin. Orthop.* **110**, 177–96.

SIKORSKI J.M., PETERS J. & WATT I. (1979) The importance of femoral rotation in chondromalacia patellae as shown by serial radiography. *J. Bone Jt Surg.* **61B**, 435–42.

SMILLIE I.S. (1960) *Osteochondritis Dissecans*. Edinburgh: Churchill Livingstone.

The foot

BECKLEY D.E., ANDERSON P.W. & PEDEGANA L.R. (1975) The radiology of the subtalar joint with special reference to talo-calcaneal coalition. *Clin. Radiol.* **26**, 333–43.

BLACK E.E. (1977) Congenital club foot. Pathomechanics, radiographic analysis, and results of surgical treatment. *Clin. Orthop.* **125**, 119–30.

BRADLEY G.W. & COLEMAN S.S. (1981) Treatment of calcaneocavus foot deformity. *J. Bone Jt Surg.* **63A**, 1159–66.

CONWAY J.J. & COWELL H.R. (1969) Tarsal coalition: clinical significance and roentgenographic demonstration. *Radiology* **92**, 799–811.

DWYER F.C. (1963) The treatment of relapsed club foot by the insertion of a wedge into the calcaneum. *J. Bone Jt Surg.* **45B**, 67–75.

DWYER F.C. (1975) The present status of the problem of pes cavus. *Clin. Orthop.* **106**, 254–75.

EYRE-BROOK A.L. (1967) Congenital vertical talus. *J. Bone Jt Surg.* **49B**, 618–27.

FREIBERGER R.H., HERSH A. & HARRISON M.O. (1970) Roentgen examination of the deformed foot. *Semin. Roentgenol.* **5**, 341.

HEYMAN C.H., HERNDON C.H. & STRONG J.M. (1958) Mobilisation of the tarso-metatasal and intermetatarsal joints for the correction of persistent adduction of the fore part of the foot in congenital club foot. *J. Bone Jt Surg.* **40A**, 299–310.

HOUGHTON G.R. & DICKSON R.A. (1979) Hallux valgus in the younger patient. *J. Bone Jt Surg.* **61B**, 176–7.

KITE J.H. (1967) Congenital metatarsus varus. *J. Bone Jt Surg.* **49A**, 388.

OZONOFF M.B. (1979) *Pediatric Orthopedic Radiology*, pp. 275–324. Philadelphia: W.B. Saunders.

SILK F.F. & WAINWRIGHT D. (1967) The recognition and treatment of congenital flat foot in infancy. *J. Bone Jt Surg.* **49B**, 628–33.

SIMONS G.W. (1978) Analytical radiography and the progressive approach in talipes equino varus. *Orthop. Clin. N. Amer.* **135**, 157–206.

The arm

AHMADI B. & STEEL H.H. (1977) Congenital pseudarthrosis of the clavicle. *Clin. Orthop.* **126**, 130.

ASH J.M. & GILDAY D.L. (1980) The futility of bone scanning in neonatal osteomyelitis. *J. nucl. Med.* **21**, 417–20.

BARNES J.C. & SMITH W.L. (1978) The vater association. *Radiology* **126**, 445–9.

ELLIS R.W.B. & CREVELD S.V. (1940) A syndrome characterised by ectodermal dysplasia, polydactyly chondrodysplasia and congenital morbus cordis. *Arch. Dis. Childh.* **15**, 65–84.

FELMAN A.H. & KIRKPATRICK J.A. (1969) Madelung's deformity. Observations in 17 patients. *Radiology* **93**, 1037–42.

FIELD J.H. & KRAG D.O. (1973) Congenital constricting bands and congenital amputation of the fingers—placental studies. *J. Bone Jt Surg.* **55A**, 1035–41.

FISHER R.M. & CREMIN B.J. (1976) Limb defects in the amniotic band syndrome. *Paediat. Radiol.* **5**, 24–9.

JANCU J. (1971) Radio-ulnar synostosis. A common occurrence in sex chromosomal abnormalities. *Amer. J. Dis. Child.* **122**, 10–11.

KELIKIAN H. (1974) *Congenital Deformities of the Hand and Forearm*. Philadelphia: W.B. Saunders.

LANDING B.H. (1975) Syndromes of congenital heart disease with tracheo bronchial abnormalities. *Amer. J. Roentgenol.* **123**, 679–86.

LLOYD ROBERTS G.C., APLEY A.G. & OWEN R. (1975) Reflections upon the aetiology of congenital pseudarthrosis of the clavicle. *J. Bone Jt Surg.* **57B**, 24.

POZNANSKI A.K. (1974) The *Hand in Radiologic Diagnosis*. Philadelphia: W.B. Saunders.

RICKHAM P.P., LISTER J. & IRVING I.M. (1978) *Neonatal Surgery*, 2nd Edition, pp. 246 and 471. London: Butterworth.

SALTER R.B. & ZALTZ C. (1971) Anatomic investigations of the mechanism of injury and pathologic anatomy of 'pulled elbow' in young children. *Clin. Orthop.* 77, 134–43.

SPRANGER J.W., LANGER I.O. & WIEDEMANN H.R. (1974) *Bone Dysplasias: An Atlas of Constitutional Disorders of Skeletal development.* Philadelphia: W.B. Saunders.

TAYBI H. (1983) *Radiology of Syndromes and Metabolic Disorders*, 2nd Edition. Chicago: Year Book Medical Publishers.

TEMTAMY S. & McKUSICK V. (1978) *The Genetics of Hand Malformations.* New York: The National Foundation March of Dimes.

Osteogenesis imperfecta

BAUZE R.J., SMITH R. & Francis M.J. (1975) A new look at osteogenesis imperfecta. A clinical, radiological and biochemical study of 42 patients. *J. Bone Jt Surg.* 57B, 2–11.

CAFFEY J. (1979) *Pediatric X-ray Diagnosis*, 7th Edition pp. 1208–13. Chicago: Year Book Medical Publishers.

HOUANG M.T.W., BRENTON D.P., RENTON P. & SHAW D.G. (1978) Idiopathic juvenile osteoporosis. *Skeletal Radiol.* 3, 17–23.

MAROTEAUX P. (1979) *Bone Diseases of Children*, pp. 102–9. Philadelphia: J.B. Lippincott.

SILLENCE D.O., SENN A. & DANKS D.M. (1979) Genetic heterogeneity in osteogenesis imperfecta. *J. med. Genet.* 16, 101–16.

SPRANGER J., CREMIN B. & BEIGHTON P. (1982) Osteogenesis imperfecta congenita. Features and prognosis of a heterogenous condition. *Paediat. Radiol.* 12, 21–8.

Arthrogryposis

FISHER R.L., JOHNSTONE W.T., FISHER W.H. & GOLDKAMP O.G. (1970) Arthrogryposis multiplex congenita. *J. Pediat.* 76, 255–61.

POZNANSKI A.K. & LA ROWE P.C. (1970) Roentgenographic manifestations of the arthrogryposis syndrome. *Radiology* 95, 353–8.

SWISCHUK L.E. (1980) *Radiology of the Newborn and Young Infant*, 2nd Edition, pp. 727–30. Baltimore: Williams & Wilkins.

Neurofibromatosis

BOYD H.B. & SAGE F.P. (1958) Congenital pseudarthrosis of the tibia. *J. Bone Jt Surg.* 40, 1245–70.

CASSELMAN E.S. & MANDELL G.A. (1979) Vertebral scalloping in neurofibromatosis. *Radiology* 131, 89–94.

DAVIDSON K.C. (1966) Cranial and intracranial lesions in neurofibromatosis. *Amer. J. Roentgenol.* 98, 550–6.

FIENMAN N.L. & YAKOVAC W.C. (1970). Neurofibromatosis in childhood. *J. Pediat.* 79, 339–46.

HALPERN M. & CURRARINO G. (1965) Vascular lesions causing hypertension in neurofibromatosis. *New Engl. J. Med.* 273, 248–52.

KLAME E.C., FRANKEN E.A. & SMITH J.A. (1976) The radiographic spectrum in neurofibromatosis. *Semin. Roentgenol.* 11, 17–33.

LEEDS N.E. & JACOBSON H.G. (1976) Spinal neurofibromatosis. *Amer. J. Roentgenol.* 126, 617–23.

MENA M., BOOKSTEIN J.J., HOLT J.F. & FRY W.F. (1973) Neurofibromatosis and neurovascular hypertension in children. *Amer. J. Roentgenol.* 118, 39–45.

Haemophilia

AHLBERG A. (1975) On the natural history of haemophiliac pseudotumour. *J. Bone Jt Surg.* 57A, 1133–6.

BOLDERO J.L. & KEMP H.S,. (1966) The early bone and joint changes in haemophilia and other blood dyscrasias. *Brit. J. Radiol.* 39, 172–80.

CAFFEY J. (1978) *Pediatric X-ray Diagnosis*, 7th Edition, pp. 1520–4, Chicago: Year Book Medical Publishers.

JENSEN P.S. & PUTNEUS C.E. (1975) Haemophilic pseudotumour. Diagnosis, treatment and complications. *Amer. J. Dis. Child.* 129, 717–19.

Rickets

CAFFEY J. (1978) *Pediatric X-ray Diagnosis*, 7th Edition, pp. 1443–53. Chicago: Yearbook Medical Publishers.

DENT C.E., RICHENS A., ROWE D.J.F. & STAMP T.C.B. (1970) Osteomalacia with long term anticonvulsant therapy in epilepsy. *Brit. med. J.* 2, 69–72.

LEONIDAS J.C. (1973) Antiepileptic therapy and rickets in children. *Radiology* 109, 409–12.

SPRANGER J., LANGER L.O. & WIEDEMANN H.R. (1974) *Bone Dysplasias. An Atlas of Constitutional Disorders of the Skeleton*, pp. 74–7. Philadelphia: W.B. Saunders.

Diaphyseal aclasis

GIDEON A., KEDSTLER R. & MUGGIASCA F. (1975) The widened spectrum of multiple cartilaginous exostosis. *Paediat. Radiol.* 3, 93–100.

LIBSHITZ H. & COHEN M. (1982) Radiation induced osteochondromas. *Radiology* 142, 643–9.

MAROTEAUX P. (1979) *Bone Diseases of Children*, pp. 88–93. Philadelphia: J.P. Lippincott.

OZONOFF M.B. (1979) *Pediatric Orthopedic Radiology*, pp. 371–80. Philadelphia: W.B. Saunders.

Fibrous dysplasia

BERGSMA D. (ed.) (1979) *Birth Defects Compendium*, 2nd Edition, p. 444. The National Foundation March of Dimes. McMillan Press.

LEEDS N. & SEAMAN W.M.B. (1962) Fibrous dysplasia of the skull and its differential diagnosis. A clinical and roentgenographic study of 46 cases. *Radiology* 78, 570–87.

STEWART M.J., GILMER W.S. & EDMONDSON A.S. (1962) Fibrous dysplasia of bone. *J. Bone Jt Surg.* 44B, 302–18.

Malignancy

BAKER M., SIDDIQUI A.R., PROVISOR A. & COHEN M. (1983) Radiographic and scintigraphic skeletal imaging in patients with neuroblastoma. Concise communications. *J. nucl. Med.* 24, 467–70.

BLOOM H.J., LAMERLE J., NEIDHERDT M.K. & VOUTE P.A. (eds.) (1975) *Cancer in Children.* Berlin: Springer–Verlag.

BOUSUAROS A., KIRKS D.R. & GROSSMAN M. (1986) Imaging of neuroblastoma: an overview. *Paediat. Radiol.* 16, 89–107.

CAFFEY J. (1985) *Pediatric X-ray Diagnosis*, 8th Edition, Chicago: Year Book Medical Publishers.

Juvenile chronic arthritis

ANSELL B. (1972) Skeletal growth anomalies resulting from Still's disease. *J. Bone Jt Surg.* **54**, 199–200.

BARBARIC Z.L. & YOUNG L.W. (1972) Synovial cysts in juvenile rheumatoid arthritis. *Amer. J. Roentgenol.* **116**, 655–60.

CAFFEY J. (1978) *Pediatric X-ray Diagnosis*, 7th Edition, pp. 1572–81. Chicago: Year Book Medical Publishers.

Chapter 10
Orthopaedic Problems in the Tropics

G. F. WALKER

Introduction

Any U.K.-based doctor, whether orthopaedic surgeon, radiologist or other, who has an opportunity of visiting and working in the tropics is almost certain to be exposed to the clinical problems of the developing countries. While there are centres of wealth and medical excellence in the oil-rich areas and elsewhere, the majority of people in the tropical and as yet undeveloped areas exist at a subsistence level. The visiting doctor will be amazed at the plethora of disease and this always includes a vast amount of very fascinating orthopaedics. Although many of the problems can be considered the direct result of poverty and ignorance, there are some conditions endemic in the tropics which are relatively uncommon in the so-called developed world. Not only does poverty almost certainly lower people's resistance to disease, but it also results in very inadequate or even no medical facilities either preventative or curative (Fig. 10.1a, b). Recently, these problems have been augmented by the epidemic of road traffic accidents and gunshot wounds which appear to be a direct result of the advance of civilization. Orthopaedic and other medical facilities, already stretched, are in danger of being swamped with injured patients when the number of motor cars and lorries, often in the first instance using very inadequate roads, increases as a result of economic improvement, whether this follows local effort or overseas aid. While the solution to many of

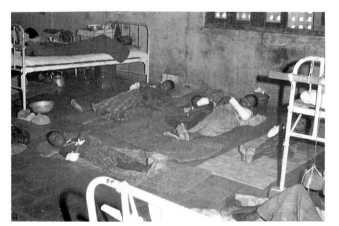

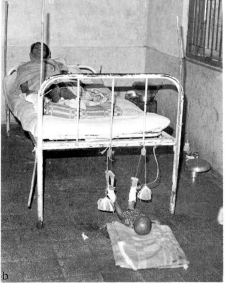

Fig. 10.1.   (a) Part of an orthopaedic ward. (b) One bed being used to manage two patients.

365

these problems depends on politics, most doctors strive to do as much as they can for all the patients who present and for whom they then become responsible. Even so, this care and attention has to be tempered by the available facilities and resources, and, alas, these are only too often in short supply.

During a recent trip abroad the author visited a hospital which still receives more than 200 children arriving as new cases of poliomyelitis each month. At another hospital there were over 500 children with clubfeet under treatment, and a short while was spent in the clubfoot clinic which coped with 40 children in the one hour which could be set aside each week for this work. However, it is surprising how much can be achieved under these circumstances by enthusiasm and the use of locally trained assistants. In the clubfoot clinic there were four plaster technicians who seemed skilled in the application of appropriate casts. Likewise, where poliomyelitis is still rampant the provision of simple calipers and footwear may make all the difference between worthwhile mobility and a totally dependent life (often as a beggar). Although an orthopaedic surgeon usually depends heavily on radiology the author has worked for as long as five weeks at a stretch without any electricity; it is surprising what can

be done with a tape measure. In both major teaching hospitals and those in the districts and rural areas, it is rare to find more than 30–50% of the X-ray machines in working order. Often they are old, but even new machines may be unserviceable through lack of spare parts or adequately trained service personnel. The most useful X-ray machine is usually of simple and robust construction and may well have been producing reasonable quality radiographs for 20 or more years. Often there are problems with films which may be 'time-expired', or stored in far from ideal conditions. Chemicals may be imported from many sources or manufactured locally, and these can be unreliable. There are often great variations in voltage, and some dark rooms have neither temperature control nor air-cooling facilities (Fig. 10.2). All this makes the production of satisfactory radiographs somewhat hazardous. This may be exemplified by the standards of some of the illustrations in this chapter, but they are the sort of films that in practice have to be used. Specialist X-ray examinations are rarely possible, although occasionally one is very surprised at what can be done by an enthusiastic radiologist with a loyal staff. Unfortunately doctors such as this may be subject to the whims of Government posting, or may simply be spending a few years in a de-

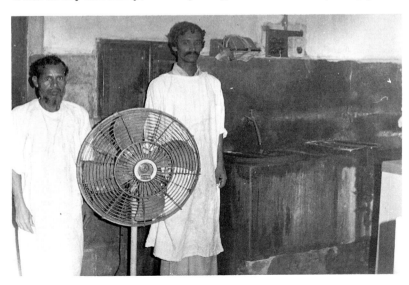

Fig. 10.2. Part of an X-ray department.

veloping country before moving elsewhere. This applies not only to expatriates, but also to national doctors who are unable to live on the relatively meagre salaries offered, and emigrate to the oil-rich areas or to more developed countries. Again these are largely political problems but they do have a direct bearing on orthopaedic and radiological practice.

In this chapter an attempt has been made to select some of the conditions which will be found not only by doctors travelling abroad, but which can on occasion turn up in the U.K. It is impossible to deal in full with each and every condition, and for detailed descriptions of radiological and pathological changes the reader will have to turn elsewhere.

While there must be considerable overlap it is practical to consider orthopaedic problems which are common in the tropics, and then follow this with diseases and deformities which are relatively rare in the U.K. and more developed areas. These may present not only in patients arriving specifically for medical attention, but also from time to time they occur in people of immigrant stock or in those who have travelled and lived extensively in the tropics. This is followed by a very short section on conditions which have proved undiagnosable by the author, certainly with the facilities available in the hospitals and clinics where they have presented.

Infections

LOCAL AND GENERAL INFECTIONS OF BONES, JOINTS AND SOFT TISSUES

These are common. 'Acute' bone and joint infections usually present late, but from time to time an ill neonate arrives with a massive thigh or limb containing a large quantity of pus which has arisen from either a septic joint or osteomyelitis. The management is primarily incision and drainage followed by splintage, in abduction when the hip is involved in order to keep the femoral head within the socket.

Radiology is useful in monitoring the development of the hip and the presence and then gradual absorption of any sequestrae (Fig. 10.3). These will frequently disappear in infants and children, particularly when sinus formation can be avoided by relatively open early surgery, skin closure over drainage, and antibiotics. The possible associated haemoglobinopathy problem is discussed later in this chapter.

Chronic pyogenic bone and joint infections seem to be very common, but a part of this apparent high incidence may be due to the chronicity of the infections, with the patients always turning

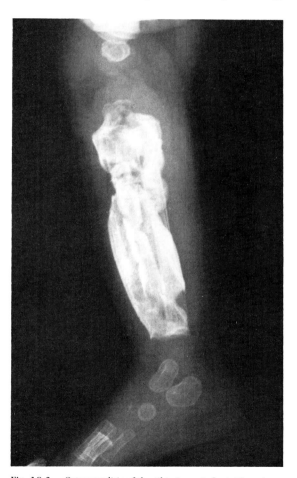

Fig. 10.3. Osteomyelitis of the tibia in an infant. There is every probability that the sequestrum will absorb at this age.

up in the clinic, and when admitted remaining in hospital for long periods (Fig. 10.4). The principles of managing chronic osteomyelitis are to remove sequestrae and dead material, to eradicate dead space, and to achieve skin cover. This can be more difficult than it sounds, and in particular sequestrae must never be removed before adequate involucrum has formed, as otherwise the periosteal tube collapses with the development of the very tenuous shaft (Fig.10.5). Some bone infections follow elective surgery (Fig. 10.6). Antibiotics play little part in the long-term management of chronic bone infection but may be useful as a cover during surgery. Simple drainage after primary skin cover following sequestrectomy, where this is possible such as with the femur, is wise, but in other areas delayed split skin grafting on to granulating healthy bone is often the best that can be achieved. Chronic septic arthritis usually results in a stiff and often deformed joint. If the ankylosis is sound then corrective osteotomy may be helpful, and this should always be done by osteotomy/osteoclasis using plaster, rather

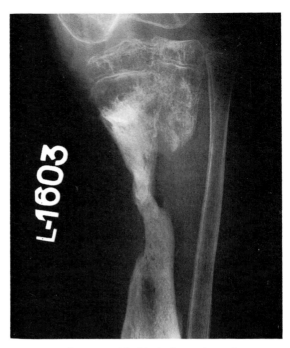

Fig. 10.5.   The narrow 'shaft' which may form after too early removal of a sequestrum in chronic osteomyelitis.

than with metallic internal fixation. Chronic bone infection can occur without the apparent formation of sequestrae; the whole bone then appears enlarged and there may be multiple minute cavities, possibly containing very small fragments of dead bone.

The Guinea worm, *Dracunculus medinensis*, as well as producing skin ulceration and soft-tissue abcesses may cause a septic arthritis, particularly of the knee. The worm may appear with the pus when the joint is incised, but on other occasions its calcified remains are an incidental finding in an X-ray taken for some other reason.

Tuberculosis can turn up anywhere, and certainly in the U.K. it is now sufficiently uncommon to be forgotten when considering the differential diagnosis of a painful bone or joint (Walker 1968). It may present in strange ways, particularly in immigrants. In the tropics the diagnosis is usually obvious from clinical and radiological examination (Fig. 10.7a, b). Histological confirmation is usually more helpful

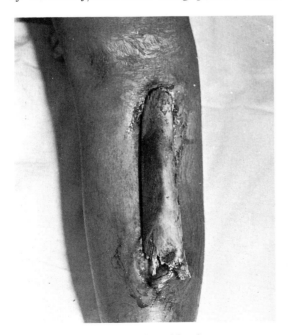

Fig. 10.4.   Chronic osteomyelitis of the tibia at presentation.

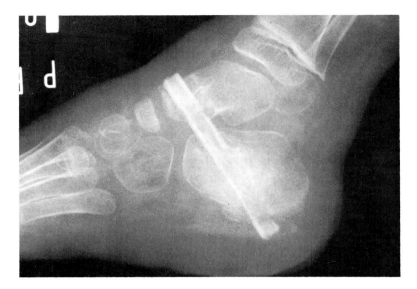

Fig. 10.6. An infected graft in a Grice subtalar arthrodesis.

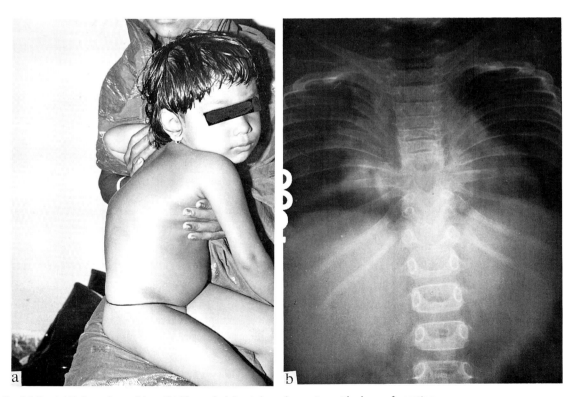

Fig. 10.7. (a) Tuberculous gibbus. (b) The underlying tuberculous spine with abscess formation.

than culture, and a therapeutic trial can help to settle any remaining doubt (Fig. 10.8). The management of skeletal tuberculosis is primarily medical with exhibition of suitable antibiotics and chemotherapy for a long enough period.

Syphilis, both congenital and acquired, remains relatively common in some parts of the world, although the only example that the author has seen (or recognized) was in fact shown to him by a radiologist in India (Fig. 10.9).

Anterior poliomyelitis. Although this crippling condition has largely disappeared from the more developed countries, it is still rife in many parts of the world (Fig. 10.10). This is really an international political tragedy, as the disease should be controlled if not totally eradicated by ensuring that the correct amount of suitably

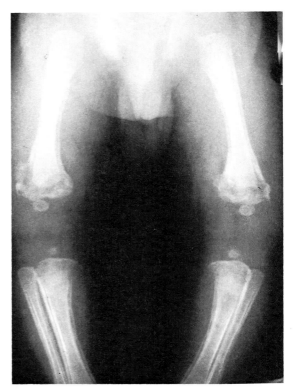

Fig. 10.9. Neonatal syphilis.

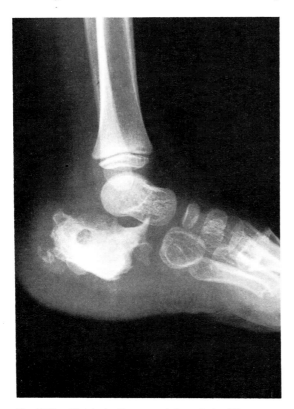

Fig. 10.8. Histologically proven tuberculosis of the os calcis.

stored vaccine goes down the correct number of throats at appropriate intervals, as well as by improving standards of hygiene. Very often children present with 'whole limb paralysis', the story being that following a fever the child receives an injection in the market, and provocative paralysis then follows. More educated parents complain of a sciatic palsy following the buttock injection of their child, but very rarely is there sensory evidence to support this; the diagnosis is nearly always poliomyelitis. While a great deal can be done by correcting contractures and deformities, followed by provision of adequate but simple calipers and footwear, the place of reconstructive tendon surgery is limited. Very often in these whole-limb problems no useful functioning muscles remain.

It is feared that children with polio paralysis will continue to appear at medical units

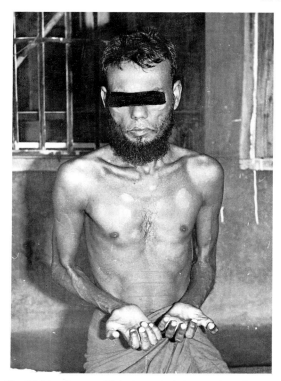

Fig. 10.11. Leprosy. Note the typical skin patches, thenar wasting and contractures of the digits.

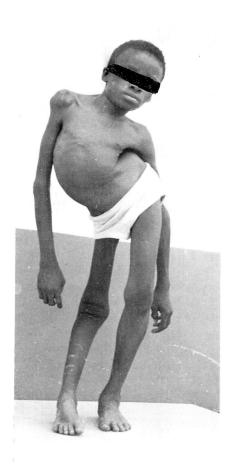

Fig. 10.10. Severe poliomyelitis.

throughout the world for many years to come, and where a caliper service is organized the number attending always rapidly increases. With lesser degrees of weakness, the basis of management must be to attempt to improve function, and this may involve overcoming contractures and possibly dislocations by surgery, and then trying to restore muscle balance and stability around joints by tendon transfer and stabilizing operations.

Leprosy. This fascinating disease remains widespread, and the figure of 13 million lepers in the world is often quoted, although whether it is, in fact, accurate is uncertain (Fig. 10.11).

Lepers tend to be paupers, and are still shunned by society in most parts of the developing world. Often they spend their life either as beggars or occasionally, if they are lucky, within special communities. In fact, the latter have largely been abandoned by the leprosy experts as unnecessary, because out-patient drug therapy proves efficacious in the majority of cases. This seems another political disease which should be controlled by ensuring that an adequate number of the correct pills go down the correct throats for long enough. Orthopaedic surgery has a small part to play in overcoming deformities, as the combination of fixed deformity and anaesthesia is extremely likely to be followed by pressure problems (Fig.10.12). The provision of really adequate protective and well-fitting footwear should go a long way towards protecting these anaesthetized feet, and similarly the hands can be safeguarded by educating the patient and providing suitable tools and utensils. The diagnosis is made on clinical grounds reinforced by laboratory investigations, and radiology really does not have a major role, although many lepers also have pulmonary tuberculosis.

Fungal infections such as maduramycosis and actinomycosis occur, but seem to be much commoner in some areas than others (Fig. 10.13). Madura foot is endemic in the Sudan, and as yet there does not seem to be any really adequate systemic antifungal medicine available, although reports are appearing of success with ketoconazole in some fungal infections (Haapasaari *et al.* 1982). While much of the secondary infection in fairly advanced cases can be controlled by antibiotics, ablative surgery is often necessary to rid the patient of an evil extremity. Again the diagnosis can usually be made in advanced cases on clinical grounds, and there are X-ray changes with bone destruction and new bone formation. In an ideal situation the fungus may be cultured and examined microscopically.

Smallpox is currently considered to have been eradicated, but this condition is of great interest as a true viral infection of bone. It has a propensity to involve the epiphyses around the

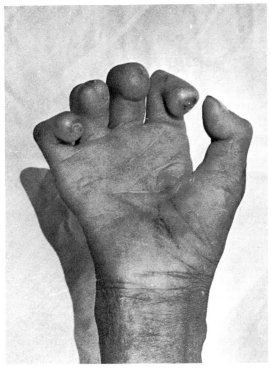

Fig. 10.12. Loss of the distal portion of the anaesthetic digits in leprosy.

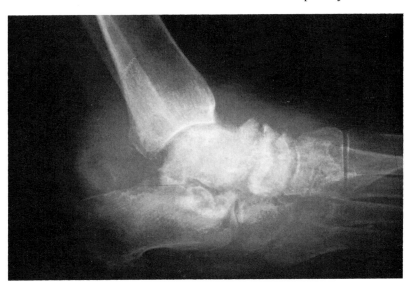

Fig. 10.13. A Madura foot.

elbow, but other bones and joints, certainly in the hands, can be affected. Joints may either be destroyed with a resulting flail pseudarthrosis, or bone ankylosis can follow the fairly acute septic arthritis (Fig. 10.14). It is not uncommon to see patients with one or two stiff elbows and the typical pox scars on their faces. Radiology of these affected joints is of interest but little practical value.

The author has never seen a case of *yaws*, although X-rays with evidence of a periostitis and this diagnosis are demonstrated from time to time. However, it apparently does still occur in some parts of the world and in the acute stage responds well to penicillin. Its old X-ray changes turn up from time to time in X-ray departments in the U.K. and elsewhere.

Tropical ulcers may be acute or chronic. There is some thought now that many of the ulcers, in fact, relate to insufficiency of the communicating veins, and it would seem that dealing with this vascular problem allows the ulcer to heal rapidly. If untreated they may become chronic and, in time, malignant. At this stage there is very likely to be bone destruction underlying the ulcer, whereas in the chronic phase there is often only a periosteal reaction without bone destruction. These carcinomas metastasize with fatal results.

Gas gangrene turns up in the tropics as elsewhere; the diagnosis should be clinical, but bubbles of gas can be recognized in radiographs (Fig. 10.15).

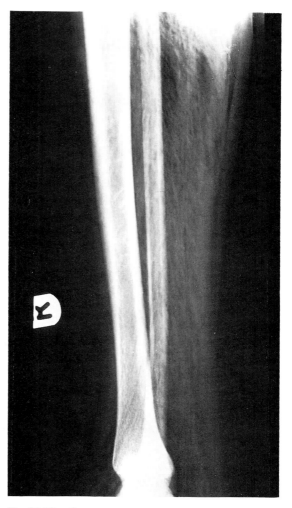

Fig. 10.15. Gas gangrene.

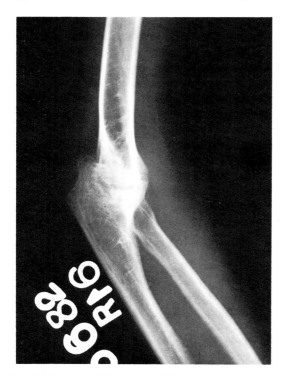

Fig. 10.14. An ankylosed elbow following smallpox.

Tetanus remains all too common in the developing world; it may be neonatal following application of cow dung to the umbilicus, or complicate wounds and compound fractures. Again this terrible disease should be controlled if not eradicated throughout the world by active immunization.

Trauma

In many respects the sequelae and management of trauma are the same everywhere in the world. However, in less-developed areas a great number of injured patients present after the optimum time has passed for the ideal management of their injuries. In major cities in the tropics there may be adequate roads, ambulances and accident and emergency departments, but these facilities are relatively rare, and most patients with closed and open fractures tend to arrive days rather than hours after their injuries. This may not be of great importance with closed fractures, providing that there have been no vascular complications and that the fracture has not united in a bad position. (Fig. 10.16) but with open fractures the results can be catastrophic. Many simple fractures are managed quite well by local 'bone setters' but even these people do not always appreciate the dangers of tight splintage, and it is not uncom-

mon to have a child present with a gangrenous arm firmly supported in a locally made splint such as split bamboo (Fig. 10.17). However, most patients who survive with open fractures eventually trickle through to a recognized hospital, and their treatment can mean months of hospital care and attention.

Acute injuries should, where possible, receive the usual management of careful assessment on arrival, resuscitation, and then active treatment. Many of the patients will be in poor general condition with low levels of haemoglobin, and there can be associated skin sores. Unless really first-class facilities are available, it is wisest and safest to treat simple fractures conservatively, as far as possible eschewing all metal implants and operation.

Patients arriving with compound fractures within a very few hours of injury can be treated by primary closure if their general condition allows, and if there are adequate facilities. If not then it is far better to clean and pack the wound and close it later by either delayed primary or secondary methods. The fracture can usually be rested, either by traction in the lower limb, or by a padded plaster gutter and elevation in the arm. More usually, patients arrive with open fractures after six or eight hours have passed. Indeed they may attend several months after

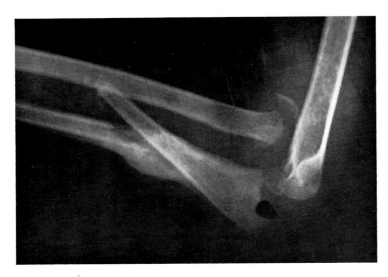

Fig. 10.16. Late presentation of a Monteggia fracture in a child with a totally stiff and virtually untreatable elbow.

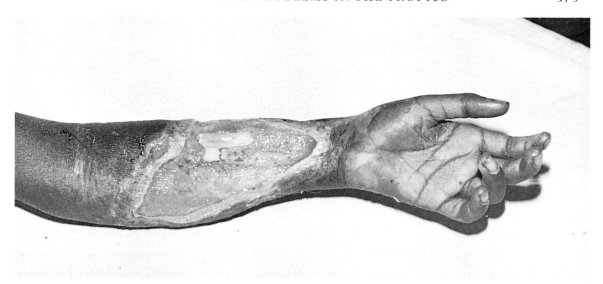

Fig. 10.17. A partly gangrenous forearm revealed on removal of a traditional split bamboo splint used to treat a simple greenstick fracture.

the injury. These problems tend to gravitate to the major centres, and on one ward round the author found five children with late-presenting and infected severe compound fracture separations of the epiphysis of the lower end of the radius, a condition rarely seen in the U.K. (Fig. 10.18). These old compound fractures will often unite in time and with an improvement in the patient's general condition, resulting from adequate food, oral iron, reinforced if necessary by intramuscular therapy, and possibly by attention to intestinal parasites. Often it is important not to remove dead bone too early, and here radiology has a major part to play when it is available, as good-quality penetrating films show the formation and eventual separation of sequestrae. By the time this has occurred and the dead bone can be removed easily, the fracture may well have joined (Fig. 10.19). If the limb has been splinted or rested in a position of function, then after the dead material is removed it is often relatively easy to produce skin closure by split skin grafting or other means, and this allows the patient to mobilize local joints either in hospital, or at home after he has run away.

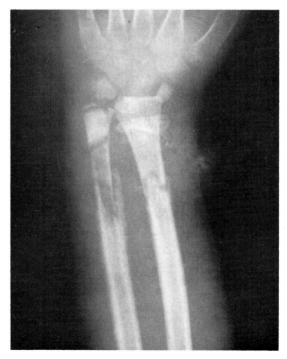

Fig. 10.18. A late-presenting compound fracture – separation of the lower end of the radial epiphysis with severe bone infection.

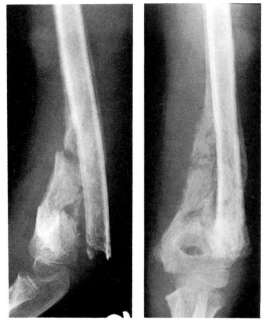

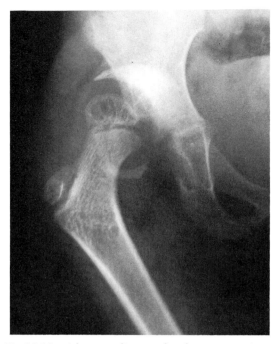

Fig. 10.19. A late-presenting compound fracture at the lower end of the humerus in a child. In time the lower end of the humeral shaft will sequestrate and separate, and the final result is likely to be a reasonably satisfactory elbow and upper limb.

Fig. 10.20. A long-standing unreduced post-traumatic dislocation of the hip in a child.

Patients with *late dislocations* are also relatively common (Figs. 10.20 & 10.21). Sometimes it is as well to leave these alone provided function is acceptable. In the hip, a Girdlestone excision arthroplasty is preferable to an arthrodesis, or even to the stiff fibrous ankylosis which follows open surgery or closed reduction by heavy femoral pin traction. This is particularly true in patients who need to squat. Many attempts have been made to produce an effective arthroplasty for late dislocations of the elbow, but the long-term results as yet have not been startling. Late dislocations of the jaw find their way to orthopaedic clinics where there are no dental services. Sometimes closed reduction by manipulation can help, but in others it is tempting to excise the condyles. This may allow the patient a little more movement of the jaw and help with feeding, but the long-term results are not sensationally good.

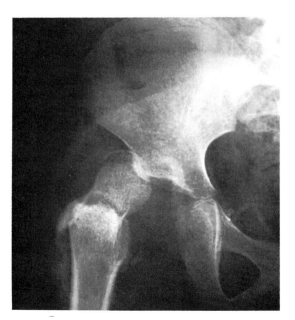

Fig. 10.21. Attempts 'elsewhere' to reduce this child's old dislocated hip had resulted in a trochanteric fracture which in the illustration can be seen to be uniting although the dislocation remains unreduced.

Non-union of closed fractures presents the same problems abroad as in the U.K. Most do very well with simple bone grafting using iliac slivers followed by plaster immobilization. Rarely is internal fixation necessary as it is only too often complicated by infection (Figs 10.22 & 10.23).

Infected non-unions present a greater problem, particularly when there is associated skin loss, joint stiffness and evidence of damage to nerves and vessels (Fig. 10.24). These sort of injuries often follow gunshot wounds, particularly with high-velocity missiles (Fig. 10.25). Again basic

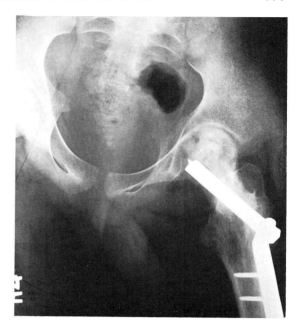

Fig. 10.23. An infected 'pin and plate'.

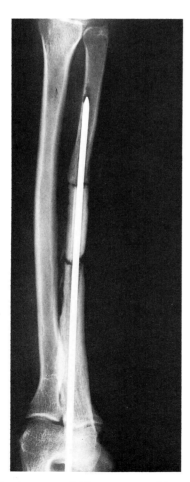

Fig. 10.22. Attempts to bridge an un-united fracture of the ulna with a bone graft and internal fixation failed on account of sepsis.

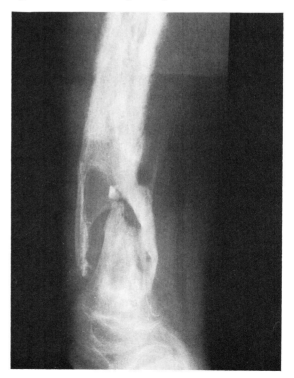

Fig. 10.24. An infected non-union of a lower femoral fracture with a totally stiff knee.

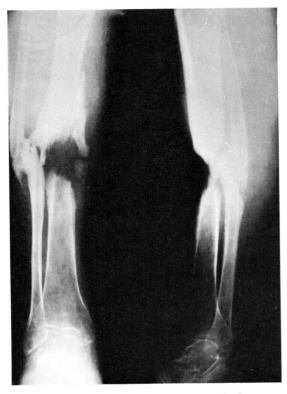

Fig. 10.25. 'Missing bone disease' following a high-velocity missile injury. The foot was stiff and anaesthetic.

which would otherwise have to be sacrificed. In the management of non-unions, whether infected or closed, it is important to improve the patient's general condition by good feeding, attention to the level of circulating haemoglobin, and possibly eradication of most if not all intestinal parasites. In practice, some of the high-velocity gunshot injuries producing large areas of 'missing bones' (Fig. 10.25) will provide a severe test of orthopaedic skill. However, when the supply of prostheses is inadequate or even non-existent, a stiff deformed limb, particularly if there is some protective sensibility, may be preferable to amputation.

Paraplegia. When travelling in the developing countries a small section of every hospital is found to contain patients with paraplegia. Most of these follow trauma, but a few are the end result of tuberculous spine infection or neurological disease. Their management, or rather lack of management, is often extremely distressing both to the patient and to all his attendants and family. However, it has been shown that simple care given by devoted staff, often relatively untrained, reinforced by family support can prevent the development of pressure sores, contractures and significant bladder infections, even in extremely poor areas. This type of work, as with the care of lepers, calls for dedication, but this can be found just as much among nationals as in expatriates, and the author has had the opportunity of seeing both good units and, alas, those where no interest is taken. It is surprising what can be done by relatives and ward orderlies given encouraging leadership. When the patients have recovered from the initial trauma, they can often be retrained to lead a useful self-supporting life from a wheelchair. For £50 sterling a paraplegic in Bangladesh can be trained and equipped as a village tailor.

orthopaedic principles must be followed. Infection will usually subside with rest and the removal of sequestrae and dead material. Skin cover can sometimes be achieved by split skin grafting, but if there is a large defect then full-thickness skin transfer, by either pedicle or cross-leg flap, may be essential. Bone grafting using chips or slivers can be performed once the area has been soundly healed for at least a month. Again internal fixation is best avoided, particularly in these potentially infected areas, and sufficient support can nearly always be achieved with plaster immobilization, or rarely by traction. It is very occasionally possible to pack small cancellous bone chips into a clean granulating cavity which presumably must be potentially if not actually infected. These grafts will often incorporate, and this technique can expedite union, and may even save a limb

Deformities

Nicholas André in 1741 coined the word 'orthopaedic' from the Greek and it means loosely 'to straighten children'. This implies that there must have been bent children seeking medical aid two centuries ago. While many of the conditions producing cripples and deformities have now disappeared from the more advanced parts of the world, they are unfortunately only too common in the developing tropical countries.

In the previous two sections it has been mentioned that inadequately treated fractures and joint injuries and infections—followed by stiffness and contractures—may produce deformities which will interfere with function as well as producing a cosmetic blemish. There are other deforming conditions which commonly occur, such as clubfeet, cerebral palsy, poliomyelitis, the metabolic bone disorders (particularly rickets), and conditions which are perhaps less important numerically such as arthrogryposis, spina bifida and the absence or duplication of limbs or parts of limbs.

Congenital talipes equinovarus often presents late. As is the case with so many conditions where medical facilities are strictly limited, it is rarely possible to supervise the management of these children's twisted feet during the whole of their growth, as parents simply do not bring them for regular follow-up appointments. It is therefore important to try to develop a technique which can be performed during one or, at most, a small number of attendances and yet have a reasonable chance of resulting in a corrected and moderately mobile foot at skeletal maturity; anyone can produce a rigid hoof. Various methods of achieving this have been tried in different parts of the world, and unfortunately there is no one technique which may be used in every instance, and for children of every age. While in many parts of the world clubfeet children do not attend until they are several months or even years old, in other more enlightened parts, and in particular if there is a clubfoot clinic available, babies are now being seen within a few weeks, if not a few days, of birth. Whatever method is chosen it is important to train and use ancillary workers as much as possible, and to limit the indications for operation, as usually there is insufficient operating time and operating skill available. Children over a few months of age presenting with significant foot deformity will almost certainly require corrective surgery. The timing of this procedure does seem important, and there are some experienced surgeons who leave well alone until the child is four or five years of age, at which time they produce complete apparent correction by extensive soft-tissue surgery and then immobilize the foot and ankle in serial plasters for several months. Others like to operate earlier, and then treat recurrences as they arise. The older child with a deformed symptomatic foot usually merits triple fusion at about the skeletal age of 12 years. Adults presenting with severe talipes equinovarus may be better with a Syme's amputation, but it is important never to correct a significant deformity in a beggar unless it is possible to provide an alternative occupation. Correcting the beggar's deformity may cost him his livelihood.

Children of all ages present with *cerebral palsy* of all types. It is rarely possible to help significantly by orthopaedic surgery alone, and physiotherapy resources are usually even more limited than surgical facilities. Occasionally, lengthening a heel cord helps, and the author has assisted hemiplegic teenagers to walk for the first time by arthrodesing their hip. In the same condition a foot which moves into varus during the second growth spurt can be significantly improved by triple fusion. More exotic tendon procedures, such as Eggar's hamstring transfer, can occasionally be helpful, but careful post-operative re-education is essential to achieve good results and, unless one has intelligent and co-operative parents who can give the necessary exercises, surgery may be followed by the rapid appearance of deformity and, even worse, decreased mobility. In spastic cerebral palsy paraplegia it is worth remembering that the hip may be 'pulled out of joint' by muscle imbalance during the early part of the second growth spurt if not before, and this can nearly always be avoided by preventing contracture of the adductors by regular hip stretching into abduction in flexion. Where an adduction contraction has occurred then closed or open tenotomy, possibly combined with partial obturator neurectomy, may prevent the hip from dislocating. Obviously, hip instability is of less importance in a child of low intelligence with no physical prospect of attaining independent walking.

Congenital dislocation of the hip. This problem is seen very little in the tropical countries in which the author has worked. Very often children are shown to an orthopaedic surgeon as examples of congenital dislocation, but on going into the history and examination carefully they are nearly always the result either of a septic arthritis of infancy, or of an underlying neurological problem. Congenital dislocation of the hip is probably worldwide, but the incidence varies a great deal from area to area.

Deformed knees. Bow legs, knock knees and windswept legs seem to be particularly common in parts of Africa and probably elsewhere (Fig. 10.26a, b, c). While many of these are of unknown aetiology, there is a feeling that many of the children with windswept legs are in fact suffering from the late result of rickets (Fig. 10.27). It is always worth remembering the possibility of an underlying metabolic bone disorder; in one young lady with asymmetrical knock-knee deformities X-rays, including a skeletal survey, raised the possibility of hyperparathyroidism, and eventually a parathyroid tumour was successfully excised. When the deformities are bizarre, and interfere with function, then correction by osteotomy/osteoclasis is usually successful. Tibia vara, Blount's disease, seems more common in the West African than the European, and if deformity is severe and progressive then early corrective osteotomy which may have to be repeated is essential (Fig. 10.28a, b).

Scoliosis certainly occurs throughout the world and may be congenital, paralytic or idiopathic as seen elsewhere. With the lack of facilities it is rarely possible to treat these unfortunate children with their progressive deformities.

Tumours
While there may well be a different incidence of soft-tissue and bone tumours in various parts of the world, there seems little doubt that any type may in fact turn up anywhere. Be that as it may, in the tropics tumours do tend to be very large by the time the patients present, unless of course they are sufficiently malignant to have proved fatal before the patient attends (Fig. 10.29). There are a few types which are probably more common in parts of the tropics than elsewhere. These include Burkitt's lymphoma, primary hepatoma which can metatasize to bone, and ameloblastoma (adamantinomas). Giant osteoclastoma in the classical sites seems common in orthopaedic centres in the tropics and developing countries (Fig. 10.30), and unfortunately local surgery is only too often followed by a recurrence. Various heroic surgical procedures have been devised using massive bone grafts and often sacrificing involved joints. The results can be encouraging. There seems to be an increase in the incidence of malignant fibrosarcomas and so-called synoviomas. However, one of the great problems in the management of bone tumours in the developing countries is from the sparcity of experienced bone pathologists. These people are rare enough in the developed world, but in the author's experience are almost non-existent in the developing areas. Bone pathology is nearly always extremely difficult, and experienced consultants are often unwilling to give an opinion on small sections of tissue sent to them, preferring to have full clinical details and the radiographs available before giving a final opinion. When the tumours are rapidly growing and peripheral, amputation is often the only practical line of treatment but this may be refused.

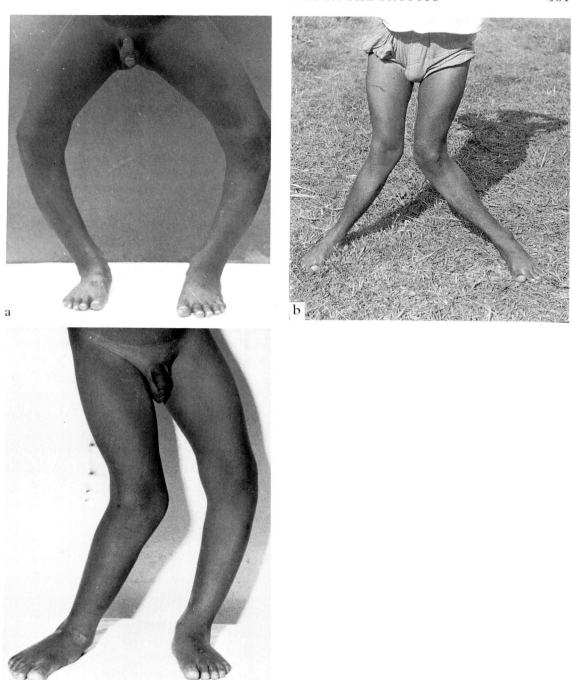

Fig. 10.26. (a) Severe bow legs. (b) Severe knock-knees. (c) Windswept legs.

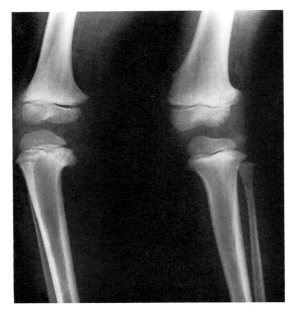

Fig. 10.27. 'Windswept legs'. Note the suggestion of possible partly healed rickets.

Other assorted conditions

Rheumatoid arthritis. This is very common in the Indian subcontinent but is rare in parts of Africa (Fig. 10.31). The clinical and radiological diagnosis is usually not difficult, but long-term medical treatment is rarely practical. Severe rheumatoid arthritis produces terrible crippling—one 22-year-old lady was only able to move two fingers of one hand. With these, sitting in a locally made wheelchair, she was able to illustrate Christmas greeting postcards.

Rickets and *osteomalacia* are seen from time to time in the tropics as well as in immigrants in the U.K. The children are irritable and show the classic swellings in the region of their joints and elsewhere. Treatment with vitamin D is usually arranged, but alas follow-up often does not occur with any satisfactory regularity. Osteomalacia, too, can follow an inadequate diet, and responds extremely well to vitamin D with calcium (Fig. 10.32).

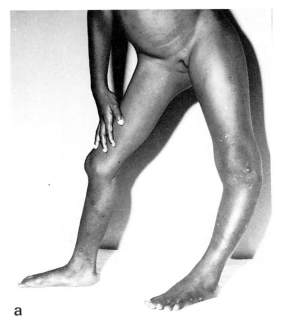

a

Fig. 10.28. (a) A child with Blount's disease in one leg and considerable polio weakness in the other. (b) X-ray of the same child's lower limbs.

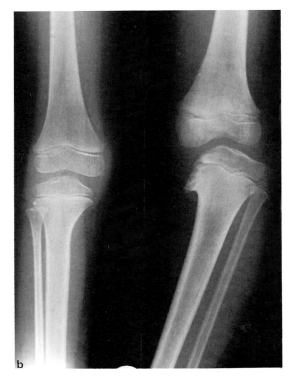

b

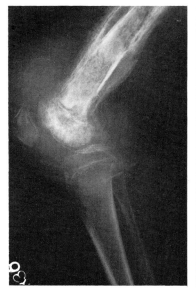
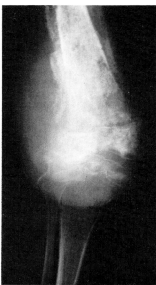

Fig. 10.29. A huge mass in the lower thigh. Differential diagnosis between infection and malignancy. This one turned out to be malignant.

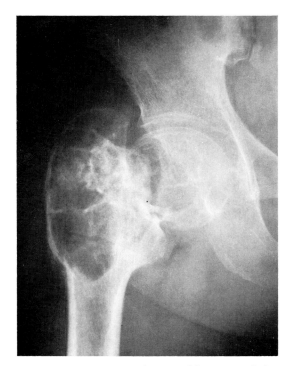

Fig. 10.30. A proven osteoclastoma of the upper end of the femur and greater trochanter with a fracture of the femoral neck.

Scurvy must appear from time to time, but the author has, in fact, never seen, or at least recognized, this condition in any tropical country. Its possible occurrence should be remembered when clinical and radiological examination raise the possibility of non-accidental injury, the battered baby syndrome.

The haemoglobinopathies. As is well known the presence of abnormal haemoglobin appears to be genetically related, and different types with their associated problems occur in different parts of the world. From the orthopaedic angle sickle haemoglobin, which is very common in West Africa, produces symptoms, signs and X-ray changes. In the bones these are the result of increased erythropoiesis, and the occurrence of infarcts (Fig. 10.33a, b). The latter, while often sterile and symmetrical, may become infected as part of a *Salmonella typhi* septicaemia. Children with homozygous SS disease (probably 2% of all births in West Africa) exist with a haemoglobin at about 8 g%. This is their normal level and it is unwise to attempt to raise this before undertaking essential surgery

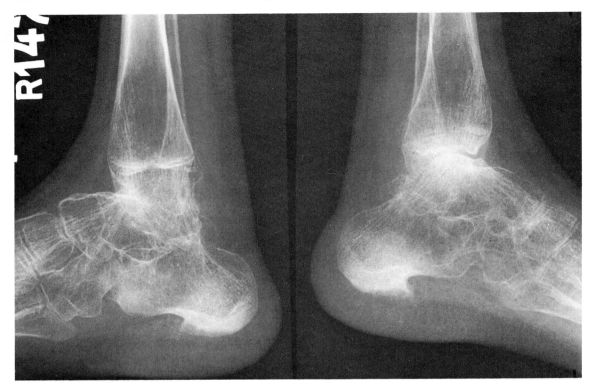

Fig. 10.31. Severe rheumatoid arthritis in an Indian young lady.

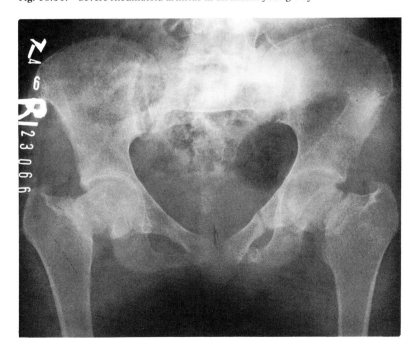

Fig. 10.32. Classical osteomalacia with bilateral femoral neck and pelvic rami fractures.

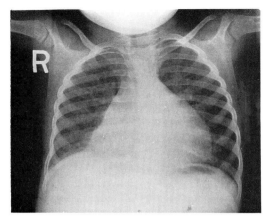

Fig. 10.33a. Homozygous sickle cell disease with haemoglobin of 8 g%, positive blood culture of *Salmonella typhi*, and X-ray evidence of infarction in the upper end of the left humerus.

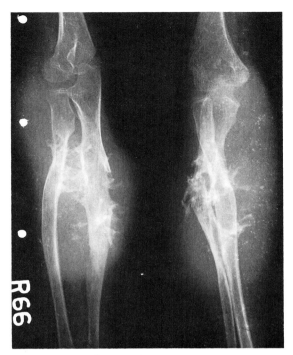

Fig. 10.34. Possible neurofibromatosis. Histology of the partly resected tumour revealed 'fibrous type-tissue'.

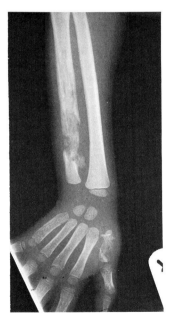

Fig. 10.33b. X-ray changes in homozygous sickle cell disease.

(although pre-operative exchange transfusion may be helpful). Tourniquets have a bad reputation with sickle cell trait and disease, but there is no real evidence for this, particularly if an exsanguinating technique is employed. Much has been written about the need to maintain high concentrations of oxygen during general anaesthesia. There is no specific therapy yet available, genetic counselling is not really practical in many parts of the world, but supportive and symptomatic treatment should not be denied. There are a sufficient number of people now resident in the U.K. with West African blood in their veins to make it essential that all doctors remember the possibility of the presence of the abnormal haemoglobins.

Undiagnosable conditions

Wherever one travels in the world, particularly in the tropics, patients and their X-rays are presented with fascinating, but often bizarre, and nearly always undiagnosable, conditions (Figs. 10.34, 10.35a–d). Interesting and unusual combinations also occur (Fig. 10.28a, b). While some of these could probably be diagnosed without any great difficulty with good laboratory, radiological and histological support, these

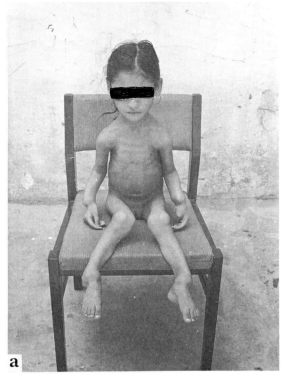

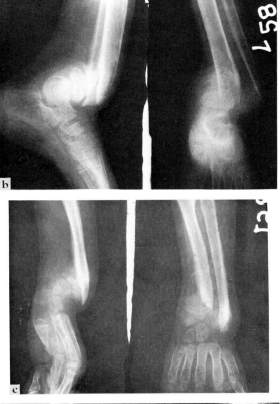

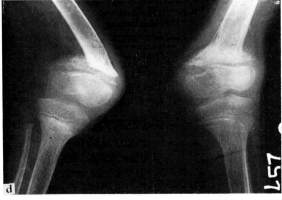

Fig. 10.35 (a) A young lady with multiple joint 'anomalies'. (b) X-rays of the same young lady's knee joints. (c) X-rays of the same young lady's ankle joints. (d) X-rays of the same young lady's wrist joints.

fairly sophisticated techniques are rarely available locally, and one has to depend on an often grossly inaccurate history, careful clinical examination and straight X-ray films, frequently of dubious quality. However, it is well worth remembering the maxim of 'going for function', particularly when the disorder does not appear

to be progressive, the patient is mentally normal and there is adequate inner drive and family support. However, always remember that the beggar may depend on his deformity for his continuing existence, and rarely is it advisable to talk anyone into elective corrective surgery. There is a one-legged gateman at a certain orthopaedic hospital, and therein hangs a tale.

Many of the orthopaedic diseases and problems which present in the developing tropical countries have been briefly described. Some of these patients, and their descendants, will, of course, appear from time to time in the U.K. and in other more developed countries. While there are a small number of conditions which are more or less restricted to the tropics, and to people with their origins in these areas, such as the haemoglobinopathies, some overseas traditions and diets when continued in the U.K. and elsewhere will result in disorders such as rickets. Skeletal tuberculosis in the immigrant population (as well as in the indigenous) may present in an unusual fashion (Fig. 10.36a, b, c), and some of these unusual manifestations have been well documented by Goldblatt and Cremin (1978). Perhaps the most important point is for all clinicians and laboratory personnel to remember the possibility of the so-called tropical diseases occurring in the U.K. Tropical conditions (e.g. malaria) can, of course, occur in people who were born in the U.K. and have been abroad for periods of varying lengths, and this too must be borne in mind.

Acknowledgements

I am most grateful to all the colleagues, too numerous to mention individually, who have allowed me to use their X-rays and photographs as illustrations. I am also most grateful to my secretary, Miss Susan Wadd, and to Miss Mary Pugh of Queen Mary's Hospital for Children, Carshalton, for producing the illustrations.

References

GOLDBLATT M. & CREMIN B. J. (1978) Osteo-articular tuberculosis: its presentation in coloured races.*Clin. Radiol.* **29,** 669–77.

HAAPASAARI J., ESSEN R. V., KAHANPAA A., KOSTIALA ANJA A. I., HOLMBERG K. & AHLQUIST J. (1982) Fungal arthritis simulating juvenile rheumatoid arthritis. *Brit. med. J.* **285,** 923.

WALKER G. F. (1968) Failure of early recognition of skeletal tuberculosis. *Brit. med. J.* **1,** 682–3.

Further reading

COCKSHOTT P. & MIDDLEMASS H. (eds.) (1979) *Clinical Radiology in the Tropics.* Edinburgh: Churchill Livingstone.

SCHWARTZ S. I., ADESOLA A. O., ELEBUTE E. A. & ROB C. G. (1971) *Tropical Surgery.* New York: McGraw-Hill Book Co.

SUTTON D. (ed.) (1980) *A Textbook of Radiology and Imaging,* 3rd Edition. Edinburgh: Churchill Livingstone.

REEDER M. M. & PALMER P. E. S. (1981) *The Radiology of Tropical Diseases, with Epidemiological, Pathological and Clinical Correlation.* Baltimore: Williams & Wilkins.

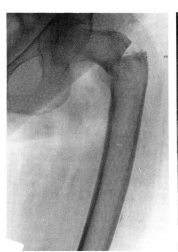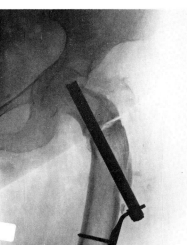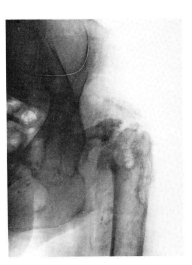

Fig. 10.36 A pathological fracture of the femoral neck with ensuing destruction of bone which eventually turned out to be tuberculous in origin.

Chapter 11
The Spine

I. W. McCALL

Anatomy and biomechanics

The spine is a composite of similar, repeated, bony units, composed of a vertebral body, pedicles, lamina, articular processes and a spinous process. These bony units are interlinked anteriorly by the intervertebral disc and posteriorly by articulating synovial facet joints. The ligaments of the spine, namely the anterior and posterior longitudinal ligaments, and interspinous and interlaminar ligaments, make a major contribution to the overall stability and mechanical function of the back, while the muscles attached to the spinal column provide the external forces. The articulating column of units is thus capable of different elastic and mechanical properties, such as flexion, extension, rotation, and lateral flexion, and is also capable of transmitting and sustaining loads. The intervertebral disc is composed of an outer annulus fibrosus comprised primarily of collagen, elastic microfibrils, proteoglycans and a water content of 69–70%. The nucleus pulposus provides the hydrostatic component to the disc with a water content of 80–90% in early life, and a high proteoglycan and low collagen component. The transition between the annulus fibrosus and the nucleus is smooth and gradual. It is likely that the collagen is responsible for the tensile strength of the annulus, and the proteoglycans for the hydrodynamic properties of the nucleus. Acid aminoglycans are responsible for the high water content of the disc and they form pathways by which nutrition diffuses through the annulus to the nucleus. On vertical loading, the nucleus exerts forces of equal magnitude on the innermost layers of the annulus. Normal compressive forces, similar to those occurring in flexion and extension, push the nucleus in opposite directions as part of the hydrostatic process. Rotation and torsional stresses are borne by the annulus where adjacent layers of collagen which are inclined at constant angles to each other give the annular fibre a high tensile resistance in all directions. The fibre layers attached to the vertebral body undergo stretching and tensile stress, which is communicated to the vertebral rim.

The ageing process of the disc is a normal process. A gradual decrease in hydration with age directly correlates with a decrease in the relative and absolute amounts of acid aminoglycans within the disc. Reduction of hydration with age causes the gel-like nucleus to become increasingly firm. This leads to the loss of the normal hydraulic properties of the nucleus and a greater percentage of the total strain is then transmitted to the annulus. Loss of fluid from the annulus also leads to change in the angle of origin of the collagen fibres which considerably reduces its torque strength. In the severely degenerated disc, the nucleus is dessicated and contains splits and clefts parallel to the endplate. Nuclear material is not present in these clefts, but inflammatory ingrowth may occur, suggesting an element of trauma and a repair reaction.

Mechanical disorders of the back occur at sites where strains are abnormally high and at points where tissues are weak. On compressive loading, the end-plates fail rather than the disc, except at L5/S1, where the wedge-shape may lead to protrusion of the posterior parts of the annulus. Abnormal rotational stresses lead to radiating fissures, which are usually posterola-teral and result from tensile failure, starting in the nucleus and propagating across the concentric layers of the annulus. The collagen content of the posterolateral part of the annulus is significantly less than anterolaterally, and this may be in part responsible for the high frequency of prolapse posterolaterally.

In the degenerated discs, the fibrotic nucleus acts non-hydrostatically under axial compression loading, and the annulus is squeezed out and therefore bulges posteriorly. The same changes also prevent movement of the nucleus, thus increasing the tensile strains on sections of the disc wall in flexion and extension.

The posterior elements transmit a substantial part of the compressive loading, especially in extension. The pars has a small cross-section but a thick cortex and so can take strain. Stress fractures may occur, however, if repeated excessive forces are applied in extension. The posterior joints regulate the degree of mobility by the alignment of the planes of articulation. The horizontal cervical joints allow greater mobility, especially in flexion and extension. The vertical thoracic facets allow some rotation but no lateral movement. In the lumbar spine the alignment varies from vertical and sagittal orientation above to an oblique coronal one in the lower segments. These allow extension, flexion and lateral bending but limit axial rotation.

Tropism and asymmetry of facets in the lower lumbar spine is not uncommon and leads, on sustained loading, to a rotational stress, putting strain on the ligaments and joints of the less oblique facet. Lumbar facets are subjected to both compression and shear forces. The tendency to slide is obviated by cupping of the facets.

The degeneration or traumatic processes that affect the spine may pass unheeded throughout life. On the other hand, the changes may be recognized in a number of ways and the most common manifestation is the production of pain.

Spinal pain

Pain is an abnormal affective state that occurs if mechanical and/or chemical changes in the tissues of the body activate the normally quiescent afferent systems. This activity is altered by a variety of somatic or visceral reflex responses and by hormonal changes that may be simultaneously evoked. Whether a stimulus is painful or not is determined by the extent to which the afferent activity is channelled into and through the central pathways. Pain is produced by a stimulation of a morphologically distinct system of receptor nerve endings which are sensitive to mechanical and chemical tissue dysfunction. This plexiform mesh of unmyelinated nerve fibres is normally inactive but becomes active when depolarized by abnormal forces or substances.

Pain has a dual nature, with a cognitive and an effective component, and sensation and reaction to pain are closely interlinked. Tolerance is affected by the mental state of the patient and the response is thus regulated centrally.

It has recently been shown that pain response is also affected by an intrinsic system of opiate production called the endorphins. The presence and actions of this system may help to explain, at least in part, the placebo effect of many forms of treatment. Because pain is a personal psychological experience and direct measurement is impossible, indirect methods have been devised. The subjective method of the visual analogue scale is the most useful and widely used. Objective methods such as changes in respiratory function, hormonal measurement or comparison of analgesic requirements are only of value in treatment comparisons.

NEUROANATOMY

Afferents from the limbs pass to the cord via the ventral rami of the spinal nerve and the dorsal nerve root, while those from the dermatomes to the lower back are conveyed through the lateral branches of the posterior primary ramus of the spinal nerve (Fig. 11.1). Afferents from the apophyseal joints, SI joints, vertebral arches, cancellous bone, periosteum, and interspinal ligaments enter the medial branches of the posterior primary rami and this innervation is plurisegmental (Fig. 11.2). The capsules of the apophyseal joints are also innervated by primary nerve filaments passing directly from the spinal nerves as they emerge from the intervertebral foramen. The ventral rami and posterior primary rami unite to form the dorsal root with their cell bodies situated in the dorsal root ganglion, which lies within the intervertebral foramen.

In the cervical spine, the dorsal and ventral nerve roots have a short course, running either horizontally or mildly obliquely upwards from the intervertebral foramen to the cord. In the thoracic spine, the roots travel upwards by the side of the cord for at least two vertebral body heights before entering the cord. In the lumbar spine, the roots have a long ascent in the cauda equina.

Afferents from the posterior longitudinal spinal ligaments, the dura, the epidural vessel walls and fat, and the periosteum and vessels of the vertebral bodies traverse branches of the sinovertebral nerve to reach the spinal nerve just distal to the dorsal root ganglion (Fig. 11.1). The synovertebral nerve is closely applied to the posterior surface of the annulus fibrosus and reaches the canal within which it is distributed intersegmentally through ascending and descending branches. The synovertebral branch of the second lumbar nerve gives off a long descending collateral branch as far as the fifth lumbar, hence its extensive referral.

Thus pain in the spine and limbs may arise from two main sources. Irritation or compression of the roots within the spinal canal or as they emerge through the intervertebral foramen produces dermatomal pain, which is sharp, often electric in quality (Fig. 11.3). The second source occurs from activation of the nerve endings in the many tissues that make up the spinal segment. This produces distribution patterns of

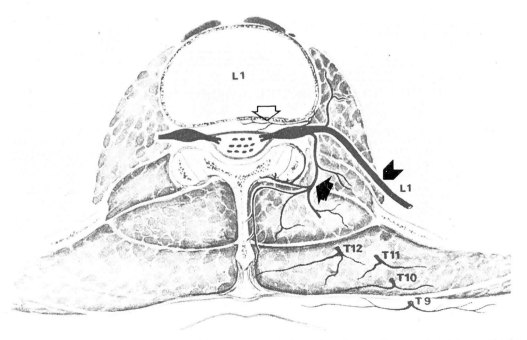

Fig. 11.1. Neuroanatomy. The distributions of the nerve supply to the various tissues of the spine is demonstrated (after Kellgren). ⇨ sinovertebral nerve. ➡ posterior primary ramus. ➢ ventral ramus.

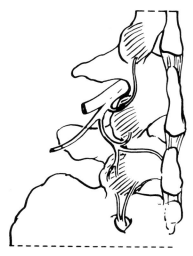

Fig. 11.2. Facet innervation. The multiple levels of innervation from the medial branch of the posterior primary rami are demonstrated.

pain described by Kellgren as sclerotomal (Fig. 11.4) and which is of a dull, deep, often aching or cramp-like quality. Distally referred pain of this type may often cause diagnostic confusion, as it may be fairly constant but does not correspond to the area of supply of any specific peripheral nerve. The significance of these two types of pain lies in the clinical and therapeutic differences. The two groups will, therefore, be described separately, although many of the pathological processes are interrelated.

DERMATOMAL PAIN

Nerve root compression
The nerve root is compressed either by prolapse of nuclear material from the intervertebral disc, or by narrowing of the spinal canal or lateral recess through which it passes. The former tends to occur in the 20–40 age group. The

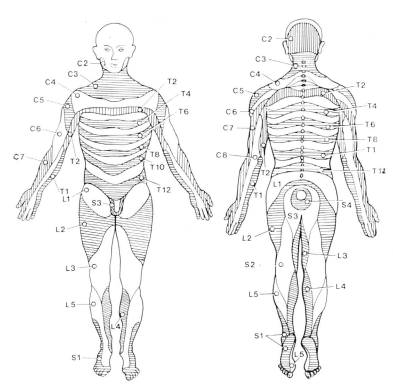

Fig. 11.3. Dermatomal distribution of pain referral.

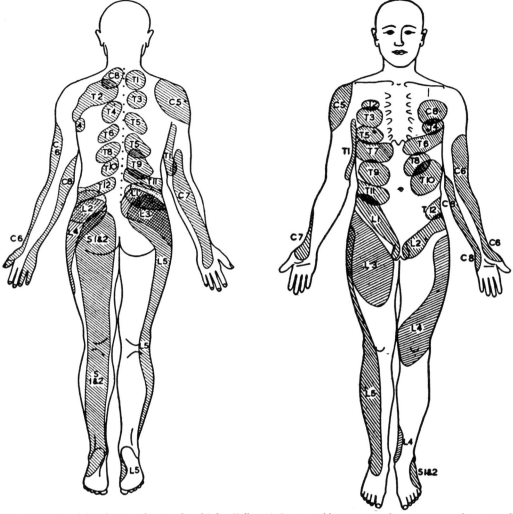

Fig. 11.4. Sclerotomal distribution of pain referral (after Kellgren). Segmental hypertonic saline injections adjacent to the midline produced the pattern of pain referral demonstrated. There is considerable similarity to dermatomal referral.

latter usually develops from the age of 40 onwards, but congenital stenosis may manifest earlier. Nerve root compression due to acute nuclear herniation predominates in the lumbar spine. In the cervical spine, acute disc prolapse is unusual and is commonly related to a traumatic episode. Nerve root compression due to disc degeneration, lateral recess stenosis or reactive osteophyte formation occurs in both cervical and lumbar spines. Nerve root compression in the dorsal spine is infrequent.

CLINICAL FEATURES

Disc herniation
Acute intervertebral disc prolapse initially causes a centrally situated ache due to irritation of the nerve endings of the posterior longitudinal ligaments. On compression of the dorsal nerve root the central pain is accompanied by dermatomal pain and this may be reinforced by reflex muscle spasm and voluntary immobilization. In the cervical spine, localization of the

nerve involved by pain distribution is less accurate than in the lumbar spine due to the greater degree of overlap in the former. Movement tends to increase pain, and coughing and sneezing may lead, in the lumbar spine, to sharp painful impulses. Paraesthesiae and numbness can occur initially, but the areas of sensory change may not be contiguous with those of referred pain. If nerve root compression continues, leading to chronic ischaemia, the pain becomes continuous with little relief from previously helpful resting positions.

Examination reveals evidence of muscle spasm causing torticollis in the cervical spine and a sciatic scoliosis in the lumbar spine. The side of the scoliosis may partly depend on whether the disc is lateral or medial to the nerve. Palpation may elicit tenderness in the midline at the level of the disc prolapse. Movement patterns show limitation of flexion and selective restriction of lateral flexion which may be accompanied by exacerbation of limb pain on the side of the lesion. Extension and rotation may not be restricted. A total loss of neck or back movement, however, is suspect as a non-organic sign. In 90% of proven lumbar disc herniations, there is restriction of straight-leg raising of between $30°$ and $70°$. The compressed nerve root cannot accommodate the stretching force and the pain induced occurs in the distribution of the affected nerve. Weakness of muscle groups and reduction or absence of reflexes, particularly the ankle reflex, may occur.

Lateral recess stenosis

Bony compression of the nerve roots produces more chronic change in both the cervical and lumbar spine. The history of pain is more prolonged with exacerbations and remissions. The pain is commonly aggravated by motion, twisting being important in the cervical spine and walking or standing in the lumbar spine. Weakness and numbness are common. On examination, muscle weakness and wasting may well be present. This is particularly noticeable in affection of the cervical spine with atrophy of the deltoid or intrinsic muscles of the hands. In the lower limb a difference in circumference of muscle masses may indicate chronic nerve compression. Sensory loss occurs but is of limited value in localization of nerve roots involved. In this group of patients, the straight-leg raising test is of less value, being normal in up to one-third of patients.

Spinal stenosis

Severe spinal narrowing leads to neurogenic claudication. This usually presents in the fifth decade and may be developmental, due to a narrow lumbar canal, which is accentuated by degenerative changes in the posterior joints and posterior bulging of the annulus. Vague pains with dysaesthesia and paraesthesia occur on ambulation. Walking tolerance becomes restricted and the lordotic stance of walking, particularly downhill, increases the symptoms. Relief occurs at rest, particularly in spinal flexion. Neurogenic claudication must be differentiated from peripheral vascular insufficiency which is made worse by walking up gradients. The absence of pulses confirms the diagnosis. As stenosis increases, the symptoms occur at rest with muscle weakness, atrophy and asymmetrical reflex change.

Severe compression of the cauda equina may occur with disc disease. Back or perianal pain predominates, and radicular symptoms cause leg pain which progresses to numbness and difficulty with walking. Problems with urination may develop early and there will be perianal numbness and loss of the anal reflex.

EMG studies

Electrodiagnosis may be used as a diagnostic test in nerve root compression. It is helpful in either distinguishing between or ruling out lesions in the spinal cord, nerve root, brachial plexus or peripheral nerves. The standard procedure involves the observation of muscle response to galvanic stimulation of peripheral nerves or electromyographic recording of the muscles themselves. If normal function in a

resting muscle is partially or completely in-
hibited by a lower motor neurone disorder, the
electrode discloses spontaneous wave forms
called fibrillation potential. By careful analysis
of different muscles, cervical and lumbar root
compression can be diagnosed. Pitfalls in interpretation occur, however, in the post-laminectomy group where previous damage may affect
the results. Early diagnosis is also restricted by
the fact that Wallerian degeneration may take
three weeks to develop following nerve damage
and the injury may not be severe enough to
cause degeneration.

Radiological studies
In the presence of clinically suspected nerve root
compression, plain radiographs of the affected
part of the spine are usually requested. In many
cases of acute disc prolapse these will be normal. Features that may be present, however,
are confirmation of a deformity due to spasm
and evidence of segmental stress or narrowing
of a particular disc space. Segmental stress of
one vertebra on another may be manifest by
loss of alignment of the spinous processes due
to rotation on the AP view, or by forward or
retrolisthesis of individual vertebrae (Fig. 11.5).

Horizontal shift can be confirmed by performing
flexion and extension films which will accentuate the abnormality of movement. In severe
cases, however, spasm may mask abnormal
movement patterns. Disc space narrowing may
occur alone or in association with degenerative
osteoarthritis of the posterior intervertebral and
uncovertebral joints. Hypertrophic bone formation in the joints and marginal osteophyte formation will lead to narrowing of the lateral
recesses in the lumbar spine and the
intervertebral foramina in the cervical spine. Degenerative spondylolisthesis may further compromise the root outlet, especially in the presence of developmental spinal stenosis. The
dimensions of the spinal canal may be roughly
assessed on the plain films. On the lateral film
an anteroposterior diameter of less than 13 mm
in the mid-cervical spine, and less than 15 mm
in the lower lumbar spine, is considered abnormally small. In the lumbar spine, apophyseal
joints lying medial to the pedicle and inclined
towards the midline also suggest stenosis. Plain
films are of little value in isolating a particular
level of nerve compression. A single diseased
level may be suggestive, but this does not pre-
clude the presence of a hidden lesion, at an

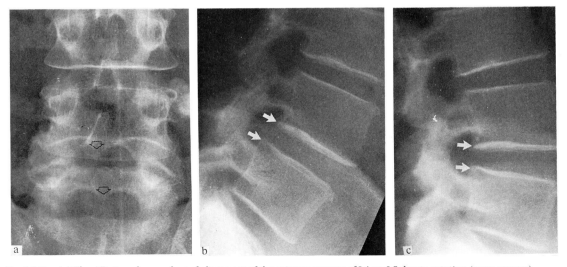

Fig. 11.5. (a) The AP view shows a loss of alignment of the spinous process of L4 on L5 due to rotation (open arrows).
(b) Flexion lateral view shows mild forward displacement of L4 on L5 (closed arrows) which resolves on extension (c).

apparently normal level, being the cause of nerve compression. Chronic changes are often present at two or more levels, which significantly reduces the specificity. In the presence of clinically suggestive nerve root compression, the clinician is therefore recommended to proceed to contrast studies. The techniques involved have already been described. In the cervical spine there will be amputation of the affected nerve root. This may be due to disc material (Fig. 11.6) but more commonly is due to osteophyte formation from the uncovertebral joints extending into the intervertebral foramina (Fig. 11.7). Oblique views will demonstrate the lesion satisfactorily and lateral views are essential to assess the degree of embarrassment of the cervical cord due to disc or osteophyte formation. Flexion and extension views in the lateral plane assess the contribution to narrowing by the ligamentum flavum posteriorly. Displacement of the roots is unusual due to the close proximity of the cord to the foramen. The radiological appearances of disc prolapse in the lumbar spine vary depending on the size of the prolapse. In

mild cases, only enlargement of the root due to swelling may be demonstrated. More extensive compression causes failure of the root sleeve to fill with contrast and the asymmetry will be clearly demonstrated on the radiculogram (Fig. 11.8a).

Finally, displacement and compression of the nerve roots may occur due to a large extradural defect which, in severe cases, causes complete obstruction of the dural sac. The extradural defect is demonstrated by the smooth nature of the contrast border without any evidence of re-entrant angles (Fig. 11.8b). Intradural lesions, such as neurofibromas, with sharp re-entrant angles, will appear surrounded by contrast media (Fig. 11.9). It should also be remembered that extradural defects may be caused by tumours, such as lipomas, within the spinal canal.

The presence of degenerative disease in the apophyseal joints will lead to nerve compression which is shown to be posterior on the lateral films. Lateral flexion/extension films will differentiate between disc bulge or posterior annular

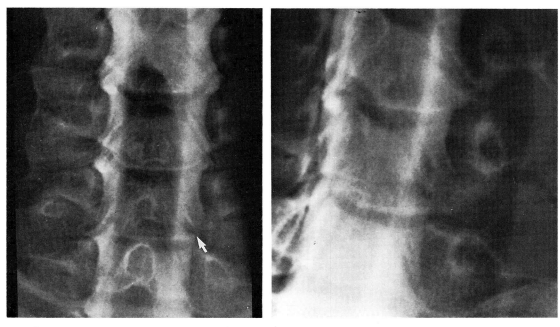

Fig. 11.6. Acute cervical disc prolapse—the nerve root sleeve is amputated and the proximal part of the nerve roots are widened (arrow). The uncovertebral joints are normal.

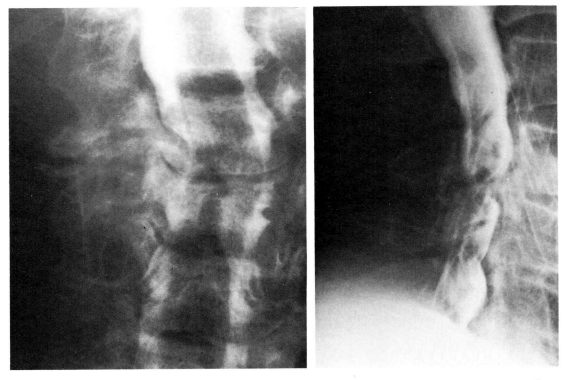

Fig. 11.7. Severe osteophyte formation from osteoarthritis of the uncovertebral and facet joints causes compression and distortion of the dural sac and nerve root. There is also stenosis of the canal on the lateral view.

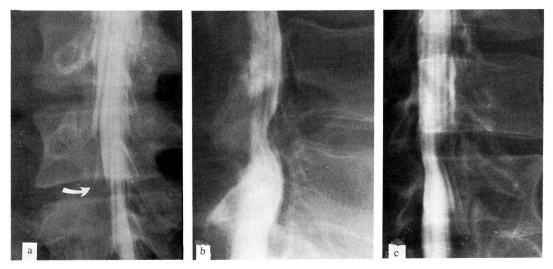

Fig. 11.8. Acute lumbar disc herniation (a) Case 1. The nerve root sleeve of L5 does not fill with contrast but no extradural mass is seen (curved arrow). (b) Case 2. The lateral view demonstrates a smooth extradural impression of the anterior margin of the dural sac by the disc prolapse. (c) The oblique view shows the L5 nerve root compressed and deviation of S1.

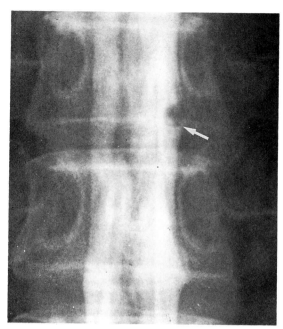

Fig. 11.9. The sharp re-entrant angles of contrast medium indicate an intradural neurofibroma (arrow).

tear and a true disc prolapse. The latter will remain substantially unchanged between flexion and extension, whereas the former will become less obvious in flexion and accentuated by extension (Fig. 11.10). The differentiation is important as laminectomy and decompression performed for disc bulges and posterior annular tears without prolapse of nuclear material are a common cause of failure to relieve symptoms. These dynamic films will also accentuate posterior compression in extension and demonstrate why forward flexion in spinal stenosis relieves symptoms.

Developmental spinal stenosis will be confirmed by generalized narrowing of the contrast column on both lateral and AP films, or indentation or occlusion of the dural sac at multiple disc levels (Fig. 11.11). A high degree of accuracy is possible in the diagnosis of root compression by disc prolapse using water-soluble radiculography.

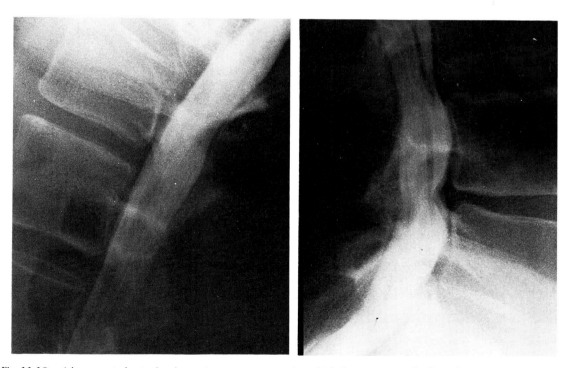

Fig. 11.10. A large central extradural mass is present on extension which disappears completely on flexion.

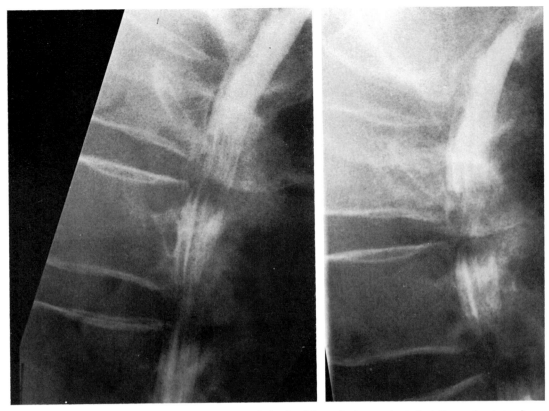

Fig. 11.11. The dural sac is completely compressed at each disc level due to both posterior indentation and anterior disc bulging. On flexion the narrowing is reduced allowing some contrast to demonstrate the nerve roots in the lateral view.

Nerve compression in the lateral recess may be missed if the root sleeves are short and limit the contrast flow. In these cases and in those with an equivocal radiculogram for disc prolapse, lumbar venography has proved valuable. The more lateral position of the anterior epidural veins and the presence of radicular veins provide an indirect assessment of the space available in the nerve root canal. Compression of the vein indicates, indirectly, compression of the nerve (Fig. 11.12). Care, however, must be taken to fill all supplying veins adequately to avoid false-positive results. False-negative results are rare.

Epidurography may be used in these circumstances also and failure to fill the root indicates compression. A technical failure of filling must, again, be excluded before diagnosis of compres-

sion is made. The advent of transaxial computerized tomography has allowed the size and shape of the lateral recess and intervertebral foramina in the cervical and lumbar spine to be assessed directly. The state of the disc and the nerve root can also be shown and this is the initial examination of choice where it is available. Finally, where there is persistent doubt about whether the patient's symptoms are due to nerve root compression, or which nerve is involved, an injection of local anaesthetic into the nerve root may resolve the dilemma.

Treatment of nerve compression
The degree of physical impairment varies enormously despite the similarity of pathology. Treatment of nerve root compression due to disc disease is still a matter of trying various tech-

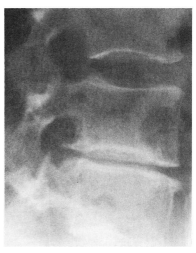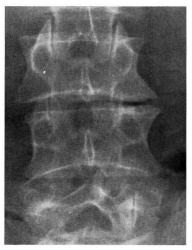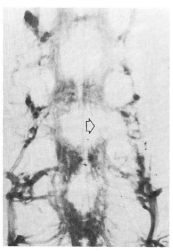

Fig. 11.12. The plain films show marked disc narrowing at L3/4 with marginal osteophyte formation. There is failure of filling of the anterior epidural veins on the left at this level, indicating lateral recess stenosis due to the posterior osteophytes.

niques. A period of conservative therapy is usually attempted. This may include a plaster jacket in mild cases, or a period of traction in more severely affected patients. Epidural anaesthetics and steroids with or without manipulation have also been successful in alleviating symptoms. If evidence of neurology is present or if pain proves intractable, confirmation of the lesion by radiculography is performed. Chymopapain injection into the nucleus has a 70% success rate, and is favoured by some surgeons prior to resorting to surgical treatment. Surgical relief of symptoms by decompressing the nerve root requires a variable degree of disruption of normal anatomy. If there is a small quantity of disc material present, decompression can usually be achieved by a fenestration technique, removing the ligamentum flavum. The prolapsed or sequestrated nuclear material is removed and the nucleus of the disc may then be evacuated with pituitary rongeurs. Part of the lamina may require removal if visibility is restricted and a more extensive disc evacuation is required. The nerve root must be seen to be free following nuclear removal of the prolapsed disc material and a probe should pass easily through the lateral recess. Preoperative evidence of lateral recess stenosis requires a more extensive

decompression of the nerve root canal with partial removal of the articular processes of the facets.

Following laminectomy, posterior fusion of the vertebral segments may be performed. This may be as a posterolateral or intertransverse fusion. Dispute still rages as to whether laminectomy should be automatically accompanied by fusion. It is probably unnecessary in the simple cases of prolapsed or sequestrated intervertebral disc disease in the younger patient. If an extensive lateral decompression has been necessary, however, or if preoperative films showed a significant movement abnormality of the motor segment, fusion at the time of decompression is likely to be beneficial.

Post-operative complications are rare. Infection of the disc occurs in less than 1% of operations. Continued and increasing pain and a raised sedimentation rate precede radiological changes by a few weeks. Vascular complications involving major vessels have occurred. The dura and arachnoid may be accidentally opened at operation with CSF leakage. Repair by suture usually suffices, but occasionally pseudocysts occur. In many cases they resolve spontaneously but they may occasionally be persistent and require surgical excision.

SCLEROTOMAL PAIN

Pain caused by irritation of nerve endings of the spinal motor segment is most commonly caused by mechanical stress due to degeneration or low-grade injury to the spinal motor segment. Other causes include infection, inflammation and tumours. Each cause has its own clinical and radiological features which will be described.

MECHANICAL DISRUPTION

The manifestations of mechanical causes of pain differ in different parts of the spine and will, therefore, be described separately.

CERVICAL SPONDYLOSIS

The onset of neck pain is insidious and is situated in the mid-part of the neck. It may extend to the interscapular area, across the shoulders and into the suboccipital region. The pain is dull and boring, often aggravated by motion, especially extension and twisting. It is seldom affected by coughing or sneezing. Movement of the neck is often restricted, but as the normal range varies with age care should be taken in interpretation. Flexion and extension diminish before rotation, although a total loss of neck movement is rare. Nerve root compression may occur secondarily due to foraminal stenosis by osteophyte formation at the uncovertebral joints.

Differential diagnosis of shoulder and neck pain includes subacromial bursitis, tendonitis and tears of the rotator cuff. Degenerative disease of the cervical canal may involve cord compression. This presents as lower extremity neurology with disturbances of gait, spasticity and hyperflexion of the deep tendon reflexes and extensor plantar responses.

Finally, vertebral artery compression due to osteophytes from the facet and uncovertebral joints may lead to symptoms of dizziness and unsteadiness, especially with head rotation.

Radiology

Plain radiographs reveal narrowed intervertebral discs. These are most frequently the C5/6 level with 6/7 and 4/5 affected less commonly. The normal lordotic curve may be reduced or even reversed. In the cases with significant narrowing, sclerosis of the vertebral end-plates is often present and osteoarthritis of the uncovertebral joints and facet joints occurs. Sclerosis and irregularity of the joint surfaces is seen on the lateral films. Osteoarthritic changes in the uncovertebral joints are best seen on the AP view with the resultant osteophyte formation being demonstrated on the oblique views (Fig. 11.13). Joint arthrosis, as an isolated finding without associated disc narrowing, is unusual. The majority of cervical spines over the fourth decade show some of these changes at one or more disc level, and over 70 years of age they are often severe. No clear relationship, however, has been established between plain film changes and symptomatic pain.

Conservative therapy of pain from cervical spondylosis is effective in most patients. The disorder tends to be self-limiting, and rest in the acute phase, with support and immobilization from a cervical collar, usually suffices. Local heat, muscle relaxants, and even traction, may help. Manipulation in the acute phase may give relief, although controlled trials have failed to establish a significant value of this procedure in chronic neck pain.

If pain is intractable and surgery is contemplated, it becomes necessary to define the level concerned. The radiographic demonstration of abnormal segmental movement patterns in full extension and flexion more accurately reflects the level of symptoms and increases the selectivity of plain films. There is increased horizontal movement, on the lateral films at the extremes of movement, from forward to retrolisthesis, and this is sometimes associated with increased tilt. The use of cineradiography to record the whole movement cycle has been claimed to provide a 90% accurate localization. Limitation of the gliding component and an exaggerated tilt or a

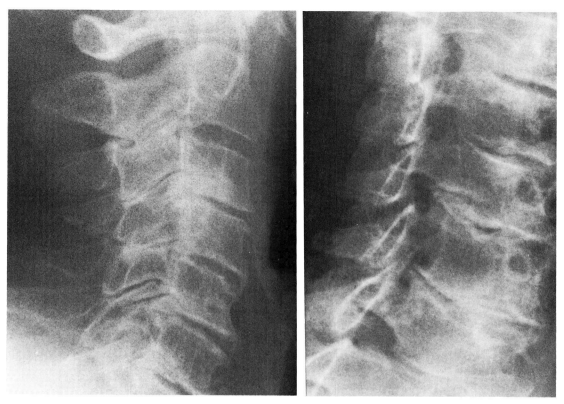

Fig. 11.13. Lateral view. The disc spaces are narrowed and vertebral margin osteophytes are present, both anteriorly and posteriorly. The posterior joints are sclerotic. The osteophytes on the uncovertebral joints extend into the foramen causing considerable narrowing.

or a double rocking motion indicate the symptomatic levels.

In order to confirm a symptomatic disc, however, discography is necessary. For patients in their twenties or thirties, a normal contained nuclear injection may be expected and posterior tears indicate disc damage. Posterolateral annular fissuring occurs early in the cervical disc and the contrast of a nuclear injection can be expected to extend to the uncovertebral joints in most cases after this age period (Fig. 11.14). The morphology is of considerably less importance at this stage.

Symptom reproduction by the injection of contrast is of major diagnostic importance in this investigation, and if symptoms are induced their relief by injecting local anaesthetic pro-

vides further diagnostic confirmation. Some patients have difficulty localizing the induced pain at cervical discography, as overlap of referral is commonly present. However, symptomatic levels of discogenic pain can be isolated by this method, particularly if only a single level is abnormal and symptomatic. The specificity decreases with multiple levels of disc degeneration. The examination may be uncomfortable for the patient, and chemical discitis and infection have been reported as sequelae. Antibiotic treatment is required only when infection is confirmed and the outcome of both is usually spontaneous cervical interbody fusion.

Surgical treatment of cervical spondylosis is performed either for the relief of pain or for progressive neuropathy. The most common

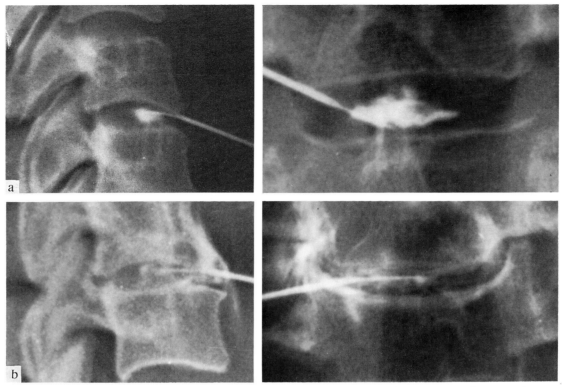

Fig. 11.14. (a) Normal cervical discogram. The contrast is contained in the nucleus. (b) Symptomatic discogram. Contrast extends into the uncovertebral joints on the AP view. The lateral shows contrast contained in a small collar-stud prolapse into the canal as well as extravasating forwards through an anterior annular tear.

approach for pain is anterior disc removal and interbody fusion. Different approaches and procedures have been described but the variations mainly involve the type of graft and extent of disc clearance. Greater debate surrounds the treatment if cervical myelopathy is the main problem. Extensive laminectomy and clearance of osteophytes has been advocated with good results. Late flexion deformity is uncommon in adults. Anterior discectomy and interbody fusion is now the more popular approach, and gradual resorption of posterior osteophytes has been noted after a satisfactory fusion.

Radiographic assessment of the fusion site is necessary to check the satisfactory position of the grafts and subsequently to confirm fusion. Failure of fusion is directly related to a poor symptomatic result. Flexion and extension films may prove valuable in demonstrating non-union.

DORSAL SPINE

Disc disease in the dorsal spine appears to cause significantly less clinical disability than in the cervical or lumbar spine. Disc degeneration regularly occurs in later life and is often associated with substantial osteophyte formation, but pain is unusual and kyphotic deformity is often the more prominent clinical feature. The most common disorder involving the dorsal spine in the earlier decades is Scheuermann's disease. This is usually a radiographic diagnosis as the disorder is commonly asymptomatic. The features include narrowing of a number of thoracic disc spaces, wedging of the thoracic vertebral bodies, and irregularity of the vertebral end-plates (Fig. 11.15). A mild kyphosis occurs which may progress significantly in a few patients. An ache in the dorsal spine may occur

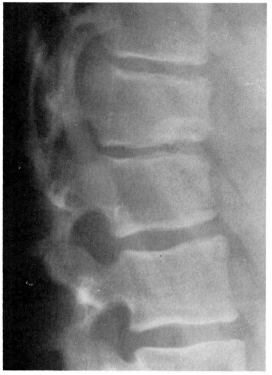

Fig. 11.15. Scheuermann's disease. There is narrowing of T11/12 and T12/L1 disc spaces. The end-plates are irregular and there is an anterior Schmorl's defect of the vertebral end-plates. A localized kyphosis is present.

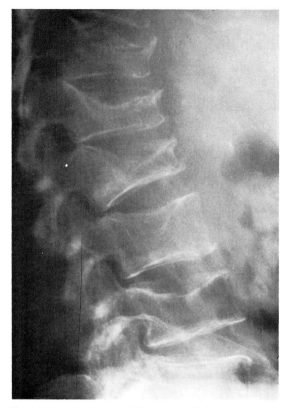

Fig. 11.16. Osteoporosis. The upper end-plates have collapsed leading to severe wedging of the vertebral bodies.

but the incidence of this symptom is difficult to establish as the diagnosis often goes undetected. Surgery is rarely required and only for steady deterioration of the kyphosis. Differential diagnosis from an infective spondylitis may sometimes be difficult.

In later life the dorsal region is frequently the site for the spinal manifestation of metabolic bone diseases. These are primarily osteoporosis and, less commonly, osteomalacia and hyperparathyroidism. The disorder is often picked up incidentally in asymptomatic patients but if symptoms are present they take the form of pain or deformity or, occasionally, difficulty in walking. Pain in metabolic disease of the spine is a dull ache which is occasionally throbbing, poorly localized, and may be referred. It is worse on walking and weight-bearing and is often

bilateral. Collapse of the vertebra may lead to acute, lancing pain, and tenderness may be present. In general terms, pain is a prominent feature of osteomalacia and is less common in osteoporosis. Kyphosis is also a prominent feature of these disorders, becoming almost universal in later life. The curve is regular, involving most of the dorsal spine, and scoliosis is absent. Gait abnormality may be due to pain but true muscle weakness is also present. This is again most common in osteomalacia or hyperparathyroidism and conforms to the pattern of a proximal myopathy with wasting hypotonia and normal reflexes. Radiological examination primarily takes the form of lateral films, although AP views are helpful in excluding pedicular destruction in malignancy and vertebral expansion in Paget's disease. Increased radiolucency of the vertebral bodies occurs but this is difficult to assess as it is affected by a number of technical factors and is not a sensitive gauge of mineral content. Changes in shape are of greater value, with increased end-plate concavity, wedging, and vertebral compression all being features of hypomineralization. In general terms, increased concavity is more common in osteomalacia and the lesions are evenly distributed, whereas wedging and compression are the most common features of porosis and have a more sporadic distribution.

The trabecular pattern of osteomalacic vertebrae is often indistinct due to uneven mineralization of osteoid, and rarely even increased density may occur. In osteoporosis, initially there may be an accentuation of the vertical trabecular pattern due to early loss of the horizontal trabeculae, but a lack of a visible trabecular pattern is the feature of the established disorder. Bone scanning is of limited value in that it may pick up early vertebral collapse but it does not always differentiate between neoplasm and metabolic bone disease and is often normal in osteoporosis. Numerical analysis of bone mineral content has, until recently, been indirect and centred around the measurement of cortical dimensions on an X-ray of a metacarpal. More recently, the use of photon absorptiometry has shown some promise, but the use of computerized transaxial tomography offers considerable possibilities for numerical analysis of vertebral body mineralization.

Treatment of osteoporosis and osteomalacia is often difficult and involves the use of calcium supplements, vitamin D therapy and sometimes hormones. Surgery plays little part in the treatment of these disorders, although corset or brace therapy may be of value.

LUMBAR SPINE

Mechanical stress particularly affects the lumbar spine and may occur in the form of a single traumatic episode or gradual wear and tear of the soft tissues and bone components of the motor segment. These changes may lead to attacks of low back pain, which are usually self-limiting, and in 90% of acute back pain syndromes only symptomatic treatment, such as rest, analgesics and rehabilitative exercises, is required. The duration of these attacks is rarely longer than two weeks and only occasionally is an anatomical pain source isolated.

Prolongation of the initial attack or repeated episodes of pain and disability, however, require more investigation, in order that specific treatment programmes can be instituted. The emergence of treatment techniques limited to individual components of the motor segment increases the importance of identification of the pain source. Failure to do so makes assessment of treatment methods difficult and prognostication impossible. Symptoms and clinical signs consistent with nerve root irritation or compression appear in only 7·5% of patients with acute back syndromes. The majority of patients present with non-specific low back pain, with or without leg pain. Leg pain alone is unusual in this group. Back pain localization to a small area is often associated with focal pathology. In most cases, however, the area of low back pain is more extensive. Radiation into the buttocks and posterolateral part of the thighs is usually associated with disorders of the L5 or S1 motor segments.

Anterior thigh pain referral is less common and may originate from the L3 or L4 regions. There is, however, considerable overlap of pain referral from different motor segments and it is, therefore, a poor localizing and differentiating feature. Pain radiating as far as the ankle is not uncommon in association with low back pain, but radiation to the toes is likely to indicate nerve root irritation. Movement-induced exacerbation of pain provides further localizing information. Increased pain on extension, especially if there is a break in normal spinal motion, suggests a pain source in the posterior elements. Pain aggravated by forward flexion or side bending is more typical of a discogenic source. Local instability is indicated when specific mechanical stimuli, such as bending in certain directions or jerking motions, exacerbate the pain. In these circumstances rest provides relief and manipulation causes an increase in pain.

The history may reveal predisposing factors such as trauma, abnormal postural patterns or intense sport or exercise activity. In these cases stress fractures of the pars interarticularis should be considered. Physical examination often reveals limitation of straight-leg raising despite the lack of nerve root irritation. In these cases the induced pain is commonly present in the back, rather than the leg. This feature also occurs in cases of central disc prolapse. Movements are often restricted but palpation does little to localize the pain source, as most muscle tenderness is referred particularly to the para-lumbar region and buttocks. Patients with acute discogenic low backache find it difficult to sit up from a supine position. Neurological examination is usually normal but loss of ankle reflexes may occur in the absence of nerve root compression. The presence of a significant spondylolisthesis causes flattening of the lumbar curve and tight hamstrings, leading to a spastic type of gait.

Radiology
Plain radiography. Radiological examination plays little part in the management of the initial attack. However, if pain persists then further assessment of the patient is indicated and plain radiographs are usually performed. The specific abnormalities which may be a source of pain, such as a defect in the pars interarticularis (Fig. 11.17), may be demonstrated. In this condition, bone scans may also reveal the developing stress fracture, but once the defect is established increased scan uptake is less likely. A large proportion of patients, however, have normal examinations or demonstrate non-specific ageing changes. Of these, disc degeneration is the most common feature and involvement of the L5/S1 disc in this process occurs in a high percentage of patients over the age of 40.

Degenerative changes at the L4/5 level are also common and more likely to occur if the L5/S1 disc lies well down in the pelvis. The radiographic features of disc degeneration are loss

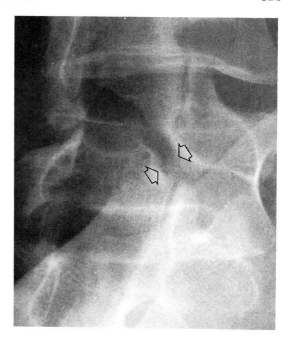

Fig. 11.17. Spondylolysis. The oblique view demonstrates the defect in the pars interarticularis which is wide and the margins well defined (arrows). Forward displacement may be present on the lateral view.

of disc height associated with small spurs of bone on the anterolateral margins of the vertebral bodies, due to elevation of the periosteum by the bulging annular attachments. As degeneration progresses there is further loss of disc height and vertebral end-plate sclerosis occurs. Fissuring in the disc at this stage may be indicated on the plain radiograph by the presence of intradiscal gas (Fig. 11.18). Horizontal shift of the vertebral bodies may be present in either the forward or backward direction, and further movement may be demonstrated by using flexion and extension films. The hypermobility demonstrated in this way is always associated with disc damage (Fig. 11.19) and experimental studies designed to create changes analogous to early disc damage lead to hypermobility in a previously normal motor segment.

Degenerative processes also occur concomitantly in the posterior facet joints, but early changes are impossible to recognize on the radiographs. When osteoarthritis is established

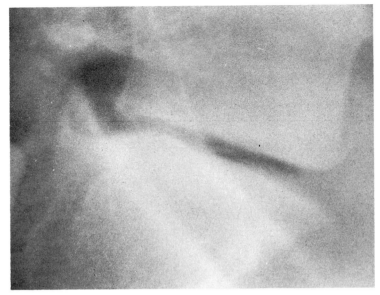

Fig. 11.18.   Isolated disc resorption. There is marked narrowing of the disc space with sclerosis of the end-plates. The vacuum sign indicates severe fissuring of the residual annulus.

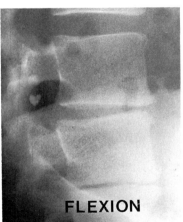

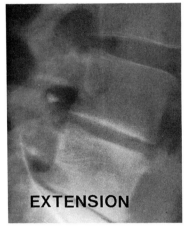

FLEXION   EXTENSION

Fig. 11.19.   The disc space is reduced in height and on flexion there is a forward rocking motion with listhesis. This resolves on extension.

there is narrowing of the facet joints with sclerosis of the articular surface. In severe cases, hypertrophic bone formation occurs around the margins of the joint. At this stage the changes are clearly demonstrated on the plain films, and evidence of foraminal narrowing may also be seen. The value of the plain film is unfortunately limted, as demonstration of degenerative processes does not mean that back pain is present. Only a 59% sensitivity and 55% specificity of back pain and sciatica with disc degeneration have been recorded. If the plain films indicate a single level of degeneration or of hypermobility, then there is a greater likelihood of this level being the symptomatic pain source. Even in these circumstances, however, pain may be originating from another apparently radiologically normal motor segment. An example is spondylolysis where the defect may be asymptomatic while the pain is arising from secondary pathological changes due to the altered mechanics. Nevertheless, the plain film in cases with back pain provides a baseline for further assessment and follow-up.

Provocation radiology. If the patient's pain fails to respond to normal symptomatic treatment and causes severe disability then further investigations prior to more radical treatment may be considered necessary. These investigations involve an injection of contrast medium which demonstrates abnormal morphology, and at the same time acts as a noxious stimulant to the area under investigation. This may or may not induce pain. If pain is produced the distribution is compared with that of the patient's symptomatic pain and a close correlation indicates the source of symptoms. Confirmation of the pain source is achieved by injecting local anaesthetic which should abolish the induced symptoms. These techniques can be used in the intervertebral discs, and the apophyseal joints, and may also be applied to locations at junctions between bone and ligament. Using these techniques various types of pain-inducing situations from both the disc and the facet joint have been demonstrated.

Discogenic pain. The use of discography has enabled certain types or stages of discogenic disease to be defined. Pain may originate from internal disruption of the disc which still has an intact outer annulus. Concentric tears occur within the annulus leading to separation of different fibre levels. At discography, radial lines of contrast medium extend from the nucleus throughout the posterior annulus but do not go as far as the outer annular border and the line of the posterior vertebral wall (Fig. 11.20). The mechanics of pain production in this group may be explained by irritation and stretching of the nerve endings which are present in the outer annulus.

More extensive disruption of the annulus occurs in the form of a radial tear. This can occur anteriorly or posteriorly. Anterior tears are less common, due to the increased thickness and thus strength of the anterior annulus, and they tend to involve the line of cleavage between the annulus and the vertebral endplate. These lesions often occur in younger patients and may be associated with a single traumatic episode. More commonly, however, they present without any clear predisposing history and probably represent similar aetiology to

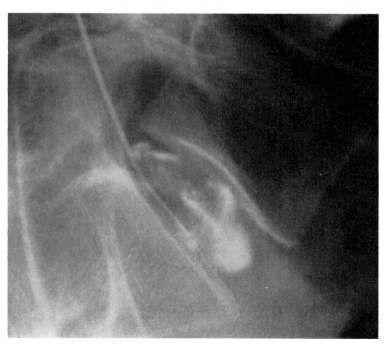

Fig. 11.20. Internal annular disruption. Contrast medium injected into the nucleus extends through the posterior annulus in a curvilinear pattern, but is contained by the posterior annular margin.

that of Scheuermann's disease. Defects in the anterior part of the vertebral end-plates are common in this group, and discography will demonstrate the contrast medium extending down into the intraosseous herniation (Fig. 11.21).

As many of these lesions are not associated with back pain and are also sometimes multiple, it is important to use discography to isolate the symptomatic level by reproduction of pain in those patients with severe disability. A more common problem is the radial tear to the posterior annulus. This occurs in the similar age group to the disc prolapse and may be related to active sport or traumatic episodes. The patients often have a long history of low back and leg pain but without evidence of neurological abnormalities. In many cases the plain films are normal, and radioculography shows no evidence of nerve root compression. Mild anterior indentation of the dural sac may be demonstrated on the lateral view and it is accentuated often by extension. Discography is necessary to identify the abnormality. Injection into the nucleus demonstrates a parallel tear

through the posterior annulus and contrast may be collected as a small central collar-stud just beyond the margin of the posterior vertebral wall. Symptom reproduction at the time of injection confirms the level of the disease (Fig. 11.22). Pain in these patients may be due to the transmission of pressures from the nucleus to the outer annulus, causing stretching of the outer annulus and the overlying longitudinal ligament. In some cases, however, inflammatory tissues may invade the tear, leading to irritation and pain. Similar types of tears can be seen in association with partly degenerate discs. These changes may be a later stage of the same original process.

The majority of patients suffering from nonspecific backache and leg pain, however, fall into the group where disc degeneration has occurred. Even in this group of patients many degenerate discs are asymptomatic and the use of discography with the induction of pain and successful Marcain blocks are essential if the symptomatic level is to be isolated. Analysis of the discographic appearance in degenerate discs has demonstrated a number of different features.

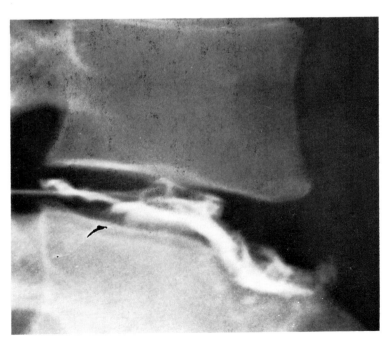

Fig. 11.21. Anterior interosseous herniation—intranuclear injection reveals leakage of contrast medium into the anterior vertebral end-plate defect through a tear in the annulus fibrosus.

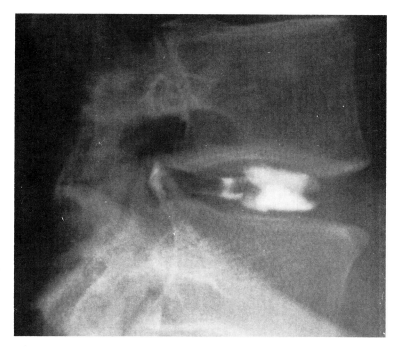

Fig. 11.22. Posterior annular tear —intranuclear injection reveals leakage of contrast through the posterior annulus fibrosus and collecting as a collar-stud under the posterior longitudinal ligament. The radiculogram was normal.

The contrast in degenerate discs extends the full width of the disc in all directions. The contrast may be contained by the annulus within the line of the posterior vertebral body wall or may bulge into the canal but still being contained as a 'collar-stud' appearance (Fig. 11.23a).

Finally, contrast may leak into the epidural space from the disc (Fig. 11.23b). Those discograms where contrast is contained and extends posteriorly beyond the line of the vertebral body produce symptomatic pain in a significantly greater number of cases than in degenerative discs where the contrast escapes through the annulus into the epidural space. It is possible, therefore, that preservation of tension of the outer annulus in a degenerate disc may be important in terms of pain production.

In conclusion, therefore, discography demonstrates the morphology of the intervertebral disc

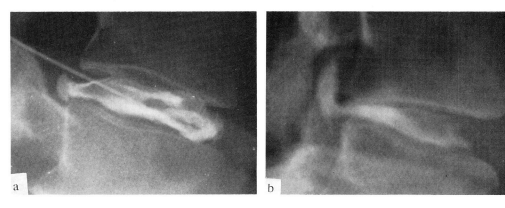

Fig. 11.23. Degenerate discs—contrast extends throughout the extent of the disc, which is also reduced in height. (a) Contrast is contained posteriorly in a collar-stud pattern. (b) Contrast leaks into the epidural space.

very accurately and is the most valuable means of diagnosing disc damage that has not caused significant nuclear herniation. It is the only means of isolating those degenerate discs that are causing symptoms. It is also of value in the preoperative assessment of patients undergoing spinal fusion in confirming the level of the first normal disc.

FACET PAIN

The facet joint as a source of backache has been recognized since the early 1930s. Its importance, however, was overshadowed by the prolapsed intervertebral disc and it has only recently returned to increasing clinical prominence. Involvement of the facets may occur in different phases of mechanical disease. In the acute phase of initial attacks of back pain, facet joints may be a pain source in as many as 60% of patients. Injections with contrast (Fig. 11.24) and local anaesthetic into the joints have defined a patient group whose pain was predominantly in the back. The onset was associated with sudden movement and trauma, such as bending and twisting, and these responded well to the local anaesthetic. The extent of spinal movement following the facet block was significantly increased and in some of the group there was long-term relief from the injections. The second group had low back pain that did not appear to be facet-orientated. The onset of pain was more insidious with an increased severity on walking and relief with sitting. Leg pain was common in this group. As the facets become part of the whole degenerative process and osteoarthritis of the facet joint occurs, the incidence with which the facet joints are the only pain source falls to 20 or 30%. Local anaesthetic injected into specific facet joints may still relieve symptomatic pain.

A study of 100 patients complaining of lumbago or sciatica, clinically indistinguishable from the disc syndrome, showed that patterns of pain referred from the apophyseal joints were produced in the back, buttocks and legs, and were then blocked with xylocaine. In this group,

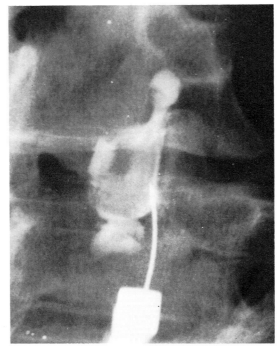

Fig. 11.24. Facet arthrogram—contrast fills the facet capsule which is circular on the AP view and oval on the oblique. Synovial pouches are present superiorly and inferiorly.

six patients with diminished straight-leg raising and three with depression of deep tendon reflexes had these changes reversed. Intra-articular steroids and local anaesthetic may give significant short-term relief and partial or complete long-term relief in 50% of patients.

The greatest difficulty in evaluation of patients with suspected facet syndrome lies in selecting those with symptomatic facets and deciding at which levels to make the injection. Referred pain distribution is not segmental, and considerable overlap occurs, even between facets four segments apart. There is also a discrepancy between the extent of pain referral in normal volunteers and in patients with low back pain, the latter consistently having a more extensive area of involvement. In most patients, however, the lower two lumbar levels are most commonly involved and individual diagnostic injections of Marcain will indicate that level which has a diagnostic degree of symptomatic improvement. The use of facet blockade continues to be of value as a simple diagnostic and treatment technique, particularly in patients with one level of disease in the early stages of symptomatology. The advent of the use of specific surgical techniques, such as rhizotomy, or Cyroprobe block of the facet innervation, makes careful preoperative assessment essential.

OSSEOUS IMPINGEMENT

Two bone masses which are abnormally close together may have an abrasive effect and may be a source of pain. The commonest example is between the spinous processes. Pain radiates from the back and is exaggerated by standing or hyperextension. Clinical examination reveals acute localized tenderness in the region of the interspinous ligaments. Radiology demonstrates impingement of the spinous processes with osteosclerosis and subcortical cysts. Local anaesthetic injected into the ligament leading to pain relief confirms the diagnosis. Osseous impingement may also occur between facet articular processes and adjacent laminae in severe disc degeneration and also in spondylolisthesis (Fig. 11.25). In these cases, also, injections of a small quantity of local anaesthetic into the joints as a diagnostic test, and further treatment by either rhizotomy or spinal fusion, may be indicated in severely affected patients.

POST-LAMINECTOMY SYNDROME

A laminectomy can be deemed to have failed if preoperative symptoms have either not been relieved or they have been made worse. Persistence of severe pain is unusual if the diagnosis of disc prolapse has been confirmed at operation. Early failure may be caused by a remnant of dessicated sequestrated disc being left beneath a nerve root, leading to continued root pressure and pain. Exploration of the wrong level may also occur, especially in the presence of transitional vertebrae. Most failures, however, occur

either when a frank prolapse has not been demonstrated preoperatively and surgery is performed for disc bulges and posterior annular tears without root compression, or when lateral recess stenosis has not been recognised, with a subsequent incomplete decompression of the bony canal. Relief of pain may last months or years. Recurrence of back or leg pain may be due to a recurrent prolapse at the operated level or a fresh disc herniation at another level. Myelography may be diagnostic but the presence of post-operative epidural fibrosis also causes distortion of the nerve roots and often the dural sac, and differentiation from a prolapse may be difficult (Fig. 11.26). Epidural fibrosis has been implicated as a cause of pain, and thus failure of laminectomy, but its exact role in the post-laminectomy syndrome has still to be clarified. In the presence of fibrosis, discography is of particular value as it assessses both disc morphology and symptom production. The higher incidence of disc degeneration in this group also makes discography the investigation of choice. The demonstration of the dimensions of the lateral recess can best be achieved using CT scanning, and this examination should accompany discography to exclude nerve compression by bone.

Finally, evidence of instability, due to either disc degeneration or the excessive removal of posterior elements, should be checked using flexion/extension films as this can also be a pain source.

In summary, pain may arise in the post-laminectomy patient from a number of sources, and discography, facet arthrography, radiculography and soft-tissue Marcain block may all be required to elucidate the problem. Despite all efforts a number of patients will still elude diagnosis and intensive therapy on a team basis will be required to provide a degree of rehabilitation.

COMPLICATIONS OF SPINAL FUSION

Early complications of posterior fusion include poor placement or inadequate quantity of graft bone. Resorption of the bone graft may occur,

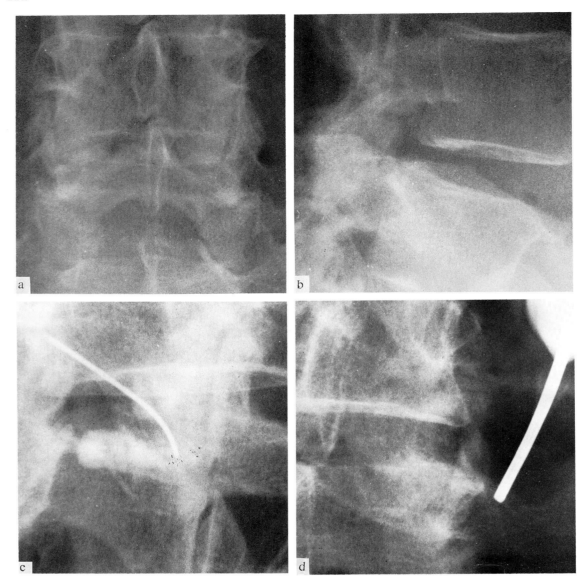

Fig. 11.25. Facet impingement. (a) The lower border of the inferior articular process is in contact with the superior surface of the lamina below. Sclerosis of bone results from the impingement. (b) There is a spondylolisthesis of the vertebral body secondary to the degenerative disease of the facets. (c) Local anaesthetic injected into the facets gave good relief of back pain. (d) Cryoprobe denervation of the medial branch of the posterior primary ramus is performed above and below the affected joint.

leading to pseudarthrosis, and this will be indicated on a bone scan as an area of increased uptake. Failure of fusion is best confirmed by tomography (Fig. 11.27). It is not clear whether a pseudarthrosis *per se* is always a cause of

pain, but localization of symptoms to the lesion can be achieved with an injection of local anaesthetic leading to the abolition of pain. Anterior interbody fusions may fail due to displacement or collapse of the graft. Movement of

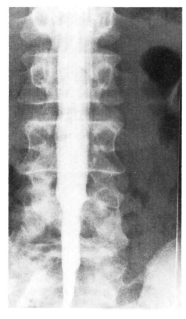

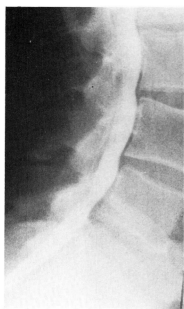

Fig. 11.26. Epidural fibrosis. There is extensive narrowing of the lower dural sac. The nerve root sleeves are obliterated. There is no significant central indentation on the lateral view.

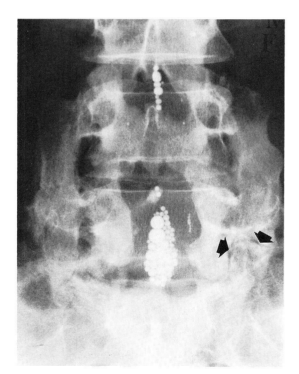

Fig. 11.27. Pseudarthrosis. Solid fusion is seen between L4 and L5 but a clear lucent line between the lower end of the graft and the sacrum is demonstrated on the left.

the fused segment may also lead to sclerosis and pseudarthrosis between the vertebral end-plate and the graft. Tomograms again confirm these findings and flexion and extension films may be helpful.

Late failure may be due to prolapse or degeneration of the disc at the level above the fusion, although the importance of this is still disputed. Discography is a valuable means of assessing the state of the disc in these circumstances. The post-operative occurrence of pain is an area of great diagnostic challenge and many investigative modalities will be required. All these examinations provide pieces of the jigsaw so that concerted help may be provided for these patients, many of whom are virtually cripples.

INFECTION

Antibiotics have radically altered the incidence of spinal infection, but it remains an important if uncommon cause of back pain. Pyogenic infection tends to occur in adults, whereas tuberculous infection has traditionally been more common in children. This age differential, however, is now less obvious. The presenting symptom of back pain, commonly situated in the dorsal region, is usually insidious in onset and aggravated by motion. There may be a delay of several months between the onset of symptoms and the visit to the hospital. The symptoms may be referred to areas distant to the spine, causing diagnostic confusion with other disorders, such as cholecystitis, renal colic or appendicitis. The presence of fever is unreliable and is found only in a minority of patients. Local tenderness is a most helpful physical sign. The white cell count may be raised in the acute phase of pyogenic infection and an elevated sedimentation rate is commonly present and is a useful screening examination. Both pyogenic and tuberculous spondylitis most commonly arise from a blood-borne organism. Predisposing factors of pyogenic infection in adults include penetrating wounds, external or urinary tract infection, pelvic surgery, or low urinary tract instrumentation or needling procedures. Patients will be submitted to plain radiography of the region of pain and the earliest radiological manifestation is a paravertebral swelling resulting from soft-tissue oedema or an abscess.

In the cervical spine, the prevertebral space will be greater than the AP diameter of the associated vertebral body. In the dorsal spine, the widened paravertebral shadow is usually clearly seen on a penetrated AP view (Fig. 11.28), and in the lumbar spine the psoas outline may bulge or become ill-defined due to inflammatory oedema of the psoas fatline. Disc space narrowing is also an early feature of pyogenic infection and this is followed by destruction of the vertebral end-plate or anterior vertebral body margins (Fig. 11.29a).

Early detection of spinal infection can be achieved with a bone-seeking isotope (Fig. 11.29b). This is especially useful in children, but the characteristic pattern may not occur initially if only the disc is involved. Scanning early during the blood-pool phase may indicate hyperaemia before the bone phase becomes positive. Gallium-67 localization has been used in infection, but uptake by liver and inadequate

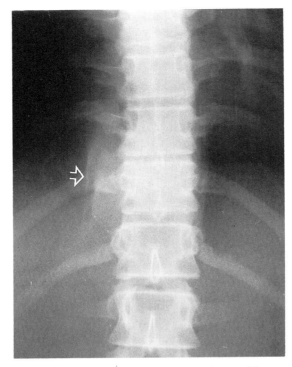

Fig. 11.28. Infection. There is localized widening of the paravertebral shadow on the right at T10/11 (arrow). The disc space is also narrowed on this view.

bowel clearance makes diagnosis in the spine unreliable. Radiological features may not allow differentiation between pyogenic and tuberculous infection. Rapid evolution, lack of osteoporosis and reactive sclerosis favour a pyogenic aetiology. Calcification in the soft-tissue abscess is a delayed feature of tuberculosis, and involvement of the spinal appendages is rare.

Needle biopsy via a posterolateral approach enables the organism and its sensitivity to be identified. Healing may involve bony ankylosis with a narrowed disc space and consolidation of damaged bone. Tuberculous infection responds to suitable antibiotics but anterior decompression and drainage of the abscess is commonly necessary in severely affected cases. Ankylosis is less common and anterior interbody strut grafts will usually be required, especially if a secondary kyphosis has occurred.

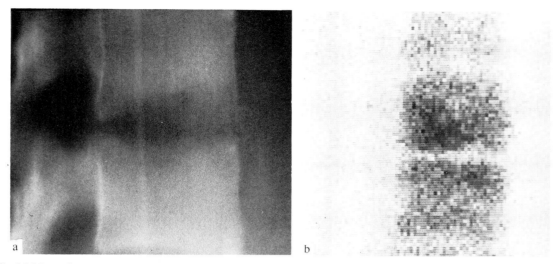

Fig. 11.29. Infection. (a) Irregular destruction of the vertebral end-plates and narrowing of the disc space is demonstrated on the lateral tomograms. (b) The isotope scan shows increased activity at the same level.

INFLAMMATORY DISEASE

Spinal pain may originate from a number of clinically related disorders which cause an inflammatory reaction in the ligaments, joints and intervertebral discs of the spine. Inflammatory changes also occur in other joints and the ratio of involvement between the axial and the non-axial skeleton varies from one disease to another. The distribution of pain is dependent on the area of spinal involvement, but sacroiliac disease is common to most of the disorders and leads to pain symptoms in the low back, hips and buttocks. Stiffness is a prominent feature, particularly in the morning. Stressing the pelvis and sacroiliac joints will increase symptoms. The extent of spinal involvement varies with the disease process. Ankylosing spondylitis may affect the whole spine, whereas Reiter's disease and psoriasis have patchy spinal lesions of a few segments and rheumatoid arthritis mostly affects the cervical spine. Pain is due to the inflammatory process but secondary neurological compression may occur. The presence of a raised sedimentation rate is common and serological and leucocyte histocompatability tests are also of value in diagnosis. Associated features such as conjunctivitis, urethritis, psoriasis, or the classical characteristic peripheral joint involvement of rheumatoid arthritis help with differentiation.

Ankylosing spondylitis
Radiological changes in ankylosing spondylitis may not be evident in the initial symptomatic period. At this stage, scanning the sacroiliac joints with technetium-labelled methyldiphosphonate has been reported to be sensitive. There is some overlap between normal and diseased joints, but clearly abnormal isotope uptake may be present in the absence of radiological changes, and the test, therefore, is of value. Prone PA views of the sacroiliac joints demonstrate patchy osteoporosis, irregularity and erosion of the joint surface, and increased joint width. In the spine, the lateral view may initially demonstrate vertebral squaring due to erosion at the enthesis (Fig. 11.30) and later the development of syndesmophytes which are typically vertically orientated and cause intervertebral bridging. Ossification of the longitudinal ligaments and apophyseal joints follows, and this process may lead to a marked kyphosis

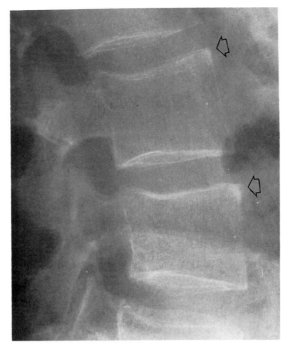

Fig. 11.30. Ankylosing spondylitis. There is squaring of the anterior border of the vertebral bodies due to small erosions at the enthesis (Romanus lesions) (arrows).

of the dorsal and lumbar spine. Atlantoaxial instability also occurs.

Involvement of the orthopaedic surgeon in this disorder is primarily due to these complications. The kyphotic deformity may be extremely restricting and lordotic osteotomies of the lumbar spine are performed to re-establish a horizontal visual field.

Pseudarthrosis may occur in ankylosing spondylitis and is associated with secondary discitis which presents as recurrent pain in patients with a solid fusion and is best demonstrated by increased isotope uptake and confirmed by tomography (Fig. 11.31). Discitis may, however, be present in the active phase, prior to complete fusion, as an extension of the disease process. This is often asymptomatic. Reunion is likely with adequate rest, although surgical fusion may be necessary.

Finally, there is an increased likelihood of spinal trauma following minor injuries. Chalk-stick fractures of the cervical spine may occur and the prognosis is often poor. Union usually occurs without surgical intervention.

Rheumatoid arthritis

The high proportion of neck involvement in rheumatoid arthritis makes radiological examination of this area essential. Weakening of the ligaments and erosion of the apophyseal joints, due to synovial inflammation, and discitis due to invasive rheumatoid granulitis, may lead to destabilization of the motor segment and subluxation. This occurs commonly at the atlantoaxial articulation but is also present subaxially (Fig. 11.32). The abnormal hypermobility will be demonstrated on flexion and extension films. Upward subluxation of the axis on the atlas may lead to compression of the medulla or the upper cervical cord, although concomitant erosion of the odontoid peg will avoid these neurological problems.

Impairment of vertebral artery blood flow due to compression, especially if the neck is rotated, is a rare complication. Lateral radiographs in flexion prior to any general anaesthesia are therefore vital in rheumatoid patients, and vertebral arteriography may occasionally be necessary. Despite the high incidence of cervical involvement neurology is unusual and only rarely is fusion necessary. The level depends on the site of instability. In rheumatoid arthritis satisfactory fusion is often difficult to achieve due to the softness of the bone. This is accentuated by long-standing steroid treatment. Instability may not be the only cause for neurological change. Pannus formation from the posterior joints may add to the cord compression and this is not visible on plain films. Myelography may be performed prior to surgery to assess the position of the neck which produces maximal canal diameter and minimum cord compression.

NEOPLASM

Spinal neoplasm is an uncommon cause of pain. Most tumours, however, present with pain which is generally persistent and not relieved

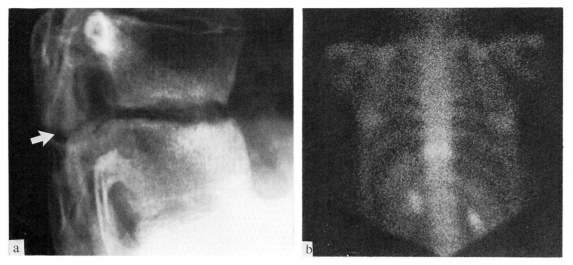

Fig. 11.31. Ankylosing spondylitis. (a) Erosions of the vertebral end-plate with sclerosis and disc narrowing are similar to changes of infection. The pseudarthrosis of the posterior elements (arrow) is the cause of this change. (b) The bone scan is a sensitive method of diagnosis.

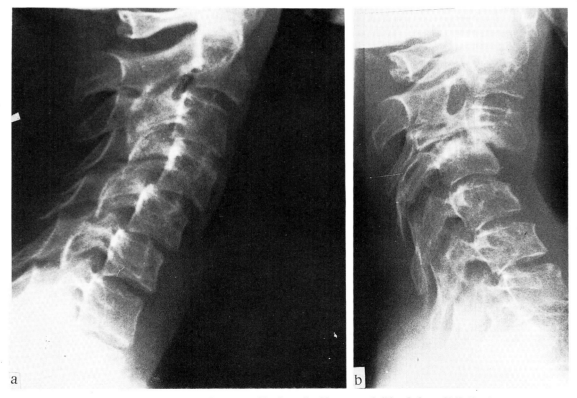

Fig. 11.32. Rheumatoid arthritis. (a) Early changes. Mild subaxial subluxation of all levels from C2/3. Erosions are present in the posterior joints and the disc spaces are reduced in height. (b) Late changes. Severe subluxation at C3/4 is now present. Extensive erosive destruction of the posterior joints is now present.

by rest. Radicular pain may occur secondarily and localizes the anatomical level. Local tenderness, muscle spasm, deformity and limited motion may all be produced. Neurological signs are unusual and occur late in the disease process. It is in the circumstances of spinal neoplasm that plain roentgenological examination is extremely valuable. The age group of the patient is important in the differential diagnosis of spinal tumours. In the young patient, benign conditions are more common and include aneurysmal bone cyst, eosinophilic granuloma, osteoblastoma and osteoid osteoma. Malignant tumours in this age group include osteogenic sarcoma and Ewing's tumour. Metastatic disease is uncommon, and neuroblastoma, lymphoma or Wilm's tumour are likely primary sites.

Metastatic deposits are by far the most common lesion in the older age groups. Primary sites include breast, prostate, lung, kidney and thyroid. Primary tumours include giant-cell tumours and haemangioma and malignant lesions, multiple myeloma, chondrosarcoma and chordomas. Bone destruction is the characteristic feature of malignant disorders but there may be both lytic and blastic features. Lysis of the vertebral bodies as in multiple myeloma may not be detectable in the initial stage but eventually leads to vertebral collapse. Sclerosis is usually visible at an earlier stage. Destruction of the pedicles viewed on the AP film is a sensitive radiological feature of malignant disease and may be accompanied by a paraspinal mass (Fig. 11.33). The main primary malignant disorder, osteosarcoma, produces expansion and bone production in association with destruction.

Benign tumours such as aneurysmal bone cysts and giant-cell tumours cause lucent expansile lesions confined by a thin rim of reactive bone (Fig. 11.34) and involve the vertebral body or posterior elements. Vertebral collapse occurs later, but in eosinophilic granulomas it is an early feature of the classical vertebra plana (Fig. 11.35). Osteoid osteoma and osteoblastoma affect the posterior elements, and scoliosis

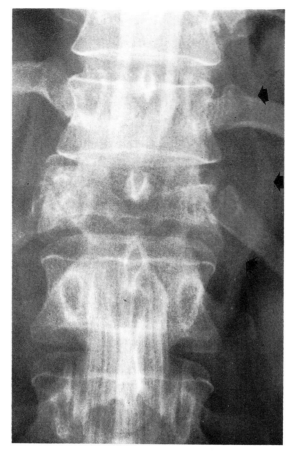

Fig. 11.33. Malignant destruction. The vertebral body of T12 has collapsed. Destruction of both pedicles has occurred and there is a large paravertebral mass (arrow). There is marked constriction of the dural sac.

is a common presenting radiographic feature. These lesions may be difficult to isolate and technetium scanning has proved a valuable localizing examination. Tomography of the active area may be required to demonstrate the lesions, the former being more sclerotic and the latter more expansile (Fig. 11.36).

Isotope scanning may also indicate the presence of disseminated metastatic lesions which usually show increased uptake. Extensive destruction in some malignant processes, however, may produce a negative scan and multiple myeloma often fails to generate increased activity. Myelography may be necessary to assess

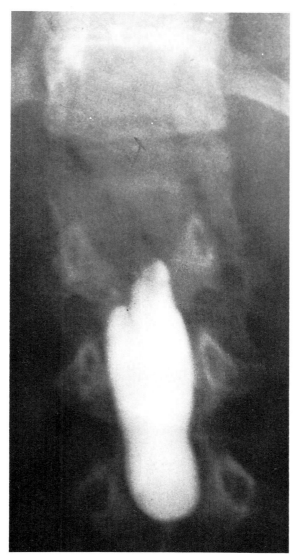

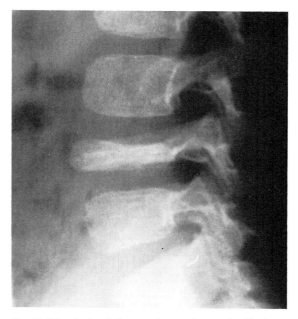

Fig. 11.35. Eosinophilic granuloma—the vertebral body is evenly flattened without end-plate destruction. The posterior elements are normal, and the disc spaces widened.

Fig. 11.34. Aneurysmal bone cyst—the lamina and spinous process of T12 have been expanded and destroyed by the tumour. A complete block of the spinal canal is indicated by the obstruction of the Myodil.

the degree of compression or invasion of the spinal canal and neurological tissue. Computerized transaxial tomography, however, combines both these investigations and demonstrates lesions in the posterior elements while simultaneously assessing the effect of tumour spread on the spinal canal and neurological tissue.

Finally, selective angiography may be required to assess the degree of vascularity and the site of supplying vessels. If the tumour is vascular, embolization may be a valuable preoperative procedure. Although the radiological appearances usually allow a precise diagnosis, confirmation of the pathology is important for appropriate treatment.

Trocar biopsy under biplane X-ray imaging provides sufficient tissue for a pathological diagnosis, although open biopsy may occasionally be required, particularly in anterior lesions of the sacrum. Malignant disease is treated by either radiotherapy or drugs. If surgery is required, resection of vertebral body or posterior elements, with subsequent bone grafting and fixation, either with Harrington or Luque instrumentation, often provides good stabilization of the spine. Surgical removal of benign tumours is usually required to alleviate pain or neural compression. A clear preoperative assessment of the extent of the lesion is vital to enable total

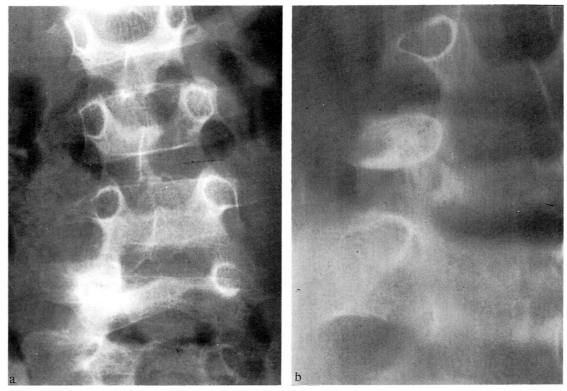

Fig. 11.36. Osteoid osteoma. (a) Scoliosis is present, and there is some sclerosis and loss of definition of L5 pedicle. (b) Tomography confirms the presence of an expanded sclerotic pedicle.

resection where possible. Simple resection without fusion may be applicable, but instrumentation may also be required to provide for future stability. In some cases, such as aneurysmal bone cyst, radiotherapy may prove a reasonable alternative.

TRAUMA

Modern technology has provided increasingly convenient and sophisticated forms of travel. One unfortunate result, however, has been a greater susceptibility to osseous and ligamentous injury of the spine. As a result, there is a need for knowledge of the clinical and radiological aspects of spinal injuries in emergency departments. In general terms, the abnormal forces applied to the spine may be vertical, either through compression or distraction;

horizontal, which includes rotational shear; and bending, either forwards, backwards or sideways. In most traumatic circumstances a combination of these forces occurs. Because the spine varies in both design and function in different regions, the vulnerability to trauma is likely to be determined by the modes and types of forces applied. The atlas and the axis together form a combination which is strong enough to carry the weight of the skull and still has considerable horizontal and rotational mobility. The atlas has large lateral articular masses which transmit the weight of the skull to the axis and, lacking a vertebral body, is ring-shaped. It is particularly vulnerable to abnormal vertical loading and splits easily. The weak points of the axis lie at the base of the odontoid process, which may fracture with horizontal stress loading of the axis, and the pedicles which appear to be vulnerable to a traction type of injury. The mid and low parts of the neck are the most mobile regions and are particularly susceptible to hyperflexion and hyperextension injuries, often in association with a rotational element.

Hyperflexion injuries involve a compressive effect on the vertebral bodies anteriorly associated with stretching and tearing of the posterior soft tissues. Conversely, hyperextension injuries will lead to tearing of the anterior longitudinal ligament and compression posteriorly. Unlike fractures which heal by apposition of new bone, ligamentous damage tends to be replaced by weaker scar tissue and is, therefore, more liable to cause longstanding instability of the spine. Biomechanical analysis of the neck in cadavers indicates that significant instability in adults may be expected when there is more than 3·5 mm of horizontal displacement or more than 11° of rotational difference between the adjacent vertebral levels. The appearances can occur with complete rupture of either the anterior or the posterior ligament complex. When rotational forces are added to the flexion forces, or are present alone, overriding of the apophyseal joints tends to occur. The horizontal alignment of the cervical apophyseal joints, which are designed primarily to accommodate flexion and extension movements, makes the cervical spine particularly vulnerable to rotational injury. Unilateral facet dislocation often occurs and may be accompanied by articular fracture.

In the thoracic and lumbar regions, hyperflexion and rotation forces are the commonest to cause injury. The predominant effect is to produce a crush injury of the vertebral body accompanied by distraction of the posterior ligament complex. In the dorsal spine, rigidity imposed by the rib cage minimizes rotational injury, but predisposes to injury of the sternum or ribs. Fractures of both must, therefore, be excluded in dorsal injury. At the thoracolumbar junction, the vertical orientation of the posterior articular processes retricts rotation, and significant twisting or lateral forces lead to fracture

of the posterior elements rather than simple dislocation. Extensive damage to the posterior ligament complex predisposes to residual instability.

In the clinical examination, the physician or surgeon will be looking for any clue which will help to localize the site of extensive injury. The presence of bruising, lacerations or local tenderness may be helpful. However, care must be exercised in the interpretation of these features, since the correlation between clinically evident injury and demonstrable radiological damage may not always be absolute. An eye witness's description of the circumstances of the accident may be of great importance in determining the likely forces involved. Spinal cord and nerve root involvement in spinal injuries may be overlooked when associated with head injuries and loss of consciousness, or when multiple injuries, which may initially be life-threatening, are present. Difficulty in neurological assessment of unresponsive patients and misinterpretation in the presence of drunkenness or unconsciousness are common problems. Fractures may not initially be accompanied by any definite neurological signs. These patients are thus vulnerable to a failure of diagnosis of the true nature and extent of injury. In addition to local signs of vertebral damage, neural injuries produce loss of movement and sensation and paraesthesia in the appropriate dermatomes. The level of neurological damage may assist in indicating the site of trauma.

Radiological examination should not be performed until a comprehensive neurological examination has been undertaken to determine the exact extent of deficit. All vital function should also have been stabilized. The radiographic examination should completely assess the damage that has occurred to avoid the consequences of misdiagnosis such as persistent pain, late deformity or further neurological damage. Many fractures and dislocations will be obvious on simple AP and lateral views provided that the site of injury has been demonstrated. Failure to do so may be due to an inappropriate request, or to poor radiographic quality. Particular care should be taken to demonstrate the junctional zones.

In the cervical spine, clear definition of the atlantoaxial and cervicodorsal regions are required, and initial radiological examinations often fail to reveal either C6/7 or C7/T1 levels (Fig. 11.37a). Films of lumbar spine examinations should always include the lower thoracic vertebrae. Supplementary radiographic manoeuvres may be necessary to demonstrate the cervicodorsal junction. A lateral film with arm traction may increase the visibility of this area, but thick-set patients or those with severe injury may make this manoeuvre unsuccessful. A swimmer's view is often, therefore, essential to provide a good lateral visualization of C7/T1 (Fig. 11.37b). The lateral views can be supplemented by performing 45° supine oblique views which avoid the need for unnecessary movement of the patient and allow visualization of

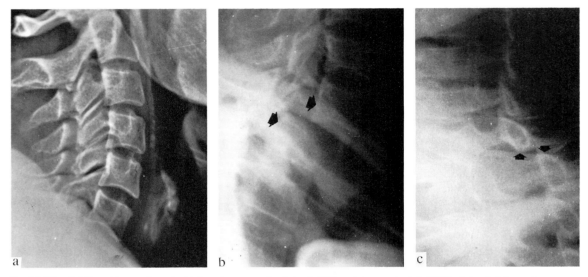

Fig. 11.37. (a) No evidence of cervical injury is seen on the lateral. C7 is not demonstrated. (b) The lateral oblique view shows a 50% forward slip of C7 on T1 (arrows). (c) The supine oblique view shows overriding of the C7 facets on T1 (arrows).

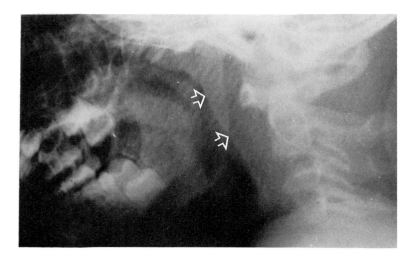

Fig. 11.38. The prevertebral soft-tissue line is widened (arrows). A traumatic rotational subluxation of the atlas is also present.

the facet joint alignment throughout the cervical spine, including the cervicodorsal junction (Fig. 11.37c). Ten-degree lateral oblique projections clearly demonstrate the articular surfaces of each facet joint and are of particular value in hyperextension injuries. On the initial radiographs there may be no obvious trauma demonstrable. Bleeding or oedema of the prevertebral soft tissue may lead to widening of this shadow and be the only initial sign of trauma. The presence of this sign should make the clinician study the films closely for indications of other damage (Fig. 11.38).

Hyperextension injuries. Hyperextension injuries may be particularly difficult, as clear radiological abnormalities may not be present. A careful search for more subtle signs is, therefore, necessary. The features of importance are small avulsion fractures of the anterior margin of the vertebral bodies or compression fractures of the posterior joints (Fig. 11.39). These latter are rare and the X-ray beam must be tangential to the joint surface for them to be demonstrated. Tomography in the lateral plane may be necessary for complete evaluation.

Hyperflexion injuries. In hyperflexion injuries, there may be localized angulation of the vertebral body with or without forward displacement. Localized widening of the interspinous distance is a crucial sign and this can be observed on both the lateral and AP views (Fig. 11.40). Hyperflexion fractures of the cervicothoracic and upper thoracic spine may be difficult to visualize, as these areas are difficult to radiograph satisfactorily in an emergency. The AP view to show increase in the interspinous distance is particularly valuable to draw attention to an injury in these areas. A sternal fracture should be excluded when this type of injury occurs in the thoracic spine. Alternatively, the presence of this fracture may be the only indicator of dorsal spine injury. A compression fracture of the anterior margin of the vertebral body completes the quartet of signs. Rigidity of the spine due to spasm may give the impression of

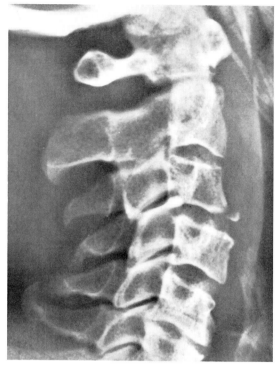

Fig. 11.39. Hyperextension injury. There is a retrolisthesis of C3 on C4. The anterior joint space of the facets is widened at this level and there is an avulsion fracture of the anteroinferior corner of the body of C3.

stability and mask the torn posterior ligaments. Flexion and extension films a few days following injury or under sedation may reveal the unstable nature of the lesion, and failure to perform these views may result in delayed dislocation (Fig. 11.41).

Atlantoaxial trauma. Fractures of the atlas or axis may easily be missed. Compression fracture of the atlas, the so-called 'Jefferson' fracture, requires good quality AP views to show that both lateral masses of the atlas have been displaced laterally and AP tomograms may be required for confirmation (Fig. 11.42). Rotation of the head causes overlap of one lateral mass, but the opposite side will be seen to lie within the line of the axis and this should not be misdiagnosed as a Jefferson fracture. The odontoid peg may be observed on the AP view by over-

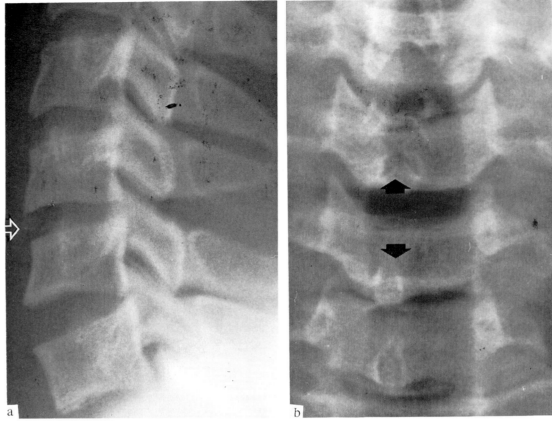

Fig. 11.40. Hyperflexion injuries. (a) Lateral view. There is widening of the interspinous distance. The vertebral body is displaced forward slightly and there is a crush fracture of the ring apophysis anteriorly (open arrow). (b) The AP view confirms the widened interspinous distance (closed arrows).

lying teeth or the arch of the atlas and the edge effect may mimic or obscure a fracture line (Fig. 11.43). A fracture line, when present in the absence of significant displacement, may be invisible. Autotomography is of value in diagnosis, and linear tomography may be necessary for confirmation (Fig. 11.44).

Flexion and rotation injuries
Fracture–dislocations are often clearly visible on the initial lateral radiographs as a forward displacement of one vertebra on another. This displacement can result from a combination of varying degrees of subluxation or dislocation of the two facet joints and it is important that this is analysed so that the appropriate treatment can

be instituted. Assessment of the degree of vertebral displacement may provide some of this information. If less than one-half of the depth of one vertebral body moves forward on the vertebra below, then this suggests a unilateral facet dislocation, whereas if forward displacement is greater than 50% a bilateral dislocation must exist (Fig. 11.45). Displacement of less than 50% may, however, occur in bilateral facet subluxation without facet overriding, and dislocation of one facet may be associated with subluxation on the opposite side. Unilateral dislocation can be recognized by separation of the facets into a 'bow-tie' appearance as opposed to the normal complete superimposition. On the AP film a unilateral facet dislocation produces

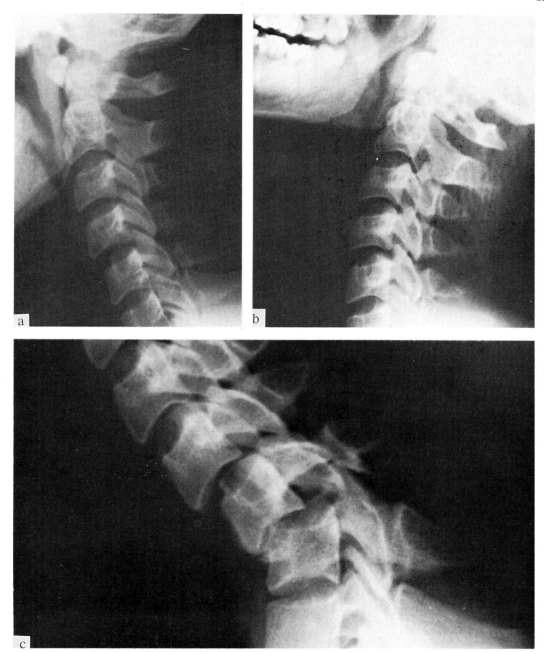

Fig. 11.41. Hyperflexion injuries, late instability. (a) and (b) Flexion and extension films suggest movement but all movement has occurred at the atlanto-occipital joint. The lower spine is rigid due to spasm. (c) Three months later, a complete dislocation has gradually developed due to instability caused by the posterior tear at the time of the original accident.

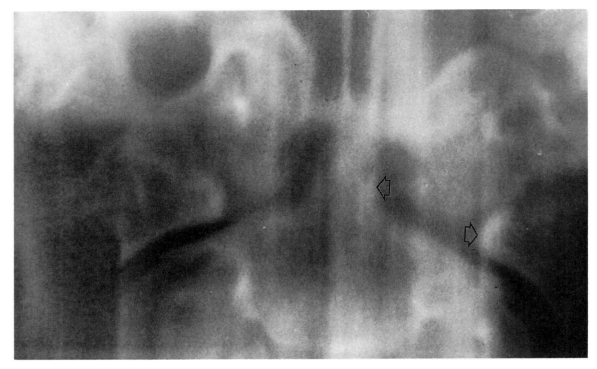

Fig. 11.42. Jefferson fracture. The lateral mass of the atlas lies outside the line of the body of the axis. The gap between the lateral masses and the odontoid is greatly increased (arrows).

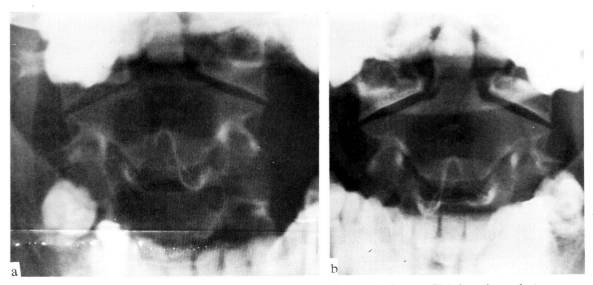

Fig. 11.43. Odontoid fracture. (a) The tooth overlies the odontoid and obscures the fracture. (b) A through-mouth view demonstrates the fracture clearly.

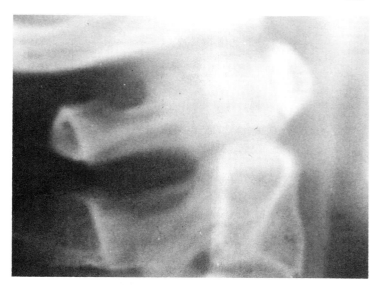

Fig. 11.44. Odontoid fracture. The side-to-side movement of the head blurs out all but the midline structure which includes the odontoid.

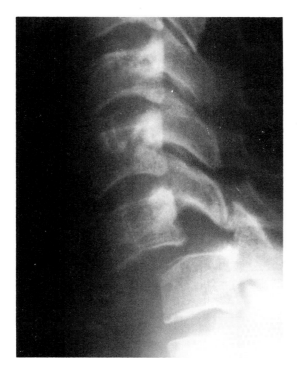

Fig. 11.45. Bilateral facet dislocation. The vertebral body is displaced forward by more than 50% of the body below. Both inferior articular processes have overridden their superior counterparts of the vertebra below.

rotation with loss of alignment of the spinous processes (Fig. 11.46). If there is a significant degree of contralateral subluxation, then the effect of this rotation is less obvious on both the lateral and AP views.

Oblique views at 45° are of considerable further value in elucidating the degree of apophyseal joint disruption. Awareness by the clinician of the distinction between facet subluxation and dislocation will prevent excessive traction being applied in subluxation and converting it into a complete dislocation. The lateral AP and AP views should be scrutinized also to exclude fractures of the pedicles or articular processes (Fig. 11.47). If these are suspected, the 45° obliques and also the 10° off-lateral obliques will provide clear demonstration of the lesions. This is important, as fractures may lead to failure of reduction or incomplete realignment and their demonstration will avoid a long unrewarding period of traction.

Thoracolumbar spinal injuries may be purely flexion but more commonly involve a rotational or side-swipe force. Excess force causes fractures of the laminae or pedicles. Widening of the interpedicular distance on the AP film is the poin-

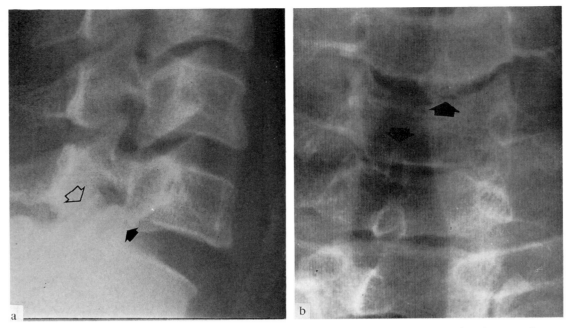

Fig. 11.46. Unilateral facet dislocation. (a) Lateral view shows mild forward displacement. Only one facet has overriden (arrows) causing rotation of the vertebra above. (b) The rotation is also seen on the AP view (arrows).

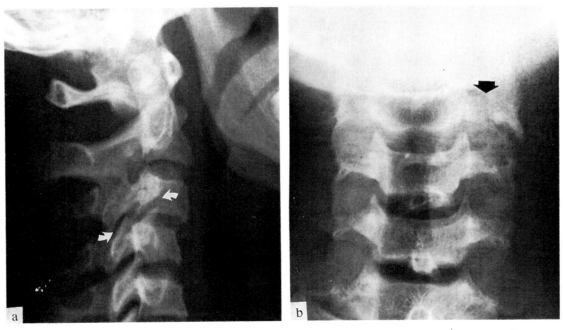

Fig. 11.47. Pedicular fracture. (a) Both C3/4 facet articular processes are aligned normally with each other but there is forward displacement and rotation at this level (arrows). A pedicular fracture must, therefore, be present and this is confirmed on the AP view (arrow).

ter to the presence of neural arch fractures, but even when suspected they may not be clearly evident. In these cases, AP tomography is of particular value in demonstrating the content of the injury (Fig. 11.48).

In most cases of dislocation, reduction is attempted. Gradual traction is undertaken, but manipulation under sedation, or anaesthesia, may be necessary. Repeated plain films are performed in the former and screening in the latter. Active reduction should not be delayed if traction fails as later attempts are less rewarding.

The ligamentous injury associated with dislocation or subluxation often fails to repair and leads to late instability. Careful assessment of the degree of anterior bone bridging is necessary to confirm the long-term stability of repair. This is of particular importance in those cases of hidden hyperflexion injury where the degree of posterior trauma has not been recognized. The importance of performing flexion and extension films after the initial spasm has resolved cannot be stressed too highly. Delayed healing may also occur in fracture of the odontoid and this will lead to atlantoaxial instability. In the lumbar spine, continued instability due to fracture of the posterior elements may lead to increase in neurological damage. Failure of satisfactory fusion is also a source of persistent pain and discomfort.

The role of the surgeon in the acute phase of injury has been the subject of continued dispute. There is little evidence that decompression of the cord in the immediate post-operative period provides any improvement in the final neurological outcome, and the removal of part of the posterior elements in the presence of anterior trauma without fusion may lead to considerable instability at a later time. Open reduction of dislocated facets in theatre may be performed in cases when closed reduction or traction has failed. If no, or partial, neurological deficit is present, this may prove hazardous, and leaving the spine unreduced may be a more preferable course. Fusion of the spine with or without reduction is a more common surgical role. In the acute stage, reduction and fusion

with either Harrington rods or a segmented wire and rod system, as described by Luque, may be performed. There is no evidence to indicate that neurological recovery is enhanced by this procedure, but its supporters claim a less stormy post-injury period, with reduction in pain, early ambulation and more rapid rehabilitation. Surgery is particularly indicated in the presence of extensive fractures of the posterior elements of the thoracic and lumbar spine due to the likelihood of instability.

In the cervical spine, evidence of delayed intervertebral union in hyperflexion injuries may make a posterior fusion necessary. Similarly, nonunion of the odontoid necessitates an occipitoaxial posterior fusion. Anterior cervical interbody fusion may also be performed in cases of delayed cervical instability.

Myelography is seldom required for the evaluation of acute injury of the spine, and the examination is difficult and may carry with it certain risks to the patient. The principal indication for this investigation has been the onset of neurological deterioration after trauma when a potential remediable compressive lesion is suspected. The assessment of both the presence and extent of root damage in brachial plexus injuries by water-soluble myelography has proved useful in the present climate of active treatment for these cases (Fig. 11.49).

The introduction and advent of CT has added a new and important dimension to the radiographic examination. Where this examination is available, it has proved valuable in the assessment of fractures of the posterior elements, and particularly in the demonstration of canal encroachment by bone or disc with subsequent cord compression. There is little indication for myelography or oblique views if CT is available, and CT with intrathecal contrast outlines neural encroachment and dural trear well.

DEFORMITY

Scoliosis is defined as a lateral curvature of the spine, and as the spine is normally straight the presence of any lateral curvature is abnormal.

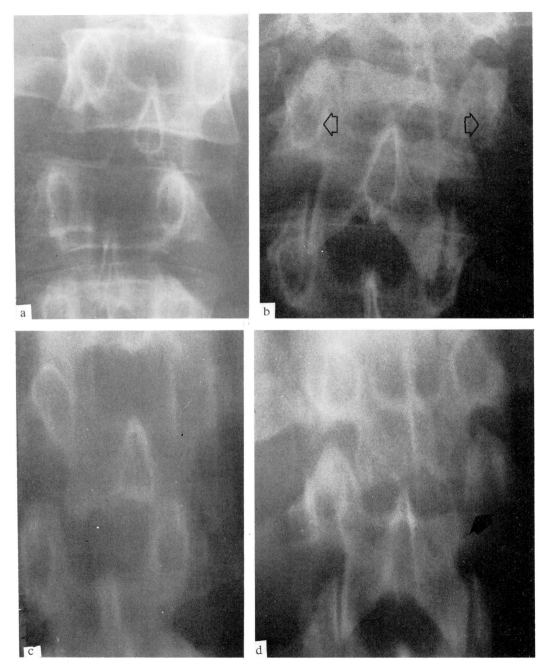

Fig. 11.48. (a) There is lateral displacement of the body of T12 on L1. The interpedicular distance is normal. (b) A similar lateral displacement has occurred but the interpedicular distance is widened (arrows). (c) Tomogram of case (a) shows that there is dislocation of joints without lamina fracture, whereas (d) shows that in case (b) a fracture of the pars (arrow) and pedicle has occurred.

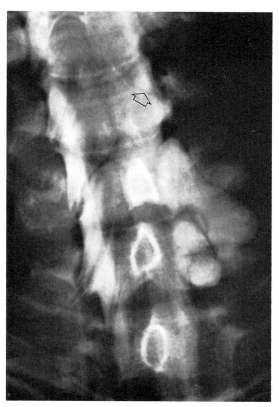

Fig. 11.49. Contrast has collected in a large traumatic meningocele under the pedicles of C6 and C7. The C7 and C8 roots have been avulsed at these levels. A single strand of the C6 root remains (arrow) associated with a small meningocele. The remaining roots are normal.

Kyphosis and lordosis differ in so far as they are normal and are only pathological where they become exaggerated. Kyphosis is normal in the thoracic spine, with a posterior convex angula-

tion of between 20 and 40°. Increase in the posterior convex angulation above this level is pathological and the increase may be generalized or localized. In the lumbar and cervical spine, concave posterior angulation produces a normal lordosis.

Aetiology

Spinal deformity has many causes and the major groups are classified in Table 11.1. Most congenital abnormalities are formulated in the first eight weeks of embryological development. Hemivertebrae are probably due to uneven pairing of the somite, and segmentation anomalies arise at the time of sclerotomal separation and the formation of the intervertebral disc. Spina bifida defects occur early during development of the notochord. Developmental defects of the anterior vertebral bodies are due to chondrification and ossification anomalies and, therefore, occur in the later period of fetal development. Multiple vertebral anomalies are often hereditary but isolated single anomalies are usually sporadic.

The aetiology of idiopathic scoliosis remains unclear. It is likely to be multifactorial with a genetic tendency to deformity. Eighty per cent of cases occur in adolescence and are regarded mainly as dominant and sex-linked to the X-chromosomes with incomplete and variable expressivity. The sex distribution is equal in minor curves, but females predominate in the progressive curves. Causative roles have been ascribed to abnormal muscular action; differing types of muscle fibres on either side of the curve;

Table 11.1. Scoliosis.

Idiopathic	Congenital	Neuromuscular
Infantile	Hemivertebra	Cerebral palsy
Juvenile	Unsegmented bar	Poliomyelitis
Adolescent	Vertebral body fusion	Muscular dystrophy
		Arthrogryposis
		Syringomyelia
Mesenchymal	Post-irradiation	Tumours
Marfans		Osteoid osteoma
Ehlers–Danlos	Neurofibromatosis	Osteoblastoma

a degree of denervation of the spinal muscles in the region of the apex; or disturbances in neurology from peripheral nerves to the deepest levels of the brain. All these, however, may be a consequence rather than a cause of the curvature. In the rare infantile group, the posture of the infant may also be important, causing a gravitational effect on the spine. The common association of plagiocephaly would support this. The remaining types of scoliosis are secondary and the onset and pattern of the disorder are related to the primary disease.

Clinical presentation

Deformity of the spine may present clinically at any age from six months to adulthood. The time of presentation is partly dependent on the aetiology, but is also related to growth patterns which vary from periods of relative quiescence to those of considerable activity.

Deformity is most commonly recognized by parents. They may see the spinal curvature, notice prominent and uneven shoulder blades, or realize something is amiss when clothes fail to fit. Examination of children by general practitioners or school doctors is also a source of diagnosis. Congenital curves are often diagnosed in early life by paediatricians. Occasionally, back pain may be the presenting feature, although this is more common in the adult population. Deformity may also be recognized during assessment of a generalized disorder which has abnormal spinal curvature as one of its many features. Delay in recognition may occur by these methods, resulting in progression to severe deformity which is intractable to treatment. A system of screening school-children during the years of greatest risk, i.e. 11 to 14, has therefore been advocated. Special curvature or shoulder inequality is noted. Unevenness of waistline, unequal hip and arm levels may also indicate deformity. A plumb-line dropped from the neck can be used to measure the compensation of the trunk in relation to the pelvis. The back is also observed horizontally, bent forward at the waist with knees straight. Asymmetry of the rib cage producing a rib hump indicates deformity and spinal rotation, although this test may be too sensitive, as the normal range has yet to be clearly defined. Finally, evidence of pelvic tilt due to leg length inequality should be assessed, as the latter may be a common cause of minor lumbar curves.

Patients with suspected deformity may be referred for radiographic assessment. Screening programmes have produced early detection and treatment of scoliosis both by the diagnosis of screened patients and by raising the awareness of scoliosis in the community. The presence and extent of pain should be clearly delineated, and in all congenital and the more pronounced idiopathic cases a full neurological examination should be performed. Neurological abnormalities either in conjunction with congenital scoliosis or causing the curve will thus be isolated. It also provides a baseline in case of deterioration of the curve, and will assist in recognition of any complications of treatment.

Radiological assessment

Children found clinically to have a deformity should undergo a single low-dose PA radiograph, ensuring that the entire spine from lower cervical to S1 is included on the film. The iliac crests should also be visible. The child should be standing with knees straight. The AP view may be used as this reduces the radiation dose to the breast but leads to magnification of the spine. The curve is measured as the angle subtended by the end-plates of the last vertebra tilted into the concavity of the curvature.

Idiopathic scoliosis

Most cases will have a mild adolescent idiopathic scoliosis which is unlikely to progress, and regular clinical review is all that is required (Fig. 11.50). Approximately three per thousand, however, will have a curve of 20° or more. These patients and those with a congenital anomaly will require more extensive radiography prior to treatment, and a full scoliosis series is undertaken. The PA view or supine view will dem-

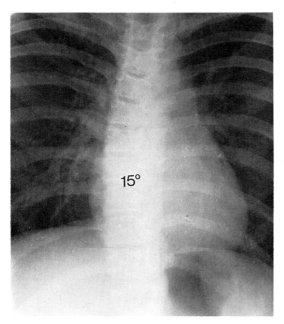

onstrate the type of curve, the most common being a right-sided single thoracic extending from T5 to T12. Curve flexibility is measured by comparing an erect film with one taken either by traction or with the patient suspended, and predicts the degree of improvement with treatment. Lateral bending films differentiate the structural compensatory curves and will also assess flexibility (Fig. 11.51). Finally, the degree of lordosis or kyphosis should be measured on the lateral film. Again, screening may be necessary to perform a true lateral film if significant rotation is present (Fig. 11.52).

As the curve progresses significant rotation occurs and in these circumstances underestimation of the true curve may result. A film in line with the ribs to account for the rotation may be performed or, alternatively, a true AP of the apical vertebra can be achieved by rotation under fluoroscopy (Fig. 11.53).

Fig. 11.50. Idiopathic scoliosis. A right-sided 15° curve of the mid and lower thoracic spine is demonstrated.

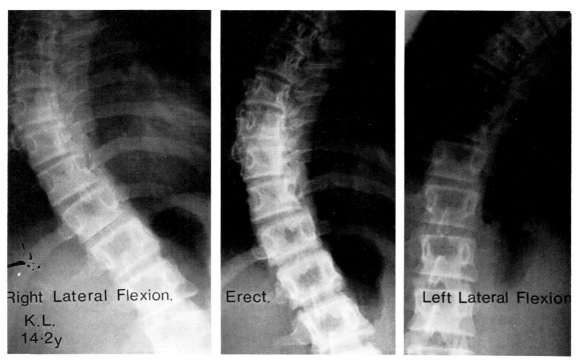

Fig. 11.51. Idiopathic scoliosis. The lateral bending films show a persistence of the thoracic curve which is the primary curve. The lumbar curve resolves on left lateral flexion and is compensatory.

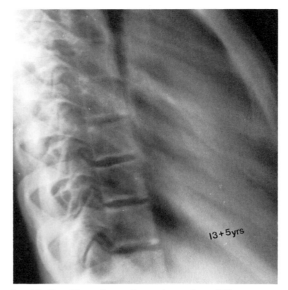

Fig. 11.52. Idiopathic scoliosis. A true lateral film demonstrates that the thoracic spine is in lordosis as well as being scoliotic.

The demonstration of wedging of both vertebral bodies and discs is an important prognostic feature. Reversal of vertebral wedging may take place following brace therapy provided there is still sufficient growth potential. If the disc is also significantly wedged then structural recovery is less likely.

Untreated idiopathic scoliosis often deteriorates rapidly through the growth spurt period, whereas deterioration after maturation of the spine is unusual, unless the curve is severe. Prognosis without treatment is, therefore, dependent on a balance between the severity of the curve and the amount of growth potential remaining. The skeletal age of the patient should, therefore, be assessed. A radiograph of the hand for comparison with known standards is helpful. The extent of ossification of the iliac crest apophysis also indicates the residual spinal growth potential (Fig. 11.54).

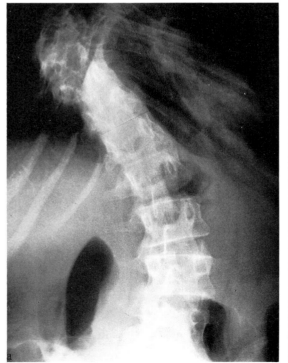

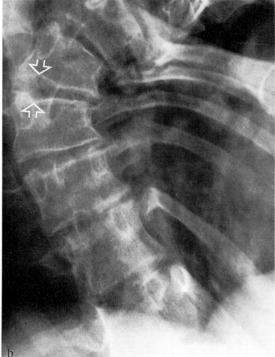

Fig. 11.53. Idiopathic scoliosis. (a) A severe sharp curve with rotation is present on the AP film. The severity and aetiology of this curve is not clear. (b) The curve is screened and rotated confirming the idiopathic curve with marked wedging of the vertebra and a shift of the disc nucleus to the convexity (arrows).

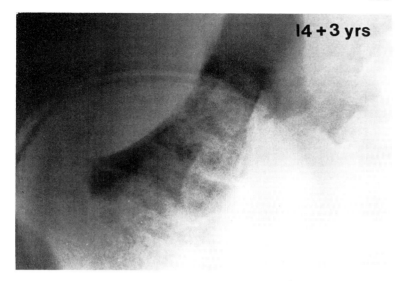

Fig. 11.54. Risser's sign. The iliac apophysis has traversed the iliac crest. Spinal growth ceases when the apophysis unites medially with the crest.

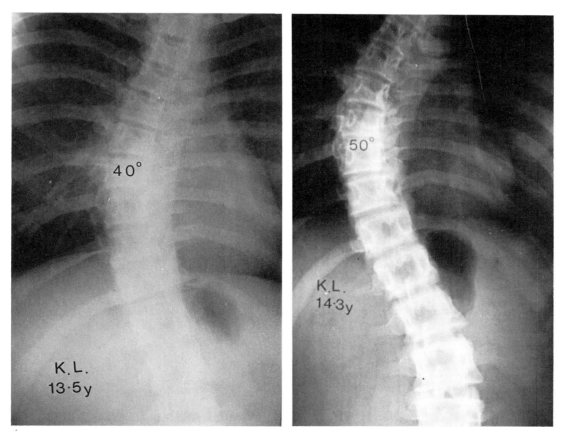

Fig. 11.55. Idiopathic scoliosis. The curve has progressed from 40° to 50° over a 10-month period despite conservative therapy and there is still a period of spinal growth remaining.

The type of therapy of idiopathic scoliosis is dependent on the degree of the curve and the skeletal age of the patient. Bracing is indicated in curves of 20° which are progressing, and 30° curves with rib hump must be braced. Curves of this degree with limited primary growth are likely to have a satisfactory outcome in conservative treatment. Even curves of 40° in patients with a skeletal age of 11 may be improved greatly by bracing. Those patients with curves over 45° are rarely candidates, especially if structural changes are present at the apex (Fig. 11.55).

Curves over 45° require fusion. The standard procedure is posterior facet fusion over the length of the curve with distraction and stabilization provided by the Harrington rod. With early brace treatment, however, few patients require fusion. Radiographs are required in the post-operative period to check the position of the hooks and rods and to measure the degree of correction. The latter is important, as a loss of correction, or pain occurring at a later stage, may indicate a pseudarthrosis, and comparison with the immediate post-operative films will enable confirmation. A break in the rod or dis-

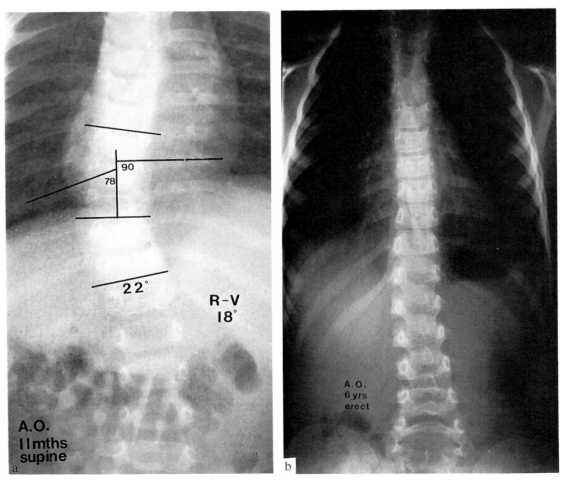

Fig. 11.56. Infantile idiopathic scoliosis. (a) A 22° curve is present at 11 months. The rib–vertebral angle is below 20° and spontaneous resolution can be anticipated (b).

placement of the hooks may also predispose to a loss of correction and pseudarthrosis. Bone scans may be helpful in isolating a pseudarthrosis, but surgical exploration is the most sensitive method of diagnosis. The natural history of infantile idiopathic scoliosis differs from that in adolescents, as the majority resolve over a time-scale varying from one to as long as twelve years (Fig. 11.56). A small proportion, however, become progressive and these may be predicted by measuring the rib/vertebral angle on the AP view. This is a measurement of both curve and rotation. Angles greater than 20° on two examinations performed three months apart are strongly suggestive of progression (Fig. 11.57). Treatment aims at minimizing the curve until the child matures. Initially, body casts are used until a Milwaukee brace can be fitted at the age of three years. This should effectively control the curve, but most children with progressive curves will eventually require fusion, and a few, not satisfactorily controlled, with curves progressing beyond 50–60° should be fused regardless of age.

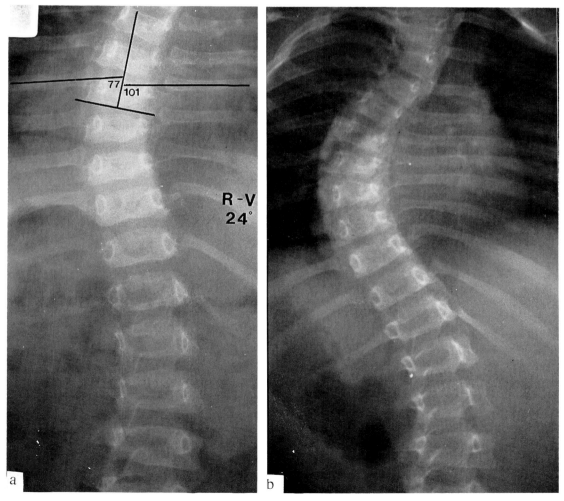

Fig. 11.57. (a) Infantile idiopathic scoliosis. The rib–vertebral angle is over 20°. (b) One year later a severe progressive curve has developed.

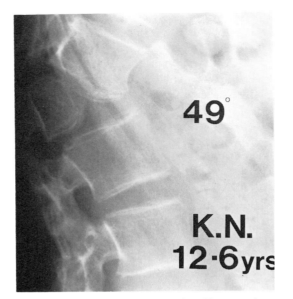

Fig. 11.58. Congenital deformity. A dorsal hemivertebra is present at C1. The body of T12 has pivoted during growth causing a marked kyphosis.

Congenital scoliosis

These curves tend to present early in childhood, and the key role of clinical and radiological assessment is to predict and monitor their progression. This is dependent on the deforming capabilities due to the arrest or promotion of unilateral growth in any plane. Hemivertebrae free to grow will cause a progressive curvature, the severity being dependent on the number present and whether they are unilateral or bilateral. Dorsal hemivertebrae, however, have a much greater deforming potential and a single level may cause a severe kyphosis (Fig. 11.58).

Defects of segmentation also vary in degree and deforming capabilities. Complete fusion of vertebral bodies causes little deformity, and even an anterior unsegmented bar extending over a few vertebral bodies will lead to only a mild kyphosis. On the other hand, a short failure of segmentation unilaterally in the posterior elements leads to a severe curve (Fig. 11.59).

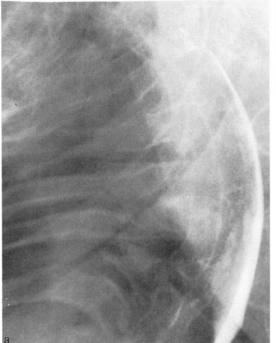

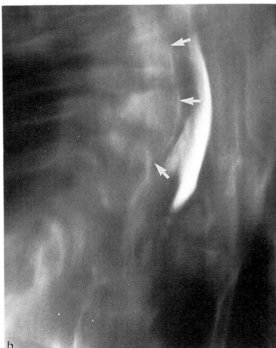

Fig. 11.59. Congenital scoliosis. (a) A long severe thoracic curve with marked rotation is demonstrated. The exact aetiology is unclear. (b) Tomography demonstrates the failure of segmentation of the posterior elements over five segments on one side (arrow). Myodil is present, delineating the cord stretched over the concavity.

Hemivertebrae fused to normal vertebrae or other hemivertebrae will have a much reduced growth and thus a milder scoliosis. Progression of congenital curves follows a similar time-scale to normal spinal growth, with increase in deformity during periods of rapid growth. These occur in the first three years of life and in adolescence. A steady deterioration, however, of 5–6° per annum occurs during the interim period.

The initial radiographs will usually reveal a relatively short, sharp curve which will be rigid on traction and bending films. There may be a compensatory curve which will be of greater length and may be confused with an idiopathic curve if the causative congenital lesion is not recognized. This occurs particularly with lesions at the cervicodorsal junction associated with compensatory thoracic curves (Fig. 11.60). The compensatory curves are normally flexible. Tomography confirms the congenital aetiology and, more importantly, allows careful analysis of the extent of the segmentation and formation defects (Fig. 11.59). Both AP and lateral tomography may be required to assess lesions completely, and if significant rotation is present

screening into the true AP plane prior to tomography is desirable. Careful follow-up assessment by erect low-dose radiographs is essential in congenital scoliosis, especially in those-at-risk groups. Comparison of each new film with the original film is essential, as a slow but steady yearly deterioration may not otherwise be appreciated.

Myelography

Neurological problems are not uncommonly associated with congenital scoliosis and also occur in severe idiopathic scoliosis. They arise either from bony compression of the cord on the concavity, particularly if it is a short segment deformity, or from associated anomalies such as diastematomyelia, or spina bifida and meningomyelocele. Diastematomyelia occurs in approximately 5% of congenital scoliosis. Splitting of the cord may occur with or without a bony spur, and only in the latter case is it demonstrable on AP tomography. Cord tethering may occur with or without diastematomyelia. Both lesions may lead to increased neurology as growth proceeds and are particularly dangerous

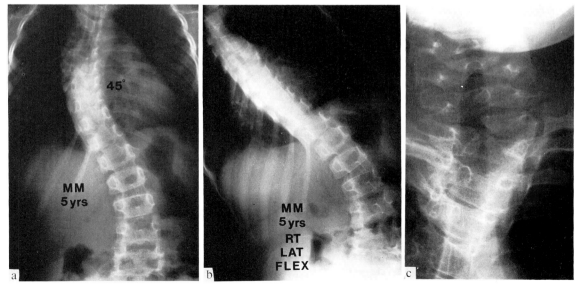

Fig. 11.60. (a) A right-sided thoracic curve is present which appears idiopathic. (b) Lateral bending films show that there is, surprisingly, considerable flexibility. (c) Careful scrutiny of the cervicothoracic junction reveals a hemivertebra. The thoracic curve is compensatory.

during treatment if traction is applied to the spine. Myelography is, therefore, essential for all congenital curves before traction or fusion is contemplated. Water-soluble contrast delineates clearly the cord and nerve roots and demonstrates the split in the cord (Fig. 11.61). The diagnosis of cord tethering is more difficult. A clearly thickened hilum may be seen, but confusion with the nerve roots may occur. The filum is posteriorly placed in the lower lumbar dural sac and is seen to extend to the lower limit of the subarachnoid space. Diagnosis may be achieved by showing limitation of cord movement during changes in position, but this is technically difficult with water-soluble contrast.

Myelography is also indicated if significant cord compression is suspected in idiopathic scoliosis. This only occurs in the severe cases, and it is important to demonstrate the extent of bony compression. In both situations the diagnostic quality of the examination is enhanced by screening for the maximum curve and then performing tomography (Fig. 11.62). CT scanning has been shown to be of considerable value in diastematomyelia and may be the examination of choice in patients suspected of having this disorder. This, however, is considered in a separate chapter (Chapter 4).

Finally, there is a clear association between congenital spinal and renal anomalies, the overall incidence being 20%. An intravenous pyelogram is, therefore, often required. Types of anomalies include unilateral renal agenesis, renal duplication, ectopia and obstruction (Fig. 11.63).

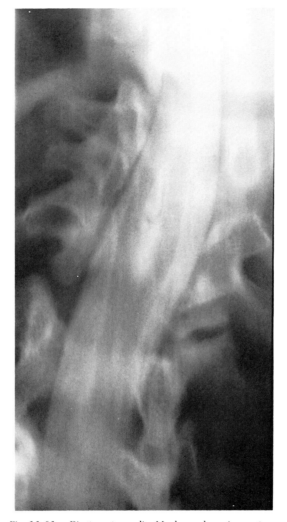

Fig. 11.61. Diastematomyelia. Myelography using water-soluble contrast media outlines the cord being split by a bony spur. Tomography enhances the detail of the investigation.

Surgical considerations

Treatment of congenital deformity depends on the type of lesion and the yearly rate of deterioration. Unilateral unsegmented bars, with or without contralateral hemivertebrae, especially in the lower thoracic and thoracolumbar regions, deteriorate rapidly and require early fusion of the deformed segment. Double hemivertebrae progress more slowly, but usually require fusion. Single hemivertebrae and wedged vertebrae may, in the upper thoracic and lumbar regions, progress slowly and rarely require surgical intervention, but those in the lower thoracic and thoracolumbar regions may require fusion during the adolescent growth spurt. Posterior fusion *in situ* is usually performed if the lesion is diagnosed and treated early. If correction is required, then a combined approach of anterior disc removal and fusion, combined with posterior fusion and, if neces-

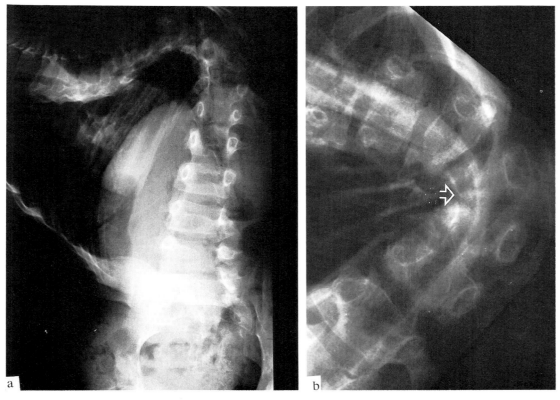

Fig. 11.62. (a) A severe idiopathic scoliosis is present. (b) Myelography with water-soluble contrast medium associated with rotation and tomography demonstrates the cord being stretched over the concavity of the curve (arrow).

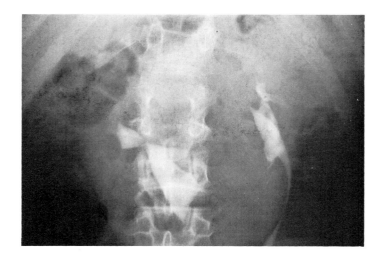

Fig. 11.63. Congenital scoliosis. An intravenous pyelogram has demonstrated a horseshoe kidney with marked rotation of the pelvicalyceal systems. An increased incidence of hydronephrosis occurs in this condition but it is not present in this example.

sary, osteotomy or removal of hemivertebrae, may be required. In the presence of diastematomyelia, it may be sufficient to remove the discs and fuse the spine *in situ*, without distraction. On the other hand, removal of the spur and release of the tethered cord is often performed and is essential if distraction is required for a subsequent spinal fusion.

Neuromuscular scoliosis

Neuromuscular scoliosis can be divided into those diseases which are neuropathic, such as poliomyelitis, cerebral palsy and syringomyelia, and those which are myopathic such as progressive muscular dystrophy, amyotonia congenita and Friedreich's ataxia. The spinal deformity develops in 96% of patients whose spinal cord injuries occur before the growth spurt and is a major problem in patients with muscular disorders. The neuromuscular curve

is a single curve, often involving the whole spine to the pelvis, and is progressive (Fig. 11.64). Secondary pelvic obliquity results, and may cause subluxation and dislocation of the hip on the high side (Fig. 11.65). The spinal curvature is often combined with a considerable degree of kyphosis. The curve is usually flexible and radiographs with suspension will indicate the degree of correction (Fig. 11.64b). Bracing may be used initially but tends to be less successful, and surgical intervention is often required. Dwyer instrumentation anteriorly followed by posterior fusion with Harrington instrumentation has proved to be a most successful method of correcting both the pelvic obliquity and the spinal curvature (Fig. 11.66). A lumbar kyphosis may be reproduced, however. More recently, the Luque procedure has been used in this group of patients with considerable success. This system involving double rods with

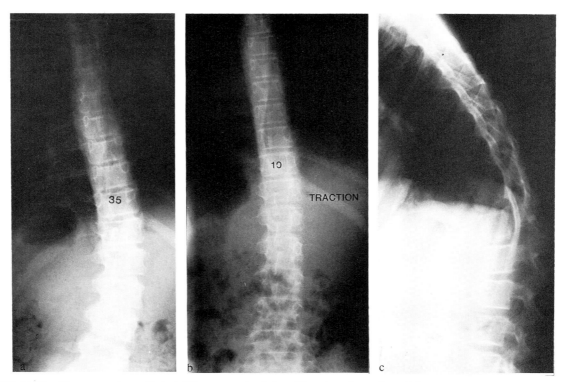

Fig. 11.64. Neuromuscular scoliosis. (a) The curve extends from T8 to the pelvis and is still flexible, as almost complete resolution occurs on traction (b). A thoracolumbar kyphosis is commonly associated (c).

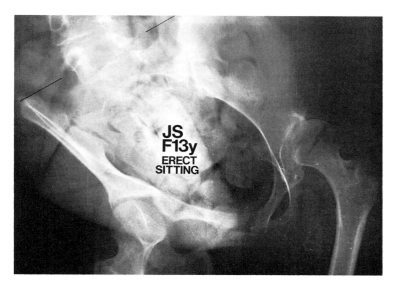

Fig. 11.65. Paralytic scoliosis due to spina bifida has produced significant pelvic obliquity. The upper femoral head is only partly covered by the acetabulum and is lateralized with a fixed adduction deformity.

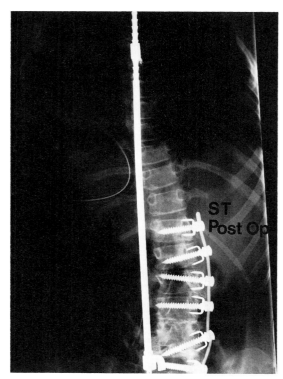

Fig. 11.66. Paralytic scoliosis. Dwyer fusion—the removal of the discs, and the reduction and compression with the screws and cable have allowed complete correction of the curve. Posterior fusion with Harrington rod instrumentation provides initial stability and a solid long-term fusion.

wires around each lamina can be shaped more accurately, producing a more balanced spine (Fig. 11.67). Rapid post-operative mobilization is also possible, thus reducing the respiratory problems, pressure sores and infection via the urinary system so common in this group of patients.

Neurofibromatosis

This generalized mesenchymal disorder is a rare case of scoliosis. The average age of presentation is 14 years. The curve is usually a short sharp curve and any part of the spine may be involved. Dystrophic changes in the spine include vertebral wedging, often with marked rotation of the apical vertebra and scalloping of the posterior vertebral margin. Neurological abnormalities may be due to either the deformity or tumour formation. Scoliosis alone does not lead to neurological deficit, but when scoliosis is combined with a kyphosis it is common. Foraminal enlargement may indicate a neurofibroma but dural ectasia may also produce these changes. This can be demonstrated on myelography (Fig. 11.68).

Other causes

Non-structural scoliosis may be due to sciatica, nerve root compression, inflammatory disease

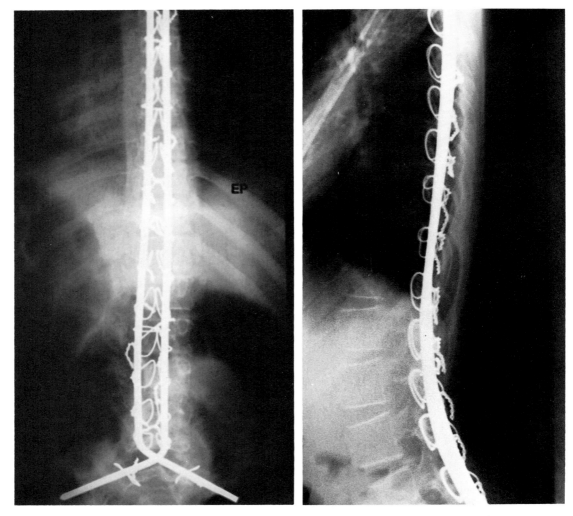

Fig. 11.67. Muscular dystrophy. The double rod and segmented wiring system of fusion is demonstrated. There is excellent correction of the scoliosis and the lordosis of the lumbar spine is preserved.

in the spine or in the paraspinal tissues, or, finally, to painful tumours such as osteoid osteoma or osteoblastoma. Bone scans are valuable in inflammatory disease and tumours to isolate an active area, and tomograms and CT scans may be necessary to show up the tumours in the posterior elements.

Non-structural scoliosis can be recognized by symmetrical side-bending films. They are usually lumbar or thoracolumbar and are mild. There is no rotation and no rib hump.

Conclusion
The clinical and radiological investigation of patients with spinal pain should be influenced by the individual features of the case. Following exclusion of specific pathological causes, back pain of sufficient severity to warrant surgical treatment should be investigated comprehensively. The radiological investigations should not, however, be considered routine, and the aim should be to choose those procedures that provide the necessary information for management.

In cases of trauma, care in interpretation of the X-rays is important to avoid the diagnostic pitfalls and to provide the maximum information for treatment.

Finally, accurate delineation of the cause and severity of spinal deformity is essential using all the necessary investigative modalities. Particular vigilance is required during periods of active spinal growth in order that severe deterioration of the curve can be avoided.

Reference

KELLGREN J.H. (1939) On the distribution of pain arising from deep structures with charts of segmental pain areas. *Clin. Sci.* **4**, 35–6.

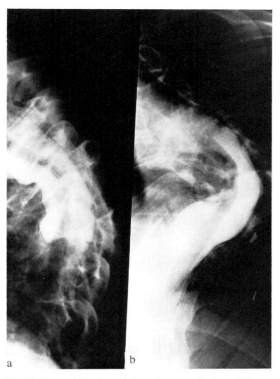

a   b

Fig. 11.68. (a) The lateral view shows scalloping of the posterior vertebral margins due to the dural sac ectasia. (b) There is a very acute scoliosis with ectasia of the dural sac. The cord is stretched tightly over the apex of the curve.

Chapter 12
The Upper Extremity
D.W. LAMB & I.M. PROSSOR

Introduction

The function of the upper extremity depends upon a series of mobile articulated levers with movement at the shoulder, elbow and wrist allowing for the positioning of the hand.

Charles Bell (1833) in his classical book on the comparative anatomy, embryology and development of the upper extremity emphasized that the dominance of man results from the twin functions of the hand arising from its movement to allow grasp or prehension and its sensation, 'that exquisite organ of sensibility'.

The importance of the function of the hand in the development of man to his pre-eminent position is emphasized by its representation in the cerebral cortex.

In order to position the hand, the upper extremity is structured to provide the freest possible range of movement at the three major proximal joints.

1 THE SHOULDER

Elevation of the arm from the side of the body to the overhead position through an arc of 180° in either the coronal or sagittal plane results from the free mobility of the ball and socket shoulder joint and also from the gliding of the scapula round the rib cage at the scapulothoracic joint.

Approximately two-thirds of this movement takes place at the glenohumeral joint, initiated in its early 20–30° by the action of the rotator cuff muscles. The term rotator cuff is used to describe the four small muscles which surround the glenohumeral joint, holding the head of the humerus firmly into the glenoid notch of the scapula. They consist of the subscapularis anteriorly, the supraspinatus superiorly, the infraspinatus posterosuperiorly and the teres minor posteriorly. Once abduction has started the deltoid muscle is the main prime mover at the glenohumeral joint. The remaining third of the combined movement that takes place occurs due to the rotation of the scapula on the chest wall. The two main muscles providing this action are the trapezius and the scalenus anterior.

2 THE ELBOW

For more precise localization of the hand in the area of the head, face and mouth, elbow flexion is of great importance. This results from the hinge joint action of the trochlear fossa of the ulna rotating on the lower end of the humerus at the trochlea, so that at full extension the tip of the olecranon rests in the olecranon fossa on the posterior surface of the humerus, and in full flexion the coronoid process rests in the coronoid notch on the anterior surface of the humerus.

Because of the shape of the lower end of the humerus and the carrying angle of the elbow, the hand is flexed towards the mouth and face, rather than to the point of the shoulder. This is obviously of great functional importance and means that the hand can be brought to the mouth simply by elbow movement, without requiring any rotation or deviation of the shoulder. When rotation of the wrist–hand unit is greatly limited or abolished, as can occur after a malunited fracture of the forearm or after unreduced dislocations of the radioulnar joints, congenital radioulnar synostosis, or single-bone forearms, such as in the absence of the radius or ulna, the value of normal movement which allows positioning of the hand between full supination and full pronation becomes evident.

Prosthetic replacement following amputation seldom allows active pronation and supination. Power-assisted prostheses, for example gas-powered limbs used in children born with limb deficiency, showed the marked improvement in function which was obtained by the active introduction of this movement.

3   THE WRIST AND HAND

Movement of the wrist is all important in hand function. It is the key joint for the positioning of the hand. The basic prehension patterns of the hand can be divided into:

(i)   Precision pinch.
(ii) Power grasp.

Precision pinch
This takes place between the pulps of the thumb, index and long fingers. It is essentially due to active movement of the thumb to oppose the other fingers, which occurs at the carpometacarpal joint. The stabilizing effect of the abductor pollicis longus attachment to the base of the metacarpal allows full mobility of the first metacarpal from the action of the thenar muscles. This pinch movement allows the pulp sensation to judge the shape, size and texture of objects, and to obtain the fine manipulative movements required in picking up small objects, holding tweezers or forceps, manipulating a fine screwdriver and other such precision functions. The stability of the radiocarpal joint and the radial longitudinal arch of the hand subserved by the second and third metacarpals with their immobile carpometacarpal joints is necessary for this function.

Power grasp
While precision grip is orientated to the radial side of the hand, power grasp is due to the strong grip provided by active flexion of the ulnar two digits into the palm and mobility of the fourth and fifth metacarpals at the carpometacarpal joints. This ulnar-orientated power grasp into the palm is improved by the transverse carpal and metacarpal arches which are shaped concave volarwards.

The shoulder joint

DISLOCATION

Because of the very free range of movement of the glenohumeral joint, the capsule, especially anteriorly and inferiorly, has to be slack. Post-traumatic dislocations of the shoulder are therefore common, particularly after a fall on the outstretched hand. The head of the humerus usually displaces in an anterior and inferior direction, stripping the capsule off the neck of the glenoid. This may tear the anterior attachment of the labrum glenoidale to the rim of the glenoid and forms the basis of the lesion described by Bankart which so often occurs in those cases which go on to recurrent dislocation. The pain and tenderness is felt anteriorly and the displacement of the head can usually be located clinically quite easily (Fig. 12.1). Following reduction it is important that a period of immobilization is carried out to allow the anterior structures to heal.

Posterior displacement of the humeral head is unusual following trauma, and the pain and tenderness is posterior and the head may be felt lying posteriorly. If there is any doubt about the clinical displacement, X-rays to show the position of the humeral head are taken (Fig. 12.2).

Posterior displacement of the humeral head is frequently missed due to inadequate views being taken.

Recurrent subluxation usually occurs after acute dislocation which has been inadequately immobilized. The commonest type is the recurrent anterior displacement, and the humeral head may show a defect in the posterior part of the head.

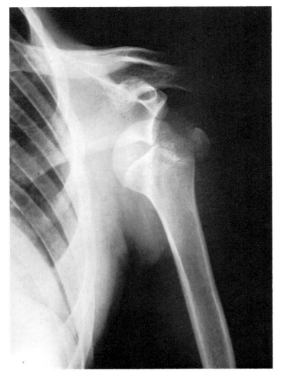

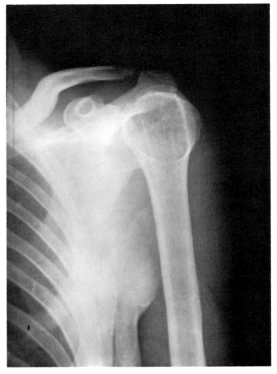

Fig. 12.1. Anterior dislocation of the shoulder with an associated fracture of the greater tuberosity extending to surgical neck and a lipohaemarthrosis.

Fig. 12.2. Posterior dislocation of the shoulder. AP view showing the classical loss of parallelism between the humeral head and the glenoid fossa. Injuries of this type may be difficult to diagnose on a frontal view alone. The axial view is a valuable supplementary examination.

OSTEOARTHRITIS

Osteoarthritis of the glenohumeral joint is unusual, but may occasionally follow a previous injury.

RHEUMATOID ARTHRITIS

The glenohumeral joint is seldom one of the early joints to be affected in rheumatoid arthritis. As the disease progresses, however, it is not infrequent for both shoulders to become affected, presenting with pain and progressive limitation of movement. This may initially be more in keeping with the changes of adhesive capsulitis around the shoulder and there may be a little in the way of radiographic change. Eventually, however, narrowing of the joint,

with associated osteoporosis and erosive changes, becomes evident.

ACROMIOCLAVICULAR JOINT

Dislocation of the acromioclavicular joint is caused by a fall on the point of the shoulder. The capsular ligament is weak and the main supports of the joint are the conoid and trapezoid components of the coracoclavicular ligament. It is only if these are damaged that there is marked displacement upwards of the outer end of the clavicle (Fig. 12.3).

Treatment will depend upon the severity of the ligamentous damage and the degree of displacement. When there is mild displacement, treatment other than symptomatic relief may

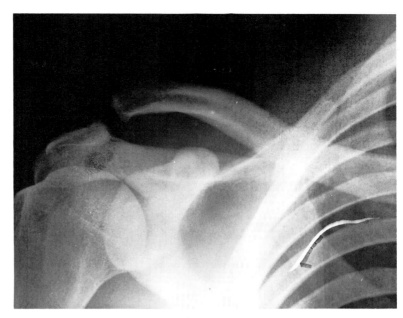

Fig. 12.3. Dislocation of the acromioclavicular joint. This is best shown if, at the time of the exposure, the arm is abducted.

not be required and the pain usually settles within two or three weeks, and full function commonly returns.

With more severe displacement of the outer end of the clavicle persistent pain, tenderness and swelling are frequent. It is usually wise to reduce and stabilize the joint. This can be secured by passing a K-wire across the joint along the medullary cavity of the clavicle, or by inserting a screw through the clavicle into the base of the coracoid process.

Degenerative arthritic changes are uncommon in this joint. Sometimes derangements of the intra-articular fibrocartilaginous disc may occur. If symptoms are persistent, excision of the outer centimetre of the clavicle is effective.

In recent years it has been suggested that minor arthritic changes in the region of this joint and osteophyte formation may be associated with degenerative changes in the rotator cuff, producing the painful arc syndrome.

ROTATOR CUFF

Rupture of one or other of the tendons of the rotator cuff near to the musculotendinous junction may occur in association with trauma to the shoulder or result spontaneously from degenerative changes of these tendons (Fig. 12.4). Rupture is unusual in the healthy tendon, but may occur in association with dislocations of the glenohumeral joint and is most likely in the supraspinatus. This injury may be suspected when the shoulder is incapable of abduction.

Hesitation and pain in abducting the shoulder, particularly in the middle-aged, may be indicative of the early changes of degeneration in the rotator cuff. This may be complicated by rupture of the tendon, making the range of movement even more limited.

Routine views of the shoulder may show no abnormality, and it is in these circumstances that arthrography may have value.

Arthrography

The methods available include single- or double-contrast arthrography, and specific indications include rotator cuff tears, damage to the articular cartilage and tears of the joint capsule. For all these indications the double-contrast method will give information not necessarily available on positive-contrast studies. For details of these techniques *see* Chapter 2.

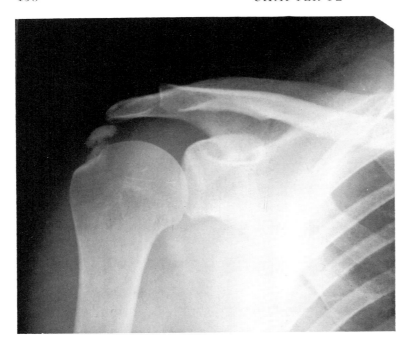

Fig. 12.4. Supraspinatus calcification.

If a rotator cuff tear has been demonstrated on the initial films, the examination can be terminated, but if the initial films appear normal the patient should be asked to exercise the shoulder joint and repeat views taken when a partial or complete tear may be demonstrated (Fig. 12.5).

If a definite tear in the continuity of one of the rotator cuff tendons can be demonstrated, consideration should be given to exploration and repair. This is easier in the normal musculotendinous unit associated with acute trauma, but may be difficult in the rupture that occurs with degenerative changes, where a gap may develop and the tissues are of poor quality for holding sutures.

Fracture of the neck of humerus

Fractures of the neck of the humerus are common and are usually the result of a fall on the outstretched hand. Depending upon the direction of violence transmitted along the humeral shaft they can be classified into abduction and adduction fractures.

1   ABDUCTION FRACTURES

These tend to occur in the older age group and to be associated with comminution of the outer aspect of the humeral shaft and greater tuberosity. Fortunately, impaction usually occurs, which prevents displacement and rotation of the humeral head by the rotator cuff muscle. It is seldom that reduction is required and simple immobilization for symptomatic relief is usually all that is needed.

2   ADDUCTION FRACTURES

Adduction fractures are more common in the younger age groups. The medial aspect of the epiphyseal plate may be involved in the impaction and cause growth supression. In addition to the varus angulation there is commonly a forward angulation at the fracture site which may be marked and can only be seen adequately on a good lateral X-ray. In view of local pain and swelling it is often necessary to take a transthoracic view. Minor degrees of angulation can be accepted and treated without

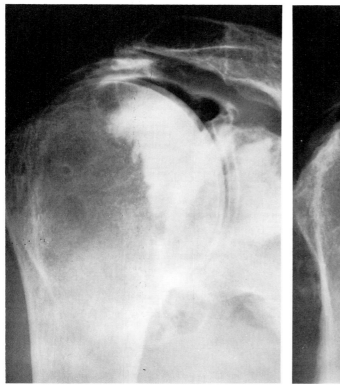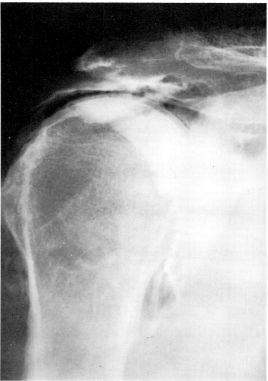

Fig. 12.5. Double-contrast shoulder arthrogram showing a complete tear of the rotator cuff with abnormal collections of air and contrast in the subacromial subdeltoid bursa below the acromion and lateral to the humeral head. (Courtesy of Dr Dennis Stoker, Royal National Orthopaedic Hospital, London.)

reduction. More severe angulation requires correction. The most stable position is one in which the upper end of the humerus is immobilized in abduction and external rotation.

Neer has produced a classification of shoulder fractures which is based upon the degree of displacement and separation of the fragments (Fig. 12.6).

The elbow

FRACTURES AROUND THE ELBOW

Fractures around the elbow are commonly caused by falls on the outstretched hand and occasionally on the point of the elbow. They may be classified into (a) those which involve the lower humerus and (b) those which involve the upper forearm bones.

(a) *Fractures of the lower humerus*

Radiological interpretation in the young child may be very difficult because of late ossification of the lateral condylar and epicondylar areas. Comparison with the non-injured side is advisable.

Common fractures in the small child include the supracondylar fracture, the lateral condylar injury—usually associated with marked rotation of the fragment from the pull of the extensor origin—and the epicondylar injuries.

The supracondylar fracture commonly occurs following a fall on the outstretched hand. Characteristic displacement is posterior. It is a worrying fracture to treat because of the displacement and associated swelling which may lead to impaired circulation distally. This is the fracture that is commonly associated with the development of Volkmann's ischaemic contrac-

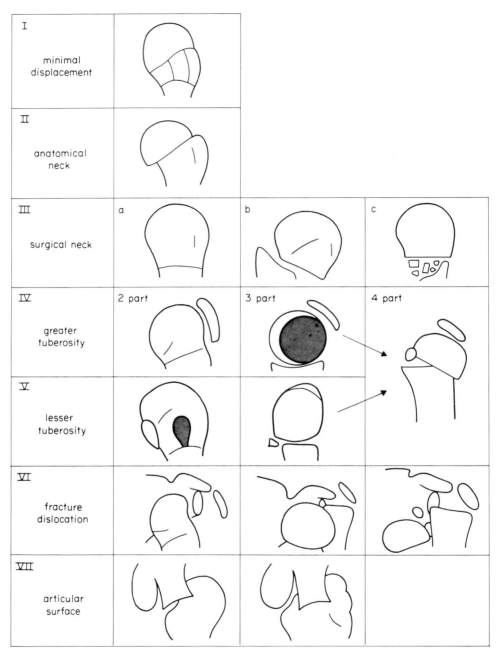

Fig. 12.6. Classification of fracture of the surgical neck of the humerus (after Neer 1970).

ture. Reduction of the displacement may be easy but the maintenance of this without compromising the circulation may be more difficult. Acceptance of some deformity may be necessary. Fortunately in the small child remodelling occurs readily.

Fracture of the lateral condyle (Fig. 12.7). Marked displacement of the lateral condylar epiphysis may be difficult to determine on X-ray in a young child, due to the cartilaginous component. The gross displacement that readily occurs is now well known, and forewarned with this knowledge the displacement can often be identified, particularly in comparison with the normal side. As a result, the severe late deformities which were common in the past and liable to lead to compression of the ulnar nerve in the post-condylar groove are now rare.

Separation of the medial epicondyle is commonly due to avulsion by the common flexor origin or the medial collateral ligament or both. This injury may be associated with subluxation of the elbow. The elbow may displace at the time of injury but reduce spontaneously before X-ray is carried out but with entrapment of the medial epicondyle fragment. With a history of a fall on the outstretched hand and findings of pain, swelling and tenderness on the medial side of the joint, particularly in a young person, this injury must be suspected. Unless looked for carefully the inclusion of the medial epicondyle in the joint can be missed easily (Fig. 12.8).

The damage to the soft tissues on the medial side of the joint is often considerable, and stress films will readily demonstrate the instability.

T- and Y-shaped fractures of the elbow occur from falls on the point of the elbow or as a result of a direct blow to the elbow. They usually involve fractures across the supracondylar area with extension into the joint. Wide displacement of the fragments may occur, and some form of internal fixation is usually required.

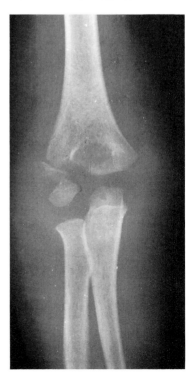
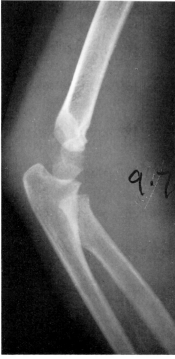

Fig. 12.7. Elbow. Fracture of the lateral epicondyle.

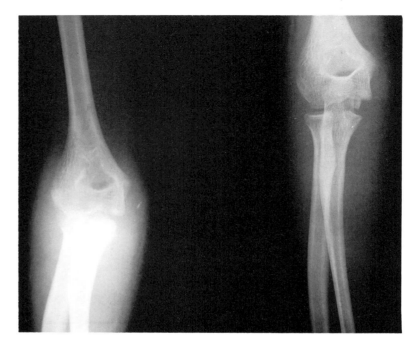

Fig. 12.8. Avulsion of the medial epicondyle. Following dislocation of the elbow, the medial epicondyle has become displaced into the joint.

(b) *Fractures of the upper end of the forearm bones*
Fracture of head of radius.   Fractures of the head of radius are usually due to a fall on the outstretched hand. The force is transmitted through the head of the radius to the capitellum. Damage to the capitellum often occurs as well and is not easily seen on X-ray.

The severity of the fracture of the head of the radius varies widely from the minor crack without displacement to the severe comminution of the head. The less severe fractures are treated conservatively (Fig. 12.9). Where there is gross comminution, excision of the head of the radius is indicated. Excellent results can follow this procedure in the adult, but it is unwise to excise the radial head in a child. The head can be replaced by a silastic cap, but there seems to be no particular functional advantage from this.

Fractures of the olecranon.   These may occur from direct injury, when they tend to be comminuted with involvement of the articular sur-

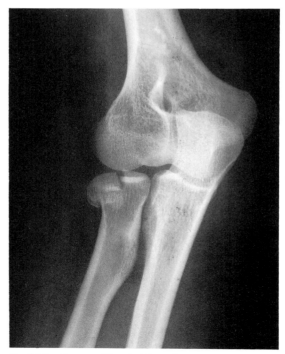

Fig. 12.9.   Fractured head of the radius.

face, or may be due to avulsion by the triceps attachment.

In younger people every effort should be made to reconstitute the bone fragments and restore the normal articular surface of the olecranon fossa. This may be achieved by internal suturing, usually with wire or by screw or other medullary fixation.

In elderly patients, particularly with comminution and where the portion of the olecranon is small, excision can be carried out with repair of the triceps. Early movement is essential.

ARTHRITIS OF THE ELBOW

This is usually associated with pain and restriction of movement and there are two main types.

1 *Degenerative arthritis* which commonly follows severe injuries with disruption of the joint surfaces. This may lead to fibrous ankylosis with very limited movement or there may be extensive para-articular ossification (myositis ossificans).

2 *Rheumatoid arthritis.* The elbow joint is frequently affected by rheumatoid arthritis with progressive limitation of movement.

In the early stages the disease affects mainly the humeroradial component of the joint. Localized synovectomy with excision of the head of radius may relieve symptoms and improve rotation of the forearm.

If the joint is more extensively involved a replacement arthroplasty can provide a painless satisfactory range of movement compatible with stability. The alternative is arthrodesis, which is usually performed with the elbow at a right angle, but this leads to considerable functional disability as well as relief of pain.

Replacement arthroplasty. The search for a satisfactory arthroplasty has continued for some years. Most of the early joints were of the hinge variety, which commonly resulted in loosening of the humeral component; these have been largely abandoned. Considerable bone needs to be removed from the lower part of the humerus, and if the prosthesis has to be removed the elbow is left very unstable.

A search has been made for types of joint replacement with more limited resection of bone and preservation of the collateral ligaments.

The most satisfactory prosthesis of this type to have been produced is the Souter arthroplasty. This consists of a metal component shaped to the normal lower end of the humerus and inserted at the lower end of the humerus with preservation of the supracondylar ridges and the collateral ligaments. A polythene replacement for the olecranon part of the joint is carried out. Both components are cemented in place (Fig. 12.10).

The wrist

Minor injuries of the wrist from sprains, strains and falls are not uncommon. The complaint is usually of pain and localized swelling with some restriction of movement. A history of the mechanism of any injury and the presence of localized tenderness may be the only features. Routine radiographs are commonly negative. Symptomatic treatment by immobilization for 3–4 weeks is usually all that is required. In those that have had no treatment, or where the injury was of greater severity than was first anticipated, symptoms may become more pronounced. Further X-ray may show evidence of ligamentous disruption of which scapholunate dissociation is the commonest (Fig. 12.11). The normal gap between the scaphoid and lunate increases when ligamentous disruption is present. A lateral view will show some rotation of scaphoid, so that the angle between the lunate and the scaphoid is greater than the normal 40°.

Rotary subluxation of the scaphoid is a more severe example of ligamentous damage. As a result the scaphoid often rotates until the tuberosity is pointing volarwards and the angle between scaphoid and lunate is as great as 90°.

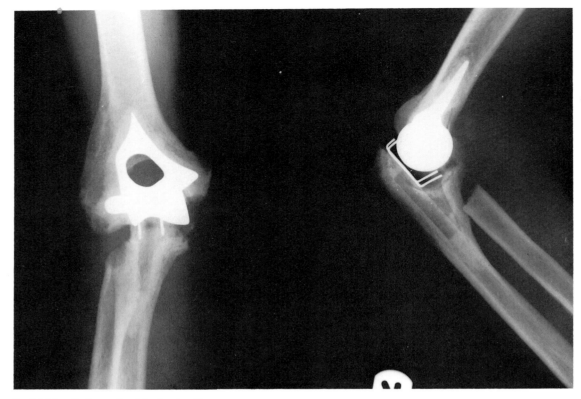

Fig. 12.10.   Radiographs of the Souter elbow.

Other examples of ligamentous disruption between the carpal bones may become evident but are much less frequent.

BONY INJURIES OF THE CARPUS

These injuries are common and the most frequent bone to be injured is the scaphoid, because falls on the outstretched hand with the wrist in dorsiflexion transmit the force to the scaphoid which lies as a strut across the intercarpal joint. A complaint of pain on the radial side of the wrist with localized swelling and tenderness in the anatomical snuff-box following such injury usually means a fracture of the scaphoid. In these circumstances scaphoid views (i.e. AP, lateral and two obliques) should be carried out but radiographic confirmation of the fracture may not always be present at the initial examination and should be repeated after 7–10 days. Failure of union in the fracture which has been ignored, missed or not treated is common and is often associated with cystic change at the fracture site or established non-union with sclerosis of the margins. Bone grafting or internal fixation with a screw (Fig. 12.12) is usually required in these circumstances to promote union and to avoid the likely development of degenerative arthritic changes.

More severe injuries of the carpus include the following:

1   Dislocation of the lunate. This is usually associated with a history of a fall followed by severe pain and swelling of the wrist. As the lunate usually rotates anteriorly into the carpal tunnel, acute symptoms of median nerve

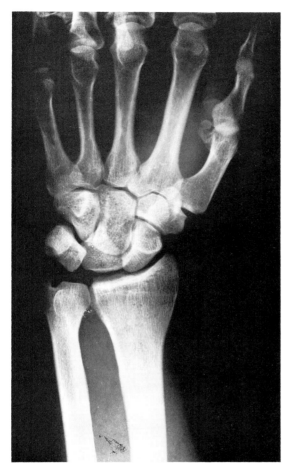

Fig. 12.11.   Scapholunate dislocation.

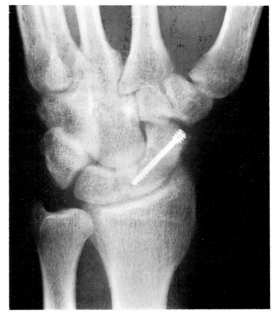

Fig. 12.12.   A Herbert screw inserted into the scaphoid to compress the fracture.

compression are not unusual (Fig. 12.13). The displacement can usually be reduced by manipulation but may require open reduction.

2   Trans-scaphoid perilunar dislocation. In more severe injuries the displacement of the lunate may be associated with a fracture of the waist of the scaphoid. The lunate and half the scaphoid may be displaced, or more frequently the rest of the carpus is dislocated around them. The displacement may have reduced by the time X-ray is taken, but the presence of a fracture of the tips of both radial and ulnar styloids should make one suspicious of the underlying nature of the injury.

Where displacement is present, manipulative reduction is often unsatisfactory and X-ray interpretation may be difficult. Operative reduction and internal fixation of the scaphoid fragment by a screw is the most satisfactory way of achieving carpal stability. If this is not obtained there is a great liability to avascular changes in the scaphoid, and late arthritis is common.

Kienböck's disease

It is generally assumed that this is an ischaemia of the carpal lunate. There may or may not be a preceding history of injury. The patient is usually a young adult complaining of pain and limitation of wrist movement. Physical examination confirms the limitation of wrist movement and there is localized tenderness over the lunate. In the early stages there may be very little X-ray abnormality to be detected apart from a slight change in the shape and density of the bone. As the disease progresses, there is

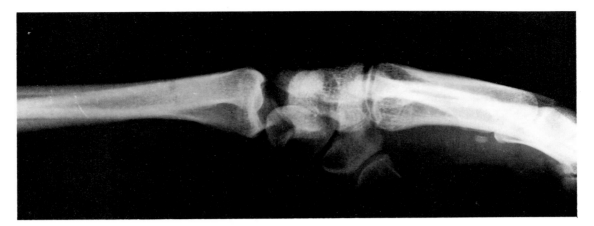

Fig. 12.13. A dislocated lunate which compressed the median nerve.

a tendency for the bone to collapse (Fig. 12.14). Immobilization of the wrist may lead to revascularization of the bone and relief of symptoms, but once collapse of the bone has taken place it is unlikely that conservative management will help. Treatment will then depend on the severity of the symptoms. Where there is considerable pain and restriction of movement, replacement of the lunate by a silastic model may be indicated.

The aetiology of Kienböck's disease is unknown. An interesting hypothesis suggests that it is due to an ulnar minus variant. In some cases it has been noted that the ulna is shorter than is usual. This theory has been most prominent in the Scandinavian and Japanese literature. The short ulna is 17 times more common in Kienböck's disease than in the normal Japanese population. Shortening of the radius has been suggested as a treatment to prevent the continuing collapse of the lunate.

A not infrequent complaint in young women is of pain in the wrist, sometimes associated with clicking. The cause of this is obscure and it is often self-limiting. A certain number may be associated with a dorsal ganglion which is not clinically visible or palpable. Injection of radio-opaque material into the wrist joint may

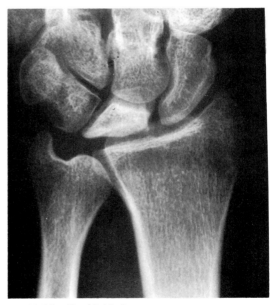

Fig. 12.14. Kienböck's disease.

show evidence of communication with the ganglion. Another possible cause may be derangement of the inferior radioulnar joint triradiate cartilage. This is also difficult to diagnose clinically and, as with the ganglion, routine X-rays are negative. Arthrography of the wrist may confirm damage to the triangular cartilage, justifying its surgical repair or excision.

This may be degenerative arthritis following extensive injury or due to rheumatoid arthritis. The presence of severe pain and restriction of movement in the wrist from arthritis may require arthrodesis or arthroplasty. In the single wrist affected by post-traumatic arthritis, and particularly where stability is required for any heavy manual work, an arthrodesis of the wrist can give very satisfactory relief of pain and good hand function. The wrist is usually arthrodesed in neutral position or in slight dorsiflexion.

In rheumatoid arthritis, where both wrists are usually involved, arthrodesis is much less satisfactory. If arthrodesis should become necessary because of pain and instability, it is usual to fix the wrist on at least one side in some slight flexion.

Progressive destructive rheumatoid disease of the wrist leads to a tendency to volar subluxation of the carpus from the lower end of the radius. In order to provide stability and retain some slight movement, dorsal shelf stabilization may be very satisfactory.

Fractures of the hand

Fractures of the hand can be divided into two main groups, stable and unstable.

Stable fractures

Most fractures of the neck of the metacarpal, isolated fractures of the shafts of the metacarpals, long oblique undisplaced fractures of the phalanges, and fractures of the terminal phalanx are stable. They do not require immobilization and the principal aim is to restore early active movement and disperse swelling.

Unstable fractures

As a general rule multiple metacarpal fractures, fractures of the base of the first metacarpal (Bennett's fracture), fractures of the base of the fifth metacarpal, transverse fractures of the proximal and middle phalanges, and fractures which involve the articular surface are likely to be unstable.

They require immobilization either by external fixation, usually on a splint, or by internal fixation. The commonest method of internal fixation is by Kirschner wire. Occasionally, fractures require more stable fixation by the use of small screws from the mini AO set. Plates are not justified in fractures of the hand.

Most fractures of the hand can be displayed adequately by routine anteroposterior and lateral views. It is important, however, that the lateral should be accurately localized on the site of the injury. Small dental laterals for the individual fingers may be valuable.

Where fractures involve the metacarpals it may be difficult to visualize the fracture adequately due to the overlap of other metacarpals. An oblique view can be valuable.

Characteristic displacements may occur with various fractures. At the base of the first metacarpal (Bennett's fracture) displacement is common due to the pull on the insertion of the abductor pollicis longus (Fig. 12.15a). On the opposite side of the hand a similar displacement occurs at the base of the fifth metacarpal due to the pull of the extensor carpi ulnaris insertion. As already stated, both these fractures are unstable and require fixation with Kirschner wires (Fig. 12.15b).

Transverse fractures of the metacarpal shaft are liable to dorsal angulation. In the long, oblique type of fracture, angulation is uncommon, but shortening of the bone and some degree of malrotation can readily occur. It is almost impossible to tell that there is malrotation on the X-ray, and this has to be a clinical assessment.

Fractures of the proximal and middle phalanges tend to angulate volarwards. The characteristic displacement of the transverse fracture of the proximal phalanx is due to the pull of the intrinsic muscles. As a result, the proximal fragment flexes and the distal fragment is extended.

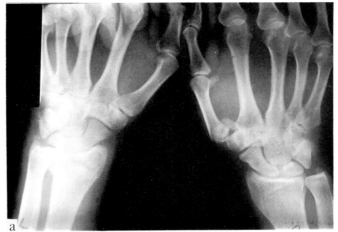

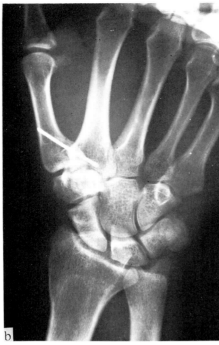

Fig. 12.15. (a) Bennett's fracture. (b) After reduction and internal fixation.

This deformity in the proximal phalanx is most easily corrected by immobilization with the intrinsic relaxed, so that the metacarpophalangeal joint is flexed.

Immobilization of the hand for fractures is seldom required for longer than three weeks. This will allow clinical union in most cases, whereas radiological union is likely to take up to three months. Immobilization of the hand for more than three weeks is liable to lead to iatrogenic stiffness of uninjured parts. The hand should always be immobilized so that the joints are in a position of safety, i.e. with the metacarpophalangeal joints flexed and the interphalangeal joints almost fully extended.

If the metacarpophalangeal joint is immobilized in extension, particularly in the presence of swelling, an irrecoverable extensor contracture may occur. In the case of the proximal interphalangeal joint, immobilization in flexion is likely to lead to flexion contracture which is difficult to correct.

Swelling with oedematous fluid is the enemy of the function of the hand and is liable to lead to adhesion and stiffness of the joints and limitation of gliding of tendons. Oedema must be controlled by elevation and active movement if this is possible, or where immobilization is required this must be done with a compression bandage in the safe position.

OSTEOARTHRITIS OF THE SMALL JOINTS OF THE HAND

Osteoarthritis involves mainly the distal interphalangeal joints, where Heberden's nodes are the classical clinical feature, and the carpometacarpal joint of the thumb. This latter joint is one of the commonest joints involved in the body, probably secondary in incidence only to the hip joint. The carpometacarpal joint is a saddle joint with the wide range of movement necessary for positioning the thumb. The characteristic changes of osteoarthrosis are seen in the joint, with narrowing of the joint and subchondral sclerosis, and lateral subluxation of the base of the metacarpal on the carpal saddle is common. The first intermetacarpal space is widened and there may be evidence of a large osteophyte filling this area.

Pain and disability are common and joint replacement is often required. Various types of joint replacement are used, the most frequent being a silicone implant. Other types of joint are being evaluated, and one in frequent use is the Caffinière prosthesis in which a metal component is cemented into the base of the first metacarpal (Fig. 12.16).

Involvement of distal interphalangeal joints is also frequent in psoriatic arthropathy and is usually characterized by greater destruction than in osteoarthrosis. As the destruction continues, the base of the distal phalanx becomes excavated and the middle phalanx becomes thin.

RHEUMATOID ARTHRITIS OF THE HAND

Rheumatoid arthritis frequently affects the wrist and hand. The earliest joints involved are often the metacarpophalangeal joints of the index and long fingers. The typical X-ray changes are seen, i.e. gradual joint destruction preceded by some joint narrowing and osteoporosis around

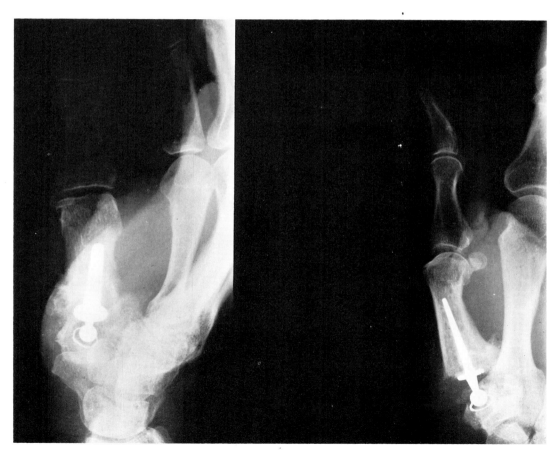

Fig. 12.16. Caffinière prosthesis for osteoarthritis of the 1st metacarpal joint.

the joint. The metacarpophalangeal joints frequently become affected severely (Fig. 12.17).
The earliest changes are due to the synovial
proliferation, which tends to burrow into the
sides of the metacarpal heads deep to the metacarpal attachment of the collateral ligaments.
This may not be seen on routine anteroposterior
and lateral views, and the oblique view is recommended. As the disease advances the damage is mainly to the metacarpal head, which
may be completely destroyed. In some cases the
major damage is to the base of the proximal
phalanx which becomes ballooned, leading to
the descriptive term of 'egg cup erosion'.

Destruction of radiocarpal and intercarpal
joints is common and there is a tendency for
radial deviation to occur at the wrist. As destruction proceeds it is common for volar subluxation of the proximal row of the carpus on
the distal end of the radius to occur, and with
damage to the inferior radioulnar joint dorsal
subluxation of the ulnar head is frequent.

One of the characteristic displacements of the
hand is ulnar deviation occurring at the metacarpophalangeal joints. There are many factors

involved in the development of this deformity,
but it is usually compounded by displacement
of the extensor tendons to the ulnar side of the
joint lying in the valley between the metacarpal
heads. The intrinsic tendons, particularly the
ulnar intrinsics, become tight, which not only
aggravates the ulnar deviation but leads to
progressive volar subluxation of the proximal
phalanx.

The proximal interphalangeal joints are also
frequently involved in rheumatoid disease, but
usually later than the metecarpophalangeal
joints. In addition to destruction of the joint,
there is a tendency for deformity to occur at the
joint, due to tendon disease. Tightness of the
intrinsic tendons is frequent in the rheumatoid
hand and may lead to swan-neck deformity.
This deformity will be compounded when there
is volar plate weakness or rupture of the super-
ficialis tendon. The other characteristic deformity
is the boutonnière deformity, which arises from
the synovium of the proximal interphalangeal
joint, eroding the central slip of the extensor
tendon. Reconstructive surgery of the wrist and
hand is frequently required and can give very

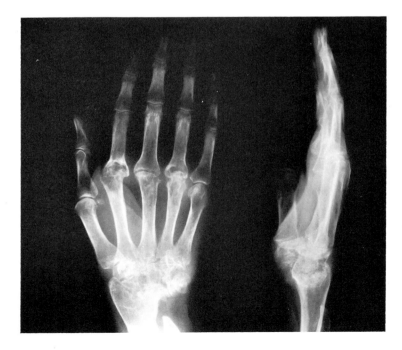

Fig. 12.17. Rheumatoid arthritis
with destruction of the MCP
joints.

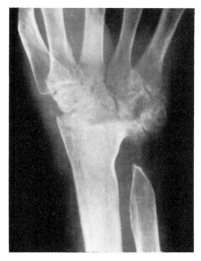

Fig. 12.18. Rheumatoid arthritis with Swanson silastic wrist replacement and excision of the lower end of the ulna.

satisfactory results in the relief of symptoms, the correction of deformity, the improvement of cosmesis, and, particularly, the improvement in function.

At the wrist joint, dorsal stabilization may be required for volar subluxation of the carpus, and excision of the lower end of the ulna is frequently required to relieve pain and improve radioulnar rotation. Replacement arthroplasty of the wrist is still at an early stage in development, but several types of prosthesis are available. These are by no means free of complications and have to be approached with caution. The most satisfactory at present is the silastic spacer (Fig. 12.18).

Interpositional arthroplasty with silicone rubber spacers is the most frequent method at the metacarpophalangeal joints (Fig. 12.19). They

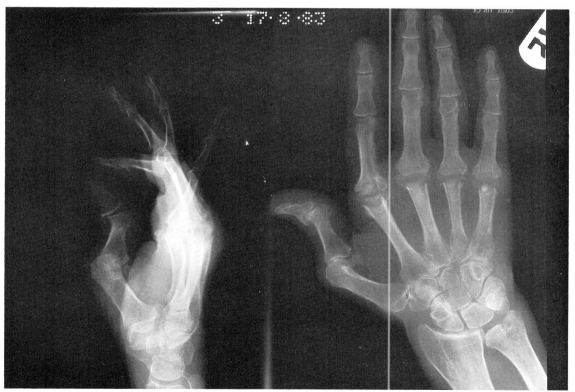

Fig. 12.19. Silastic spacers inserted into the MCP joints in a patient with rheumatoid arthritis. Note the deformity as the thumb at this stage is not yet corrected.

have a limited amount of hinge movement but are essentially spacers inserted after resection of the metacarpal heads. Movement takes place mainly by sliding of the distal part of the prosthesis in the proximal phalanx.

Joint replacement at the proximal interphalangeal joint is at a very unsatisfactory stage of development and there is no reliable prosthesis. Soft-tissue release may give an increased range of movement with relief of pain in the early stages of the disease, but when there is considerable joint destruction arthrodesis is the most frequent method of treatment.

References

BELL, SIR CHARLES K.G.H. (1833) *The Hand. Mechanism and Vital Endowments as Evincing Design.* London: William Picking.
NEER C.S. (1970) Displaced proximal humeral fractures. 1 Classification and evaluation. *J. Bone Jt Surg.* **52A**, 1077–89

Chapter 13
Pelvic Girdle

M.F. MACNICOL

Pelvic girdle

The pelvic girdle includes the iliac, ischial and pubic components of the pelvic ring, the posterior articular relationship with the sacrum and, indirectly, the coccyx, and the hip joints. Pathological conditions that affect these structures will be discussed, insofar as they produce problems for the orthopaedic surgeon. Abnormalities of the hip joint in the adult will also be described, with the inclusion of fractures of the proximal femur as far distally as the trochanteric region.

PELVIC FRACTURES

The degree of force required to fracture components of the pelvis will vary, and depend greatly upon the strength of the bone (and thus the age of the patient), and the site of injury. Falls from a standing position or against furniture may be sufficient to fracture the anterior pelvic ring or lateral pelvic wall in the elderly, whereas much greater violence is necessary to produce a fracture of significance in a young adult. Motor vehicle collisions, crushing injuries and falls from a considerable height are therefore encountered in this younger group of patients, and often the stabilizing ligaments of the pelvis will have sustained damage in addition to the skeleton.

Since most of the structural integrity of the pelvis depends upon the strength of the ligaments, particularly posteriorly in the shape of the sacroiliac, sacrospinous and sacrotuberous ligaments, much of the stability of the pelvis is lost when these are ruptured. Whether the fracture pattern is stable or unstable can therefore be deduced largely from the relationship between the iliac wings and the sacrum, and the orthopaedic surgeon will look to his radiological colleague for advice when establishing this fact. Stable fractures include avulsion fragments, commonly encountered in athletic individuals who subject the pelvic girdle to repetitive muscular stress, single fractures of the pelvic ring with no evidence of sacroiliac joint disruption, bilateral pubic rami fractures in the osteopenic patient, and undisplaced double fractures. Generally speaking, anteroposterior and lateral compression forces are less likely to disturb the posterior ligamentous complex than vertical shear forces (Tile 1980, Fig. 13.1).

Once stability of the fracture pattern has been established, it is usual to classify the radiographic appearances in terms of whether the pelvic ring has been breached or not. The ring is uninvolved in the following fractures:

1 Avulsions.
   (a) ischial tuberosity.
   (b) anterior superior iliac spine,
   (c) anterior inferior iliac spine,
   (d) pubic arch (adductor origin).
2 Pubic or ischial ramus.
3 Iliac wing (fracture of Duverney).
4 Sacrum.
5 Coccyx (with or without dislocation).

The presence of apophyses in the adolescent may occasionally prove to be confusing when assessing these fractures.

Breaks in the pelvic ring may be either single or double:

1 Single break.
   (a) ipsilateral rami (pubic and ischial),
   (b) fracture beside or subluxation of the pubic symphysis,

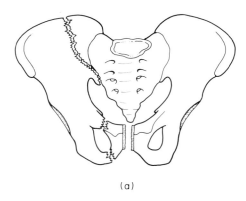

(a)

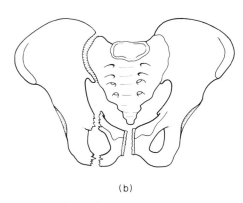

(b)

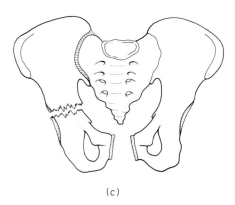

(c)

Fig. 13.1. Basic mechanisms of major pelvic disruption.
(a) Lateral compression, (b) vertical shear (may be
bilateral with pubic diastasis and sacroiliac joint
disruption, (c) anteroposterior compression.

(c) fracture beside or subluxation of the
sacroiliac joint,
2 Double break.
(a) double vertical fractures,
(i) ipsilateral involving the iliac wing
(Malgaigne type),
(ii) ipsilateral involving the sacroiliac
joint,
(iii) bilateral, usually of the anterior 'saddle' type,
(b) multiple, highly unstable pelvic injuries,
inevitably associated with severe visceral
damage.

When the acetabulum is thought to be involved it is important to enlist further radiographs so that the exact nature of the fracture
pattern can be deduced. External and internal
oblique radiographic projections (Figs. 13.2 and
13.3) are obtained by rotating the supine
patient 45° towards the injured side and 45°
away from the injured side respectively, and are
mandatory if surgical reconstruction of the acetabulum is contemplated (Judet *et al.* 1964).
Pelvic inlet and outlet views, tomography, and,
above all, CAT scanning will further define the
extent of the fracture. Classification of acetabular fractures is now relatively precise, and a
contemporary list is given below:

1 Ischial (including the ischioacetabular fracture of Waldius).
(a) posterior wall,
(i) single fragment,
(ii) multiple fragments,
(b) posterior column,
(c) posterior wall and posterior column,
(d) transverse, involving the posterior wall.
2 Pubic.
(a) anterior wall,
(b) anterior column.
3 Iliac—comprising dome fractures.
4 Medial wall (a composite of ischium, pubis
and ilium).

Stress fractures of the pelvis are now well-
recognized, particularly those involving the

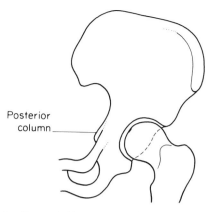

Fig. 13.2. External oblique view to show the posterior pelvic column (obtained by rotating the supine patient 45° towards the injured side).

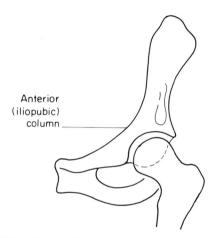

Fig. 13.3. Internal oblique view to show the anterior column (obtained by rotating the supine patient 45° away from the injured side).

pubic rami near the symphysis. These were reported first in military recruits undertaking a great deal of 'square-bashing', but are also seen in joggers, particularly women (Pavlov *et al.* 1982), and in association with obesity and after total hip replacement. The symptoms of groin, buttock or thigh pain may be non-specific, but the history is usually diagnostic, and a bone scan will localize the lesion, which may only become radiographically apparent after a few months. The infractions are, of course, entirely

comparable to Looser zones in osteomalacia, although the fracture line is less easily seen. Pathological fractures of the pelvis are less of a problem orthopaedically than similar lesions in the proximal femur, and hence their discussion will be postponed until that section of this chapter. Finally, fractures of the sacrum, because of their relative rarity, are often missed. Neurological injury is common and may be the reason for suspecting such a fracture. Of themselves, neither sacral nor coccygeal fractures require active treatment, although a per-rectal manipulation of an angulated coccygeal fracture is sometimes necessary.

PROXIMAL FEMORAL FRACTURES

Fractures of the head and neck of the femur often occur in association with the more severe pelvic injuries. Femoral head fractures almost invariably denote that the hip joint has sustained a traumatic dislocation, and indeed this is generally true also of anterior and posterior rim fractures of the acetabulum. Fractures below the round ligament (fovea) are produced by a posterior dislocation of the femoral head, while those above this level are considered to be the result of an anterior dislocation. Once again, tomography and CAT scans may be helpful in elucidating the nature of the injury, and also whether the fractured segment is significantly displaced. As a rule, the larger the fragment and the more it involves the weight-bearing segment of the femoral head, the worse will be the prognosis. Although surgical fixation of a fragment may produce a relatively satisfactory short-term result, osteoarthritis is likely later, particularly if there is comminution, or if the acetabulum is involved. Avascular necrosis is almost inevitable if the femoral head fragments are widely displaced or if there is an additional femoral neck fracture.

Fractures of the neck of the femur (Waldenstrom 1924) are as common as fractures of the femoral head are rare, and of course the former are usually the result of minimal force in the elderly. Standard anteroposterior and lateral radiographic projections usually suffice, the lateral view indicating the degree of displacement of the femoral head far more effectively. The quality of this film must therefore be good, and this is not always easy to ensure in a patient in pain, or where obesity complicates the exposure time required. Even when the patient is anaesthetized and positioned upon the orthopaedic table, the lateral projection may be difficult to interpret, particularly on the image-intensifier. If full abduction of the 'good' leg does not allow an adequate view, then it may have to be flexed to 90° at the hip and knee in order to position the X-ray tube or image-intensifier correctly. In crack fractures of the neck and trochanteric region of the femur the surgeon may request further radiographic views of the possible fracture site and, as with scaphoid fractures, the diagnosis may not be confirmed until oblique views or later radiographs are obtained.

Incomplete fractures of the femoral neck may either be acute, especially in osteoporotic bone, or as a result of fatigue secondary to repetitive stress. Occasionally, the bone may be a site of a pathological process with lesions evident elsewhere in the skeleton if these are sought. Complete fractures may be either:

1 Impacted.
2 Partially displaced.
3 Completely displaced.

Garden (1964) introduced a grading system based upon the degree of displacement, as described above, although no radiographic classification can be expected to predict accurately the extent of soft-tissue damage, or the subsequent survival of the femoral head. The principal concern of the orthopaedic surgeon is the patency of the retinacular vessels encompassing the femoral neck, and the displacement of the two fragments at the time of injury largely dictates this. Complete but 'impacted' fractures (Garden grade II) lead to a later avascular necrosis rate, manifest by segmental collapse of the femoral head, of approximately 15%; the partially displaced grade III fractures result in late segmental collapse of 30–50%, and grade IV

fractures to a rate of over 50%, particularly in the young and very old patients.

Although it is unlikely that the radiologist will be asked for a detailed assessment of the nature of a subcapital fracture, an opinion is regularly sought as to whether avascular necrosis is developing. The changes may take months to appear radiographically, with a diffuse radiodensity evident in the ischaemic segment when compared with the relative osteopenia of the surrounding vascular bone. Radionuclide imaging is often helpful in the early stages when the radiographs are equivocal, and it is at this stage that treatment, whether by conservative non weight-bearing physiotherapy, or by redirectional femoral osteotomy, holds out some hope of success. The extent of the avascular change is variable, but a progressive scale has been described (Marcus et al. 1973):

Superior marginal (crescentic).
Segmental.
Partial.
Quadrantic (producing a 'roller-bearing' joint).
Subtotal.
Total.

A further influence upon the outcome of these fractures may be the inclination of the fracture line. This 'Pauwels' angle' (Pauwels 1935, Fig. 13.4) is measured on the anteroposterior projection and was originally described by Waldenström (1924). It has been suggested that angles greater than 30° will fare poorly, since these adduction fractures are unstable, and malunion or non-union is more likely. However, the error inherent in attempting to interpret a spiral or comminuted cervical femoral fracture in terms of an 'angle' on a single radiographic view has rightly led to the value of this measurement being questioned. Basal cervical fractures and fractures in very weak bone yield poor results, as do high subcapital fractures; in these cases, as with any displaced fracture in the very old (generally accepted as over the age of 70 years), replacement arthroplasty is to be preferred to fixation after reduction using a sliding screw

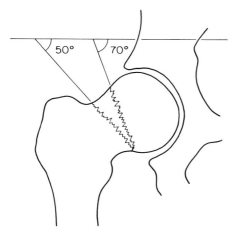

Fig. 13.4. Pauwels' angle (using an anteroposterior projection).

device or double screws or nails. The Moore (1952) and Thompson (1954) prostheses, the latter requiring complete resection of the femoral neck prior to insertion with cement, are still the most commonly encountered, but there are now a range of newer implants which attempt to reduce the wear that occurs in the acetabulum subject to the biomechanically and biologically unsatisfactory articulation of metal upon cartilage. A conventional total hip replacement is not particularly suitable in these cases, since there is a considerable risk of dislocation, but in rheumatoid patients with a subcapital femoral fracture, or in cases with malignant deposits in the acetabulum and proximal femur, a standard low-friction arthroplasty is indicated.

Trochanteric fractures can be arbitrarily divided into the following groups:

1 Avulsion of the lesser trochanter.
2 Avulsion or comminution of the greater trochanter.
3 Stable trochanteric fractures, with an undisplaced intertrochanteric fracture line.
4 Stable trochanteric fractures, but with a displaced intertrochanteric line or fractured lesser trochanter.
5 Unstable trochanteric fractures, with a displaced intertrochanteric line and often an asso-

ciated greater trochanteric (three-part) fracture; although there is no posteromedial comminution, posterolateral support is deficient and hence a varus deformity may occur.
6 Unstable four-part trochanteric fractures where there is additional posteromedial comminution, and often a subtrochanteric extension making fixation difficult.

Complications of trochanteric fractures include malunion, with implant failure and sometimes nail penetration into the acetabulum, non-union on rare occasions, infection, deep venous thrombosis and pressure sores, and a mortality rate of 10–15%.

PATHOLOGICAL FRACTURES

The exceedingly common proximal femoral fracture in the elderly is generally 'pathological' to the extent that it occurs in osteoporotic or osteomalacic bone, but the term pathological fracture is confined clinically to fractures through bone weakened by tumour, infection or some other localized process. Nevertheless, the conditions predisposing to such fractures are extensive and it is of interest to list those that may lead on to a fracture in the region of the pelvic girdle.

1 Congenital abnormalities, including enchondromatosis, fibrous dysplasia and osteogenesis imperfecta.
2 Metabolic bone disease, including rickets, osteomalacia, scurvy, hyperparathyroidism, and of course osteoporosis.
3 Inflammatory conditions, particularly osteomyelitis and rheumatoid arthritis.
4 Avascular necrosis.
5 Neoplasia, which is rarely primary and usually secondary to disseminated carcinoma from breast, bronchus, kidney, prostate, thyroid and the other glandular tissues of the body.
6 Disseminated bone disorders, such as the reticuloses.
7 Neuromuscular diseases such as poliomyelitis, paraplegia and spina bifida, resulting in disuse osteoporosis.

The characteristics of such fractures include whether they are osteolytic or osteosclerotic, whether the fracture line extends completely across the bone or not, and whether a joint surface is breached. Enlarging metastatic or primary lesions should alert the radiologist and oncologist to the probability of eventual fracture (Figs. 13.5–13.7), at which stage the orthopaedic surgeon should be consulted. While local irradiation and chemotherapy may control the spread of metastases for many years, once the strength of the bone is significantly weakened a prophylactic fixation of the skeleton is advised (Harrington 1972). Apart from the risk of complete fracture, necessitating an emergency admission, surgical fixation usually provides excellent pain relief and certainly improves the quality of life. The patient becomes more mobile

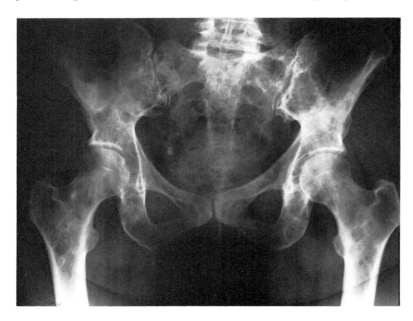

Fig. 13.5. Initial view of the pelvis of a woman with metastatic breast carcinoma. Note the deposits in the femoral necks.

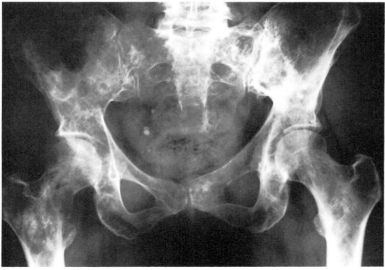

Fig. 13.6. The metastatic deposits have enlarged and fracture is imminent.

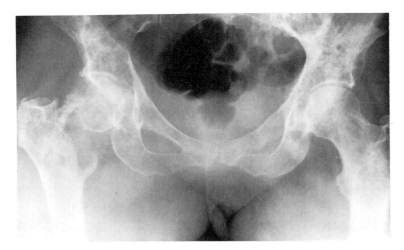

Fig. 13.7. A pathological fracture has occurred. The pain and anxiety of an emergency admission might have been avoided by prophylactic replacement of the proximal femur at an earlier stage. A total hip arthroplasty was performed.

and can thereafter attend for further medical treatment if that is considered advisable. Survival times in this group of patients, approximately 12–15 months, may be increased as they exercise and eat more after surgical intervention, and several remarkably long-term survivors have been reported.

Methylmethacrylate cement is an important adjunct to the metal implant, since it makes good any major loss of bone structure and improves the hold of screws in weakened bone. Periosteal callus forms remarkably quickly, despite the presence of cement, and most fractures show evidence of union by three months after the stabilization. When the acetabulum and surrounding pelvis are extensively involved there may still be a place for mesh or custom-built implants, augmented by cement, and the long-stem femoral prosthesis can be used as part of a total hip replacement when metastatic deposits are present in the middle and distal femoral shaft. Consequently, it is very important that the full length of bones is reviewed radiographically prior to any major surgery.

ARTHRITIS OF THE HIP JOINT

The hip joint is commonly the site of an arthritic process, whether osteoarthritis, rheumatoid arthritis or an infective arthritis. Pain, stiffness and a limp are the cardinal clinical features,

and the stigmata of arthritis may be evident elsewhere in the body. Further investigation may reveal metabolic abnormalities, as in gout or crystal synovitis (pyrophosphate arthropathy), or systemic disease, such as Reiter's syndrome, gonococcal infection, sarcoidosis or leukaemia.

When assessing the extent of rheumatoid involvement radiographs will be requested not merely of the hips, but also of the hands, other weight-bearing joints and also of the cervical spine if a general anaesthetic is to be considered. Atlantoaxial subluxation, indicated by an anterior odontoid gap of more than 4 mm, and any other evidence of cervical spine instability must be known prior to any stress being applied to the neck of an unconscious patient.

Radiographic features of rheumatoid arthritis include:

1 Soft-tissue swelling and capsular distension.
2 Periarticular osteoporosis.
3 Narrowing of the articular space.
4 Subarticular erosions.
5 Loss of mass and a narrowing of long bones.
6 Deformity.
7 Eventual ankylosis.

Osteoarthritis differs from rheumatoid arthritis in a number of important respects (Arnoldi & Reiman 1979) and represents a final common pathway of cartilage loss and bone hypertrophy following a number of inflammatory, metabolic and mechanical abnormalities of the hip joint (Solomon 1976). The causes of 'secondary' osteoarthritis are listed in Table 13.1, and a very extensive catalogue it is. Whether there is truly a 'primary' or idiopathic form of osteoarthritis is disputed (Harris 1977), but until genetic, clinical, biochemical and, indeed, radiographic studies gain more precision it does appear that there is a small group of patients in which no underlying cause can be identified to account for the pathological process. The classical radiographic changes are (Fig. 13.8):

1 Narrowing of the joint space.
2 Subchondral sclerosis.
3 Osteophyte formation.
4 Periarticular cysts.

Involvement of the hip joint may be confined to the upper segment, the medial segment or may be concentric (total) (Wroblewski & Charnley 1982), and crude definitions of severity have been suggested (Cooperman *et al.* 1983) such as:

1 Mild—less than 25% of joint space affected.
2 Moderate—25–75% of joint space affected.
3 Severe—more than 75% of joint space affected.

Changes in the normal skeletal architecture occur, such as eccentricity or flattening of the femoral head (Fig. 13.9), thickening and loss of the normal inferior concavity of the femoral neck, and osteophytes enlarging from various sites (Bombelli 1976) (Fig. 13.10). In osteoarthritis secondary to acetabular dysplasia the femoral head may displace laterally (Fig. 13.11) and subsequently sublux (Severin 1941), although a medial migration, particularly in the rheumatoid arthritis patient, may also occur and is termed 'protrusio acetabuli' (Figs. 13.12 & 13.13).

Osteoarthritis secondary to inflammatory conditions of the hip in childhood will be characterized by other radiographic features. Damage to the growth plate will produce an associated shortening of the femoral neck, often

Table 13.1. Causes of secondary osteoarthritis of the hip joint in the adult.

Biochemical
  Congenital dysplasia
  Perthes' disease
  Slipped upper femoral epiphysis
  Iatrogenic 'pressure lesion'

Inflammatory
  Rheumatoid arthritis
  Juvenile chronic arthritis
  Ankylosing spondylitis
  Psoriasis
  Other spondyloarthropathies

Traumatic
  Fracture–dislocations
  Dislocations (with avascular necrosis)
  Fractures (with avascular necrosis)

Infective
  Pyogenic arthritis
  Tuberculous arthritis
  Rare viral and fungal arthritides

Haematological
  Haemophilia
  Haemochromatosis
  Sickle cell anaemia

Avascular (necrosis)
  Traumatic ischaemia
  Caisson disease
  Chronic alcoholism
  Steroid therapy
  Gout
  Collagen diseases
  Haemostatic disorders
  Haemoglobinopathies

Metabolic
  Paget's disease
  Ochronosis
  Synovial chondromatosis
  Pseudogout

Neuropathic
  Syphilis
  Other causes of Charcot joint

Skeletal
  Epiphyseal dysplasias
  Spondyloepiphyseal dysplasia
  Metaphyseal dysplasias
  Various forms of dwarfism
  Mucopolysaccharidoses
  Altered bone development and texture

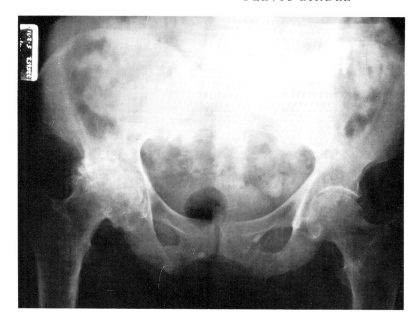

Fig. 13.8. Typical radiographic features of osteoarthritis of the hip.

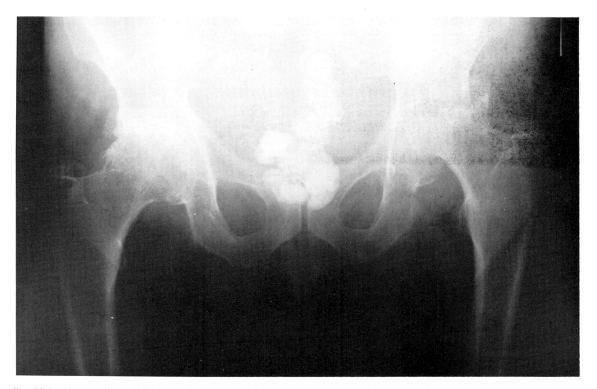

Fig. 13.9. Osteoarthritis of the hip with an associated avascular necrosis of the femoral head.

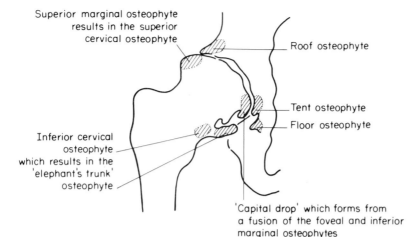

Superior marginal osteophyte
results in the superior
cervical osteophyte

Roof osteophyte

Tent osteophyte
Floor osteophyte

Inferior cervical
osteophyte
which results in the
'elephant's trunk'
osteophyte

'Capital drop' which forms from
a fusion of the foveal and inferior
marginal osteophytes

Fig. 13.10. Patterns of osteophyte formation around the hip (after Bombelli 1976). Osteophytes form around the hip joints as a result of plastic deformation and bone metaplasia of the capsule and synovium.

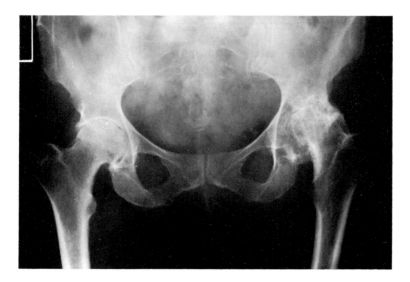

Fig. 13.11. Osteoarthritis of the hip with an associated lateral subluxation of the femoral head.

interpreted as a varus deformity although a partial lateral physeal arrest is fairly common and induces a valgus alignment. The greater trochanter will appear to have 'overgrown' and the abductor mechanism is thereby compromised. Similarly, injury to the capital epiphysis, whether from an inflammatory process or from pressure, will flatten and deform the femoral head, resulting in coxa magna or coxa plana. Previous episodes of growth cessation may be evident in the form of 'Harris' lines, and in the haemophiliac patient there may be enlargement

of the ossified portions of the epiphysis, periarticular soft-tissue thickening, and calcification and loss of bone formation, exemplified by generalized osteoporosis and cysts.

Congenital dysplasia (Sharp 1961) or subluxation of the hip accounts for approximately 25% of all adult cases of osteoarthritis of that joint, and various means of classifying the extent of the pre-existing deformity have been proposed. The Severin grading (Severin 1941) is widely accepted (Fig. 13.14), although its correlation with later arthritis or, indeed, symptoms, is not

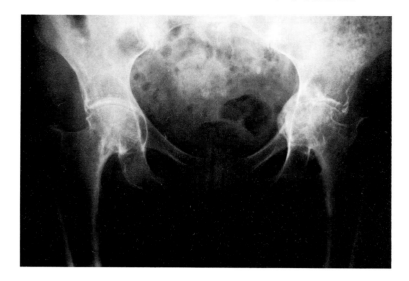

Fig. 13.12. Osteoarthritis of the hip with an associated protrusio acetabuli. Protrusio acetabuli describes both a medial and an upward movement of the femoral head, which should be contained within the triangle outlined below.

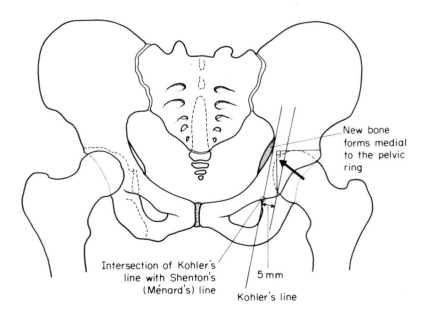

Intersection of Kohler's line with Shenton's (Ménard's) line

5 mm

Kohler's line

New bone forms medial to the pelvic ring

Fig. 13.13. A diagram to show Kohler's line and the medial and upward movement of the femoral head in protrusio acetabuli.

close (Cooperman *et al.* 1983). The extent of femoral head subluxation has also been quantified as follows (Crowe *et al.* 1979):

Class I   Less than 50% subluxation.
Class II   50–75% subluxation.
Class III Greater than 75% subluxation.
Class IV   Total dislocation.

Once again, it is stressed that these radiographic indices may bear little relationship to the clinical problem encountered; but the need to compare results of surgery using some identifiable criteria makes the use of these measurements acceptable.

The presence of calcification or heterotopic bone around the hip joint is also of interest to

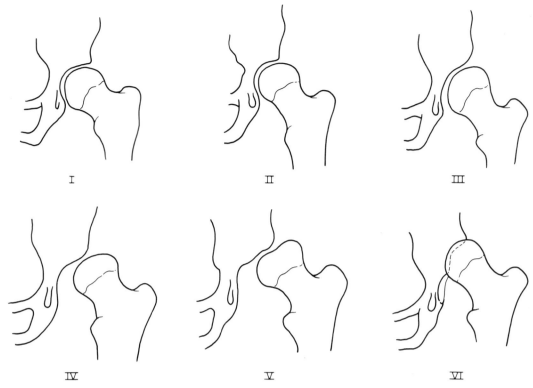

Fig. 13.14. Severin's grading of the dysplastic and subluxated hip joint.
Grade I: CE (centre-edge) angle more than 25° (or more than 15° in the child).
Grade II: CE angle more than 25° but the femoral head is slightly uncovered and deformed.
Grade III: Hip dysplasia without subluxation (CE angle less than 20° but no significant break in Shenton's line).
Grade IV: Subluxation with associated valgus and/or anteversion of the femoral neck and femoral head deformity.
Grade V: Deformed femoral head articulating with the upper portion of a deformed acetabulum.
Grade VI: Dislocation of the femoral head which articulates with a false acetabulum.

the clinician, and may have some bearing upon the treatment elected, and upon the outcome of surgery. There may, for instance, be a familial tendency to form heterotopic bone, and if one total hip replacement has been compromised in its function by the presence of periarticular bone, then it is likely that the opposite hip, if operated upon, will suffer a similar fate. Low-dose irradiation of such hips post-operatively may be justifiable, since this treatment has a significantly inhibitory effect upon this unwanted process. Brooker et al. (1973) classified the extent of heterotopic bone formation abritrarily into four groups:

Group I   Small bone islands.

Group II   Spurs of bone more than 1 cm apart.
Group III   Spurs of bone less than 1 cm apart.
Group IV   Ankylosis.

This grading is of some value to the orthopaedic surgeon when following the radiographic appearances of a total hip replacement compromised in this fashion.

Soft-tissue calcification in the region of the hip should be differentiated into periarticular and intra-articular processes. The former includes heterotopic bone and myositis ossificans progressiva, and is regularly seen in dermatomyositis, other connective tissue disorders, hypercalcaemia, and following trauma or infection. Intra-articular calcification, resembling a thin, curvilinear arc of density in parallel with the head of the femur, characterizes gout, pseudogout and hyperparathyroidism, and is sometimes apparent in the substance of degenerating articular cartilage. This 'chondrocalcinosis' differs from the other form of intra-articular calcification where separate loose bodies are seen, occurring as a result of synovial chondromatosis or after the fracturing of osteophytes.

The surgical treatment of painful dysplasia or osteoarthritis of the hip in an adult does not revolve entirely upon which total hip replacement prosthesis to insert, although it is true that an artificial joint offers the greatest chance of producing a pain-free hip. In adolescents and young adults the long-term complications, dealt with later in this chapter, are simply too great following a total replacement, and hence a variety of ingenious, and usually mechanically sound, osteotomies have been devised. Proximal femoral osteotomies may include the head and neck into more varus or valgus, in an attempt to improve femoral head cover, and perhaps congruity, within the acetabulum. Rotation of the proximal femoral segment can be combined with this initial realignment, particularly internal rotation if there is a residual and significant anteversion. Abduction, adduction and internal rotation positions of the femoral head should be scrutinized preoperatively, before embarking on this major surgery, and the additional information provided by arthrography and CAT scanning is of value in the more complex case. When there is angulation of the femoral head (Figs. 13.15–13.17) or a segmental collapse consequent upon avascular necrosis (Fig. 13.18), alterations in the weight-bearing configuration of the head may delay the progress of the osteoarthritis.

Previously, arthrodesis was commonly employed for patients with advanced degenerative conditions of the hip, but now the operation is less popular, at least in the developed countries. Nevertheless, in the younger adult with no symptoms from the lumbar spine and the other major lower limb joints, arthrodesis is an effective solution, and allows the option of a 'con-

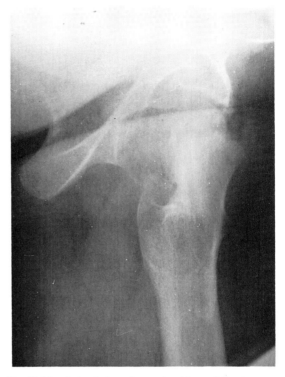

Fig. 13.15. Lateral view of a proximal femur following posteromedial slipping of the capital epiphysis with resultant 90° (severe) displacement of the femoral head.

version' to a total arthroplasty in later life (Figs. 13.19 & 13.20).

The Chiari pelvic osteotomy is reasonably effective as a salvage procedure in young adults with painful dysplasia of the hip (Fig. 13.21), and various other pelvic and acetabular redirectional osteotomies are appropriate if osteoarthritis is not evident radiographically.

Radiographic appearances of total hip replacement
Surgical replacement of the hip joint is the most common arthroplasty procedure in orthopaedic surgery, and probably the most successful. A few years ago it was hoped that surface replacement of the hip (Wagner 1978) would outmode conventional arthroplasty which requires a greater removal of proximal femoral bone stock. However, the early promise of surface replacement has not been sustained, and, paradoxi-

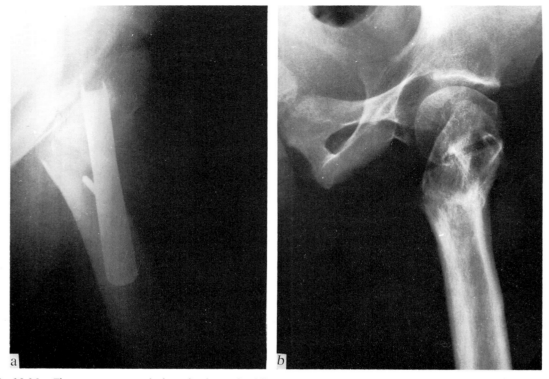

Fig. 13.16. The appearances on the lateral radiographs following a corrective intertrochanteric osteotomy and subsequent removal of the plate. Both the hyperextension and external rotation deformities were reversed.

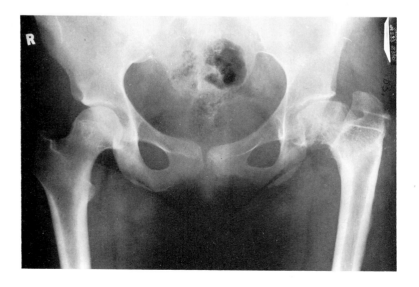

Fig. 13.17. The comparable anteroposterior radiographic projection following surgery. The varus deformity of the femur is more apparent than real, and congruity of the hip joint is good. Note that the left proximal epiphyseal plate has closed, whereas on the right side it has yet to obliterate.

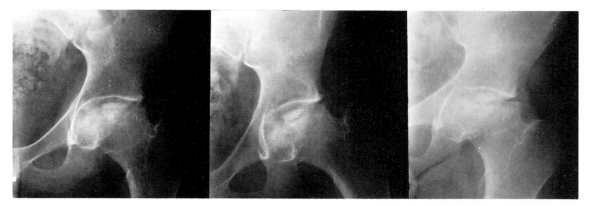

Fig. 13.18. Neutral, abduction, and adduction views of the anteroposterior projection of this hip show that congruency is improved by adduction. This symptomatic and severe avascular necrosis of the femoral head in a young adult was treated by an abduction (valgizing) proximal femoral osteotomy.

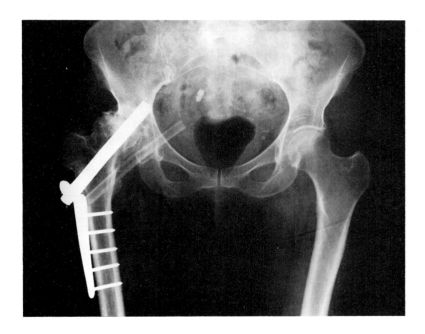

Fig. 13.19. Arthrodesis of the right hip using an ischiofemoral fibular strut graft (Brittain's method).

cally, more acetabular bone removal is required by this procedure. Problems associated with ischaemia of the residual head and neck of the femur, with resultant fracture of the femoral neck, and a loosening of the acetabular component after relatively short periods of time, have meant that conventional arthroplasty is still the preferred operation in most orthopaedic units.

The enormous demand for total hip replacement in countries that can afford the financial outlay of such surgical treatment has led to a commensurate increase in complications from the operation. Undoubtedly the major concern is with infection of the prosthesis, generally in the early stages after surgery, and with component loosening after some years. Unlike the less frequent complications of dislocation and

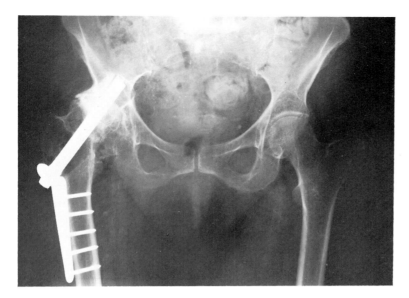

Fig. 13.20. The attempted arthrodesis failed and not only is loosening evident from the 'windscreen wiper' sign/ but the fibular graft has been resorbed. A total hip replacement relieved the patient's pain.

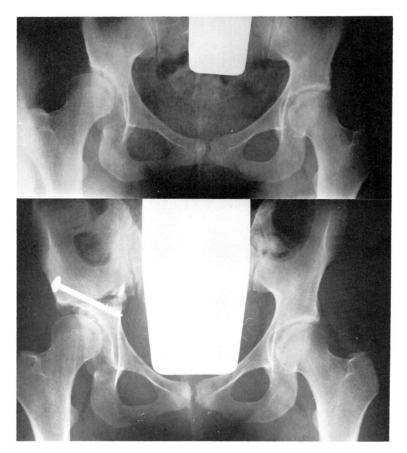

Fig. 13.21. Femoral head cover in this dysplastic right hip was increased by a Chiari pelvic osteotomy. Pain is relieved in the majority of these cases by this procedure, and a later hip arthroplasty is made easier owing to the improved pelvic bone stock.

fractures of the femoral shaft, infection and loosening may be quite difficult to establish clinically, and the pain felt by the patient is generally non-specific. The radiographic aspects of loosening have been described in great detail in the orthopaedic literature, and therefore most attention will be directed towards this, possibly inevitable, complication. However, Table 13.2 lists the other complications of total hip replacement, and a short account of the problem of infection is appropriate.

The control of infection depends upon sterile operating conditions and careful surgical technique. Standardized regimes of preoperative patient preparation, skin cleansing and draping, and wound care are widely practised. The insertion of a foreign body, however sterile, poses further problems in effective prevention of infection, particularly as methylmethacrylate

Table 13 2. Complications of total hip replacement.

Early
  Local
    Dislocation
    Wound haematoma
    Wound infection
    Arteriovenous fistula
    Bladder fistula
    Sciatic nerve damage
    Fracture of femoral shaft (if penetrated by the reamer or femoral stem)
    Avulsion of greater trochanter (either if fractured or after inadequate wiring technique following trochanteric osteotomy)

  General
    Chest infection
    Urinary tract infection
    Deep venous thrombosis
    Pulmonary embolism
    Other medical complications in the aged

Late
    Infection (often low-grade)
    Dislocation
    Loosening
    Heterotopic bone
    Pain over the trochanteric wires (bursitis)
    Fractured femoral component
    Fracture of femoral shaft
    Stress fracture of pelvis
    Calcar resorption
    Acetabular component wear or deformation

cement is also required. Thus, further precautions are recommended by many of the pioneers of this surgery, particularly the use of laminar air flow in operating theatres and the separation of surgical personnel from the wound by means of special tents. Prophylactic antibiotics are also freely advised, whether in the cement or blood-borne following parenteral injection. These antibiotics should be capable of penetrating bone effectively, and should be active against *Staphylococcus aureus* and *albus*, streptococcus and certain of the Gram-negative organisms. Host immunity, which may be diminished in the old or in those with debilitating conditions such as carcinomatosis, is also being studied more extensively, so that the immunodeficient patient may be recognized more precisely in future, and effective therapy directed towards making good any abnormalities. Hence, early and late infection, which currently occurs at a rate of 2–3%, should eventually be much reduced. An increasing use of uncemented prostheses should also lower this rate.

Loosening of the femoral and acetabular components of a hip arthroplasty occurs either at the bone–cement interface, which is more common, or between the implant and the cement mantle (Figs. 13.22 & 13.23). Stauffer (1982) has reviewed both forms of loosening and has recently confirmed that femoral loosening is greater during the first 5–10 years after surgery than acetabular loosening (Fig. 13.24). However, acetabular loosening continues inexorably, whereas the femoral rate of loosening tends to plateau, so that the rates may become equal in the longer term. Permeation of the trabecular surface of bone by the cement should be as complete as possible, preferably over a zone of several millimetres. This is achieved by careful surgical clearance of the articular cartilage and some of the subchondral bone of the acetabulum, by the insertion of keying holes, and by a thorough cleansing of the raw bone surface, using water under pressure to clear debris from the crevices. Cement in fairly liquid form, and uncontaminated by blood, is inserted under

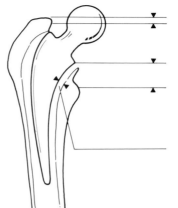

Sinking is measured by the increase in
the distance between the tip of the
greater trochanter and the centre of
the femoral head or the inferior margin
of the collar (or neck) and
the lesser trochanter.

Tilt (horizontal migration) is measured
from the medial margin of the proximal
femoral stem and the endosteal surface
of the proximal femoral shaft.

Fig. 13.22. Radiographic
measurements of femoral stem
loosening (from Sutherland *et al.*
1972).

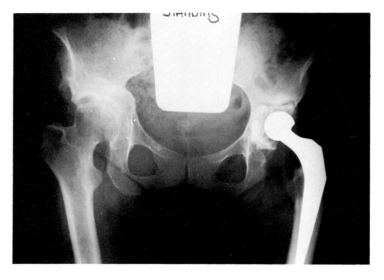

Fig. 13.23. Loosening of the hip
prosthesis is evident, with obvious
displacement of the acetabular
component.

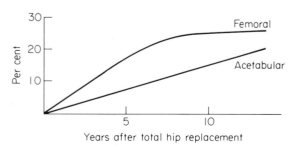

Fig. 13.24. Graph showing the rates of loosening of the
femoral and acetabular components (after Stauffer 1982
and Sutherland *et al.* 1972).

pressure. Various special introducers are available to achieve this in the acetabulum, and for the femoral component a cement, bone or plastic plug is inserted in the femoral shaft approximately 2 cm below the tip of the prosthesis. Cement is pressurized in the femur using a hand-powered gun.

Femoral loosening appears to be more common if the prosthetic stem does not fill the marrow cavity as fully as possible, if a varus position of the component is accepted, and in the younger, heavier and male patient, particularly if the replacement is unilateral. Hence, loosening is an expression of both poor technique and the activity of the subject. If osteoporosis is marked, and this can be quantified by the Singh indices (Singh *et al.* 1970), then loosening of both the acetabular and femoral components is more likely. Poor bone stock around the acetabulum will also lead to problems with the cup anchorage, and this is seen in cases with acetabular dysplasia, protrusio acetabuli and metabolic bone disease or tumour deposits.

Migration of the prosthesis may be difficult to detect, and in these instances an arthrogram may be helpful, in that it sometimes shows tracking of radio-opaque medium between the implant and the bone. However, in many cases the loosening is more subtle, and may be secondary to a low-grade infection. In these patients bone scanning with both technetium and gallium may help to differentiate the pathological processes, as should the different phases of the scan. Routine screening for infection is also recommended, but the erythrocyte sedimentation rate is often indeterminate and the specific tests for infection in joint aspirates or the blood are regularly negative. Once loosening has become more gross, lucent lines appear around the cement mantle, which is often cracked, and between the prosthesis and the cement. The appearance, or the extension of this lucent line (Delee & Charnley 1976), which should be one or more millimetres thick, can be assessed reasonably accurately on a radiograph. However, comparison from one film to another is bedevilled by the usual problem of projection and exposure. As the lucencies increase in size the component begins to move, tilting or sinking, and subsequently shifting position completely. Such movement wears away the surrounding bone rapidly, and is invariably painful.

Pain may be experienced in a hip arthroplasty where there is no evidence of loosening, heterotopic bone or other radiographic abnormality. In some cases the symptoms may be caused by immune reactions to the wear products of the prosthesis, by the toxicity of the unpolymerized cement monomer or barium sulphate or as a result of a low-grade inflammation at the cement–bone interface secondary to micromovement. These processes are hard to prove, and in many instances no convincing reason for the pain is forthcoming.

Technical difficulties arise when hip replacement is carried out in patients with a dysplastic acetabulum or protrusio acetabuli. When there is insufficient bone stock for the acetabular component to sit within the lateral wall of the pelvis, the depth of the acetabulum may be increased either by a controlled medial fracture of its inner wall or by the medial displacement pelvic osteotomy of Chiari. Alternatively, the femoral head may be used as a superior buttress, thus increasing the capacity of the acetabular dome. Narrow stem femoral components are required for the anteverted and slim proximal femoral shaft, and the femoral head can only be brought down to the level of the acetabulum after an extensive soft-tissue release.

When significant protrusio acetabuli is encountered, the deficient medial acetabular wall should be reinforced with cancellous bone graft. A convenient source of such bone is the excised femoral head. Further buttressing with wire mesh may be prudent, but cement alone, as a means of supporting the acetabular component, is not recommended. The whole mass of cement and the contained cup may in time prolapse medially as the stresses of weight-bearing continue. To guard against this eventuality further special circumferential flanges or rings have been devised; these are incorporated around the acetabular component and spread the load from the femoral head over the lateral pelvic wall.

Revisional surgery of symptomatically loose or infected hip arthroplasties is now regularly practised. Instruments have been designed to remove completely cement from the femoral canal, and every effort must be made to clean out the acetabular and femoral bone. Obviously the cortical bone becomes weaker with the extensive clearance necessary, and fracture or further loosening is an extremely worrying complication of this difficult endeavour.

MISCELLANEOUS CONDITIONS

Coccydynia is an ill-understood condition which may eventually be referred to the orthopaedic surgeon with the request that excision of the apparently offending bone be considered. The pain may not be relieved by this radical approach, although other remedies are even less effective. The radiographic characteristics of the coccyx may be of some predictive value (Postacchini & Massobrio 1983):

Type I   Slight forward curve.
Type II   Marked forward curve, pointing anteriorly at the tip.
Type III Sharp forward angulation (of approximately 90°).
Type IV   Subluxation at the sacrococcygeal or intercoccygeal joints.

According to the authors of this classification, symptoms are more likely with the types II to IV coccyx.

Increased density of the pelvic bones may be seen particularly on contiguous sides of a joint. Thus osteitis pubis and osteitis condensans ilii are recognized radiographic diagnoses, although the clinical cause of the altered bone texture is not always obvious. Neoplasia and infection should be excluded, and the use of radionuclide scanning and CAT scanning is advised. Ankylosing spondylitis should always be considered, and indeed is the most common cause of sacroiliac sclerosis in the younger patient.

The appearance of the various apophyses of the pelvis has already been mentioned in the section dealing with trauma. The iliac apophysis is of value in assessing the skeletal maturity of the patient. This finds particular use in assessing whether a scoliotic curve will progress, since the increase in a scoliosis is dependent upon the growth of the skeleton. 'Risser's sign' describes the extent to which the iliac apophyses have appeared, starting anterolaterally and growing backwards towards the posterior iliac spines. Completion of this excursion marks the end of growth, and with it the likelihood

that a spinal curve will progress significantly.

Finally, it should be remembered that the texture of the pelvic bones will mirror the effects of metabolic bone disease. Osteoporosis, osteomalacia (with the possibility of inferior pubic ramus infractions), Paget's disease and less common conditions such as hyperparathyroidism alter the appearance of the pelvis, as will the infiltrative disorders. Skeletal dysplasias produced characteristic alterations (Wynne-Davis & Fairbank 1976) and the superimposition of soft tissue-shadows and calcification may add puzzling abnormalities which may confuse the inexperienced clinician.

References

ARNOLDI C.C. & REIMAN I. (1979) The pathomechanism of human coxarthrosis. *Acta orthop. scand.* Suppl. **181**.

BOMBELLI R. (1976) *Osteoarthritis of the Hip.* Berlin: Springer-Verlag.

BROOKER A.F., BOWERMAN J.W., ROBINSON R.A. & RILEY L.H. (1973) Ectopic ossification following total hip replacement. Incidence and a method of classification. *J. Bone Jt Surg.* **55A**, 1629–32.

COOPERMAN D.R., WALLENSTEN R. & STULBERG S.D. (1983) Acetabular dysplasia in the adult. *Clin. Orthop.* **175**, 79–85.

CROWE J.F., MANI V.J. & RANAWAT C.S. (1979) Total hip replacement in congenital dislocation and dysplasia of the hip. *J. Bone Jt Surg.* **61A**, 15–23.

DELEE J.C. & CHARNLEY J. (1976) Radiological demarcation of cemented sockets in total hip replacement. *Clin. Orthop.* **121** 20–32.

GARDEN J. (1964) Fractures of the neck of the femur. *J. Bone Jt Surg.* **46B**, 355.

HARRINGTON K.D. (1972) The use of methylmethacrylate as an adjunct in the internal fixation of malignant neoplastic fractures. *J. Bone Jt Surg.* **54A**, 1665–76.

HARRIS W.H. (1977) Idiopathic osteoarthritis of the hip — a twentieth century myth? *J. Bone Jt Surg.* **59B**, 121.

JUDET R., JUDET J. & LETOURNEL E. (1964) Fractures of the acetabulum; classification and surgical approaches for open reduction. *J. Bone Jt Surg.* **46A**, 1615–46.

MARCUS N.D., ENNEKING W.F. & MASSAM R.A. (1973) The silent hip in idiopathic aseptic necrosis. Treatment by bone grafting. *J. Bone Jt Surg.* **55A**, 1351–66.

MOORE A.T. (1952) Metal hip joint—a new self-locking vitallium prosthesis. *Sth. med. J.* **45**, 1015–18.

PAUWELS F. (1935) *Der Schenkenhalsbruch. Ein Mechanisches Problem.* Stuttgart: F. Enke.

PAVLOV H., NELSON T.L., WARREN R.F., TORG J.S. & BURNSTEIN A.H. (1982) Stress fractures of the pubic ramus. *J. Bone Jt Surg.* **64A**, 1020–5.

POSTACCHINI F. & MASSOBRIO M. (1983) Idiopathic coccydynia (analysis of fifty-one operative cases and a radiographic study of the normal coccyx). *J. Bone Jt Surg.* **65A**, 1116–24.

SEVERIN E. (1941) Contribution to the knowledge of congenital dislocation of the hip joint. Late results of closed reduction and arthrographic studies of recent cases. *Acta chir. scand.* Suppl. **63**.

SHARPE I.K. (1961) Acetabular dysplasia: the acetabular angle. *J. Bone Jt Surg.* **43B**, 268–77.

SINGH M., NAGRATH A.R. & MANI P.S. (1970) Changes in trabecular pattern of the upper end of the femur as an index of osteoporosis. *J. Bone Jt Surg.* **52A**, 457–67.

SOLOMON L. (1976) Patterns of osteoarthritis of the hip. *J. Bone Jt Surg.* **58B**, 176–83.

STAUFFER R.N. (1982) Ten-year follow-up study of total hip replacement. *J. Bone Jt Surg.* **64A**, 983.

SUTHERLAND C.J., WILDE A.H., BORDEN L.S. & MARKS K.E. (1972) A ten-year follow-up of one hundred consecutive Nuller curved-stem total hip replacement arthroplasties. *J. Bone Jt Surg.* **64A**, 970–82.

THOMPSON F.R. (1954) Two and a half years' experience with a vitallium intramedullary hip prosthesis. *J. Bone Jt. Surg.* **36A**, 489–500.

TILE M. (1980) Pelvic fractures: operative versus nonoperative treatment. *Orthop. Clin. N. Amer.* **II**, 423–64.

WAGNER H. (1978) Surface replacement arthroplasty of the hip. *Clin. Orthop. rel. Res.* **134**, 102–30.

WALDENSTRÖM J. (1924) Fractures recentes du col femoral – traitement operative en orthopedique. *J. Chir.* **24**, 129–36.

WROBLEWSKI B.M. & CHARNLEY J. (1982) Radiographic morphology of the osteoarthritic hip. *J. Bone Jt Surg.* **64B**, 568–9.

WYNNE-DAVIES R. & FAIRBANK T.J. (1976) *Fairbank's Atlas of General Affections of the Skeleton.* Edinburgh: Churchill Livingstone.

Chapter 14
Knee Joint

D. H. R. JENKINS

The knee joint

ANATOMY AND FUNCTION

There is a tendency, in the author's view, for clinicians to come to rely too heavily on investigative procedures, rather than to rely on clinical examination of a particular problem. Notwithstanding that, the multiplicity of radiological techniques now available makes at least some of them absolutely essential in orthopaedic problems about the knee joint. Since this chapter is on practical clinical problems, unusual or expensive investigations shall not be dwelt on where there are thoroughly reasonable, less expensive alternatives, but which of the investigations should be the most useful in any particular practical problems will be outlined. Thus, while there is considerable interest in nuclear magnetic reasonance and computed tomography, neither of these techniques will be discussed in depth because, by and large, the same information can be gleaned from simpler investigative methods.

Soft-tissue problems

LIGAMENTS

The ligamentous stuctures of the knee are the anterior and posterior cruciate ligaments and the medial and lateral collateral ligaments. In addition, the capsular structure of the knee will normally be damaged to some extent if there is a disruption of any one of these structures. Certain syndromes have now become classical. The O'Donoghue triad (O'Donoghue 1950) of

a tear of the anterior cruciate ligament, the medial collateral ligament and medial meniscus is so well known that it behoves every examiner when faced with a suggested medial meniscal tear to examine for the integrity of the other two structures. In acute injuries gross disruption of any ligament will be obvious on clinical examination, but it is in the minor disruptions that radiographic examination has great value. Clearly, plain X-rays of the knee in such injuries will only be of value in demonstrating avulsions of the attachments of the ligaments, but a more reliable index of ligamentous instability is obtained by stress views. For medial and lateral collateral ligament disruptions, the knee should be stressed medially and laterally, while screening takes place in an AP direction. It is preferable to do this under general anaesthetic in acute injuries. Chronically unstable knees can be examined without anaesthetic, but frequently, except in cases of marginal instability, there is very little to be gained from this examination.

The anterior cruciate ligament is a double structure. When the anterior part is disrupted, the tibia can be lifted forwards away from the distal femur within a few degrees flexion (Latchman's sign). Disruption of the posterior part of the anterior cruciate is detected by the anterior drawer sign with the knee in $90°$ flexion. Pure disruption of the anterior cruciate leads to anterolateral instability as determined by the anterolateral jerk test (Galway *et al.* 1972). There is no single reliable radiological technique which will always accurately determine the presence or absence of a disruption of the anterior cruciate ligament, nor is there a single technique which will demonstrate the pivot shift test. One has to rely on clinical examination, with the addition of arthroscopy. Arthrography will certainly demonstrate avulsions of the anterior tibial spine, as will plain X-rays, but it will also demonstrate a total disruption of the anterior cruciate ligament in many cases (*see* Chapter 3).

The posterior cruciate ligament is less commonly injured. This is fortunate, because while there are a multitude of repair procedures which are all reasonably adequate for the anterior cruciate ligament (Ireland & Trichey 1980, Tilbery 1977, Cho 1975, Knoyes & Sonstegard 1973 D'arcy 1978, Jenkins 1978) there is, as yet, no one single procedure which adequately replaces the posterior cruciate. The author has had some experience in replacement of the posterior cruciate in its anatomical position using carbon fibre, and of a series of 14 posterior cruciate replacements over the last five years has been successful in eight, i.e. normal function has returned and has remained in a stable knee in the period six months to four years after implantation. All failures have occurred in the first six months following implantation. Arthrography can occasionally demonstrate the disruption of the posterior cruciate, but usually the most valuable sign is an avulsion of the tibial attachment of the posterior cruciate and this is seen on plain X-rays.

Pellegrini–Steida disease is characterized by calcification of the medial collateral ligaments. It is probably incorrect to regard this as a disease syndrome, since it is now thought to be a radiological sign which appears following trauma and partial avulsion of the femoral insertion of the medial collateral ligament. Occasionally, arthrography will demonstrate contrast medium which has leaked from the knee up on the inside aspect of the medial collateral ligament. More commonly the condition is diagnosed on plain AP views of the knee itself.

In Pellegrini–Steida disease an initial examination is obviously required. One should attempt to establish on clinical grounds whether or not there is true instability and ignore the radiological signs of Pellegrini–Steida disease, relying totally on clinical examination. The X-rays, as in all orthopaedic problems, are an adjunct to, not an essential part of, the investigation. Again, arthrography comes into the category of an adjunct investigation. None would suggest that an operation should be carried out on radiographic findings, but the whole emphasis should be on the clinical appreciation of whether the instability is present or not. Clearly, the radiographic signs of instability should be used as a valuable pointer towards surgery.

CAPSULE

It would in incorrect to make a distinction between capsular injuries and medial and lateral collateral ligament injuries, since stress injuries on either side of the knee will inevitably produce a disruption, partial or otherwise, of the capsule if either one of the two major ligaments is disrupted. Stress views with or without the addition of arthrography are the only useful investigations.

BAKER'S CYSTS

Large Baker's cysts (popliteal cysts) can cause calf pain, but small ones are generally considered to be asymptomatic. One of the problems associated with improved arthrographic techniques is that popliteal cysts are frequently diagnosed when in fact they may have nothing to do with the pain in and around the knee. Symptomatic Baker's cysts will always be clinically readily diagnosable. They may sometimes be seen on soft-tissue films, and will always be outlined arthrographically, particularly if they rupture (Fig. 14.1). Other techniques such as ultrasound scans will, of course, outline such cysts, but this is one condition where the diagnosis is almost exclusively clinical in its nature (Butt & McIntyre 1969, Lapayowker *et al.* 1970). It must be remembered that an absolute contraindication to arthrography, or for that matter any invasive technique involving the knee, is infection.

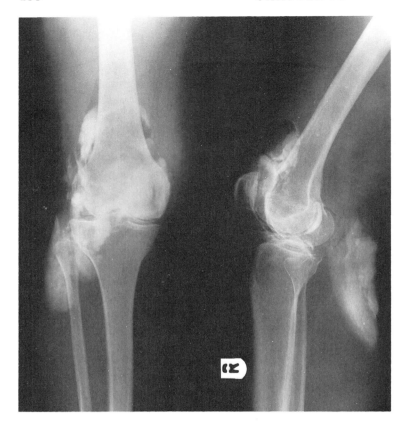

Fig. 14.1. An X-ray of a Baker's cyst.

MENISCAL LESIONS

A major advance in recent years in the management of suspected meniscal lesions has been the development of arthroscopy (O'Connor 1977, Dandy 1981) (Figs. 14.2 & 14.3). Following the initial enthusiasm by surgeons to arthrotomize a painful knee, with subsequent removal of a meniscus, on the assumption that the meniscus was an unimportant appendage, more accurate diagnosis of a suspected meniscal lesion is now possible (Fig. 14.3). Coupled with the development of arthroscopy, as both a diagnostic and a surgical tool, the improvements in arthrography (Freiberger *et al.* 1966) have meant that it is now possible to achieve a diagnosis before a knee is arthrotomized (Fig. 14.4).

In the author's experience in Cardiff, it is pos-

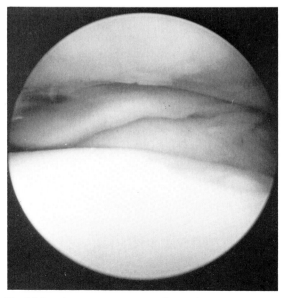

Fig. 14.2. A torn meniscus viewed on arthroscopy.

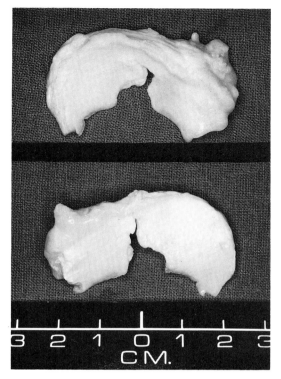

Fig. 14.3. A parrot-beak tear of the medial meniscus.

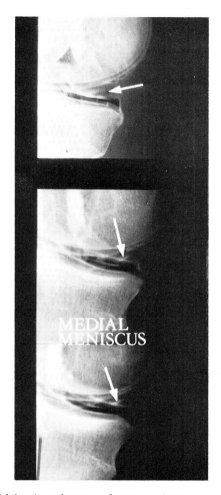

Fig. 14.4. An arthrogram of a torn meniscus.

sible to achieve arthrographic diagnostic accuracy rates approaching 95% for tears of the medial meniscus and about 85% for tears of the lateral meniscus. It has also been the author's experience that arthrography does not produce false-positive results, but can indicate that there is not a tear when in fact a tear is present. This has lead some surgeons to view arthrography as a technique which should be used when there is a considerable doubt about the presence or absence of a lesion within a joint. Where there is little doubt in the surgeon's mind that there is some form of internal derangement of the knee, many will prefer to avoid the mild discomfort and use of expensive radiological time in favour of an arthroscopic diagnosis. The reasonably logical argument in favour of this approach is that if the patient is going to come to surgery anyway there is little point in a

time-consuming exercise which can never be 100% accurate. The author has, however, found arthrographic examinations to be particularly useful in the teenager whose symptoms simulate a meniscal tear and where the actual diagnosis may be the presence of a loose body or an osteochondritic fragment, or the synovial shelf syndrome (Aoki 1973). While arthrography is valuable in the exclusion of meniscal lesions it is actually, in the author's experience, of little use in the diagnosis of problems associated with the medial and lateral synovial folds.

With the exception of infections involving gas-producing organisms, radiography has little place in the diagnosis of soft-tissue infections. Plain X-rays are, of course, a valuable tool when there is a suspicion of infection involving bone, and this is dealt with below.

PATELLAR TENDON INJURIES

Total disruption of the patellar tendon leads to total inability to extend the knee. Plain lateral views of both knees will demonstrate a high-riding patella on the side of injury. Again, arthrography is of value here. The author has found that plain X-rays and clinical evaluation of patellar ligament lesions are of greater value than arthrography. Arthrography will do no more than tend to confirm what the clinical examiner already knows.

In both the acute and chronic situations, the patellar tendon should be repaired. In the acute injury it is essential to try and repair the patellar tendon using the standard techniques of primary tendon suture. So often one finds that patellar tendon injuries arrive late for examination. In those situations, the patella will be seen to be riding high, and clinical examination will tend to demonstrate that a lag sign is present. Once the knee is opened and the patellar tendon exposed, what appears initially to be an intact patellar tendon will, more often than not, be a mass of disorganized scar tissue in which the patellar tendon has healed in an elongated manner. It is the author's view that the patellar tendon should be incised and shortened and the patella brought down to its normal anatomical position. Whether the patellar tendon is repaired using the standard anatomical techniques of carbon fibre will depend entirely on whether the patella can be brought down to its normal position. In the author's view, carbon fibre lends itself well to this situation. The technique is to drill a hole through the distal pole of the patella and through the tibial tubercle.

Lesions involving bone

PATELLA

Variations of the normal need to be considered in all aspects of knee pathology, and nowhere is this more relevant than in the case of the patella. The bipartite patella is frequently, but not invariably, bilateral, and accessory ossicles may be seen. They are occasionally multicentric, and are usually considered to be without clinical significance. Wide comment on this and other variants can be found in *An Atlas of Normal Roentgen Variants that may Simulate Disease* (Keats 1973). By the age of 10 the patella should normally be well formed and radiologically visible. Rarely, the patella may be congenitally absent. Usually, however, the patella is hypoplastic and may be the first indication of the nail–patella syndrome (Fong's syndrome) (Fong 1946, Valdueza 1973). True fractures of the patella can frequently be diagnosed by the presence of a gap between the two fractured halves and the inability of the patient fully to extend the knee. If this condition is anticipated, plain lateral views of both knees are required. The fracture is repaired using cerclage wire and tension banding (Fig. 14.5).

Subluxations and dislocations of the patella are either congenital in origin or post-traumatic. When congenital the dislocation or subluxation is almost always to the lateral side, and is usually associated with hypermobility of the patella (Fig. 14.6). Other precipitating causes include genu valgum and hypoplasia of the lateral femoral condyle (McDougall *et al.* 1968). The axial skyline view of the patella is valuable, particularly if the view is taken firstly with the knee flexed at 30° and then fully flexed. In this way a comparison can be made of the two positions of the patella as it advances forward over the distal femur. There are several operations available for this condition, including lateral release with medial plication and patellar tendon transfer.

Post-traumatic necrosis of the patella is similar to Kienböck's disease of the lunate,

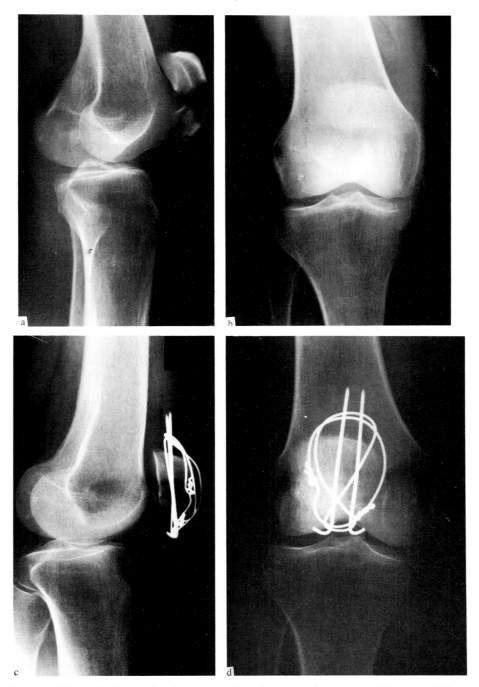

Fig. 14.5. (a) A lateral X-ray. (b) AP view showing a fractured patella. Tension band wiring, (c) lateral and (d) AP views.

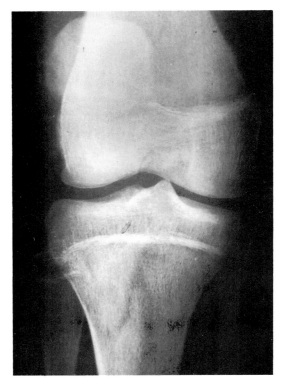

Fig. 14.6. A subluxing patella. It is displaced superiorly and laterally.

Perthes' disease of the hip, Köhler's disease of the navicular and Freiberg's disease of the metatarsal head. The ossification centre becomes fragmented and dense and, like all similar conditions, settles within a period of 1–2 years if rested.

Chondromalacia
Pain in the femoropatellar joint is common, and especially so in teenage girls. Frequently the clinical findings are unimpressive and radiological examination is unrevealing. The characteristic X-ray changes are those of subarticular translucencies in the centre of the patella. It has been suggested (Murray & Jacobsen 1977) that AP tomograms may demonstrate characteristic multiple translucencies in the patella, and that if employed there is likely to be an increase in positive findings. Since the medial facet articular

cartilage of the patella is affected more than the lateral side, skyline views may demonstrate asymmetry of the femoropatellar joint. Radiological examination, however, is often disappointing, and relevant abnormalities are detected in only about 20% of cases (Leading Article 1972). Because of this the surgeon has to rely on a clinical history, frequently assisted by the finding of articular cartilage fibrillation when arthroscopy is performed. On the whole there is a limited role for surgery, which includes shaving the affected area, lateral release and either tangential or coronal osteotomies of the patella.

FEMUR

Injuries
Plain X-rays are essential not only in the acute stage of management of injuries of the distal femur, but also to assess progression of the fracture.

Epiphyseal fractures
It is imperative to be able to make a distinction between epiphyseal fractures with and without separation. Occasionally, epiphyseal separation may take place and spontaneous reductions occur before radiographs are taken. Then the radiological appearance is only of a slightly widened epiphyseal plate. The importance of recognition of such an injury is that growth disturbance may result, and this will only be noticed as progressive photographs are taken over the months and years that follow. As in all cases of injuries in children, both sides should be radiographically examined.

Chronic stress
Blount's disease (congenital tibia vara) (Fig. 14.7) is now thought to be due to chronic stress. The lateral portion of the epiphyseal plate of the tibia is abnormally wide and the lateral portion of the metaphysis is partially resorbed. Stress thickening of the medial tibial cortex de-

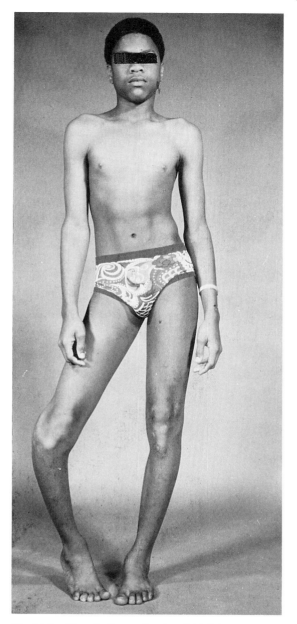

Fig. 14.7. Blount's disease showing right tibia vara. From Hughes & Sweetnam (1981) with permission.

Dislocations

Chronic dislocations of the knee are rarely diagnosed clinically. The major value in the post-reduction films lies in the demonstration of ligamentous damage associated with the dislocation. Stress views, as mentioned above, will demonstrate.

Fractures and internal fixation

While preoperative X-rays are of value in determining the nature of the particular injury, and incidentally in assessing whether or not a fracture should or should not be fixed, and whether such a fracture is indeed fixable, the author has some doubt about the value of immediate post-reduction films. The reason is that if the fracture has been opened and all fragments seen, the X-rays will largely confirm what the clinician already knows. X-rays are, of course, of value in assessing the progression or otherwise of the rate of healing.

Osteochondritis dissicans (Konig's disease)

Areas of subarticular post-traumatic necrosis are only encountered on convex articular surfaces. The medial femoral condyle is the most common site. Frequently there is no frank history of injury, although Aichroth (1971) established support for the theory of traumatic origin. While osteochondritis dissicans is the commonest cause of loose bodies in the knee, it is particularly important to establish whether or not such an osteochondritic fragment is in fact loose. Early radiological diagnosis will lead to early treatment, either by immobilization of the knee in plaster, or by arthrotomy and internal fixation, which will then prevent the potentially loose body from becoming totally loose.

Loose bodies

The characteristic behaviour of a loose body within the knee, with episodic locking and the occasional appearance of a readily palpable lump in the suprapatellar pouch, is well known. The loose bodies are frequently difficult to visualize. Special techniques, including intracondylar tunnel views with or without rotation of

velops. Evidence for the stress concept as a cause of the condition has been provided by Golding (1963) and Bateson (1968). Correction of the varus deformity is by upper tibial osteotomy.

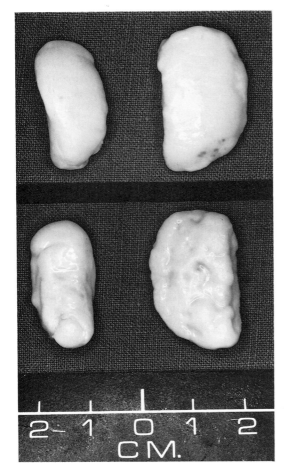

Fig. 14.8. Loose bodies removed from the knee joint.

the knee, usually demonstrate the position of the body. Having demonstrated the loose body, removal via the use of the arthroscope or via arthrotomy (Fig. 14.8) will restore the knee to normal. It is important to be aware of the presence of the fabella behind the knee; this is not a loose body.

Non-accidental injury

In recent years non-accidental injury to children has become recognized as a definite clinical syndrome. Described first by Caffey in 1946 and Silverman in 1953 the syndrome is recognized by ecchymoses, abrasions, broken bones, bruising and skeletal trauma. Usually long bones and epyphyses are involved. The later manifesta-

tions are of cortical hypostosis seen as the subperiosteal haematomas calcify (Leading Article 1973).

Osgood–Schlatter disease

Osgood–Schlatter disease is only seen in the teenage child. It presents as pain over the insertion of the patellar tendon. It is thought to be a chronic avulsion injury of the tibial tuberosity. Radiological appearances are those of an apophyseal plate which is abnormally wide, with irregularity and flattening of the tibial tuberosity (Fig. 14.9). Less penetrative soft-tissue films will demonstrate thickening of the distal end of the patellar tendon near its insertion. The treatment is essentially directed towards the symptoms, using analgesics and rest as required.

Progressive deformities affecting the knee

The value of radiographs in the assessment of the nature of the deformity of the knee joint lies

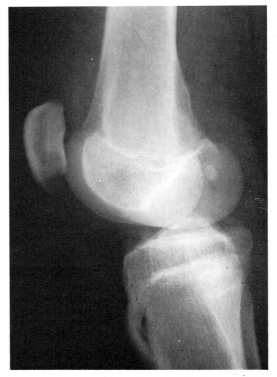

Fig. 14.9. Osgood–Schlatter disease, with elevation of the tibial tubercle.

in the fact that it gives one the facility to measure increasing or decreasing deformities. Nowhere is this more important than in assessment of growth. Premature epiphyseal fusion has already been mentioned. Scanograms are the most accurate measurement of limb length. By a comparison of the lengths of the two lower limbs, a decision can be reached over whether leg equalization should be achieved by lengthening the short limb or by shortening the normal limb. The alternative choice of epiphyseodesis or stapling may be appropriate, depending on the patient's age.

Bone quality

Osteomalacia
Osteomalacia and osteoporosis are conditions that affect the knee as other parts of the body. These conditions are dealt with elsewhere.

Metabolic conditions
Scurvy and gout are generalized conditions affecting the whole of the body and are dealt with elsewhere.

Caisson disease (dysbaric osteoporosis)
A medullary infarct resulting from occlusion of the vascular supply to an articular segment by the formation of nitrogen bubbles within the capilliaries is a characteristic sign of this condition. It is difficult to distinguish the radiological features from those of medullary osteochondromata, unless there is a history of deep-sea diving and of pain commonly known as 'the bends' (McCallum 1966).

Infections of the knee joint

Pyogenic
The usual organism involved in pyogenic osteomyelitis is the staphylococcus but streptococcus, pneumococcus, coliforms and pseudomonas can all result in pyogenic infections. The classical clinical presentation is one of an acute onset of severe pain in the knee in which even the slightest movement causes extreme distress. In the child, pyogenic osteomyelitis and pyogenic arthritis should head the differential diagnosis where there is pain in the joint without associated trauma. Frequently, the radiological signs never appear, because the condition is suspected and treated blindly with broad-spectrum antibiotics. A skeletal lesion normally takes 7–10 days following its pathological inception to become radiologically visible. The first manifestations are obliteration of the usual planes between bone, muscles and fat, with the early formation of periosteal new bone. The Codman triangle follows, but the development of radiologically visible sequestra is a late event. Chronic infection, seen as areas of translucency surrounded by dense reactive sclerosis, is an unusual event in western Europe and North America. The Brodie's abscess, however, must always be considered when there is pain associated with the characteristic lucent area on plain radiographs. Bone scanning is of value but cannot be completely diagnostic of osteomyelitis, since a high uptake of any of the commonly used bone-seeking radionuclides such as technetium diphosphonate is associated just as commonly with neoplasia as with infection (Genant *et al.* 1974).

Tuberculosis
Tuberculosis more commonly affects the spine than any other bony area. Involvement of joints, however, comes a close second. The hip and the knee account for 75% of all tuberculous joint involvement. The cartilaginous epiphyseal plate offers no resistance to the spread of infection, with the result that articular surfaces rapidly become involved. Like all infections, the initial presentation is one of an effusion, followed by the development of abscesses, sinus formation and secondary infection. The radiological characteristic is one of irregular areas of destruction with late marginal sclerosis. Periosteal reaction is minimal. The triad of slow cartilage destruction, periarticular bone atrophy and peripheral erosive defects of the articular surface is characteristic of the condition. Only

in the very late stages of the disease do joints ankylose spontaneously. It is frequently difficult to distinguish, radiologically, tuberculosis from rheumatoid arthritis. However, rheumatoid disease characteristically affects multiple joints, whereas tuberculosis frequently affects one joint only.

Fungal infections

Fungal infections characteristically involve the metaphysis of the long bones and therefore rarely involve the knee joint. When they do the radiological changes are those of other chronic bone infections.

Neuropathic disease of the knee

Neuropathic lesions of the knee follow injuries where the pain normally associated with that injury is not appreciated. There is mechanical disintegration of the joint surfaces. Frequently fractures are unrecognized and progress to a comparatively painless non-union because of the failure to appreciate pain, and infections may develop.

Congenital causes include congenital indifference to pain (asymbolia), and spina bifida. The acquired causes include diabetes, leprosy, neurosyphilis (Charcot's joints) and syringomyelia. Iatrogenic causes include any injuries which occur whilst the patient is taking analgesics or anti-inflammatory agents such as indomethacin or steroids.

The radiological findings are similar in all groups. They are of florid damage to the knee joint. Characteristically the clinical and radiological findings do not match: the destruction seen would normally produce far more discomfort (Johnson 1967).

Arthritis

OSTEOARTHRITIS

Osteoarthritis, whether primary or secondary to injury or other diseases such as gout or infection, always presents with similar radiological features. The main abnormalities are joint space narrowing due to actual collapse and thinning of the cartilage, marginal osteophyte formation, post-traumatic subarticular cyst formation, subchondral reactive sclerosis and the development of osteocartilaginous intra-articular loose bodies (Fig. 14.10). The main value of radiological investigation, from the clinical point of view, is to determine the degree of the condition within the knee, and to demonstrate the degree of deformity presenting. It is, however, frequently disappointing that the radiological and clinical features do not always match. Following failure of conservative management, which includes the use of anti-inflammatory agents, physiotherapy and occasionally intra-articular steroid injections, the only remaining satisfactory treatment is that of surgery. Surgery of the knee in osteoarthritis includes the removal of loose bodies, and occasional synovectomy, the realignment of the joint by femoral or tibial osteotomy, and arthroplasty. It is generally agreed that where there is a gross valgus or varus deformity that preserves one half of the femorotibial joint, then osteotomy will bring adequate pain relief in approximately 70% of patients. Where all compartments of the knee are involved, osteotomy appears to offer little relief of pain. In that situation total knee joint replacement is normally preferred (*see* Arthroplasty, p. 498).

RHEUMATOID ARTHRITIS

Rheumatoid arthritis is common and frequently affects the knee. In Britain 2·4% of the population are affected. Clinically, the condition usually occurs in the fifth, sixth or seventh decades and is more common in females (Figs. 14.11 & 14.12). Following the development of synovial inflammation, there is localized tissue hypertrophy, followed by nodulogranulomatous formation and erosive bone destruction at the synovial attachments. Treatment options are similar to those in osteoarthritis, but greater emphasis should be placed on the medical management of the condition. In children, juvenile rheumatoid arthritis (Still's disease) usually

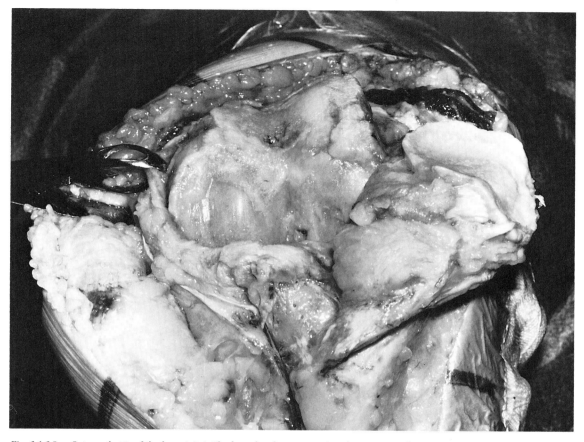

Fig. 14.10. Osteoarthritis of the knee joint. The knee has been opened as there is gross destruction of the femoral condyles.

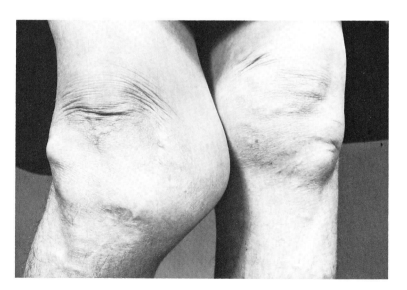

Fig. 14.11. A patient with rheumatoid arthritis of the knee.

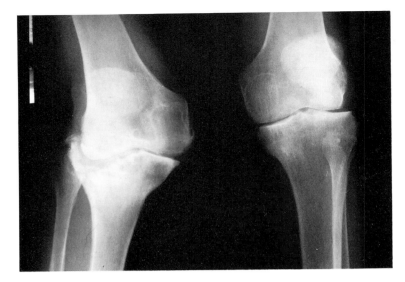

Fig. 14.12. An X-ray of rheumatoid arthritis of the right knee.

causes acceleration of maturation and consequent epiphyseal enlargement. After the rheumatoid activity has subsided, the progression of rheumatoid arthritis continues.

The earliest radiological changes include periarticular soft tissues, periosteal reaction and erosion of synovial attachments with subarticular demineralization as a result of localized hyperaemia. Arthrography may demonstrate the amount of synovial hypertrophy before bone involvement becomes obvious. The smooth contour of the synovium may be replaced by an irregular cobblestone appearance. These tiny nodules may proliferate and separate, producing the so-called 'melon-seed loose bodies'. Once established, rheumatoid arthritis leads to total erosion of the cartilage, producing narrowing and subluxation; para-articular destruction may lead to complete bony ankylosis. The characteristic changes associated with the knee are the development of early erosions, usually evident on the inner aspect of the medial tibial condyle, and then the progression of the changes described above.

PSORIATIC ARTHRITIS

Approximately one-third of patients with psoriasis develop radiological evidence of classical psoriatic arthritis (Avilar *et al.* 1960). Rarely does psoriatic arthritis develop before the dermatological manifestations of the disease.

While the clinical features of psoriatic arthritis are similar to those of rheumatoid arthritis, the radiological appearances are quite different. It is unusual for the knee to be involved first. More usually there is destruction of the interphalangeal joints of the hand and the feet. Abnormally wide joint spaces with sparsly defined articular margins are initially seen, followed by erosion of the articular surfaces. It is worth remembering that Reiter's syndrome has similar radiological appearances. The treatment options open are similar to those in osteo- and rheumatoid arthritis.

ARTHROPLASTY

The main knee arthroplasties in use in the 1980s are: the anametric total knee arthroplasty (Thinnerman *et al.* 1979); the Marmor knee replacement (Marmor 1982); the Oxford knee (Fig. 14.13; O'Connor & Goodfellow 1982); the duo patellar knee and duo condylar knee (Sledge & Ewald 1979); the porous-coated anatomical knee and the Insall–Burstein posterior stabilized knee (Insall *et al.* 1979; Fig. 14.14); the ICLH knee replacement (Freeman *et*

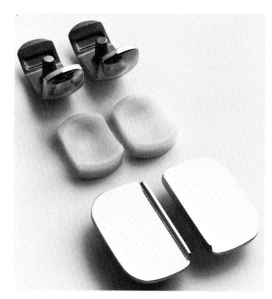

Fig. 14.13. The Oxford total knee replacement.

al. 1973); the variable axis knee prosthesis (Murray & Webster 1981); the spherocentric knee (Kaufer & Matthews 1981); the Sheehan knee (Sheehan 1978); and the Attenborough total replacement (Attenborough 1978; Fig. 14.15). The variations in knee prostheses design are that some are constrained, some semi-constrained and some totally constrained. In addition, some (the porous-coated anatomical knee for example) are designed to be fixed in place without bone cement. The place of radiology in knee arthroplasty lies firstly in the evaluation of the knee and an assessment of its suitability for a particular type of prosthesis. In knees where there is gross ligamentous laxity, for example in rheumatoid arthritis, it is frequently necessary to use a knee arthroplasty which is a semi-constrained or totally constrained hinge, whereas in others where the primary problem is osteoarthritis, with equal ero-

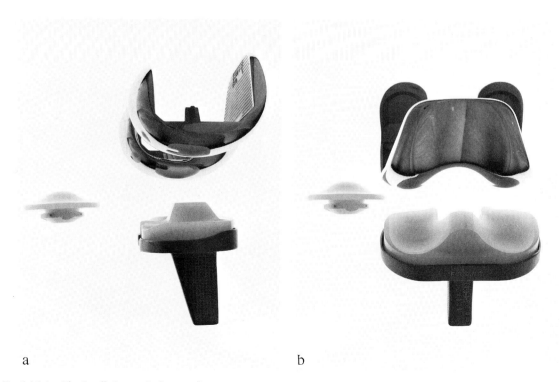

a   b

Fig. 14.14. The Insall–Burnstein knee replacement.

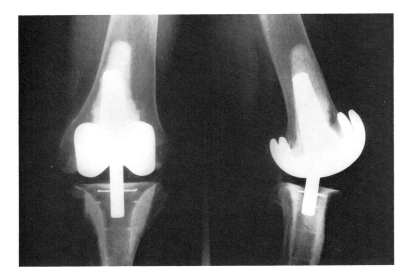

Fig. 14.15. An X-ray of an Attenborough total knee replacement.

sion of both medial and lateral femoral and tibial compartments, a totally unconstrained knee offers a great advantage in that much less bone has to be removed for fixation of the implant. The second purpose of radiological assessment is to check the femorotibial alignment, the position of the prosthetic components and to assess of the cement–bone interface. Lotke and Eckar (1977) have shown that there is a good correlation between the position of the prosthesis and the clinical result. A good placement of the prosthesis predisposes to a good clinical result. The final role of radiology in evaluation of knee arthroplasty is in recognition of stress fractures, the position of cement debris, mechanical failure of the implant, infection, loosening, instability and dislocation.

It is recommended that in the preoperative assessment of a knee, weight-bearing films should be taken (Fig. 14.16). Stress radiographs are of value since these will indicate the spacing which is required in order to take up the slack which may be present in medial or lateral collateral ligaments (Laskin 1979). It has recently been demonstrated that radionuclide bone scanning can also be helpful. When the plain films indicate unicompartmental arthritis, radionuclide scanning may show an abnormality in the other compartments of the knee joint, thus sug-

gesting that a total prosthesis is more appropriate than a unicompartmental prosthesis.

Post-operative radiographs will naturally demonstrate any malalignment. It is perhaps in the evaluation of the radiolucent zone of the cement–bone interface in an assessment of possible loosening that radiographs have their greatest place (Fig. 14.17). It is generally as-

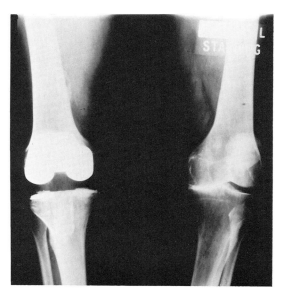

Fig. 14.16. Standing views of the left knee to obtain alignment. The right knee has been replaced.

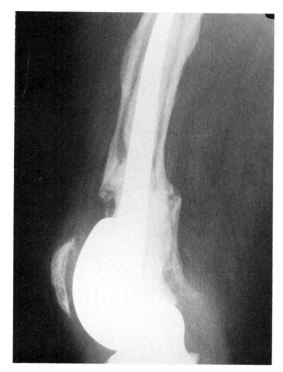

Fig. 14.17. Loosening following a hinged total knee replacement.

sumed that micromotion can cause radiolucent zones of fibrous tissue to develop between the cement and the bone (Ahlberg & Linden 1977). The radiological indices of a loose component are the actual shift in the position of the parts, or the development of the radiolucent zone at the cement–bone interface of 2 mm or more (Convery *et al.* 1980). The presence of a stable (i.e. a non-progressive) radiolucent zone of less than 2 mm, particularly around the tibial component, is thought to have no significance (Reckling *et al.* 1977).

The main role of arthrography is in the demonstration of sinus formation. The contrast material normally used (meglumine diatrizoate or meglumine iothalamate) has the same radiographic density as radio-opaque cement, and therefore it is of little value in the demonstration of the loosening of the cement–bone interface.

For reasons which are not clear, radionuclide scans will often demonstrate a mild to moderate

increase for many years after surgery without any clinical abnormality. This feature is not seen following hip replacements (Schneider *et al.* 1982). Normally technetium-99 phosphate agents are used in radionuclide scanning. When used in conjunction with gallium-67 citrate, valuable information can be acquired about the presence of infection. Because gallium-67 accumulates to a mild degree in normal bone, it is essential to scan first using technetium diphosphonate and to follow this with a gallium scan in order to compare the normal and doubtfully normal sides.

KNEE ARTHRODESIS

While knee arthrodesis was, and probably still is, the treatment of choice for the sequelae of septic arthritis, it is becoming an increasingly essential procedure for failed knee replacements. Waugh (1982) has indicated that the majority of knee replacements will last adequately for between four and six years. This suggests that as knee replacements are carried out in younger and younger individuals the incidence of failure will increase, and therefore arthrodesis will become a more common procedure. The author has found that plain films do not give an adequate assessment of a sound arthrodesis. However, stress films and image intensification can save unnecessarily long periods of immobilization, since they will demonstrate the presence or absence of movement at the site of arthrodesis.

Tumours

It is beyond the scope of this chapter to discuss the tumours which may appear around the knee, and these are dealt with in Chapter 8.

Metastatic disease of the skeleton
It is an unfortunate clinical fact that primary tumours of other parts of the body frequently

present as secondary deposits in the skeleton, and it behoves any clinician dealing with an expanding radiological lesion or a pathological fracture to achieve a tissue diagnosis as rapidly as possible. It is beyond the scope of the chapter to deal with all the various types of metastatic disease, but it is relevant to comment on the necessity for early pathological diagnosis and not to rely on radiological implications of a diagnosis if a regional treatment plan is to be instituted.

Pigmented villonodular synovitis

This is a condition frequently seen in the knee, which is thought to be a synovial tumour. The clinical features are those of a painful chronic swelling of the joint and the knee is more commonly affected than any other area. Radiological features are those of an intra-articular effusion and an increase in opacity of the synovium due to haemosiderin deposits. An interesting radiological feature is the absence of subchondral osteoporosis. Periosteal reaction is unusual and calcification of the synovium is very rare. Pneumarthrography can be valuable in the demonstration of the villonodular synovial hypertrophy. Arthrography can be similarly useful (Scott 1958).

Synovial chondromatosis

This peculiar condition is most commonly seen about the knee in males in the second and third decades. There is low-grade pain and mild swelling in association with locking of the knee. Pathologically cartilaginous masses form and cluster as discrete nodules within the synovium. Calcification occurs, leading to the typical radiological appearance of small stippled calcified nodules. The appearance of multiple small calcified bodies may lead to confusion with a post-traumatic joint degeneration and loose body formation, but the distinction is usually made because of the presence of large numbers of very small calcified nodules in synovial chondromatosis (Jeffreys 1967).

References

AHLBERG A & LINDEN B. (1977) The radiolucent zone in arthroplasty of the knee. *Acta orthop. scand.* **48**, 607.

AICHROTH P. (1971) Osteochondral fractures and their relationship to osteochondritis dissicans of the knee. An experimental study in animals. *J. Bone Jt Surg.* **53B**, 440.

AOKI I. (1973) The ledge lesion in the knee. International Congress Series 291. *Excerpta med. (Amst.)* 462.

ATTENBOROUGH C.G. (1978) The Attenborough total replacement. *J. Bone Jt Surg.* **60B**, 320.

AVILAR R, PUGH D.G., SLOCOMBE C.H. & WINKELMAN R.K. (1960) Psoriatic arthritis. A study. *Radiol.* **75**, 691–701.

BATESON E.M. (1968) The relationship between Blount's disease and bow legs. *Brit. J. Radiology* **41**, 107.

BUTT W.P. & McINTYRE J.L. (1969) Double contrast arthrography of the knee. *Radiology* **92**, 487–99.

CHO K.O. (1975) Reconstruction of the anterior cruciate ligament by semitendonosis tenodesis. *J. Bone Jt Surg.* **57A**, 608–12

CONVERY F.R., MINTEER CONVERY M. & MALCOLM L.L. (1980) The spheriocentric knee. A revaluation and modification. *J. Bone Jt Surg.* **62A**.

DANDY D.J. (1981) *Arthroscopic Surgery of the Knee.* Edinburgh: Churchill Livingstone.

D'ARCY J. (1978) Pes anserinus transposition for chronic anteromedial rotational instability of the knee. *J. Bone Jt Surg.* **60B**, 66–70.

FONG E.E. (1946) Nail–patella syndrome (Fong's syndrome). Iliac horns (symmetrical bilateral central posterior iliac processes). *Radiology* **47**, 517.

FREIBERGER R.H., KILLORAN P.J. & CARDONA G. (1966) Arthrography of the knee by double contrast method. *Amer. J. Roentgenol.* **97**, 736.

FREEMAN N.A.R., SWANSON S.A.V. & TODD R.C. (1973) The ICLH knee replacement designed by Freeman. Total replacement of the knee using Freeman–Swanson knee prosthesis. *Clin. Orthop.* **94**, 153.

GALWAY R.D., DEUPRE A. & MacINTOSH D.L. (1972) Pivot shift: a clinical sign of symptomatic anterior cruciate insufficiency. *J. Bone Jt Surg.* **54B**, 763–4.

GENNANT H.K., BAUTOVICH G.J., SINGH M., LATHROP K.A. & HARPER P.V. (1974) Bone seeking radionuclides. An *in vivo* study of factors affecting skeletal uptake. *Radiology* **113**, 373–82.

GOLDING J.S.R. (1963) Obervations on the aetiology of tibia vara. *J. Bone Jt Surg.* **45B**, 320.

INSALL J., RANOWAT C.S. & SCOTT W.N. (1979) The porous-coated anatomic knee: the Insall–Burstein posterior stabilised knee. The total condylar knee prosthesis. A report of 220 cases. *J. Bone Jt Surg.* **61A**, 172.

IRELAND J. & TRICKEY E.L. (1980) MacIntosh tenodesis for anterolateral instability of the knee. *J. Bone Jt Surg.* **62B**, 340–5.

JEFFREYS T.E. (1967) Synovial chondromatosis. *J. Bone Jt Surg.* **49B**, 530.

JENKINS D.H.R. (1978) The repair of the anterior cruciate ligament with flexible carbon fibre. *J. Bone Jt Surg.* **60B**, 520–2.

JOHNSON J.T.H. (1967) Neuropathic fractures and joint injuries. Pathogenesis and rationale of prevention and treatment. *J. Bone Jt Surg.* **49A**, 1.

KAUFER H. & MATTHEWS L.S. (1981) Spherocentric arthroplasty of the knee. *J. Bone Jt Surg.* **63A**, 545.

KEATS T.E. (1973) *Atlas of Normal Roentgen Variants that may Simulate Disease.* Chicago: Year Book Medical Publishers.

KNOYES F.R. & SONSTEGARD D.A. (1973) Biomechanical function of the pes anserinus at the knee and the effect of its transplantation. *J. Bone Jt Surg.* **55A**, 1225–41.

LAPAYOWKER M.S., CLIFF M.M. & TOURTELLOTT C.D. (1970) Arthrography and the diagnosis of calf pain. *Radiology* **95**, 319–23.

LASKIN R.S. (1979) Total knee replacement. *Orthop. Clin. N. Amer.* **10**, 223.

LEADING ARTICLE (1972) Chondromalacia patellae. *Brit. med. J.* 223.

LEADING ARTICLE (1973) Non-accidental injury in children. *Brit. med. J.* 4656.

LOTKE P.A. & ECKAR M.L. (1977) Influence of positioning of prosthesis in total knee replacement. *J. Bone Jt Surg.* **59A**, 77.

MARMOR L. (1982) The Marmor knee replacement. *Orthop. Clin. N. Amer.* **13**, 55–64.

McCALLUM R.I. (1966) Bone lesions in compressed air workers. *J. Bone Jt Surg.* **48B**, 207.

McDOUGALL A. & BROWN J.D. (1968) Radiological sign of recurrent dislocation of the patella. *J. Bone Jt Surg.* **50B**, 841.

MURRAY R.O. & JACOBSEN H.G. (1977) *The Radiology of Skeletal Disorders,* 2nd Edition, p. 1626. Edinburgh: Churchill Livingstone.

MURRAY D.G. & WEBSTER D.A. (1981) The variable axis knee prosthesis 2-year follow-up study. *J. Bone Jt Surg.* **63A**, 687.

O'CONNOR R.L. (1977) *Arthroscopy.* Philadelphia: J.B. Lippencott & Co.

O'CONNOR J. & GOODFELLOW J. (1982) Fixation of the tibial components of the Oxford knee. *Orthop. Clin. N. Amer.* **13**, 65–8.

O'DONOGHUE D.H. (1950) Surgical treatment of fresh injuries to the major ligaments of the knee. *J. Bone Jt Surg.* **32A**, 721–38.

RECKLING F.W., ASHER M.A. & DYLAN W.L. (1977) A longitudinal study of the radiolucent line of the bone cement interface following total joint replacement procedures. *J. Bone Jt Surg.* **59A**, 355.

SCHNEIDER R., HOOD R.W. & RANAWAT C. (1982) Radiological evaluation of knee arthroplasty. *Orthop. Clin. N. Amer.* **13**, 225.

SCOTT P.M. (1978) Bone lesions in pigmented villonodular synovitis *J. Bone Jt Surg.* **50B**, 306.

SHEEHAN J.M. (1978) Arthroplasty of the knee. *J. Bone Jt Surg.* **60B**, 333.

SLEDGE C.B. & EWALD F.C. (1979) The duo patella knee and duo condylar knee total knee arthroplasty experience at the Robert Breck Brigham Hospital. *Clin. Orthop.* **145**, 78.

THINNERMAN G.A.N., COVENTRY M.B. & RILEY L.H. (1979) Anametric total knee arthroplasty. *Clin. Orthop.* **145**, 85.

TILLBERG B. (1977) The late repair of torn cruciate ligaments using menisci. *J. Bone Jt Surg.* **59B**, 15–19.

WAUGH W. (1983) Knee replacement. In *Recent Advances in Orthopaedics* (ed. McKibbin B.). Edinburgh: Churchill Livingstone.

VALDUEZA A.F. (1973) The nail-patella syndrome. Report of 3 families. *J. Bone Jt Surg.* **55B**, 145.

Chapter 15
The Foot and Ankle

S.P.F. HUGHES & I.M. PROSSOR

The normal anatomy of the foot and ankle

The foot is a complex unit, composed of 26 bones that can bear the full weight of the body on standing and are also capable of transporting the human frame. It is subjected to forces of both stress and strain, can be accommodated into shoes, and permits the act of walking on hard surfaces. In addition, the foot is one of the parts of the musculoskeletal system which is most accessible to direct examination. It contains 14 phalanges, five metatarsal bones and seven tarsal bones. It can be divided into three functional portions. The posterior portion, which lies in direct contact with the tibia, contains the talus, which is part of the ankle joint, and the calcaneum, which is the hind portion of the foot, and is in contact with the ground. The middle portion contains five tarsal bones which form the middle portion of the foot and there is an anterior portion which consists of the metatarsus and phalanges.

Ligaments contribute to the arches of the foot. The medial longitudinal ligament passes from the calcaneum through the talus to the forefoot. The lateral longitudinal arches pass through the calcaneum and the cuboid to the lateral side of the foot. These are not fixed arches but are maintained in position by the action of the small muscles of the foot, along with the tendons and ligaments which are inserted in the foot.

The plantar fascia has a changing modulus of elasticity, so that with increasing load the fascia becomes stiffer and therefore is able to resist deformity.

The ankle joint has two axes of movement:

1 Dorsiflexion and plantarflexion.
2 Rotation (Barnett & Napier 1952).

In plantar flexion, the talus, which is wedge-shaped, and is wider in front than behind, rotates medially about the vertical axis, whilst in dorsiflexion it rotates laterally. The subtalar joint is a hinged joint but has an inclined axis to the ground. A torque conversion is produced by the effect of a hinge joining two segments at an angle. Hence rotation of one segment about its long axis causes a similar rotation on the other segments. The movements of inversion and eversion occur about a vertical axis and are terms applied to the foot when it is off the ground.

Pronation and supination of the forefoot are terms applied to the foot when it is weight-bearing, and these movements occur in the forefoot and in the mid-tarsal joints.

During the action of walking, the lumbricals, the small muscles in the foot, flex the metatarsophalangeal joint, and the interossei draw the metatarsal heads together, preventing the foot from spreading. Both sets of intrinsics in the foot prevent the toes from clawing.

The walking cycle

The walking cycle is the sequence of events occurring during a single step, which on a horizontal surface consists of a 60% stance phase and a 40% swing phase. The gait cycle is the the total period from the time one of the feet strikes the ground till the same foot makes contact with the ground again. At mid-stance the body weight is entirely over the foot. In the stance phase the ankle is dorsiflexed to project the heel forward to begin the initial period of contact with the ground, and this is followed by quick plantar flexion to allow early contact of the whole foot with the ground.

The foot standing

On a firm flat surface, the weight of the body is carried by the heel and forefoot. The mid-foot carries very little load. This load, which is transmitted by the body weight to the forefoot, stresses the longitudinal arch, which is then braced by the plantar ligament., The muscles are not that active.

It is helpful to have an understanding of the walking cycle, because it is useful to be able to compare different gait patterns, Hence in a patient with a contracture of the posterior calf muscles, the initial floor contact is either by the toes or with the flat of the foot. Spasticity causes the heel to be raised off the ground and may reduce the swing phase. Flaccidity, on the other hand, prolongs the swing phase.

Clinical conditions affecting the ankle and foot

The foot and ankle are integral parts of each other and are frequently involved together in orthopaedic problems. The foot and ankle joint are involved in many different clinical conditions, which will be discussed under the following general headings:

1   ORTHOPAEDIC CONDITIONS AFFECTING THE WHOLE FOOT

(a)   *Congenital talipes equinovarus* (*clubfeet*) (*see* Chapter 9)
This is a condition in which there is a fixed structural deformity of both the forefoot and the hindfoot at birth. The hindfoot and the forefoot are in varus. There is also an equinus deformity associated with a supination deformity of the forefoot (Fig. 15.1). Clubfeet are more common

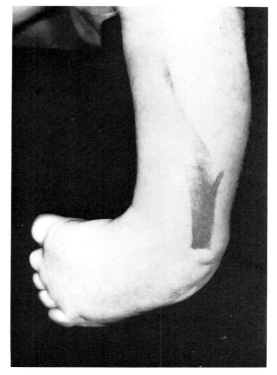

Fig. 15.1.   Congenital talipes equinovarus.

in males than in females and are frequently bilateral. As yet no cause for this condition has been found in the majority; however, several other disorders can present with clubfeet, including spina bifida, cerebral palsy, poliomyelitis and arthrogryposis. X-rays taken on the initial examination include AP and lateral views.

AP view.   The talus and calcaneum may override to form a small angle of less than 15° in the patients less severely affected. But this angle may be lost entirely in severe clubfeet, so that the talus and calcaneum are parallel (Fig. 15.2).

The mid-talar line lies lateral to the metatarsus, and the supination deformity of the forefoot is seen as a convergence of the bases of the metatarsal bones.

Lateral view.   Mid-calcaneal and mid-tarsal lines run parallel, and an obtuse angle is formed between the mid-talar and first metatarsal lines.

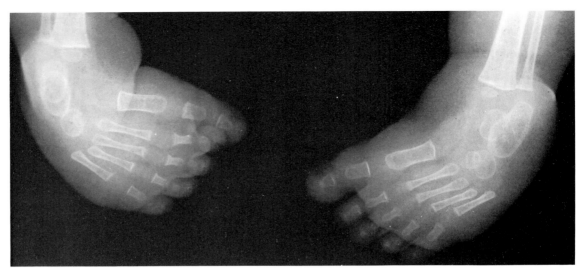

Fig. 15.2. Radiographs of CTEV.

Plantarflexion or equinus of the forefoot is recognized by an angle of greater than 90° being formed by the calcaneum and distal end of the tibia (*see* Chapter 9).

When the child is diagnosed at birth to have a clubfoot, immediate manipulation and strapping is started to correct the deformity. This is done regularly under supervision for a period of six weeks. If the correction is maintained the child can be left in Denis–Browne boots until he is walking. However, if the deformity persists, a posteromedial release is performed, in which all the tight volar tissues are divided and the subtalar and talonavicular joints are released in order to provide a correction. Serial plaster and Denis–Browne boots can then be used to maintain the correction until the child is walking.

In a few patients who do not correct, and in those children who present late, further soft-tissue release is necessary, coupled with tendon transfers, usually the tibialis anterior, in order to pronate the foot. After the age of four years a persistent clubfoot can be treated by a *calcaneocuboid* fusion, which was described by Evans (1961). The principle in this procedure is to correct the supination deformity.

In later life, particularly after skeletal maturity, a triple arthrodesis can be performed, in conjunction with wedge resections, to correct the residual deformity and to maintain a plantigrade foot.

(b)   *Pes planovalgus (flat feet)*
This common condition is due to a variety of different disorders and relates to flattening of the medial longitudinal arch (Fig. 15.3a, b).

Flat feet may be classified into mobile and stiff.

Mobile.   Up to the age of three years it is normal to have flat feet. After three years mobile flat feet may be caused by:

Posture.
Hypermobility syndrome.
Neurological conditions.

Posture.   Excessive femoral antetorsion of the femoral neck may lead to a patient presenting with genu valgum and pes planus. This condition corrects with time in the majority of patients and rarely requires surgical intervention.

Hypermobility.   Patients with significant joint laxity can present with flat feet. However, as in postural flat feet, the foot is mobile and fully correctable and the condition rarely requires surgical intervention.

Neurological. Patients with conditions such as cerebral palsy, poliomyelitis or myopathies can present with painless mobile flat feet.

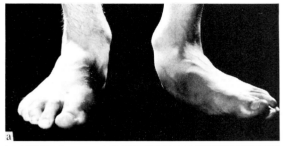

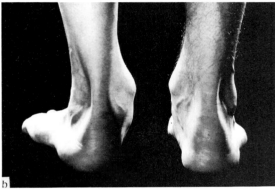

Fig. 15.3. (a) Pes planovalgus. (b) The heel is in valgus.

In a selected group of patients subtalar fusion is helpful to control the valgus drift using a Grice (1952) procedure or a tarsocalcaneal fusion with a screw and cancellous graft (Dennyson & Fulford 1976).

Mobile flat feet can best be demonstrated with weight-bearing views. The sagging of the longitudinal arch is easily recognized on the lateral film (Fig. 15.4), the basic anatomical abnormality being the valgus of the calcaneum. The mid-talar and mid-calcaneal lines produce an angle of greater than 35°. The lower border of the navicular lies below the middle third of the cuboid. The mid-talar line forms an angle to the first metatarsal bone.

Stiff flat feet. These are invariably painful and can be due to:

Infection.
Trauma.
Inflammation.
Congenital.
Osteochondritis.

Infection. Osteomyelitis due to acute or chronic infections can lead to a painful flat foot when it affects the talonavicular joint or the medial longitudinal arch.

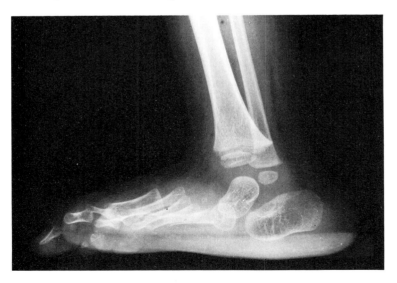

Fig. 15.4. Radiograph of a paralytic flat foot.

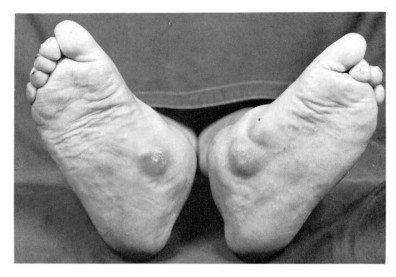

Fig. 15.5. A patient with painful flat feet due to arthritis involving the talonavicular joint.

Trauma. Fractures involving the foot can lead to pain and a stiff flat foot, particularly if the talonavicular joint is involved.

Inflammation. Rheumatoid disease or osteoarthritis can lead to destruction of the talonavicular joint with collapse of the medial longitudinal arch and a painful flat foot. These patients, who may have severe pain, are best treated by a triple fusion to remove any further movement in the subtalar, talonavicular and calcaneocuboid joint and relieve the pain.

Congenital. This group of painful stiff flat feet is caused by (i) tarsal coalition, referred to as peroneal spastic flat feet, and (ii) congenital vertical talus.

(i) *Tarsal coalition* is a relatively uncommon condition which persists in early adolescence and is due to two main types of coalition although there are others.

Calcaneonavicular.
Talocalcaneal.

Calcaneonavicular. This type is best demonstrated on oblique views of the foot (Fig. 15.6) and can be found in both feet. The actual condition may be due to bone or may be fibrous tissue (Fig. 15.7).

Talocalcaneal. This can be shown on oblique views (Fig. 15.8) or by means of tangential views of the heel (Harris views) (Fig. 15.9). The talocalcaneal articulation is obliterated.

Lateral tomography may also be of value in demonstrating the complete union. The coalition indeed may be partial or complete and can be fibrous, cartilaginous or bony.

The treatment of the peroneal spastic flat foot is directed towards symptoms, and frequently a period of rest in plaster will suffice.

Excision of the calcaneonavicular bar is helpful before skeletal maturity has occurred (Fig. 15.10a, b). (Mitchell & Gibson 1967). Occasionally, particularly if osteoarthritis of the talonavicular joint has occurred, triple arthrodesis in the adult will help.

(ii) *Congenital vertical talus.* This rare condition is characterized by a rigid flat foot. The heel is in equinus and valgus and the forefoot is in fixed dorsiflexion and pronation. The sole of the foot is convex with the head of the talus forming the lowest point on the medial side.

The treatment is to excise the talus, in order to correct the deformity.

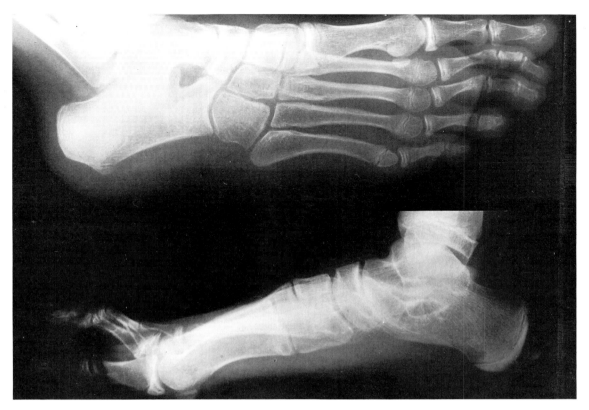

Fig. 15.6. Calcaneonavicular bar.

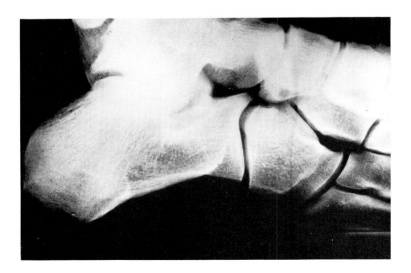

Fig. 15.7. Cartilaginous calcaneonavicular bar.

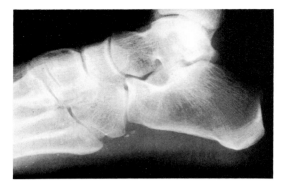

Fig. 15.8. Talocalcaneal bar.

Osteochondritis (Köhler's disease). This is a condition in which there is a disturbance in the blood supply to the navicular, and it occurs in children between the ages of three and six years. They present with pain on the inner side of the foot and the lateral X-ray shows flattening of the navicular (Fig. 15.11). This condition recovers with rest and does not appear to be a long-lasting problem.

(c) *Pes cavus*

Pes cavus, or claw foot, is a common condition which is due to a variety of different causes. The arch of the foot is raised, producing an equinus deformity, while the heel is in varus. The toes may become clawed due to the contracture of the small muscles of the foot (Fig. 15.12). The patient may proceed to develop painful callosities over the metatarsal heads (Fig. 15.13) and pain over the interphalangeal joint from clawing of the toes. There are several known causes of pes cavus (Brewerton *et al.* 1963):

Idiopathic.
Neurological.
Peroneal muscular atrophy.
Poliomyelitis.
Spinal dysraphism.
Meningomyelocele.
Muscular dystrophy.
Friedreich's ataxia.
Cerebral palsy.
Polioneuritis.

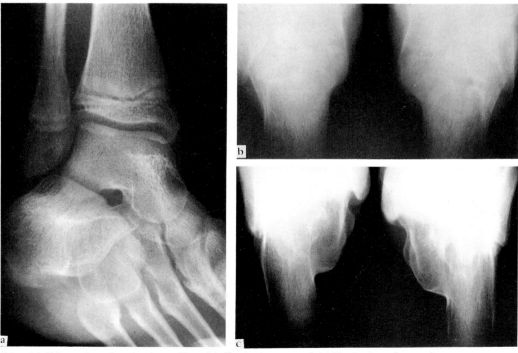

Fig. 15.9. (a) Oblique view of a talocalcaneal bar. (b) Harris view, normal. (c) Harris view, abnormal.

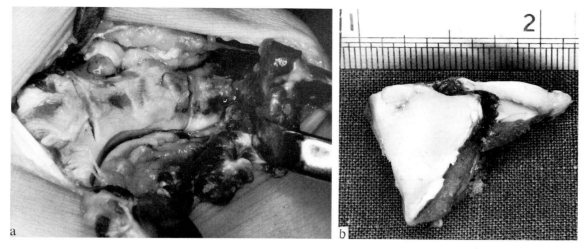

Fig. 15.10. (a) Calcaneonavicular bar at operation. (b) The amount excised.

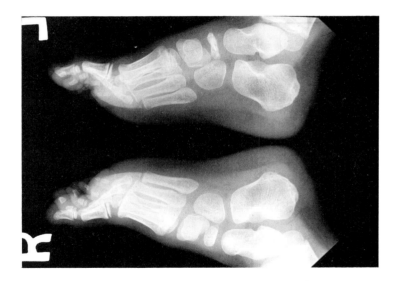

Fig. 15.11. Köhler's disease of the navicular.

The lateral X-rays demonstrate the elevation of the longitudinal arch and should be taken standing.

A line drawn through the inferior margin of the calcaneum and the inferior margin of the metatarsus is increased from the normal. Therefore the mid-talar line forms an angle with the mid-tarsal lines of the fifth metatarsal.

Treatment is directed towards (a) correcting the varus heel by plantar fascia release or osteotomy (Fig. 15.14), (b) correcting the clawing and preventing pain by tendon transfers and interphalangeal joint fusion of the hallux, and (c) a corrective osteotomy in the painful deformed foot of the adult.

(d) *Rheumatoid disease*

The foot is frequently involved in this crippling condition, and the whole of the joints may be implicated, leading to a painful flat foot.

Surgical treatment consists of triple arthrodesis of the hind- and midfoot and excision ar-

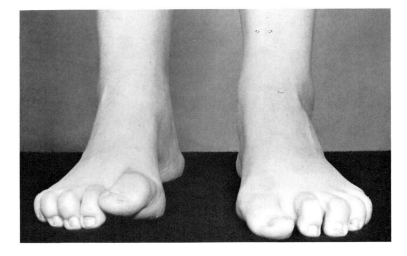

Fig. 15.12. Pes cavus.

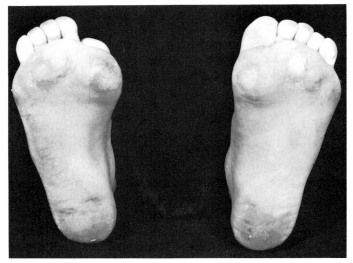

Fig. 15.13. Callosities produced
by pes cavus.

throplasty for the painful metatarsphalangeal
joints (Fowler 1959). Replacement arthroplasty
has not been used widely for this condition except replacement of the first metatarsophalangeal joint.

(e) Diabetic foot
Not infrequently the foot is involved in patients
with diabetes mellitus. This may be because of
infection or neuropathic or ischaemic ulcers.
There may be associated bone destruction and
treatment is aimed at eradicating the infection
and allowing the ulcers to heal.

Surgical shoes which are well padded are the
most appropriate form of treatment.

2   PROBLEMS AFFECTING THE HINDFOOT

Sever's disease
This is a form of osteochondritis of the calcaneum, although it may be the result of repeated
traction by the tendoachilles insertion. The condition occurs only in children and they present
with pain over the heel. The condition responds
spontaneously and does not appear in adult life.

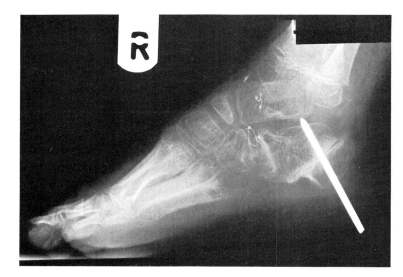

Fig. 15.14. Os calcis osteotomy
for the varus heel.

3   PROBLEMS AFFECTING THE MIDFOOT AND FOREFOOT

Metatarsus varus
This is a common condition in which the hindfoot is normal but the midfoot and forefoot are
adducted (Fig. 15.15). It presents in young
children as a cause of intoeing and may be associated with adductor hallucis tightness. The
foot, however, is not supinated as in congenital
talipes equinovarus but the forefoot is adducted
(Fig. 15.16). The angle between the mid-talar
and mid-calcaneal lines is above 35° and the
mid-talar line crosses medial to the first metatarsal shaft. The mid-calcaneal line lies lateral
to the normal position and the calcaneum is in
valgus. The majority, more than 85%, of children with metatarsus varus will have normal feet
by the age of 3, without any specific treatment
(Rushforth 1978). In those few that persist, abductor release is of benefit and corrects the deformity (Mitchell 1980).

4   PROBLEMS AFFECTING THE FOREFOOT

(a)   *Hallux valgus*
This common deformity may present in adolescents, but usually occurs in adult life and affects
women more frequently than men. It has been

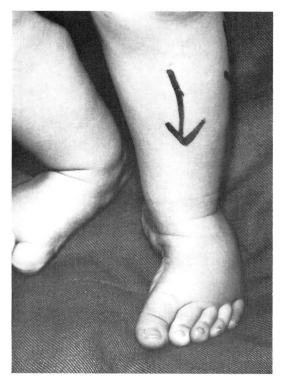

Fig. 15.15. Metatarsus varus.

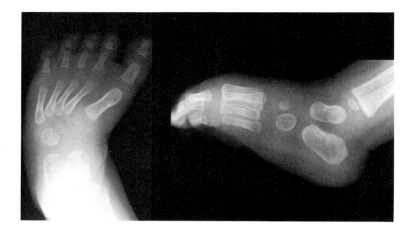

Fig. 15.16. The X-rays of a patient with metatarsus varus.

suggested that there is a familial incidence, although footwear seems to be a contributing factor. However, it is of interest that hallux valgus may be unilateral.

The deformity is a hallux valgus in association with a metatarsus primus varus. The combination produces deviation of the big toe and subluxation of the first metatarsus. Osteophytes form on the medial border of the metatarsal head, and articular erosion occurs within the joint surface. The bunion which develops consists of a callosity on the overlying skin. There is also inflammation of the underlying adventitious bursa with increased prominence of the metatarsal head from the metatarsus primus varus along with subluxation of the metatarsophalangeal joints. Later pronation of the big toe can occur, and this is due to the alteration in the action of the abductor muscle, due to its more plantar position. Because of these changes in the first toe it starts to override the second toe, or alternatively the second toe may be pushed into valgus itself overriding the third toe, resulting in subluxation of the joint. This effect tends to cause increasing pressure on the fourth and fifth toes, producing a bunionette on the fifth toe.

Hallux valgus may be divided into two main clinical types:

(i) *Adolescent.* Patients with adolescent hallux valgus can present at any age, but usually at about 12 years onwards. The patients are frequently female and the condition is bilateral (Fig. 15.17).

Adolescent hallux valgus is sometimes only a cosmetic problem, and the patient and her parents are concerned about her developing painful feet in later life.

In order to be able to answer this, Piggott (1960) classified adolescent hallux valgus into three different types: congruous; deviated; subluxed. He was able to show that in the congruous type where the base of the proximal phalanx was congruous with the first metatarsal head, the deformity was, in general, non-progressive. In contrast, in the deviated and subluxated group, where the base of the proximal phalanx is deviated or subluxed on the metatarsal head, the deformity tends to progress. On the basis of this classification management could be planned.

Another technique is to use standing X-rays which can demonstrate any increase in the metatarsal angle. This angle is developed from a line drawn through the axis of the first metatarsus and a similar line drawn through the second metatarsus. Normally, this angle is less than 10° (Fig. 15.18).

There are a variety of surgical operations for this condition and these include McBride's (1928) abductor hallucis tendon transfer, and osteotomies on the shaft of the first metatarsus.

Probably the best known are Mitchell's distal

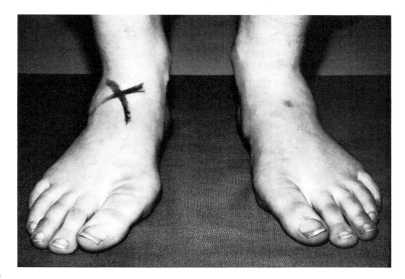

Fig. 15.17. Adolescent hallux valgus affecting the right foot in particular.

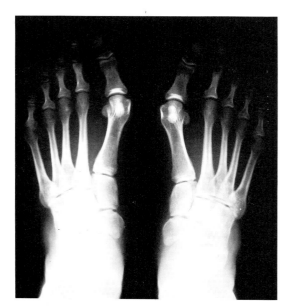

Fig. 15.18. X-rays of a girl with adolescent hallux valgus.

osteotomy (Mitchell *et al*. 1958), where the shaft of the metatarsus is divided below the head of the bone which is displaced laterally (Fig. 15.19), and Wilson's osteotomy (1963), whereby the metatarsal shaft is divided and the distal end displaced laterally and superiorly.

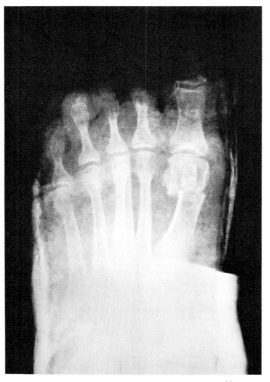

Fig. 15.19. Mitchell's osteotomy for hallux valgus.

(ii) *Adult.* This is a different clinical problem, because the patient now presents not first with deformity, but with pain, particularly if the joint is involved.

There is obvious deformity from subluxation or dislocation of the metatarsophalangeal joint, and the foot may be broadened due to loss of the transverse arch.

The radiological diagnosis of hallux valgus is made on standing AP views.

The surgical treatment of younger adults with pain from the deformity, without degeneration of the joint, can also be an osteotomy. However, in older patients Keller's excision arthroplasty is useful (Keller 1904), whereby the proximal half of the proximal phalanx is excised and the bunion is trimmed. Replacement arthroplasty can be undertaken using silastic with the benefit of retaining the length of the big toe.

In children terminal hallux valgus may be a problem and this can be relieved by wedge osteotomies of the terminal phalanx.

(b) Hallux rigidus

This condition is seen equally in men and women and produces a painful first metatarsophalangeal joint. It has been suggested that osteochondritis of the first metatarsal head is the prime cause of this condition (McMaster 1978).

This osteochondritis leads to flattening of the metatarsal head with incongruity of the joint and subsequent osteoarthritis. Patients present with pain on walking with limitation of movement, and X-rays demonstrate the typical appearances of osteoarthritis (Fig. 15.20). The surgical treatment involves either an excision or a replacement arthroplasty.

(c) Hammer toes

These are a common cause of discomfort in the foot. The hammer toe is a fixed deformity of the proximal interphalangeal joint in the adult. Because of the shape of the toe, a corn frequently develops over the proximal interphalangeal joint.

This condition is usually found in the second toe but may involve other toes. The straight AP film will show shortening of the second toe, and this is confirmed on oblique films. The affected toe shows dorsiflexion at the metatarsophalangeal joint, plantarflexion on the proximal interphalangeal joint, and extension at the dorsal interphalangeal joint.

Surgical intervention is best, and the simplest procedure is to excise the proximal interphalangeal joint along with the overlying corn. Arthrodesis of the interphalangeal joint may be preferred, or excision of the whole phalanx, leaving a floppy painless toe, may be useful.

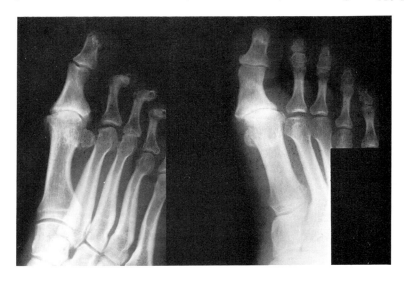

Fig. 15.20. Hallux rigidus.

(d)   March fractures

These are stress fractures affecting the second metatarsal shaft, but can also occur in the third and fourth shafts. The patients have pain and swelling in the foot which is made worse by weight-bearing. There may be a distinct swelling on palpation of the foot and the fracture is then demonstrable on X-rays. The only treatment is rest.

(e)   Osteochondritis of the metatarsal heads

Freiberg's disease is a condition found in children and adolescents in which there is osteochondritis of the head at usually the second metatarsal head (Fig. 15.21). It is demonstrable on X-ray and usually responds to rest, although it may lead to hallux rigidus in adults.

Fractures

1   ANKLE JOINT

There are several classifications of ankle joint injuries, but the two easiest to follow are:

(a) Ashhurst and Bromer (1922) defined ankle injuries into simple groups.

1   Fractures by external rotation.
2   Fractures by abduction.
3   Fractures by adduction.

All three can be further divided into 1st, 2nd and 3rd degrees.

4   Compression fractures.
5   Fractures caused by direct violence.

(b)   The other classification is by Colton (1976) and is a modification of the Lauge–Hansen (1950) classification.

1   Abduction fractures.
2   Adduction fractures.
3   External rotation injuries with diastasis of the inferior tibiofibular joint.
4   External rotation injuries without diastasis of the inferior tibiofibular joint.
5   Vertical compression injuries.
6   Unclassifiable injury patterns.

Abduction injuries

These injuries frequently result in an avulsion or fracture of the medial malleolus (Fig. 15.22). If the malleolus is fractured it should be reattached (Fig. 15.23).

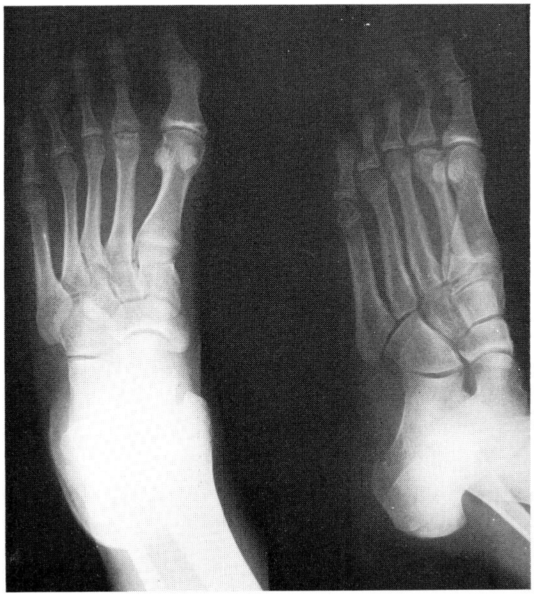

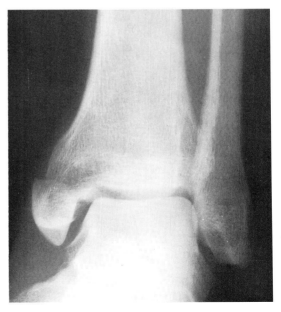

Fig. 15.21.   Freiberg's disease of the second metatarsal head.

Fig. 15.22.   Abduction injury of the ankle.

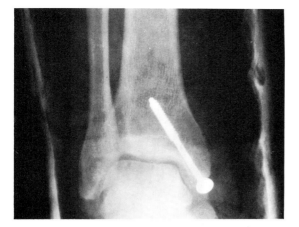

Fig. 15.23. Internal fixation of the fracture.

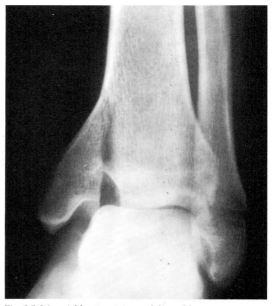

Fig. 15.24. Adduction injury of the ankle.

Adduction injuries
Here the talus is adducted within the mortise producing a compression force on the medial joint structure. There is no rotational movement of the talus and there is a shearing force through the medial malleolus sometimes in association with a transverse fracture of the fibula (Fig. 15.24).

External rotation injuries
These can occur without a diastasis and can, in fact, be more of a problem, if not correctly diagnosed, than the complete diastasis of the inferior tibiofibular ligament or Dupuytren's fracture–dislocation (Figs. 15.25 & 15.26).

The external rotational injury without diastasis can be treated conservatively provided the ankle is accurately reduced (Hughes 1977) (Figs. 15.27 & 15.28), or by internal fixation. It is essential to fix and reconstruct internally the rotating disrupted Dupuytren's injury. Occasionally an external rotational injury can occur with rupture of the deltoid ligament, talar shift and a fracture of the fibula near to the superior tibiofibular ligament. This is Maisonneuve's fracture (Fig. 15.29) and the interosseous membrane is ruptured. Treatment is to fix internally the structures that have been ruptured,

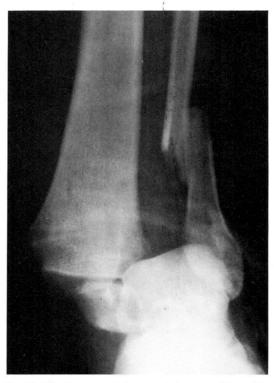

Fig. 15.25. Dupuytren's fracture–dislocation of the ankle. From Hughes (1983) with permission.

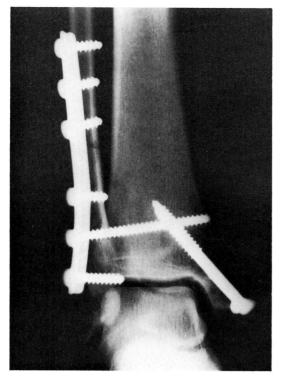

Fig. 15.26. Internal fixation of the fracture. From Hughes (1983) with permission.

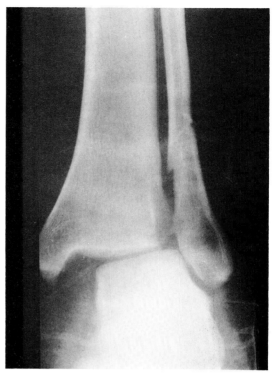

Fig. 15.27. External rotational injury without diastasis.

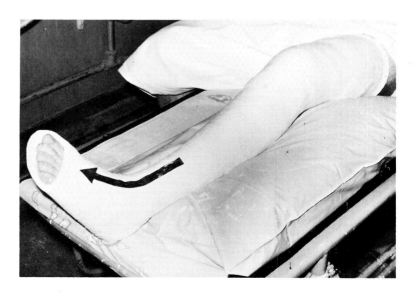

Fig. 15.28. Treated by closed reduction.

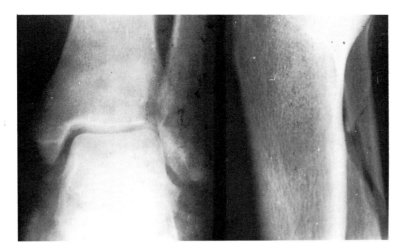

Fig. 15.29. Maisonneuve's fracture involving the fibula.

namely the deltoid ligament and tibiofibular ligaments.

2   THE CALCANEUM

Fractures of the calcaneum can occur when the patient falls from a height, landing on his feet, and pelvic and spinal injuries may also occur.

Fractures of the calcaneum can be divided into those that involve the subtalar joint and those that do not (Rowe *et al.* 1963).

Those fractures that do not involve the subtalar joint obviously carry a better prognosis than those that involve the joint (Figs. 15.30 & 15.31), as the joint destruction can lead to osteoarthritis early on.

Conservative management consists of elevation and early mobilization of the foot and ankle. Operative treatment by open reduction and internal fixation has a limited role for those patients who have subtalar joint damage.

Early posterior subtalar joint fusion has been advocated in patients with painful stiff subtalar joints (Noble & McQuillan 1979).

3   TALUS

It is fortunate that major injury to the talus is uncommon. The talus receives its blood supply distally (Kelly & Sullivan 1963), and therefore

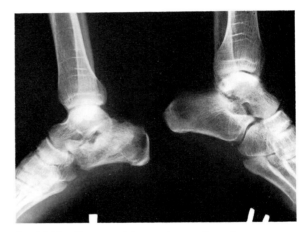

Fig. 15.30.   Fracture of the os calcis involving the subtalar joint.

avascular necrosis of the body of the talus is a notorious complication which can occur (Fig. 15.32).

Should avascular necrosis occur then ankle arthrodesis, which should include the subtalar joint, is indicated.

4   FRACTURES OF THE NAVICULAR

Fractures of the navicular are relatively uncommon (Fig. 15.33) and if undisplaced can be treated in a walking plaster. However, if the fracture is displaced closed reduction is not of

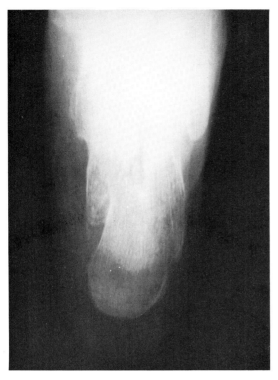

Fig. 15.31. Calcaneal view showing fracture extending into joint.

any use and the fragments are best reduced by open means and internally fixed.

Fractures of the tuberosity of the navicular can occur, and lead to quite severe discomfort and are best rested in plaster.

Fracture–dislocation of the tarsus can occur and is usually associated with extensive soft-tissue damage. A fortunately rare fracture–dislocation can occur between the tarsus and metatarsal bones, Lisfranc dislocation (Figs. 15.34 & 15.35).

Reduction must be attempted immediately and can be closed, but it is frequently necessary to open the foot to realign the bones.

5 FRACTURES OF THE METATARSUS AND PHALANGES

Inversion injuries to the foot may result in a fracture of the base of the fifth metatarsal bone, into which is inserted the peroneus brevis.

Phalangeal injuries can include dislocation and fractures and are best treated by reduction and immobilization. The commonest injury is a fracture of the big toe, as the result of a heavy weight falling on it.

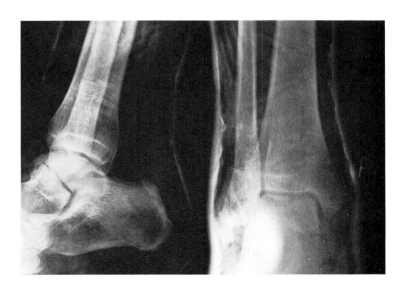

Fig. 15.32. Fracture of the body of the talus.

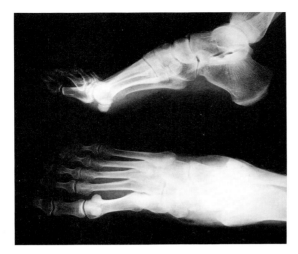

Fig. 15.33. Fracture of the navicular.

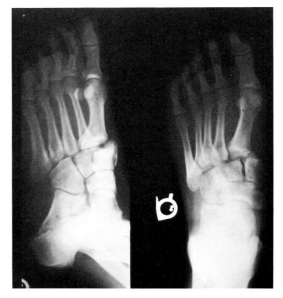

Fig. 15.34. Lisfranc's fracture–dislocation.

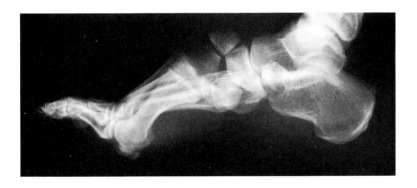

Fig. 15.35. Lisfranc's fracture–dislocation.

References

ASHHURST A.P.C. & BROMER R.S. (1922) Classifications and mechanism of fractures of the leg bones involving the ankle. *Arch. Surg.* **4**, 51.

BARNETT C.H. & NAPIER J.R. (1952) The axis of rotation of the ankle joint in man: its influence upon the form of the talus and the mobility of the fibula. *J. Anat.* **86**, 1.

BREWERTON D.A., SANDIFER P.H. & SWEETNAM D.R. (1963) The aetiology of pes cavus. *Brit. med. J.* **2**, 659.

COLTON C.L. (1976) Injuries of the ankle. In *Watson–Jones Fractures and Joint Injuries*, 5th Edition (ed. Wilson J.N.). Edinburgh: Churchill Livingstone.

DENNYSON W.G. & FULFORD G.E. (1976) Subtalar arthrodesis by cancellous grafts and metallic internal fixation. *J. Bone Jt Surg.* **58B**, 507.

DUPUYTREN G. (1874) *On the Injuries and Diseases of Bones* (translated and edited by F. le Gros Clark). London: Sydenham Society.

EVANS DILLWYN (1961) Relapsed club foot. *J. Bone Jt Surg.* **43B**, 722.

GRICE D.D. (1952) An extra-articular arthrodesis of the subastragalar joint for correction of paralytic flat feet in children. *J. Bone Jt Surg.* **34A**, 927.

HUGHES S.P.F. (1983) *Basis and Practice of Traumatology.* London: Heinemann.

HUGHES S.P.F. & SWEETNAM D.R. (1981) *Basis and Practice of Orthopaedics.* London: Heinemann.

KELLER W.L. (1904) Surgical treatment of bunions and hallus valgus. *N. Y. med. J.* **80**, 741.

KELLY P.J. & SULLIVAN C.R. (1963) Blood supply of the talus. *Clin. Orthop. rel. Res.* **30**, 37.

LAUGE-HANSEN N. (1950) Fractures of the ankle. *Arch. Surg.* **60**, 957.

McBRIDE E.D. (1928) A conservative operation for bunions. *J. Bone Jt Surg.* **10**, 735.

McMaster M.J. (1978) The pathogenesis of hallux rigidus. *J. Bone Jt Surg.* **60B**, 82.

Maisonneuve J.G. (1840) Recherches sur la fracture du perone. *Arch. gén. Méd.* **1**, 165.

Mitchell G.P. (1980) Abductor hallucis release in congenitcal metatarsus varus. *Internat. Orthop.* **3**, 299.

Mitchell G.P. & Gibson J.M. (1967) Excision of calcaneonavicular bar for painful spasmodic flat foot. *J. Bone Jt Surg.* **49B**, 281.

Mitchell C.L., Fleming J.L., Allen R., Glenney C. & Sandford G.P. (1958) Osteotomy-bunionectomy for hallux valgus. *J. Bone Jt Surg.* **40A**, 41.

Noble J. & McQuillan W.M. (1979) Early posterior subtalar fusion in the treatment of fractures of the os calcis. *J. Bone Jt Surg.* **61B**, 90.

Piggott H. (1960) Natural history of hallux valgus in the adolescent and early adult life. *J. Bone Jt Surg.* **42B**, 749.

Rowe C.R., Skellarides H.T., Freeman P.A. & Sorki C. (1963) Fractures of the os calcis—a long term follow up study of 146 patients. *J. Amer. med. Ass.* **184**, 920.

Rushforth G.F. (1978) The natural history of hooked forefoot. *J. Bone Jt Surg.* **60B**, 530.

Wilson J.N. (1963) Oblique displacement osteotomy for hallux valgus. *J. Bone Jt Surg.* **45B**, 552.

Index

Abdomen, traumatic injuries 237–8,
   258, *see also* pelvis, fracture
Abscesses
  Brodie's 94, 495
  epidural 77
Acetabular angle 183, 317
  Sharp's 186
Acetabuloplasty 316
Acetabulum
  alignment 315, 317–18
  anteversion 317–18
  fractures 466–7
  measurements 183, 185–6
  protrusio acetabuli 327, 472, 483
  realignment 316
Achilles tendon bursitis 27
Acromioclavicular joint
  arthritic changes 449
  arthrography 66
  dislocation 448–9
Acromiohumeral interval 177
Adamantinoma 284–5
Albright's disease 124
Amelia 346
Amputation, level selection,
   radionuclide imaging in 138
Angiography 90–102
  digital 170
Angiomas, spinal 97
Ankle
  arthrodesis 520
  arthrography 65–6, 254–6
  dislocation 251
  fractures 248–52, 517–20
   with dislocation 518
  instability 193
  lateral ligaments, injuries to 252–
   6
  measurements 193
  movement at 504
  stress views of 193
  traumatic injuries 248–52
Ankylosing spondylitis 415–16, 484
Annulus fibrosus
  split annulus syndrome, contrast
   medium investigation 79, 80

tears in 407–8
Antimony colloids, technetium 99m-
   labelled 107
Aortography 103
Arachnoiditis, adhesive
  contrast media and 68
  radioculography 72
Arms
  amniotic bands 347
  deformities, children 345–9
  intrauterine amputation 347
  painful 348
Arteriography 90–3
  complications 93
  digital 170
  uses 93–9
   neoplastic disease 95–6
   trauma 93–5
Arthritis
  degenerative
   elbow 455
   wrist 457
  diagnostic signs 22, 27, 29
  hip 471–7
  juvenile chronic 356–7
  periarticular osteoporosis 22
  periosteal new bone formation
   in 27
  psoriatic 498
  pyogenic
   in children 320–1
   knee 495
  rheumatoid *see* Rheumatoid
   arthritis
  septic 348, 349
   chronic 368
  subchondral cortical bone loss 23
  see also Osteoarthritis
Arthrography
  acromioclavicular joints 66
  ankle 65–6, 254–6
  elbow 65–6
  facet, lumbar spine 83–4, 85
  hip
   adults 58–60
   children 56–8, 318–19

complications 58, 60
  techniques 57–8, 58–9, 318–
   19
interphalangeal joints 66
knee 487–90
  comparison with arthroscopy
   56
  complications 46
  contraindications 46
  indications for 46
  interpretation 49–56
  techniques 47–8
metacarpophalangeal joints 66
Perthes' disease 325
shoulder
  complications 61
  interpretation 63
  techniques 61–3
subtalar joints 66
temporomandibular joints 66
wrist 64
Arthrogryposis 334, 350–1
Arthroplasty
  elbow 455
  feet 512
   toes 516
  hip 468–9, 477
  knee 498–501
  metacarpal joints 461, 463
  Souter 455
  wrist 463
Arthroscopy, knee 488–9
  comparison with arthrography 56
Athletes, stress lesions/fractures
   256–9
Atlas, fractures 423–4
Atlas–odontoid distance,
   measurement 197–8
Axis, fractures 423–4

Back *see* Spine
Baker's cysts 56, 57, 101, 169, 487

Bands, amniotic 347
Barium-135m 106
Battered baby syndrome *see* Non-accidental injury
Baumann's angle 177–8
Bends 495
Bennett's fracture 459
Biopsy, needle aspiration 172–3
Bladder, traumatic injury 238
Blount's disease 329, 380, 382, 492–3
Boehler's angle 194, 248
Bone
  age, assessment of 182, 297–8
  atrophy 14
    radiographic diagnosis 14–15
  cortical
    destruction 9, 21
    loss of 3–4, 23
  cysts *see* Cysts
  density
    measurement 14
    post-traumatic increase 7
  destruction
    by erosion 9
    by infiltration 9
  disappearing 272
  disease, premature infants 302
  disorders
    cardinal signs 3–14
    generalized, in children 349–57
  erosion 9
    synovial mass disease 17, 21
  fixation 470–1
  formation, new 11–14, 27
  grafts, radionuclide evaluation 134
  growth, abnormalities 298–300
  hypertrophy 14
  infections *see* Infections; *specific infections*
  islands, radionuclide imaging 122
  long
    deformities 330–3
    fracture of 210
    lengthening 332–3
  mass, measurement 14
  measurement
    lower limb 182–96
    spine 196–204
    upper limb 177–82
  medullary destruction 35
  minerals, measurement of 162–3, 404
  pain
    evaluation 137
    in metastases 119–20

repair 9–14
rotation, radiographic diagnosis 7–8
sclerosis 9
tumours *see* Tumours, bone
union, radiographic demonstration 35
Bone marrow, radionuclide evaluation 107
Bow legs *see* Genu varum
Brevicollis 303
Brodie's abscess 495
  arteriogram of 94
Bunion 514
Bursitis, Achilles tendon 27

Caffey's syndrome *see* Non-accidental injury
Caffinière prosthesis 461
Caisson disease 495
  radionuclide imaging 136
Calcaneocavus foot 343
Calcaneocuboid
  arthrodesis 342
  fusion 506
Calcaneonavicular coalition 344, 345, 508
Calcaneum
  Boehler's angle 194, 248
  fractures 248, 250, 520
  measurements 194
  osteotomy 342, 343
Calcification
  hip area 475–7
  joints, in diagnosis of disease 25
Cameras, gamma (scintillation) 11–12
Carcinoma, metastatic 289
Carpometacarpal joint
  osteoarthritis 460–1
  replacement 461
Carpus 238–9
  bony injuries 456–9
  dislocation 240–2
  traumatic injuries 239
    instability following 240–3
Cartilage, articular
  loss of 21–2
  oedema 22
Cauda equina
  compression of 393
  tumours, radiculography 71, 75

Cellulitis, radionuclide imaging 125, 127
Chemonucleolysis, lumbar spine 80–1
Chiari pelvic osteotomy 477
Children
  arm deformities 345–8
  foot deformities 338–45, 379–80
  generalized bone disorders 349–57
  hip
    dislocation 314–19
    pain 321
  infections 348–9
    management 349
  knee 333–8
    pain 335
  non-accidental injury 131, 300–1, 494
  normal variations 297
  Perthes' disease 321–5
  slipped upper femoral epiphysis 325–33
  spine 300–14
    cervical 302–5
    congenital disorders 302–4, 308, 309–11
    infections 306–7
    intervertebral disc disorders 305, 309
    pain 305–6
    tumours 309–11
  see also Infants
Chondroblastoma, benign 270–1
  radionuclide imaging 121–2
Chondrodysplasia, diaphyseal aclasis 267
Chondroma 267–70
Chondromalacia patellae 337, 492
Chondromatosis, synovial 55, 502
Chondromyxoid fibroma 271–2
Chondrosarcoma 9, 278–80
  arteriogram of 100
  CT scan of 150
  radionuclide imaging 120
Chordoma 285
Clavicle, congenital pseudarthrosis 347–8
Clubfeet 505–6
Cobb angle 200–1
Coccydynia 484
Coccyx, fractures 467
Codman's triangle 12–13, 275, 278
Computed tomography 144
  acute spinal injury 429
  metrizamide-enhanced 162

Computed tomography   *Cont'd.*
  musculoskeletal
    clinical applications   147–64
    infection   154
    low back pain syndrome   157–
      62
    neoplasms   147–54
    technology   145–7
    trauma   154–6
  technology   144–7
  scanners   145
Congenital anomalies
  arm   345–8
  foot   313, 338–44, 379–80, 505–
    6, 508, 513
  generalized   350–6
  hip   380
  knee   193, 194, 328, 329–30
  limb bones   330, 380
  metacarpal index and   182
  patella   333, 490
  spine   302–4, 308, 311–14, 431,
    438–42
  in tropics   379–80
  see also specific disorders
Contrast media   68
  adverse effects   68, 69
Contrast medium investigations   45
  acromioclavicular joint   66
  ankle   65–6
  children   57
  elbow   66
  finger joints   66
  hip   56–60
  knee   46–67
  shoulder   61–3
  spine
    cervical   87–90
    lumbar   67–85
    thoracic   85–6
  subtalar joint   66
  temporomandibular joint   66
  wrist   64
  see also specific techniques
Coxa vara   327–8
Cysts
  aneurysmal   286, 309, 418, 420
  Baker's   56, 57, 101, 169, 487
  juvenile   285
  meniscal   50, 334–5
  popliteal   335, 487

De Quervain's fracture   240
Diaphragm, traumatic rupture   258–9

Diaphyseal aclasis   267, 355
  wrist   179
Diastematomyelia   313
  lumbar spine, radiculogram of   72
  in scoliosis   439–40
  thoracic spine   86
Digital radiography   169–70
Diphosphonates, in radionuclide
    imaging   107
Discitis   416
  juvenile   306
Discography
  cervical   89, 401
  lumbar   75–9, 84, 407–10
    complications   79
    techniques   76–9
  post-laminectomy syndrome   411
Discs, intervertebral   *see*
    Intervertebral discs
Dracunculus medinensis   368
Dupuytren's fracture–dislocation   518
Dyschondroplasia   267
Dyschondrosteosis, wrist   179
Dysostoses   298
Dysplasia
  fibrous   287–8, 355–6
    radionuclide imaging   122
  skeletal   298–300
Dysprosium-157   106
Dystrophy, reflex sympathetic   259–
    62

Ectromelia   346
Elbow
  arthritis   455
  arthrography   66
  Baumann's angle   177–8
  carrying angle   177
  dislocation   218
  fractures around   451–5
    lateral condyle   453
    supracondylar   451
    T- and Y-shaped   453
  humeral angle   177, 178
  measurements   177, 178
  movement at   446–7
  pulled   348
  replacement   455
  subluxation   453
  supracondylar fracture   177
  ulnar angle   177, 178
Electromyography in diagnosis of
    spinal nerve compression
    393–4

Emergencies, radiographic
    examination   209–10
Emission tomography   170–1
Enchondroma   267
Enchondromatosis, multiple   270
Endosteum
  erosion   9
  repair   14
Epidural
  fibrosis   411
  venography, lumbar spine   81–2,
    85
Epidurography   398
  lumbar spine   82–3
Epiphyseal quotient   187
Epiphysis, upper femoral, slipped
    325–7
Equinovarus deformity   194
Ewing's sarcoma   274, 281–2
  arteriogram of   95
  metastases   121
  radionuclide imaging   120, 121
Exostosis
  multiple   355
  osteocartilaginous   267

Facet joints
  arthrography, lumbar spine   83–4,
    85
  disorders of   410–11
  pain   410
Fasciitis, plantar   27
Femur
  alignment   318
  anteversion   318, 331
  congenital anomalies   330
  dislocation, measurement   184,
    185
  dysplasia   327
  epiphyseal quotient   187
  fractures   211, 244–6
    epiphyseal   492
    fixation   493
  head
    avascular necrosis   321, 325,
      327
    dislocation   225–34, 316–18,
      327
    fracture   214, 467
    fracture–dislocation   229–31,
      241
    necrosis   229

Femur, head *Cont'd.*
  osteotomies 477
  subluxation 472
lengthening of 332–3
measurements 184–8
minor epiphyseal displacement 187–8
neck
  anteversion 188–9
  fractures 35, 38, 134, 467–9
  measurement 186
  osteotomies 477
proximal focal deficiency 328
slipped upper epiphysis 325–33
  radiology 325–6
torsion 330, 331
Fibroma
  chondromyxoid 271–2
  desmoplastic 272
  non-ossifying 286
Fibrosarcoma 280
  arteriogram of 98
  CT scan of 149
  radionuclide imaging 120
Fibrosis, epidural 411
Fibrous dysplasia 287–8, 355–6
  radionuclide imaging 122
Fibula
  proximal, fracture 248, 258
  spiral fracture 211
Fingers, malformations 346–7
Fluorine-18 106
Fong's syndrome 490
Foot
  anatomy 504
  arthrodesis 511
  arthroplasty 512, 516
  claw (pes cavus) 313, 343, 510–11
  deformities
    children 338–44, 379–80
    congenital 313, 505–6, 508, 513
    measurements in 194–5
    terminology 338
    tropics 379–80
  diabetic 512
  dislocations 251
  flat 338–9, 506–10
    congenital 508–10
    peroneal spastic 508
  fractures 520–1
    march 517
  measurements, forefoot alignment 194–5
  movements 504

osteonchondritis 510
painful 344–5
rheumatoid disease 511
standing 505
Fractures
  in adults 210
  – dislocations 214–19
  Bennett's 459
  bone dislocation following 35
  child abuse 131
    radionuclide imaging 131
  chip 41
  corner metaphyseal 300, 355
  CT scanning 154–6
  De Quervain's 240
  displaced, radiographic diagnosis 6
  Dupuytren's fracture–dislocation 518
  Galeazzi 214
  healing 131
    delayed 131–2
    electrical stimulation for 132
    radionuclide imaging 131–2
  Jefferson 154, 423–4
  joints 24
  Jones' 248, 253
  longitudinal 6
    radiographic diagnosis 6
  Maisonneuve's 248, 258, 518
  march 258, 517
  Monteggia 214
  non-accidental injury 300–1
  oblique 210
  pathological 469
    metastases and 470–1
  'ping pong' 7
  radiographic diagnosis 5–7, 35, 37, 209–19
  radionuclide imaging 114, 127–30
  spiral 211
  stress 130, 256–9, 293–4
    metatarsus 345
    pelvis 467
    radionuclide imaging 130
    spine 389, 405
  in tropics
    infection in 377–8
    late presentation 374–5
    management 374–5
    non-union 377–8
  undisplaced, diagnosis of 39–40
  see also sites of fracture
Freiberg's disease 517
Fungal infections 372
  knee 496

Galeazzi fracture 214
Gallium-67 107–8, 126, 127
Gamma camera 111–12
Gas gangrene 373
genu
  recurvatum 334
  valgum 329–30
    measurements relevant to 193, 194
  varum 329
    measurements relevant to 193, 194
Giant-cell tumours 272–3, 418
Glenohumeral joint 446, 447–8
  dislocation 219–225
    arthrography 225
Gorham's disease 272
Gout
  calcified tophus 25
  diagnosis 25
Granuloma, eosinophilic 287, 418
  children 310
Grasping 447
Growth, assessment of 182, 203
Guinea worm 368

Haemangioma 272
Haemangiomatosis 272
Haemarthrosis 353–4
Haemoglobinopathies 383–5
Haemophilia 353–4
Hallux
  rigidus 516
  valgus 338, 343, 513–16
Hand
  deformities 462–3
    boutonnière 462
    swan-neck 462
  flexion and extension ranges 179–80
  fractures 459–60
  immobilization 460
  malformations 346–7
  measurements 179–80, 182
  osteoarthritis 460–1
  prehension patterns 447
  rheumatoid arthritis 461–4
Hand–Schüller–Christian disease 287
Heel
  painful 344
  plantar fasciitis 27
Hemivertebrae 431, 438–9, 440

Hilgenreiner's line 183, 317
Hill–Sachs deformity, arthrography
  61, 63
Hip
  arthritis 471–7
    surgical treatment 477
  arthrodesis 477
  arthrography
    adults 58–60
    children 56–8, 318–19
    complications 58, 60
  avascular necrosis, arteriography
    98
  calcification 475–7
  congenital anomalies 474–7
    surgical treatment 477
  congenital dislocation 314, 380
    arthrography 56–8, 318–19
    measurements 317
    Ortolani test 315
    pathology 315
    radiology 316–18
    in spina bifida 312
    treatment 315–16
    ultrasonography 319
  dislocation 225–37
    congenital see Hip, congenital
      dislocation
    with fracture 229–37, 241
    late presentation 376
    measurement 184, 185
  erosion, synovial mass disease 17
  fracture, CT scan 155, 156
  infections
    children 320–1
    tropics 367
  irritable hip syndrome 321
  loose bodies, arthrography 60
  measurements 182–9
  pain, infants 320
  pinning, adolescents 326
  radiographic examination 32
  replacement
    arthrography of 58–60
    complications 481–3
    infection in 481
    loosening of 481–3
    pain in 58
    radiographic appearances 477–
      81
    radionuclide imaging of 132–4
  subluxation 474–5
  trauma, avascular disease in 134
  ultrasonography 319
  see also Acetabulum; Femur; Perthes'
    disease

Histiocytoma, fibrous
  CT scans 153
  malignant 280–1
Horner's syndrome 303
Humerus
  head
    dislocation 219–25, 447
    fracture 220, 222, 223–4
    fracture–dislocations 225
    rotation 7
  lower, fractures 451–2
  neck, fractures 450–1
  proximal, fractures 255
  supracondylar angle 177
Hyperparathyroidism 403
  brown tumour of 287

Infants
  hip
    dislocation in 314–19
    pain 320
  premature, bone disease 302
  see also children
Infections 123, 289–92
  children 348–9
    management 349
  CT scanning 154
  fungal 372, 496
  hip 320, 367
  knee 495–6
    soft tissue 490
  radionuclide imaging 124–7
  spine 291–2, 306–7, 413–14
  tropics 367–74
    chronic 367–8
    in fractures 377–8
    post-operative 368
  see also specific infections
Interphalangeal joints, arthrography
  66
Intervertebral discs
  biomechanics 388
  calcification 305
  composition 388
  CT scanning 157–8
  degenerative disease 388–9
    cervical 87–9, 400–2
    chemonucleolysis 80–1
    comparison of contrast medium
      techniques 84–5
    CT scanning 157–60
    discography 75–9, 84, 89

dorsal 402–4
  epidural venography 81–2, 85
  epidurography 82–3
  facet arthrography 83–4, 85
  lumbar 67–85, 157–60, 405–6,
    408
  myelography 87–9
  radiculography 67–75, 84
Prolapse
  acute 392–3
  in children 309
  radiography of 395–7
  treatment 398–9
Iopamidol 69
Ischaemia
  and joint growth disorder 25
  in radiological assessment 41, 43

Jaw, late dislocation 376
Jefferson fracture 154, 423–4
Joints
  calcification 24
  cartilage, loss of 21–2
  dislocation, late presentation 376
  disorders, cardinal signs 15–29
  erosion 17–18, 21
  fracture–dislocations 214–19
  fractures 24
  growth disorder 25
  haemarthrosis 353–4
  infection see Infections; specific
    infections
  lipohaemarthrosis 24
  looseness 29
  malalignment 25–7
  measurement
    lower limb 182–96
    spine 196–204
    upper limb 177–82
  prosthesis, looseness of 29, 31
  proteolysis and 21–2, 23
  replacement
    complications 132
    radionuclide imaging evaluation
      132–4
  subluxation 25–7
  synovial
    effusion 15
    mass disease 15–21
    pannus 21–2
    vacuum phenomena 31
  see also specific joints
Jones' fracture 248, 253

Kidney, traumatic injury 238
Kienböck's disease 457–9
Klippel–Feil syndrome 303
Knee
  arthritis
    osteoarthritis 496
    psoriatic 498
    pyogenic 495
    rheumatoid 496–8
  arthrodesis 501
  arthrography 487–90
    in acute injury 54–5
    comparison with arthroscopy
      56
  arthrography
    complications 46
    contraindications 46
    indications for 46
    interpretation 49–56
    techniques 47–8
  arthroscopy 488–9
  bone lesions affecting 490–5
  caisson disease 495
  capsular injuries 54–5, 487
  children 333–8
  cortical defect 338
  cysts
    Baker's 56, 57, 101, 169, 487
    meniscal 50, 334
    popliteal 335, 487
  deformities
    congenital 193, 194, 328, 329–
      30
    progressive 494–5
    tropics 328
  dislocation 214, 248, 493
  femoral angle 189–90
  fractures 244–8
  hyperextension 334
  infections
    fungal 496
    pyogenic 495
    soft-tissue 490
    tuberculosis 495–6
  ligaments
    arthrography 53–4
    damage 53–5, 486–7
  loose bodies 493–4
  measurements 189–93
  meniscus
    arthrography of 49–53
    cysts 50, 334–5
    discoid 50–1, 334
    tears 49–50, 51–3, 336, 488–9
  metabolic disorders and 495
  neuropathic disease 496

ossification variants 338
osteochondritis 335–6
osteomalacia 495
pain
  children 336, 337
  patellofemoral 337
patellar position 190
replacement 498–501
  radionuclide imaging of 132–4
rupture, arthrography 56
snapping (clicking) 334
synovial mass disease 17
synovial plicae 337
synovium, arthrography 55
tibial angle 189–90
tibial plateau angle 190
traumatic injuries 244–8
tumours 501–2
see also Patella
knock-knee see Genu valgum
Köhler's disease 510
Konig's disease 493
kyphosis 430, 431, 433
  adolescent 307
  assessment 204

Laminectomy 399
  failure of 411
Leg
  length
    discrepancy 331–3, 495
    measurement 196, 332
  windswept 380
Legg–Calvé–Perthes disease see
  Perthes' disease
Legg–Perthes disease see Perthes'
  disease
leprosy 371–2
Letterer–Siwe disease 287
Ligaments see Knee, ligaments; Wrist,
  ligaments
Limbs
  bone deformities
    reduction 330
    rotational (torsion) 330–1
  length, discrepancy 331–3, 495
Lipohaemarthrosis 24
Lipoma, CT scan of 151, 152
Liposarcoma
  CT scanning 151–4
  radionuclide imaging 137
Lisfranc dislocation 251, 521
Looser's zones 294

Lordosis 430, 431, 433
  assessment 204
Lumbar puncture, technique 69
Lunate
  dislocation 456–7
  Kienböck's disease 457–9
  subluxation 242
Lymphography 103
Lymphoma, malignant 282–4

McCune–Albright syndrome 356
McGregor's line 197
Madelung deformity 179, 347
Madura foot 372
Magnification, radiography 167
Maisonneuve fracture 248, 258, 518
Malgaigne's fracture 232, 236, 238
Marfan's syndrome, metacarpal index
  in 182
Measurement, bone and joint
  lower limb 182–96
  spine 196–204
  upper limb 177–82
Meniscus
  cysts 50, 334–5
  discoid 334
  tears 336
Metabolic bone disease
  quantitative mineral analysis by
    CT 162–3
  radionuclide imaging 116
  spine 403–4
Metacarpal index 182
Metacarpophalangeal joints
  arthrography 66
  replacement 463–4
  rheumatoid arthritis 461–2
  subluxation 26
Metacarpus
  fractures 459
  measurement 182
Metaphyseal fibrous cortical defect
  286–7
Metatarsalgia 345
  Morton's 345
Metatarsus
  adductus 339
  dislocation 252
  fractures 521
    stress 345
  head, osteochondritis 345
  osteotomy 342
  varus 513

Methylene diphosphonate (MDP) 107
Metrizamide 68, 69
    adverse effects 68–9
    contraindications 69
Monteggia fracture–dislocation 214, 217
Morquio's disease, metacarpal index in 182
Myelography 67
    acute spinal injury 429
    cervical 87–90
        disc disease 87–9
        rheumatoid diseases 90
        trauma 89–90
    lumbar 70
    in scoliosis 439–40
Myeloma 284
    multiple 121
Myelomeningocele 311–12
Myodil 68
Myositis ossificans 287, 455

Nail–patella syndrome 490
Navicular, fractures 520–1
Neck
    pain 400
    shortening 303–4
    twisted, children 302–3
Needle aspiration biopsy 172–3
Neoplasms see Tumours
Neuroblastoma
    cervical 303
    radionuclide imaging 114, 137
Neurofibroma, spinal 76, 395
Neurofibromatosis 351–2, 443
Non-accidental injury (NAI) 300–1, 494
    lesions associated with 131
    radionuclide imaging 131

Odontoid, fractures 423–4
Olecranon, fractures 454
Ombredanne line 184
Ortolani test 315
Os lunatum, subluxation 242
Osgood–Schlatter disease 336, 494
Osteitis
    condensans ilii 484

deformans see Paget's disease
    pubis 484
Osteoarthritis
    glenohumeral joint 448
    hand 460–1
    hip 471–7
    knee 496
    radionuclide imaging 114, 127
Osteoarthropathy, hypertrophic pulmonary 27
Osteoblastoma 418
    benign 265, 267
        radionuclide imaging 121
    children 310
Osteochondritis
    dissecans 335–6
        knee 493
    feet 510
        metatarsal head 345, 516, 517
        tibial tubercle 335, 336
Osteochondrodysplasia 298
Osteochondroma 267
    CT scan of 151
    radionuclide imaging 122
Osteochondromatosis 355
Osteoclastoma in tropics 380
Osteogenesis imperfecta 300, 349–50
    tarda 350
Osteolysis, massive bone 272
Osteoma, osteoid 264–5, 418
    children 310–11
    CT scan of 148
    diagnosis 265
    radionuclide imaging 121, 137
Osteomalacia 294, 382–3, 403, 404
Osteomyelitis 124, 289–92
    children 349
    chronic 291, 367–8
    haematogenous 289–91
    knee 496
    radiographic diagnosis 9
    radionuclide imaging 124–6
    tropics 367
Osteonecrosis, radionuclide imaging 136
Osteophytes
    hip 472
    spine 395, 399, 400
Osteoporosis 9, 14, 295–6
    diagnosis 35
    disuse 14, 22, 23
    dysbaric see Caisson disease
    periarticular 22–3
    spine 403, 404
    of subchodral cortex 23–4

Osteosarcoma 275–8, 418
    arteriography of 96, 97, 99
    CT scan of 148, 149
    metastases 121
        radionuclide imaging 120
    multifocal 274
    radionuclide imaging 120, 121
    subtypes 276

Paediatrics see Children
Paget's disease 292
    radionuclide imaging 116–17
Pain 389
    bone see Bone pain
    response to 389
    see also individual sites of pain
Palsy, cerebral 379–80
Pannus, joints 21–2
Paraplegia, tropics 378
Pars interarticularis, stress fracture 404
Patella
    alta 190, 334
    chondromalacia 337, 492
    congenital anomalies 333, 490
    dislocation 191–2, 333, 490
    fractures 246, 335, 490
    measurements 190–1
        Laurin's projection 191–2
        Merchant's projection 191
    patellofemoral pain 337
    post-traumatic necrosis 490–1
    radiography 333–4
    Sinding–Larsen disease 335
    tendon injuries 490
Pauwel's angle 468
Pedicles, loss of 3
Pellegrini–Steida disease 487
Pelvic girdle 465
Pelvis
    apophyses 484
    Chiari osteotomy 477
    fractures 232–8, 465–71
        associated injuries 237–8, 258
        of Malgaigne 232, 236, 238
        pathological 469–71
        prophylactic fixation 470–1
        stress 467
    miscellaneous conditions 484
    radiographic examination 32
    sprung 232
Periosteum, new bone formation 11–13, 27

Periostitis 27
  of infancy 301
Perkins' line 184, 317
Perthes' disease 29, 321–5
  arteriography 98
  arthrography 61, 325
    in children 58
  avascularity in 134
  measurements relevant to 185,
      186, 187
  nuclear imaging 324–5
  radiology 321–4
  radionuclide imaging 134–6
Pes cavus 313, 343, 510–11
Pes planovalgus 506–10
  congenital 508–10
Pes varus 313
Phalanges, measurement 182
Phlebography 102
Phocomelia 346
Phosphonates 106–7
Plantar fasciitis 27
Poliomyelitis, anterior 370–1
Polyarteritis nodosa, arteriography
  98
Polydactyly 346
Pott's disease 292
Proteolysis, joints 21–2, 23
Protrusio acetabuli 327, 472, 483
Pseudarthrosis
  radionuclide imaging 132
  spine 411–12, 416, 436–7
Pseudoparesis 348
Pseudotumours 354
Pyrophosphate 107

Radiculography 67
  lumbar spine 68–75
    complications 70–1
    contrast media 68–9
    evaluation of 84
    interpretation 71–4
    technique 69, 71
Radiography
  digital 169–70
  emergency 209–10
  errors in diagnosis 31–44
    fundamental deficiencies of
      radiography 35–44
    inadequate/incomplete
      examinations 31–4
  hazards of 3

interventional 172–3
  limitations 35–44
  magnification 167
  microfocal 34
  shortcomings 105
  standard examination 3
  technical advances 34
  xeroradiography 169
Radionuclide imaging 105–43
  blood pool scan 111
  clinical applications 118–38
    amputation level selection 138
    avascular disease 134–6
    bone tumours 119–23
    fractures 127–34
    infectious diseases 124–7
    osteonecrosis 136
    prosthetic implant evaluation
      132–4, 500–1
    soft-tissue disorders 137–8
  factors influencing quality of 112–
      13
  instrumentation 111–12
  interpretation
    false-negative 114
    false-positive 113–14
    localization and pattern
      recognition 114–17
    serial scanning 117–18
  photon-deficient areas (cold spots)
      110
  radiopharmaceuticals for 105–8
    extraosseous localizations 109
    mechanisms of skeletal uptake
      108–11, 119
    serial (sequential) scanning 117–
      18
    quantitation of tracer uptake
      in 117–18
  three-phase 111
Radius
  distal, alignment of 179
  Galeazzi fracture 214
  head
    alignment of 178–9
    congenital dislocation 345
    dislocation 214
    fracture 215, 454
  malformations 346, 347
Raynaud's phenomenon 97
Reflex sympathetic dystrophy 259–
  62
Reiter's syndrome 27
Renal tract, traumatic injury 238
Rheumatoid arthritis
  in children 356

elbow 455
glenohumeral joint 448
hand 461–4
hip 471
knee 496–8
  children 496–8
periarticular osteoporosis 22
radionuclide imaging 114, 127,
    137
spine 416
in tropics 382
wrist 459
Rib–vertebral angle 203–4
Ribs
  fractures 215
    child abuse 300–1
    radionuclide imaging 114
  in neurofibromatosis 352
  ribbon 352
Rickets 294, 354–5, 380, 382
  premature infants 302
Risser's sign 435, 484
Rotator cuff 446
  arthrography 61–3, 449–50
  injuries 61–3, 177, 449

Sacroiliac joint
  dislocation 236
  radionuclide imaging 137
Sacrum
  agenesis 314
  fractures 216, 232, 467
Sarcoma
  Ewing's 95, 274, 281–2
    radionuclide imaging 120, 121
  parosteal, CT scan of 150
  soft-tissue 290
Scaphoid
  fractures 39, 40, 213, 239–40,
    456, 457
  rotation of 455–6
  rotatory subluxation 242
Scapula, congenital high 303–4
Scheuermann's disease 204, 307,
  402
Scintigrams, interpretation 105
Scintigraphy, three-phase 111
Scintillation camera 111–12
Scleroderma, arteriography 97
Scoliosis 429
  annular tears 407–8
  congenital 438

Scoliosis, congenital *Cont'd.*
   radiological assessment 438–40
   treatment 440–2
  idiopathic 431, 432–7
   radiological assessment 432–3
   treatment 436–7
  infantile, rib–vertebral angle
    203–4
  measurement of 200–4
  in neurofibromatosis 352, 443
  neuromuscular 442–3
  non-structural 443–4
  thoracic spine 86
  in tropics 380
Scurvy 383
Sever's disease 512
Sharp's angle 186
Shenton's line 184, 317
Shoulder
  Acromiohumeral distance 177
  arthritis 448
  arthrography
   complications 61
   interpretation 63
   subdeltoid bursography 63
   techniques 61–3
  capsulitis, adhesive, arthrography
   61
  dislocation 219–25, 447
   arthrography 61–3, 225
   with fracture 225
  erosion, synovial mass disease 17
  fractures 225, 450–1
  frozen, arthrography 61
  Hill–Sachs deformities,
   arthrography, 61, 63
  movement 446
  rotator cuff 446
   arthrography 61–3, 449–50
   injuries 61–3, 177, 449
Sickle cell disease 383–5
Simon's line 317
Sinding–Larsen disease 335
Sinography 103
Skeletal
  dysplasias 298–300
  maturation, assessment 182, 203,
   297–8
  see also Bone
Skull
  fractures
   child abuse 301
   depressed 7
  haemangiomas 272
  invagination by C1 197
  in neurofibromatosis 352

Slit scanography 332
Smallpox 372–3
Soft-tissue tumours *see* Tumours,
  soft-tissue
Spina bifida 311–12, 431
  lower limb in 312
  occulta 313
Spine
  anatomy 388
  angiomas 97
  ankylosing spondylitis 415–16,
   484
  biomechanics 388
  cervical
   children, radiography of 302
   congenital anomalies 302–4
   contrast medium investigations
    87–90
   discography 89
   displacement 198–9
   instability 198
   invagination of skull by 197
   lateral masses, tomography of
    29
   myelography 87–90
   pain 400
   radiographic examination 34
   rheumatoid disease 90
   spondylosis 400–1
   subluxation in children 303
   trauma 89, 304
  cervicodorsal, in Sudeck's atrophy
   261
  children 302–14
  contrast medium investigations
   67–90
  deformities 429–42
   aetiology 431
   clinical presentation 432
   congenital 302–4, 308, 311–
    14, 431, 438–42
   idiopathic 431, 432–7
   radiological assessment 432–40
   screening for 432
   see also Scoliosis
  dislocation 424–9
  dorsal
   disc disease 402–3
   metabolic disease 403–4
   radiographic examination 34
  facet joints *see* Facet joints
  fractures 421, 423–9
   with dislocation 424–9
   stress 389, 405
  fusion, complications 411–12
  infections 291–2, 413–14

  children 306–7
   tuberculosis 414
  inflammatory disease 415
  innervation 389–90
  instability
   measurements for 198–200
   in spondylolisthesis 200
  intervertebral discs *see*
   Intervertebral discs
  lumbar
   annular tears 407–8
   chemonucleolysis 80–1
   contrast medium investigations
    67–85
   CT scan 147, 157–62
   diastematomyelia 72
   disc degeneration 405–6, 408
   discography 75–9, 84
   dysraphism 72
   epidural abscess 77
   epidural venography 81–2
   epidurography 82–3
   facet arthrography 83–4, 85
   neurofibroma 76
   pain 404–5, 407
   radiculography 68–75, 84
   radiographic examination 34
   spondylolysis 405, 406
  measurements 196–204
  mechanical disorders 388–9
  metabolic diseases 403–4
  nerve root compression 391–9
   EMG studies 393
   radiological studies 394–8
   treatment 398–9
  neuroblastoma 303
  in neurofibromatosis 352
  osseous impingement 411
  osteophytes 395, 399, 400
  pain 389, 390–1
   children 305–6
   dermatomal 391–9
   referral 391, 400
   sclerotomal 391, 400–45
  pseudarthrosis 411–12, 416,
   436–7
  pseudosubluxation 297, 304
  radionuclide imaging 136–7
  rheumatoid arthritis 416
  Scheuermann's disease 204
  stenosis 393
   CT scanning 160–2
   lateral recess 393, 398, 399
   myelography 87–9
   radiculography 69, 73, 74–5
   radiography 394, 396, 397–8

Spine *Cont'd.*
  thoracic
    contrast medium investigations
        85–6
    diastematomyelia 86
    obstruction 86
    scoliosis 86
  traumatic injuries 420–9
    clinical examination 421
    flexion 424–9
    forces causing 420–1
    hyperextension 421, 423
    hyperflexion 421, 423, 429
    ligamentous 421, 429
    radiological examination 421–
        3, 429
    rotation 421, 424–9
    surgery in acute phase 429
    see also Spine, fractures
  tumours 395, 416–20
    benign 265–7, 272, 273
    children 309–11
    metastatic 418
  see also Vertebrae
Spondylitis
  ankylosing 415–16, 484
  infective, in children 306–7
  non-specific 306
Spondylolisthesis 308–9, 411
  contrast medium investigation 80
  spinal instability in 200
Spondyloptosis, measuring
        displacement in 200
Spondylosis
  cervical 400–1
  lumbar 405, 406
Sports injuries
  knee 335
  lateral ligaments of ankle 252–6
  stress lesions/fractures 256–9
  tears in annulus fibrosus 407–8
Sprengel's shoulder 303–4
Sternum, fracture in Sudeck's atrophy
        261
Still's disease 356, 357, 496–8
Stress
  fractures 130, 257–9, 293–4
    metatarsus 345
    pelvis 467
    radionuclide imaging 130
    spine 389, 405
  injuries 256–9
Strontium-85 106
Strontium-87m 106
Subluxation 25–7
Subtalar joints, arthrography 66

Sudeck's atrophy 15, 23, 259–62,
        296
Sulphur colloids, technetium 99m-
        labelled 107
Syndactyly 347
Synovitis
  pigmented villonodular 289, 502
    arthrography of 55, 60, 67
    radionuclide imaging 127
Synovium
  mass disease 15–21
  swelling of 15
Syphilis 370

Talipes
  calcaneovalgus 339
  cavus 195
  equinovarus (TEV) 194, 339–40,
        505–6
    radiography 340–1
    treatment 341–3
    in tropics 379–80
Talocalcaneal
  angle 194–5
  coalition 344–5
Talometatarsal angle 194
Talus
  congenital vertical 339, 508
  dislocations 193, 251
  fractures 252, 520
    flake fracture of articular cortex
        251
Tarsometatarsal joint, dislocation
        251
Tarsometatarsal release 342
Tarsus
  coalition 344–5
  fracture–dislocation 521
Technetium-99
  –antimony colloid 107
  characteristics 106
  extraosseous localizations 109
  phosphate complexes 106–7, 109
  –sulphur colloid 107
  use in radionuclide imaging 106–
        7, 109
Teleroentgenography 332
Temporomandibular joint,
        arthrography 66
Tenography 102–3
Tetanus 374
Thermography 173–4

Thrombosis, deep venous,
        demonstration by venography
        100–2
Tibia
  bowing of 330
  fractures 219, 246–8, 252
    oblique 212
    in genu varum 329
    intercondylar eminence, fractures
        247–8
    proximal, fractures 246–7
    stress lesions 258
    torsion 330–1
    tubercle, osteochondritis 335, 336
    vara (Blount's disease) 329, 380,
        382, 492–3
Toes
  congenital flexion contractures
        338
  fifth, congenital dorsiflexion 338
  fracture 521
  hallux rigidus 516
  hallux valgus 338, 343, 513–16
  hammer 516
Tomography 167–9
  computed *see* Computed
        tomography
  emission 170–1
  limitations 35
  measurement of level of tomographic
        plane 29
  uses of 29
Tophus, calcified 25
Torsion 330–1
Torticollis 302–3
Traction 29, 31
Trauma
  radiographic examination in 209–
        10
  in tropics, management 374–5
  see also Fractures; *sites of trauma*
Trochanter, fractures 469
Tropics
  deformities 378–82
  infections 367–74
    in fractures 377–8
  orthopaedics in 365–87
  paraplegia in 378
  radiology in 366
  trauma 374–8
  undiagnosable conditions 385–7
Tuberculosis 22, 27, 291, 292,
        387
  knee 495–6
  spinal 307, 414
  tropics 369–70, 387

Tumour-like lesions 285–8
Tumours
  arteriography of 95–6
  bone
    benign 121–3, 264–73
    brown, of hyperparathyroidism
      287
    children 309–11
    CT scanning 147–51, 154
    diagnosis 264–85
    giant-cell 272–3
    malignant 119–21, 273–85
    metastases from 273–4, 289
    metastatic 114, 117, 119, 153,
      154, 289, 310, 356, 501–2
    radionuclide imaging 119–23
  knee 501–2
  locally recurrent, CT scanning 154
  malignant, radiographic diagnosis
    12–13
  soft tissue 289
    CT scanning 151–4
    radionuclide imaging 137–8
  spine 265–7, 272, 273, 309–11,
    395
  in tropics 380
  see also Cysts; specific types of
    tumour

Ulcers, tropical 373
Ulna
  dislocation, Galeazzi fracture 217
  distal alignment of 179
  malformations 346, 347
  Monteggia fracture 214, 217

Ultrasound 171–2
  dislocated hip 319
Urethra, traumatic injury 238
Urethrography 103
  retrograde 237, 238
Urography, excretion 237, 238

Vacuum phenomena 31
Vater anomalad 313–14
Venography 100–2
  leg 102
  lumbar 81–2, 85, 398
Vertebrae
  congenital anomalies 311–14,
    431, 438–9, 440
  fusion 303
  loss of a corner 6
  plana 418
  pseudosubluxation 297, 304
  rotation of, measurement 202–3
  spondylolisthesis 308–9
  subluxation 303
  tumours 309
Volkmann's ischaemic contracture
  451
Von Rosen projection 185

Wagner device 332–3
Walking cycle 504–5

Wiberg, centre angle of 185
Wrist
  arthritis 459
  arthrodesis 459
  arthrography 64
  carpal angle 179
  diaphyseal aclasis 179
  dislocation 240–2
  dyschondrosteosis 179
  flexion and extension ranges 179–
    80
  injuries 455–8
  instability 181
  ligaments
    arthrography 64
    injury 64, 455
  measurements 179–81
  movement at 447
  replacement 463
  scapholunate angle 181
  traumatic injuries 239
    instability following 240–3
  ulnar angle 179
  ventral angle 179

Xanthoma, fibrous 286
Xeroradiography 169

Yaws 373